Laser Surgery and Medicine

...DICINE AND ...

...RARY, TURN...

Laser Surgery and Medicine

Principles and Practice

Edited by

Carmen A. Puliafito, M.D.

Professor and Chair
Department of Ophthalmology
Tufts University School of Medicine

Adjunct Professor of Electrical Engineering and Computer Science
Tufts University

Director
New England Eye Center

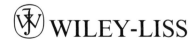 WILEY-LISS

A JOHN WILEY & SONS, INC., PUBLICATION
New York • Chichester • Brisbane • Toronto • Singapore

While the authors, editor, and publisher believe that drug selection and dosage and the specification and usage of equipment and devices, as set forth in this book, are in accord with current recommendations and practice at the time of publication, they accept no legal responsibility for any errors or omissions, and make no warranty, express or implied, with respect to material contained herein. In view of ongoing research, equipment modifications, changes in governmental regulations and the constant flow of information relating to drug therapy, drug reactions, and the use of equipment and devices, the reader is urged to review and evaluate the information provided in the package insert or instructions for each drug, piece of equipment, or device for, among other things, any changes in the instructions or indication of dosage or usage and for added warnings and precautions.

Library of Congress Cataloging-in-Publication Data:

Laser surgery and medicine : principles and practice / edited by
   Carmen A. Puliafito.
      p.   cm.
   Collection of review articles previously published in Lasers in surgery and medicine.
   Includes bibliographical references and index.
   ISBN 0-471-12070-7 (cloth : alk. paper)
   1. Lasers in medicine.   2. Lasers in surgery.   I. Puliafito,
Carmen A., 1951–   .
   [DNLM: 1. Laser Surgery—methods—collected works.   2. Lasers—
therapeutic use—collected works.   WO 511 L343 1995]
R857.L37L416   1995
610'.28—dc20
DNLM/DLC
for Library of Congress   95-36635

Printed in the United States of America

10 9 8 7 6 5 4 3 2 1

The following chapters originally appeared in *Lasers in Surgery and Medicine*. The journal is the only appropriate literature citation for the articles printed on these pages.

Chapter 1   15:315–341 (1994)
Chapter 2   16:103–133 (1995)
Chapter 3   16:2–23 (1995)
Chapter 4   16:205–214 (1995)
Chapter 5   17:201–301 (1995)
             Erratum 17:378-383 (1995)
Chapter 6   16:331–342 (1995)
Chapter 7   15:126–167 (1994)
Chapter 8   17:102–159 (1995)
Chapter 9   15:217–248 (1994)
Chapter 10   17:2–31 (1995)
Chapter 11   16:215–225 (1995)
Chapter 12   17:315-349 (1995)
Chapter 13   16:312–330 (1995)

Contents

Contributors

Gregory T. Absten, M.A., Executive Director, Professional Medical Education Association, Inc.; Chairman, Advanced Laser Services Corporation; Clinical Instructor, Ohio State University College of Medicine, Columbus, Ohio

Jeffrey R. Basford, M.D., Ph.D., Consultant in Physical Medicine and Rehabilitation, Mayo Clinic; Associate Professor, Mayo Medical School, Rochester, Minnesota

Lawrence S. Bass, M.D., Division of Plastic Surgery, Columbia University College of Physicians and Surgeons; Assistant Attending Surgeon, Manhattan Eye, Ear and Throat Hospital, New York, New York

Krishna M. Bhatta, M.D., Reddington Fairview Hospital, Skowhegan, Maine; Division of Urology, Brigham and Women's Hospital, Boston, Massachusetts

Jack A. Coleman, Jr., M.D., Assistant Professor, Department of Otolaryngology, Vanderbilt University Medical Center, Nashville, Tennessee

Mark S. Courey, M.D., Assistant Professor, Department of Otolaryngology, Vanderbilt University Medical Center, Nashville, Tennessee

Lawrence I. Deckelbaum, M.D., Medical Director, Cardiovascular Clinical Research, Merck Research Laboratories, Blue Bell, Pennsylvania

James A. Duncavage, M.D., Associate Professor and Vice-Chairman, Department of Otolaryngology, Vanderbilt University Medical Center, Nashville, Tennessee

John D. B. Featherstone, Ph.D., Professor, Department of Restorative Dentistry, Public Health and Hygiene, University of California, San Francisco, California

Anita M. R. Fisher, Ph.D., Research Specialist, Division of Ophthalmology, Children's Hospital of Los Angeles, Los Angeles, California

Daniel Fried, Ph.D., Assistant Professor, Eastman Dental Center, Rochester, New York

Charles J. Gomer, Ph.D., Professor of Pediatrics and Radiation Oncology, University of Southern California School of Medicine; Director, Research Institute, Children's Hospital of Los Angeles, Los Angeles, California

Joel M. Krauss, M.D., Mt. Sinai Hospital, New York, New York

Satish Krishnamurthy, M.D., Resident in Neurological Surgery, Milton S. Hershey Medical Center, Pennsylvania State University, Hershey, Pennsylvania

A. Linn Murphree, M.D., Professor of Ophthalmology and Pediatrics, University of Southern California School of Medicine; Head, Division of Ophthalmology, Children's Hospital of Los Angeles, Los Angeles, California

Norman S. Nishioka, M.D., Assistant Physician, Medical Services, Gastrointestinal Unit, Massachusetts General Hospital; Assistant Professor of Medicine, Harvard Medical School, Boston, Massachusetts

Robert H. Ossoff, D.M.D., M.D., Professor and Chairman, Department of Otolaryngology, Vanderbilt University Medical Center; Medical Director, the Vanderbilt Voice Center, Nashville, Tennessee

Stephen K. Powers, M.D., Professor and Chief of Neurological Surgery, Milton S. Hershey Medical Center, Pennsylvania State University, Hershey, Pennsylvania

Carmen A. Puliafito, M.D., Director, New England Eye Center; Professor and Chair, Department of Ophthalmology, Tufts University School of Medicine, Boston, Massachusetts

Richard Reid, M.D., Assistant Professor, Department of Obstetrics and Gynecology, Wayne State University School of Medicine, Detroit, Michigan; Director of Gynecologic Endoscopy, Crittenton Hospital, Rochester, Michigan

Lou Reinisch, Ph.D., Assistant Professor and Director of Laser Research, Department of Otolaryngology, Vanderbilt University Medical Center, Nashville, Tennessee

David H. Sliney, Ph.D., Chief, Laser Branch, United States Army Environmental Hygiene Agency, Aberdeen Proving Ground, Maryland

Michael R. Treat, M.D., Associate Professor of Clinical Surgery, College of Physicians and Surgeons, Columbia University; Director of Laparoendoscopic Surgery, Columbia Presbyterian Medical Center, New York, New York

Steven R. Visuri, M.S., Research Assistant, Biomedical Engineering Department, Northwestern University, Evanston, Illinois

Joseph L. Waldvogel, D.D.S., private practice, Joliet, Illinois

Joseph T. Walsh, Jr., Ph.D., Associate Professor, Biomedical Engineering Department, Northwestern University, Evanston, Illinois

Jay A. Werkhaven, M.D., Assistant Professor, Department of Otolaryngology, Vanderbilt University Medical Center, Nashville, Tennessee

Ronald G. Wheeland, M.D., Professor and Chair, Department of Dermatology, University of New Mexico School of Medicine, Albuquerque, New Mexico

Harvey A. Wigdor, D.D.S., Dental Section Chief, Ravenswood Hospital Medical Center, Chicago, Illinois

Preface

In the past decade, the application of lasers in surgery and medicine has increased dramatically. Recent advances in technology and procedures have brought many changes to the field and created a need for an authoritative, focused reference that reviews not only the basic principles of laser medicine but provides detailed coverage of specific applications in various surgical subspecialties.

Laser Surgery and Medicine: Principles and Practice assembles work from a diverse group of leading clinicians to offer a comprehensive, integrated survey of the current status and latest innovations in the biomedical uses of lasers. The text covers such general topics as laser safety, laser welding of tissue, and photodynamic therapy in addition to targeting nine distinct specialty areas. Chapters addressing surgical specialties feature illustrations showing the finer points of essential techniques, as well as reports on current clinical trials, new therapeutic techniques, and relevant aspects of laser biophysics, bioengineering, and photobiology.

Laser technology has had a profound and lasting effect upon medicine and surgery. This text provides a comprehensive review of the most important applications of lasers in medicine, surgery, and dentistry, by experienced clinicians in each specialty. We hope that it will be useful for clinicians who desire an update on laser applications in their field, as well as those physicians who desire a broad overview of the current status of laser surgery. Basic scientists and engineers interested in biomedical laser research applications will also find this work relevant.

I am grateful to the authors for their impressive contributions to this volume. I would like to express my gratitude to Alan Ball, who provided invaluable editorial assistance, and to the staff of Wiley-Liss, who provided encouragement throughout the process. Finally, thanks to my wife Janet, and children, Amy, Ben, and Sam, for their constant support.

Laser Surgery and Medicine

Chapter 1

Cardiovascular Applications
of Laser Technology

Lawrence I. Deckelbaum, MD

Cardiac Catheterization Laboratory, West Haven VA Medical Center,
West Haven, Connecticut and Yale University School of Medicine,
New Haven, Connecticut

INTRODUCTION

When laser radiation interacts with tissue, there are several potential results. The light can be absorbed and then reemitted at a longer wavelength in the form of fluorescence. Alternatively, the light can be absorbed and converted to heat with a resultant rise in the tissue temperature. As this tissue heating continues, an ablation threshold may be reached, at which point the tissue (and tissue water) undergo vaporization. Alternatively, it is possible that light absorption could result in direct bond breaking, resulting in photochemical tissue ablation. All of these potential laser interactions with tissue have been exploited to develop cardiovascular applications of laser technology. Lasers have been used to induce fluorescence, to heat biomaterials, and to ablate tissue in the cardiovascular system.

Laser technology has been evaluated for the treatment of coronary artery disease, ventricular and supraventricular arrhythmias, hypertrophic cardiomyopathy, and congenital heart disease.

Laser-based approaches are made more attractive because of the ability of fiberoptics to transmit laser radiation anywhere in the cardiovascular system that is accessible to an optical fiber. In most applications, laser radiation has been used to ablate the abnormal and disease-causing cardiovascular tissue. The major application, and the only one that has received FDA approval in the United States, has been laser angioplasty, or the use of laser radiation to vaporize obstructing atherosclerotic plaque. As an alternative to laser or balloon angioplasty, laser balloon angioplasty has used laser radiation to heat the vessel wall during balloon angioplasty to improve the vessel remodeling that balloon dilatation induces. Lasers have also been evaluated for ablation of thrombus and for photoactivating drugs that may inhibit restenosis following angioplasty. A more revolutionary approach to the treatment of coronary artery disease has been the use of laser radiation to vaporize multiple transmural channels in the ventricular myocardium to improve local perfusion. Laser ablative approaches have been used to ablate ventricular foci responsible for arrhythmias and to ablate supraventricular tachyarrhythmia pathways. Ablation of the abnormally thickened septum in idiopathic hypertrophic subaortic stenosis (IHSS) has also been performed using laser radiation. Laser-induced fluorescence spectroscopy has been used to differentiate normal and atherosclerotic tissue, as well as to assess myocardial metabolism based on NADH fluorimetry.

This review summarizes the current status of the multiple applications of laser technology to cardiovascular diagnosis and therapy. As with any new technology, there is continual evolution and change, and the various laser applications have had variable levels of development and clinical application. Laser angioplasty has been the major driving force for the evaluation of laser technology in cardiology. Since the first clinical application of lasers for the treatment of cardiovascular disease in 1983, there has been tremendous growth in laser angioplasty with > 15,000 procedures having been performed worldwide. In contrast, laser balloon angioplasty has been developed, briefly evaluated, and almost abandoned in the past 10 years. Transmyocardial laser revascularization represents the rebirth of an approach ("myocardial acupuncture") abandoned in the 1960s but now being performed with laser radiation. Laser thrombolysis, laser photochemotherapy, and laser ablation therapy of arrhythmias and hypertrophic cardiomyopathy are still in their infancy. The extent to which laser diagnostics will have a clinical utility is still unclear. The development and current status of these laser applications are reviewed.

LASER ANGIOPLASTY

Despite the widespread growth and success of percutaneous transluminal (coronary) angioplasty (PTA or PTCA), the realization of several constraints and limitations of balloon angioplasty stimulated the development of alternative revascularization approaches such as laser angioplasty.

In contrast to balloon angioplasty where the plaque material is fractured, compressed, or displaced, laser angioplasty would vaporize the plaque material and thereby have a high success rate for treating chronic coronary artery occlusions and diffuse atherosclerotic disease. It was also hoped that the bulk removal of plaque material could improve acute procedural success rates, decrease complication rates, treat "untreatable" lesions or lesions not amenable to conventional techniques, and decrease restenosis rates.

History

The ability of laser energy to vaporize atherosclerotic plaque was first demonstrated in 1963 by McGuff and colleagues [1] only 3 years after the first laser was developed by Maiman. The first intravascular recanalization using lasers was reported by Choy [2] who used argon laser radiation for thrombolysis in animals. In 1983, Choy performed the first clinical coronary laser angioplasty using an argon laser and bare fiber intraoperatively [2]. The high incidence of complications (perforation and occlusion) were in part due to the rigid catheter, the small amount of tissue ablated, and the laser-induced thermal damage. Ginsburg [3] used a similar system for the successful percutaneous laser revascularization of an occluded superficial femoral artery.

In an attempt to minimize the risk of arterial perforation due to laser ablation and mechanical trauma from the optical fiber, several approaches were pursued. Olive-shape metal tips were placed on the terminal ends of the silica fibers used for laser angioplasty. These hollow tips converted the laser light energy from continuous wave argon or Nd:YAG lasers into heat energy to achieve recanalization by tissue vaporization and mechanical compression of plaque material in a process referred to as laser thermal angioplasty. Spherical sapphire-tip optical fibers were also developed for laser thermal angioplasty, although these tips also allowed some direct transmission of the laser radiation to the tissue [4]. Percutaneous transluminal laser angioplasty was performed with these contact probes, ranging from 1.5 mm to 3 mm in diameter for peripheral arterial disease starting in 1985 [5]. Adjunctive balloon angioplasty was necessary in the vast majority of patients to achieve an adequate lumen. The initial rate of laser probe recanalization of femoropopliteal artery occlusions was 78–82% with a perforation rate of 8–14% [4]. However, a randomized trial [6] showed no showed no statistical difference in recanalization rates of femoropopliteal occlusions between conventional guidewires and laser contact probes. Although initial reports touted safety and efficacy of laser thermal angioplasty, the lack of demonstrably better acute or chronic results [7] dampened enthusiasm for this technique.

Percutaneous coronary laser thermal angioplasty procedures were performed in 1987. Despite the acute success of the system in the peripheral circulation, coronary laser thermal angioplasty was a disappointment. Of the 15 patients reported in the literature [8–10] (3 intraoperative, 12 percutaneous), only 60% (9 patients) had a successful procedure. There was one perforation, three acute occlusions, and four abrupt closures or myocardial infarctions postprocedure.

Another approach to enhancing the safety of laser angioplasty was to use a multifiber coronary laser catheter consisting of an array of fibers circumferentially arranged around a guidewire lumen. The use of multiple smaller fibers enhanced catheter flexibility over that using single larger fibers, and the passage over a guidewire decreased the likelihood of perforation from irradiation of the vessel wall. Cote [11] reported percutaneous multifiber coronary laser angioplasty in 23 patients using a four-fiber catheter coupled to an argon laser. He reported a 100% success rate with reduction in the mean stenosis from 97 to 14% following adjunctive balloon angioplasty. The continuous-wave argon laser was operated in a chopped or intermittent manner to deliver brief pulses of argon laser irradiation to minimize thermal damage.

Concerns regarding laser thermal damage as witnessed with laser thermal angioplasty resulted in the development of pulsed laser angioplasty systems. Continuous wave laser radiation, such as that emitted by the argon, Nd:YAG, or CO_2 lasers, will vaporize tissue with thermal damage to the adjacent tissue. In contrast, delivery of laser energy in the pulsed mode eliminates gross and microscopic evidence of thermal injury [12]. Linsker [13] reported the use of far ultraviolet (193 nm) irradiation from excimer laser to vaporize atherosclerotic lesions without apparent thermal damage in vitro. Isner and Grundfest reported the ability of the excimer laser at 308 nm to ablate vascular tissue with minimal thermal damage [14–16]. Deckelbaum [12] described tissue ablation with minimal thermal damage that could be achieved using a variety of pulsed lasers at ultraviolet, visible, and infrared wavelengths if appropriate parameters of pulse duration and fluence, or energy density (mJ/ cm^2), were chosen.

In 1988, Wollenek [17] reported the first percutaneous laser angioplasty performed with an excimer laser coupled to a 1-mm diameter single optical filter for recanalization of a femoral artery occlusion. Also in 1988, Litvack et al. [18] reported the first percutaneous coronary angioplasty performed with a pulsed excimer laser cou-

pled to a multifiber catheter. A pulsed dye laser coupled to a 200-µm fiber was used for initial recanalization of totally occluded ileofemoral arteries in 1989 [19]. In 1990, the first percutaneous pulsed holmium laser angioplasty (infrared wavelength 2.1 µm) was performed also with a multifiber catheter in the coronary circulation [20]. In 1992 and 1993, the FDA approved marketing of the LAIS Dymer 200 + (Advanced Interventional Systems, Irvine, CA) and Spectranetics CVX-300 (Spectranetics, Colorado Springs, CO) coronary laser angioplasty systems. In Europe, a Technolas MAX-10 (Fa. Technolas, Graefelfing, Germany) excimer laser coronary angioplasty system has been used clinically. By mid-1994, > 15,000 excimer laser angioplasties were estimated to have been performed worldwide, the large majority in the coronary circulation. Fewer holmium laser angioplasties (~ 1,500) have been performed since the holmium laser angioplasty system (Eclipse 2100, Eclipse Surgical Technologies, Palo Alto, CA) is limited to investigational use pending FDA approval.

Laser Angioplasty Procedure

Since laser angioplasty systems have not been as widely used or FDA approved for peripheral vascular applications, the following discussion focuses primarily on coronary vascular applications. Clinical excimer lasers for angioplasty contain a mixture of xenon and chlorine (XeCl) and lase at 308 nm. To facilitate fiberoptic coupling and transmission of excimer laser radiation, the pulse duration of clinical excimer lasers has been "stretched" from values used for industrial applications. Parameters employed for laser angioplasty using the LAIS [21] or Spectranetics [22] systems are pulse durations of 185 or 135 nsec, respectively, repetition rates of 20 or 30 Hz, and fluences (pulse energy density) of 30–80 mJ/ mm^2. The Technolas system operates at a shorter pulse duration of 55 nanosec, a repetition rate of 2–40 Hz, and a fluence of 42–51 mJ/mm^2 [23]. Holmium lasers for angioplasty emit radiation in the midinfrared at a wavelength of 2–2.1 µm, at a pulse energy up to 4 Joules, a pulse duration of 250 msec, and a repetition rate of 5 Hertz (data from Eclipse 2100 specification sheet).

The typical multifiber coronary laser angioplasty catheter consists of an array of 50–100-µm diameter fibers circumferentially arranged around a guidewire lumen (Fig. 1). The laser radiation is emitted from the catheter in a ring or halo shape and as a result cores out the obstruc-

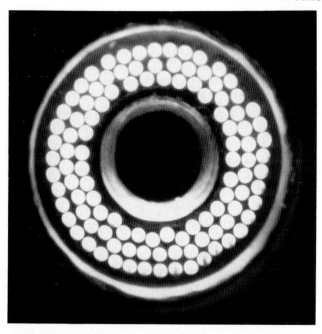

Fig. 1. The ablative face of a multifiber coronary laser angioplasty catheter (Spectranetics 1.7 mm diameter concentric) is shown above. The catheter consists of ~ 100 fifty μm fibers arranged concentrically around a guidewire lumen. The laser irradiation is emitted in a ring or halo shape.

tive plaque in the coronary artery resulting in a neolumen approximating the catheter diameter. The active area (area occupied by optical fiber) of these catheters is ~ 20–30% of the total surface area at the tip excluding the guidewire lumen. Laser catheters range in external diameter from 1.3–2.0 mm with common sizes being 1.3, 1.6, 2.0 for AIS catheters, 1.4, 1.7, and 2.0 for Spectranetics, and 1.4, 1.5, 1.7, and 2.0 for Eclipse catheters. Catheters are available in standard over-the-wire or monorail formats, as well as in concentric and recently available eccentric fiber configurations. The latter eccentric catheters are suitable for eccentric lesions and may be capable of achieving greater debulking by multiple passes through the lesion at varying orientations.

The procedural similarities between excimer laser angioplasty and balloon angioplasty are greater than their differences. Similar to balloon angioplasty, laser angioplasty requires the crossing of the lesion with a 0.014–0.18″ guidewire over which the multifiber catheter is then advanced. Laser irradiation is then initiated with catheter advancement through the lesion at a rate of 0.5–1.0 mm per sec. The guidewire is maintained taut to support the laser catheter and maintain its intraluminal orientation. Several

trains of laser pulses (e.g., of 3–5 sec each) may be performed before the lesion is crossed by the laser catheter (a "pass"). On occasion, several passes may be performed with the same or larger catheters in an attempt to maximize debulking of the lesion. Following laser ablation, adjunctive balloon angioplasty is performed in most cases. The undersizing of the laser catheter with respect to the vessel enhances safety at the expense of neolumen size and therefore requires a secondary procedure, usually PTCA. Representative angiographic frames from a laser angioplasty procedure are shown in Figure 2. Additional procedural details and nursing considerations of excimer laser coronary angioplasty (ELCA) are well described in reference [24].

Specimens retrieved by directional atherectomy immediately after laser angioplasty have documented acute pathological alterations resulting from in vivo laser angioplasty similar to that predicted by experimental studies in vitro [25]. Fine-edge disruption with infrequent foci of vacuolar injury was seen following excimer laser irradiation, whereas frequent vacuolar injury with rare thermal damage was seen following holmium laser irradiation. The absence of grossly visible thermal damage following excimer laser angioplasty has also been confirmed angioscopically [26,27].

Torre [28], Margolis [29], and Bittl [30] reported that ELCA minimal luminal diameters were comparable to the size of the catheter used (0.0–0.2 mm less), consistent with excimer laser tissue ablation. Laser ablation results in less elastic recoil than that following balloon PTCA where the final minimal lumen diameter ranges from 30–60% less than the balloon's inflated diameter [31–33]. The residual lumen diameter to device diameter (RLD/D) ratio, a measure of the efficacy of lumen enlargement, was significantly greater for excimer laser angioplasty as compared to balloon angioplasty (0.85 ± 0.30 vs. 0.71 ± 0.11) [34]. Torre and Sanborn et al. [28] reported an observation supporting the benefit of plaque debulking prior to balloon angioplasty. When comparably sized vessels were treated with ELCA and adjunctive PTCA, the degree of laser debulking correlated with the final lumen diameter. Seventy-five 3.0 mm diameter vessels with a mean stenosis of 85% were treated with 1.4, 1.7, or 2.0 diameter laser catheters prior to 3.0 mm diameter balloon catheter dilatation. The final vessel diameter was 2.0, 2.2, and 2.9 mm, respectively, demonstrating less elastic recoil in the vessels treated with the

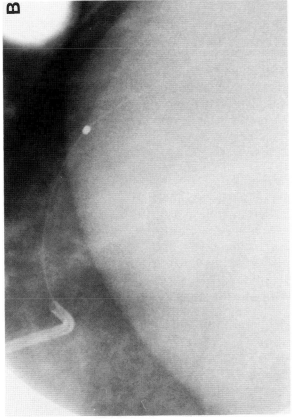

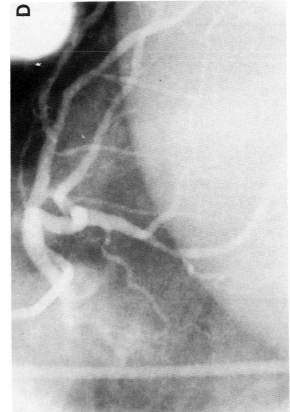

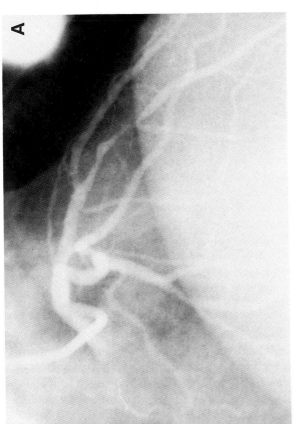

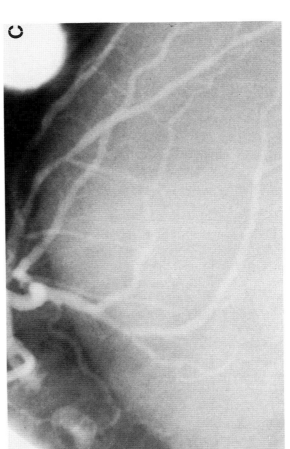

Fig. 2. Cineangiogram frames from a typical laser angioplasty procedure are shown above. **A:** The initial angiogram revealed two sequential long stenotic lesions in the left anterior descending (LAD) coronary artery. **B:** A guidewire was passed through the vessel across the stenosis and a 1.7-mm diameter, concentric multifiber catheter coupled to an excimer laser was then passed over the guidewire through the stenoses. The radiopaque distal marker of the laser catheter is seen traversing the distal lesion. **C:** Following laser angioplasty, a neolumen was created approximating the diameter of the catheter. **D:** The final result following adjunctive balloon dilatation shows minimal residual stenosis at the site of the prior lesions.

larger laser catheters with presumably greater laser ablation of plaque.

Results of Laser Angioplasty

For the analysis of laser angioplasty results, clinical success was defined as a reduction by ≥20% of the narrowing of the vessel diameter to a ≤50% residual stenosis in the absence of a major in-hospital complication (MI, death, or emergency CABG). Laser success was defined as a reduction by ≥20% of the narrowing of the vessel diameter. Lesions were graded according to the A, B, C classification of the ACC/AHA Task Force as modified by Ellis et al. [35] to include types B1 and B2, depending on whether one or more complex features were present.

The reported results using either the Spectranetics or LAIS excimer laser angioplasty systems are comparable. Overall, laser angioplasty has a procedural success rate of 86–94% with a major complication rate of 5–7% [29,30,36–40]. Laser success occurred in 82–85%. Failure of laser angioplasty occurred more often due to the inability to advance the catheter to the site of the lesion because of prestenotic vessel tortuosity than to the inability to pass the laser catheter through the lesion [41]. Based on quantitative angiographic data from the AIS [36,29] and Spectranetics [30] registries, the mean lesion % stenosis of 80–87% was reduced to 43–50% following laser angioplasty, and to a final residual stenosis of 21–29% following adjunctive balloon angioplasty. These data are consistent with the smaller series of patients undergoing ELCA using the Technolas system who experienced a mean stenosis reduction from 90% to 52% following laser angioplasty and to 25% after adjunctive balloon dilatation. Laser alone produced a residual stenosis ≤50% in only 55% of treated lesions [30]. Adjunctive balloon angioplasty was performed in 47–88% [23,30,36] of patients. The important role of adjunctive balloon angioplasty for the success of new coronary device interventions such as laser angioplasty is discussed in reference [42].

The reported results using the Eclipse holmium laser angioplasty are similar with a procedural success rate of 94–95%, a laser success rate of 79–83%, and a major complication rate of ~ 5% [43–45]. Mean % stenosis decreased from 89% to 57% following laser angioplasty and to a final residual stenosis of 22% after balloon angioplasty. Procedural success did not differ substantially for A, B, and C lesions [45]. Most patients had adjunctive PTCA. Comparable success rates with both holmium and excimer laser angioplasty have also been reported from the experience of a single center [46].

The results of excimer laser angioplasty appear to be somewhat insensitive to lesion complexity. Equivalent ELCA success rates have been reported for simple and complex lesions: 91% for type A, 91% for type B1, 89% for type B2, and 95% for type C lesions [30]. Major complication rates were also not higher in complex lesions: 6% for type A, 6% for B1, 9% for B2, and 3% for type C lesions. Similar insensitivity of success and complication rates to AHA/ACC Task Force classification was also found in the other series that addressed this question [21,41].

Multivariate analysis [30,38] identified that bifurcation lesions (odds ratio = 0.16) and tortuous vessels (odds ratio = 0.48) reduced the likelihood of clinical success. However, restenosis lesions, ostial lesions, and saphenous vein graft lesions were associated with a greater likelihood of clinical success. Yet, the multivariate model could account for only 23% of the variability in clinical success suggesting that it is still difficult to predict the clinical outcome from excimer laser angioplasty in a specific patient. In another series [36], multivariate analysis showed lesion eccentricity to be the only independent predictor for the occurrence of a major procedural complication (odds ratio = 3.32, or expressed inversely for clinical success, odds ratio = 0.30). However, in this series eccentric catheters were not utilized, and 20% of the lesions with no complications had a high eccentricity index. Although angiographic evidence of thrombus was an uncommon occurrence in ELCA treated lesions (9% of lesions), when present it decreased the clinical success rate to 58% and was associated with a 25% incidence of embolization, a 33% incidence of myocardial infarction, and a 17% incidence of abrupt closure [47]. The presence of intracoronary thrombus was the most important (negative) predictor of clinical success in this analysis. In contrast to these observations with excimer laser ablation, holmium laser angioplasty has been used successfully for recanalization in patients with acute myocardial infarction [48] where the presence of thrombus is a near universal occurrence.

Risk of myocardial infarction during the procedure or during hospitalization was 2–4% [29,30,39,40,49,50]. The risk of abrupt closure was 5–7% with 2/3 occurring in the catheterization laboratory and 1/3 occurring later in-hospital. Abrupt closure was treated with balloon angioplasty with success in more than half of cases. Bypass surgery was required at some time during hospitalization in 3–4% [30,29]. Coronary spasm was reported in 2–4% [29,51], although another study [52] suggested a much higher incidence of persistent mild vasospasm demonstrable angiographically the day following ELCA. This same study also reported a 38% incidence of vasospasm during the ELCA procedure (in 38 patients), which is a higher incidence than that reported in other series and may have resulted from longer lasing times. Complication rates were relatively independent of AHA/ACC Task Force classification [21,30]. Predictors of major complications were bifurcation lesions and eccentric stenoses [36,38]. The risk of death from ELCA was 0.4% [53]. The reported complications of holmium laser angioplasty [43] are similar to those of ELCA with an incidence of myocardial infarction of 2%, perforation 2%, emergency bypass surgery 3%, dissection 5%, and death 0.3%.

In one series [30], 5.5% of patients undergoing ELCA showed evidence of significant dissection that impaired flow, resulted in myocardial infarction, or required bypass surgery. Overall incidence of excimer laser induced dissections has been reported to be 13–16% angiographically [36,40]. Angioscopy following excimer laser angioplasty [26,27] has documented irregular recanalized channels with intraluminal flaps, tissue remnants, and plaque fractures. Intracoronary ultrasound also suggests that the incidence of dissections following laser and adjunctive balloon angioplasty may be higher than appreciated angiographically [53]. The incidence of dissection was correlated with the use of larger diameter catheters, high pulse energies, long lesions, and presence of a side branch [50]. The presence of a dissection correlated with the occurrence of an important complication (odds ratio = 3.9). A lower dissection rate following holmium than excimer laser angioplasty was reported in the small experience of a single center [46]. In vitro data [54], however, demonstrated larger dissections following holmium irradiation of aorta than following excimer irradiation.

Mechanical trauma to the arterial wall due to passage of the laser catheter might contribute to the incidence of dissection, but this was probably more a factor in the first generation of laser catheters that used larger diameter fibers and were much stiffer than current catheters. The adjunctive balloon angioplasty probably does play a major role in arterial wall dissections; however,

many of the dissections are noted after laser angioplasty alone. In vitro studies [55,56] have shown that pulsed excimer or holmium laser ablation is associated with photoacoustic effects such as rapidly expanding and collapsing cavitation bubbles and acoustic shock waves that may play an important role in causing these arterial dissections. Time-resolved photography revealed forceful vapor bubble formation during excimer or holmium laser ablation that resulted in tissue elevation up to 2.5 mm. Irradiation and vaporization of blood (as opposed to tissue) probably contribute to cavitation bubble formation and acoustomechanical trauma without any procedural benefit. In blood, each excimer laser pulse generated a fast-expanding and imploding vapor bubble whose size was proportional to the pulse energy. In vivo, excimer laser irradiation coaxially in a rabbit artery produced an antraluminal bubble that resulted in microsecond dilatation (to a 50% increase in vessel diameter) and invagination of the arterial segment [55]. This was associated with histologic dissections and extensive wall damage far beyond the penetration depth of the 308 nm laser light. Abela [56] postulated that multiple layers of dissection could cause the artery to puff up similar to a "mille-feuilles" pastry. This swelling in the arterial wall as a result of multilayered dissection planes could be the etiology of angiographic "spasm" or acute occlusion following laser angioplasty. PTCA is often effective in compressing these layers back together and restoring the vessel lumen. It is possible that this mechanical distention of the vessel is a potent stimulus for smooth muscle cell proliferation and an increase in vasomotor tone contributing to restenosis and vasospasm, respectively [57]. Minimizing the number of laser passes as well as irradiation of blood may decrease the incidence of laser-induced dissections.

Vessel perforation has been reported to occur in 1–3% of cases [22,29,36,37]. Of the patients with perforation, 39–60% had a major complication resulting directly from perforation (cardiac tamponade, myocardial infarction, or need for emergency CABG surgery), and the other 40–61% had no clinical complications after successful sealing of the puncture site. Of 2,759 patients in the AIS registry [37], 1.3% had perforation. Of these, 36% required emergency CABG surgery, 17% experienced a myocardial infarction, and 6% had a fatal outcome. Large catheter: vessel ratio was an important risk factor as vessel perforation occurred in 8.3% of lesions in which the laser catheter was ≤0.5 mm smaller than the diameter of the target vessel, but occurred only in 1.5% of lesions in which the laser catheter was > 1 mm smaller than the target vessel. In one series [22], multivariate analysis revealed that bifurcation lesions, target vessel diameter <2.25, diabetes mellitus, and female gender were associated with increased risk of vessel perforation. Long lesions and calcified lesions were not at increased risk. Follow-up angiography in 12 patients whose perforation was sealed with balloon angioplasty revealed an aneurysm in one patient (8% incidence). The incidence of perforation has declined by avoiding higher risk lesions and by careful catheter sizing such that the incidence of perforation has been decreasing, to 0.4% in the last 1,000 patients treated in the AIS registry [49].

Coronary artery aneurysm formation has been rarely reported following excimer laser angioplasty: once following balloon sealing of a laser-induced perforation [22] and once following an uncomplicated stand alone excimer laser angioplasty [58]. The authors speculated that ablation into the media may have been responsible for aneurysm formation in the latter case.

Regarding potential long-term effects, experimental and epidemiological studies have demonstrated the carcinogenic potential of UV-B (280–320 nm) at fluences comparable to those used during laser angioplasty. Cytotoxic and mutagenic effects of 308 nm irradiation are due to error-prone repair mechanisms. However, it is not known if there is any risk of a single intravascular exposure to 308 nm irradiation, or if vascular tissue is susceptible to UV carcinogenesis [59].

It was hypothesized that by ablating atherosclerotic plaque laser angioplasty could decrease the restenosis rate by diminishing elastic recoil that contributes to restenosis and by decreasing vessel injury induced smooth muscle cell proliferation. Unfortunately, there is no evidence that excimer or holmium laser angioplasty has a lower overall restenosis rate than balloon angioplasty [45,60]. Restenosis may be due to the inadequate tissue ablation or in response to the mechanical injury induced by laser dissections (see below) or adjunctive balloon angioplasty. In a subgroup of 95 ELCA-treated patients undergoing quantitative angiography, Bittl [30] reported at restudy an average of 5.2 months postprocedure that the mean minimal lumen diameter had decreased from 2.3±0.5 to 1.2 ± 1.0 mm, and the mean percent stenosis had increased from 21±14% to

56±32. Lumen diameter at follow-up did not correlate with the postlaser lumen diameter but did correlate with the postprocedural lumen diameter after adjunctive balloon angioplasty. Overall restenosis rate was 48%. However, only 31% had clinical evidence of restenosis with recurrence of angina, positive exercise treadmill test, MI, or need for revascularization. Six-month angiographic restenosis rate following holmium coronary laser angioplasty has been reported to be 44% [45].

Relative risk analysis revealed that lesion length was a predictor of restenosis, whereas adjunctive PTCA and vessel diameter > 3.0 mm were predictors of freedom from restenosis. As reported for other interventional modalities, the risk of restenosis following excimer laser angioplasty is related to the vessel diameter immediately postprocedure. The minimal lumen diameter at 3–6 month follow-up was directly related to reference vessel diameter and to minimal lumen diameter after laser and balloon treatment. The lowest likelihood of restenosis occurred when laser ablation and balloon dilatation were used in large vessels to produce a lumen that approached the reference diameter of the vessel [61,62] (e.g., vessels with the largest postprocedural minimal lumen diameters).

Current Status

The absence of any randomized clinical trial comparing PTCA and laser angioplasty makes it difficult to determine which lesions are best treated by laser angioplasty. However, comparison with historical controls suggests certain niche applications. ELCA success > 90% has been reported [21,29,30,63] in certain lesions that have responded poorly to balloon angioplasty. These include diffuse disease (lesion length > 20 mm), lesions in saphenous vein grafts > 3 years old, ostial lesions, chronic total occlusions, and type B and C lesions. PTCA results in these lesions range from 61–84% [35]. However, some investigators perceive no advantage of excimer laser over balloon angioplasty for the treatment of discrete uncomplicated lesions [21]. These comparisons must be interpreted cautiously as historical PTCA controls may differ in patient selection and do not represent what is achievable using current techniques and equipment. However, based on such comparisons, excimer laser coronary angioplasty is being predominantly used for the treatment of type B2 and C lesions [40].

The currently approved indications for exci-

TABLE 1 Indications for Coronary Laser Angioplasty

Long lesions (≥ 10–20 mm long)
Saphenous vein graft lesions
Moderately calcified lesions
Aorto-ostial lesions
Total occlusions that can be crossed with a guidewire
Lesions that cannot be crossed or dilated with a balloon
    catheter

mer laser angioplasty are listed in Table 1. Although Holmium laser angioplasty systems are still investigational and have not received FDA clinical approval, they are commonly used for comparable indications. Laser angioplasty appears to be safe and effective for the treatment of saphenous vein graft lesions, aorto-ostial lesions, long lesions, moderately calcified lesions, total occlusions that can be crossed with a guidewire, and balloon dilatation failures. These niches have been proposed for laser angioplasty because, as stated above, the success rate for ELCA treatment of these lesions appears to be higher than that with balloon angioplasty when compared with historical controls. Restenosis lesions may also be appropriate for laser angioplasty as both laser success and procedural success [38,39,64] were higher in restenosis lesions than in de novo lesions. It will be important for the greater acceptance and growth of laser angioplasty to confirm these benefits in randomized clinical trials.

With the current catheter technology, this author contends that optimal lesions are probably those causing very high grade stenoses or total occlusion in large vessels. In these cases, a large multifiber catheter can be safely used and the large overlap of the catheter face with the obstructing atheroma will result in the greatest amount of laser debulking.

Excimer laser coronary angioplasty has been successful in cases of PTCA failure [21,38,65,66]. In those instances, ELCA debulking was effective in facilitating balloon crossing of a long rigid stenosis that could not be crossed after guidewire passage through the lesion, and/or in overcoming prominent elastic recoil of the stenosis after PTCA, and/or in dilating hard lesions that resisted balloon dilatation even at high pressure.

Despite the overall clinical success of laser angioplasty, several remaining problems must be addressed. The development of the current laser angioplasty systems has reflected a compromise between efficacy and safety. However, George Abela's comments [56] may be telling: "Unless laser angioplasty can be performed safely as a stand-alone procedure that can debulk plaque with minimal mechanical and acoustic wall injury, it will not be possible to utilize lasers effectively or assess the impact of lasers." Passing the catheter over a guidewire adds safety. However, it limits the application of the procedure to lesions that can be crossed with a guidewire (which fortunately represents the majority of lesions treated with percutaneous interventional techniques). However, chronic total occlusions that cannot be crossed by a guidewire, which occurs ~ 50% of the time, cannot be treated with laser angioplasty. Second, current systems and approaches result in inadequate plaque ablation. The diameter of the laser catheter is chosen to be ~ 1 mm less than the normal vessel diameter to afford a margin of safety and minimize the risk of complications, such as arterial perforation. As a result, the achieved neolumen is usually inadequate and requires adjunctive balloon angioplasty to achieve an optimal result. Third, pulsed laser angioplasty results in arterial wall injury reflected by an incidence of coronary dissection of approximating 20% during clinical procedures. Although this dissection rate may be lower than that reported with balloon angioplasty, laser-induced dissections occur unpredictably and are associated with the major complications of the procedure. The fourth problem that laser angioplasty has still failed to address is that of restenosis. One of the hypotheses driving laser angioplasty has been that plaque ablation by laser radiation, as opposed to plaque displacement by a balloon catheter, would result in a lower restenosis rate. This hypothesis has still to be proven. Current clinical trials have not clearly demonstrated a lower restenosis rate following excimer laser angioplasty. This may be due to the inadequate plaque ablation that usually necessitates adjunctive balloon angioplasty. The unchanged restenosis rates may reflect the effect of the balloon injury.

To foster further acceptance and growth of laser angioplasty, there are several goals for the future. It is important to expand the applications of the current laser systems. The development of fiberoptic laser guidewires for the primary recanalization of chronic total occlusions by direct plaque ablation is one approach. The incidence of complications following laser angioplasty needs to be reduced, and the predictability of outcome needs to be improved. Specifically, arterial wall injury and the incidence of dissections during the procedure need to be minimized. One approach that is being investigated is the use of saline infusion into the coronary artery during laser angioplasty to displace blood and minimize acousto-mechanical injury [67,68].

In vitro experiments documented that excimer laser ablation in blood resulted in a bubble diameter of 1.2 mm and an acoustic pressure of 15 kbar as compared to no acoustic signal or bubble formation in saline [67]. A fourfold dilution of blood reduced the bubble diameter to 0.48 mm and the pressure to 0.25 kbar. The difference undoubtedly is due to the strong absorption of 308 nm radiation by blood as compared to saline. The transmission through 1 mm of saline was 100% but only 59% through a 10% blood/saline solution [68]. The magnitude of the pressure pulse was nine times greater in 1 0% blood solution and 23 times greater in 100% blood compared to saline. Pressure pulses were ever greater during excimer laser ablation in contrast media [69]. Theoretical and experimental data [70] suggest that the dimensions of the vapor bubble generated during excimer laser ablation of tissue in blood can be reduced by flushing with saline (decreasing hematocrit) or multiplexing (decreasing pulse energy and effective "fiber" size).

Another approach to reducing arterial wall injury is the use of multiplexing, or sequential firing of the laser into sections of the multifiber catheter to decrease the pulse energy, and thereby reduce acousto-mechanical damage. An 11-fold reduction in shock wave and acoustic pressure, reduction of histologic acoustic injury, and decreased neointimal proliferation in an animal model were reported following multiplexing [71,72]. Multiplexing still enabled effective ablation of fibrous atherosclerotic plaque in vitro at clinically relevant fluences [73].

The restenosis rate needs to be decreased following laser angioplasty. This may come about by newer catheter systems that are capable of achieving more complete plaque ablation. Directional or eccentric multifiber catheters may be able to achieve larger neolumens by multiple passes through the stenotic artery [74,75]. Both Spectranetics and LAIS have developed 1.7–1.8 mm diameter over-the-wire catheters with eccentric placement of the optical fibers. Preliminary experience suggests that these catheters may be effective for highly eccentric lesions and bifurcation lesions. It is possible that with multiple passes of this catheter at varying orientations, a neolumen larger than the catheter diameter might be achieved. Feedback systems based on fluorescence spectroscopy [76,77], angioscopy

[78], or intravascular ultrasound [53] may be capable of safely guiding greater plaque ablation and thereby decreasing restenosis. Fluorescence spectroscopy (see later section on Antiarrhythmic Laser Therapy) is capable in vitro of discriminating normal and atherosclerotic artery and of guiding recanalization of total occlusions [76]. Preliminary in vivo trials have begun to evaluate the efficacy of fluorescence spectroscopy in determining catheter tissue contact, guiding eccentric catheter orientation, and confirming the adequacy of saline infusion in clearing blood from the catheter–tissue interspace [77].

LASER THROMBOLYSIS

In addition to laser vaporization of atherosclerotic obstructions, laser vaporization of thrombus has been evaluated in vitro and in vivo. Argon laser dissolution of human thrombus was reported by Choy and Lee [79,80] in vitro. Marco reported that 16 thrombus-occluded canine femoral arteries were successfully recanalized using argon laser irradiation and remained patent for up to 2 weeks [81].

The differing absorption properties of thrombus and vascular tissue could afford a degree of selective laser ablation. LaMuraglia [82] correlated ablation studies with optical absorption for arterial tissue and thrombus. Hemoglobin accounted for > 10 times higher absorption by thrombus compared to inferior vena cava or pulmonary artery tissue at 482 nm. This difference accounted for threshold fluences for ablation for thrombus that were < 1/100th that for the venous or arterial tissue. Ablation efficiency of thrombus was in excess of 100 mg/J under conditions that caused no histologic injury to the pulmonary artery. The investigators suggested that laser radiation at this wavelength could be used selectively and safely to ablate venous thrombi or emboli with parameters that would not injure the endovascular tissue. This concept was applied by Gregory et al. [83] for selective laser thrombolysis of coronary artery thrombi in 18 patients with acute myocardial infarction. A pulsed dye laser was used that emitted 1 ms duration pulses at 480 nm at a fluence of 60–75 mJ per pulse and a repetition rate of 3 Hz. Laser energy was delivered via a novel flowing, fluid-core light guide using radiographic contrast as the optical core fluid. This enabled simultaneous laser radiation transmission and fluoroscopic monitoring of the establishment of vessel patency during laser thrombolysis.

Laser thrombolysis using this system successfully removed thrombi in 17 of the 18 patients and improved coronary flow following delivery of 240–600 laser pulses. Mean coronary artery stenosis decreased from 99% pretreatment to 80% after laser thrombolysis and finally to 24% after adjunctive angioplasty therapy. The absence of any perforations or acute vessel closures supported the concept of selective thrombolysis without damage to the arterial wall. There were no recurrent infarctions or deaths during hospitalization in this limited clinical study.

As discussed above, holmium laser angioplasty has been used successfully for arterial recanalization in patients with acute myocardial infarction [48]. Topaz [84] used holmium laser radiation in six patients specifically for the purpose of coronary thrombolysis. Each patient had angiographic evidence of thrombus resulting in vessel occlusion or high grade stenosis and a clinical syndrome of prolonged or recurrent chest pain in the setting of acute myocardial infarction. In each case, a guidewire was placed across the stenosis and a multifiber laser catheter was utilized with comparable parameters and technique as for laser angioplasty. All patients had a reduction in stenosis and resolution of angiographic evidence of thrombus after lasing. Adjunctive balloon angioplasty was performed in each patient without major complication.

The results of these small clinical series suggest that laser thrombolysis with a pulsed dye or holmium laser may offer an alternative treatment for patients with acute myocardial infarction, especially if there are contraindications to conventional systemic lytic pharmacotherapy. Although intracoronary thrombus correlated with complications during excimer laser angioplasty [47], excimer laser thrombolysis has been demonstrated in vitro [85] and might also be clinically effective. Whether laser thrombolysis might also have a role in the treatment of arterial thrombi complicating balloon angioplasty or other therapeutic coronary interventions is currently an unanswered question.

LASER BALLOON ANGIOPLASTY

As noted earlier in the discussion of laser angioplasty, despite the widespread growth and success of percutaneous transluminal coronary angioplasty (PTCA), several limitations remain. Abrupt coronary occlusion and long-term restenosis continue to be the major problems associated with the procedure. In addition to laser angioplasty, which attempts to ablate the offending atherosclerotic plaque, laser balloon angioplasty (LBA) is a nonablative technique that has been developed to improve the results of PTCA. During LBA, laser energy is delivered circumferentially to the arterial wall by an optical fiber that terminates in a central diffusing tip within an angioplasty balloon [86]. The Nd:YAG laser energy heats the surrounding arterial wall to subvaporization temperatures in an attempt to smooth irregular intimal surfaces, seal or weld intimal and medial dissections, dehydrate thrombi, and inhibit the elastic recoil that usually occurs with balloon deflation. The rationale behind the simultaneous application of heat and pressure was to leave a larger, less thrombogenic vessel, thereby treating abrupt coronary occlusion and possibly contributing to a better long-term result. The technique of laser balloon angioplasty is diagramed in Figure 3.

Laser balloon angioplasty developed out of the work of Dr. Richard Spears, and colleagues. In 1985, Spears demonstrated that continuous wave Nd:YAG laser radiation could fuse human atheromatous plaque-arterial wall separations in vitro [87]. A linear correlation was found between thermal weld strength and adventitial tissue temperature. Tissue temperatures > 80°C were required for tissue welding, with reliable welding occurring at temperatures > 95°C. Temperatures > 140°C resulted in tissue charring. Therefore a decremental ramped laser dosimetry was developed to maintain tissue temperatures in the range of 95–120°C. The decremental ramped power delivery used a higher power initially to rapidly achieve target tissue temperature followed by lower power levels to maintain a constant target tissue temperature.

The effects of LBA have been evaluated in several animals models. Jenkins [88] subjected the normal external iliac artery of rabbits to LBA and compared the results with balloon angioplasty of the contralateral artery. Quantitative angiography demonstrated that the iliac arteries, initially 2.1 mm in diameter, were stretched to 2.8 mm during the 3.0 mm diameter angioplasty balloon inflation, but recoiled to 2.2 mm after balloon deflation. Arteries treated with the same size balloon as well as with LBA had less elastic recoil with final luminal diameters of 2.4 and 2.6 mm following irradiation with moderate or high-dose Nd:YAG laser powers, respectively. Arteries treated with the high laser dose showed a loss of

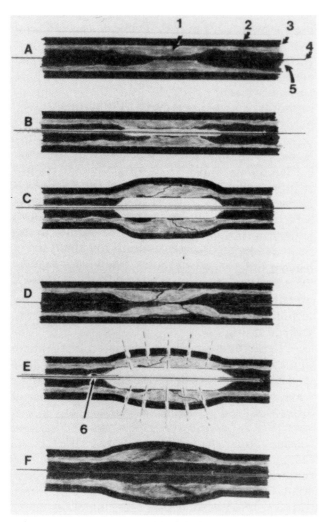

Fig. 3. Laser balloon angioplasty. **A–C** show conventional balloon angioplasty in which a guidewire (4) is inserted into the arterial lumen (5). The balloon is threaded over the guidewire to the obstructing plaque (1) and inflated, sometimes causing dissection of the arterial wall. Extensive dissection may cause abrupt reclosure or early restenosis **(D)**. In this instance, laser balloon angioplasty **(E)** may be useful in fusing dissected layers of arterial wall, resulting in a smooth, dilated lumen **(F)**. (From Hiehle JF, Bourgelais DBC, Shapshay S, et al: Nd:YAG laser fusion of human atheromatous plaque-arterial wall separations in vitro. Am J Cardiol 1985; 56:952, with permission).

the initial gain in lumen diameter by 1 month caused by both extravascular fibrosis of the artery and mild neointimal proliferation, whereas arteries treated with the moderate laser dose retained the increment in mean vessel diameter at 1 month over that of balloon angioplasty-treated arteries. Alexopoulos [89] performed a similar acute experiment in atherosclerotic rabbit iliac arteries. Laser balloon angioplasty resulted in a

greater increase in luminal diameter of 0.5 mm acutely. However, this improved lumen diameter was accompanied by increased platelet deposition measured by Indium-111 labeled platelets. Histologic evidence of laser "sealing" was present in only one artery, suggesting that abolition of vascular recoil was the most important advantage acutely of laser balloon angioplasty. In contrast, Jenkins [90] reported in a study in atherosclerotic rabbits that four of five iliac arteries with severe dissections and three of three arteries with angiographically visible perforation were sealed angiographically with LBA.

Ischinger [91] evaluated laser balloon angioplasty in the normal carotid and femoral arteries of dogs using a different fiberoptic balloon catheter than that employed by Spears and his colleagues. Using lower adventitial surface temperatures of 50–80°C during LBA, he demonstrated acute lumen enlargement that was subsequently complicated by thrombosis and neointimal proliferation on follow-up. These chronic results differ from those reported by Sinclair [92] in normal dog coronary arteries. Using a ramped decremental dosimetry calculated to give peak tissue temperatures of 125°C, Sinclair [92] reported that LBA achieved an acutely increased luminal diameter with the increment maintained long-term up to 1-month follow up. Administration of ergonovine at 1 month after LBA resulted in vasoconstriction of the coronary artery in all areas except the LBA-treated area, leaving the impression of a cast of the balloon. Sinclair referred to this as a "biologic stent." In contrast, Ischinger [91] did not observe a difference in ergonovine response in the dog femoral artery between laser-treated versus nontreated sites at 2–3 months restudy. Differences in these results may reflect the different thermal parameters employed. These studies performed in normal nonatherosclerotic canine arteries were also somewhat limited due to the absence of balloon-induced plaque dissections and therefore the inability to evaluate the potential of LBA to "weld" separated arterial layers.

Based on in vitro and in vivo animal studies, clinical trials were initiated. A 3.0-mm diameter fiberoptic laser balloon catheter with an internal 100-μm optical fiber terminating in a diffusing tip was manufactured by the USCI Division of C.R. Bard (Spears Laser Balloon Catheter). In a multicenter clinical trial of 55 patients [93], coronary artery lesions were initially treated with conventional balloon angioplasty. The Spears Laser Balloon Catheter was then introduced across the lesion and inflated. The Nd:YAG laser energy was delivered during a 20-sec exposure using a decremental power dosimetry. This dosimetry was 18–35 watts for 5 sec, 12–25 watts for 5 sec, and then 10–15 watts for 10 sec for a total of 20-sec laser dose. This duration of laser exposure was based upon in vitro experiments demonstrating that at least 10 sec were necessary for reliable welding but that > 20 sec provided no further benefit [94]. Balloon inflation was maintained for 30 sec after termination of laser exposure to ensure return of arterial temperature to baseline values before balloon deflation. Quantitative coronary angiography revealed that the minimum luminal diameter increased from 1.74 mm after conventional balloon angioplasty to 2.32 mm after laser balloon angioplasty with no significant change in diameter on 1 day and 1 month follow-up angiograms. Three patients with acute closure following balloon angioplasty were successfully treated with LBA with restoration of an adequate coronary artery diameter. However, with more patients and larger follow-up the multicenter randomized trial of 232 patients randomized to conventional PTCA or LBA did not demonstrate a reduction in restenosis at 6 months [95]. Despite a cogent theoretical basis, and some promising preliminary animal trials, laser photocoagulation did not prevent the process of restenosis.

During the performance of the LBA clinical trial, it was observed that LBA was effective in treating unsuccessful PTCA (inadequate lumen improvement or abrupt closure). Although no restenosis benefit could be demonstrated, LBA appeared to improve the acute results of angioplasty by decreasing elastic recoil and by treating abrupt closure. LBA presumably reversed abrupt closure by decreasing elastic recoil, by desiccating thrombus, and/or by sealing dissections. In 154 patients with refractory, impending, or acute vessel closure post-PTCA, LBA achieved a clinical success (< 50% diameter stenosis and avoidance of CABG and other in-hospital major complications) in 83% [96]. Despite the potential niche of LBA as a "bailout" for failed PTCA, USCI has discontinued the manufacturing and marketing of the Spears Laser Balloon Catheter, and no clinical trials are ongoing. Laser balloon angioplasty, however, is still being investigated for the application of bioprotective materials to injured arterial surfaces following angioplasty [97]. In this process, LBA is used to thermally coagulate or precipitate insoluble biocompatable materials containing pharmacologic agents onto the luminal arterial surface. Other thermal angioplasty balloons using nonlaser energy sources such as radiofrequency energy are still undergoing experimental and clinical evaluation [98,99].

LASER PHOTOCHEMOTHERAPY

An additional laser approach to the problem of restenosis is the use of laser radiation to photoactivate drugs capable of inhibiting smooth muscle cell proliferation and intimal hyperplasia. The drugs investigated for this purpose include hematoporphyrins, phyocyanin, phthalocyanine, and psoralen.

Naturally occurring porphyrins have been known to accumulate in neoplastic tissue. The fluorescence of parenterally injected hematoporphyrin derivative (HPD) has been used to localize tumors, and the cytotoxic effect of light-activated HPD has been used in cancer therapy [100]. Whereas ultraviolet light is commonly used to induce HPD fluorescence, HPD is photoactivated at a variety of wavelengths in the visible spectrum. However, light at a wavelength of ~ 630 nm is commonly used because of its greater tissue penetration. Upon HPD photoactivation, release of singlet oxygen with subsequent damage to the cell is thought to be the primary mechanism for cytotoxicity (photodynamic therapy).

Spears reasoned that HPD may be preferencially concentrated in atheromatous plaques due to the proliferation of smooth muscle cells and the hydrophobic lipid environment [101]. He demonstrated HPD localization in experimental atheromatous plaques of rabbits and monkeys by the selective HPD fluorescence in these lesions following systemic drug administration. Prevosti [102] similarly demonstrated that helium cadmium laser (325 nm) irradiation of normal and atherosclerotic rabbit aorta demonstrated fluorescence at 632 nm only in plaques from atherosclerotic rabbits pretreated with HPD. Kessel [103] demonstrated the accumulation of HPD in human atheromatous plaques in vitro. These and other data [104,105] suggested that human atheromatous plaques would take up hematoporphyrin derivative in vivo and might therefore be susceptible to photochemotherapy. Photodynamic therapy could therefore be a new approach to cause atherosclerosis regression or to inhibit restenosis following angioplasty. In in vivo animal models, administration of HPD following by 630–636 nm irradiation revealed quantitative and qualitative differences and reduction in plaque compared to nonirradiated control plaques [106–108]. A potential concern for clinical application, however, was the demonstration of coronary artery spasm following 632 nm laser irradiation of normal dog coronary arteries pretreated with dihematoporphyrin ether (DHE) [109].

Dartsch [110,111] evaluated the effect of DHE on human smooth muscle cells in vitro. He demonstrated a differential sensitivity of smooth muscle cells from atherosclerotic as compared tonon-atherosclerotic arteries. There was a greater cytotoxicity of the DHE alone or following ultraviolet light photoactivation in the cells derived from atherosclerotic plaques. Thus the localization of hematoporphyrins in atherosclerotic plaques, the ability to photoactivate them for cytotoxicity, and the greater sensitivity of atherosclerotic smooth muscle cells suggest that photodynamic therapy may be capable of specific and localized effect in the vascular wall.

The photosensitivity that occurs following systemic administration of HPD has resulted in the development and evaluation of other photosensitizing agents. Phycocyanin is a cytotoxic photosensitizer that also demonstrated specific localization in human atherosclerotic artery segments in vitro [112]. This drug can be photoactivated with wavelengths of 620–650 nm, which are minimally absorbed by blood and have reasonable tissue penetration. Ortu [113] studied the inhibition of intimal hyperplasia by photodynamic therapy in the balloon injury model of the rat carotid artery using chloroaluminum-sulfonated phthalocyanine. Phthalocyanine does not produce skin photosensitivity and has a high absorption peak at 675 nm enabling good tissue penetration. There was a significant decrease in intimal hyperplasia in the irradiated carotid artery of the phthalocyanine rats as compared to the nonirradiated control carotid artery. Lack of intimal hyperplasia was achieved without evidence of structural injury or inflammation.

8-methoxy-psoralen is another photoactivatible drug that is being investigated for cardiovascular application. Unlike the above drugs that are thought to mediate their toxicity through the photodynamic generation of singlet oxygen, the methoxypsoralen molecule inserts itself into the DNA double helix and forms monofunctional or bifunctional (cross-link) adducts with pyrmidine bases upon ultraviolet A irradiation. This DNA damage to the DNA can lead to inhibition of cellular proliferation or cell function and/or to cell death. Several studies have demonstrated that smooth muscle cell proliferation in vitro can be inhibited by the combination treatment with psoralen and light activation [114–117]. Neither low-dose light nor psoralen alone had an effect on cell proliferation. In one study [114], a single exposure to psoralen and UVA (1 mm, 1.5 J/cm^2, respectively) resulted in complete stasis of cell proliferation over a 28-day period without recurrent exposure. Although commonly activated with UVA, psoralens can also be activated with visible light [118] resulting in a greater percent of monoadduct as opposed to cross-link formation. Visible light irradiation might be preferrable for photochemotherapy because of its deeper penetration into tissue, its easier fiberoptic delivery, and its potentially lesser mutagenic and cytotoxic effects [117]. Visible light photoactivation of psoralen inhibited smooth muscle cell proliferation in vitro, although requiring greater light or drug doses than with UVA activation.

Gregory [116] demonstrated that UVA-activated psoralen reduced intimal smooth muscle cell proliferation assessed by bromodeoxyuridine incorporation in a porcine angioplasty model. Psoralen was given rectally to achieve adequate systemic drug levels, and a titanium-aluminum sapphire laser was used to deliver 365 nm irradiation through a fiberoptic balloon catheter to the arterial wall. There were no adverse vascular or system complications. Spaedy [119] similarly demonstrated a decreased proliferation of smooth muscle cells in a rabbit angioplasty model in those sites exposed to parenteral psoralen and local UVA irradiation. The decreased proliferation index correlated with decreased cellularity in the neointima of the combined light and drug treated angioplasty sites. Although only preliminary in vitro and in vivo animal data are available, the approach of systemic (or local) administration and local photoactivation of cytotoxic drugs is feasible and offers a potential potent therapy for restenosis and atherosclerosis.

TRANSMYOCARDIAL LASER REVASCULARIZATION

Laser angioplasty and laser balloon angioplasty attempt to improve myocardial blood supply by increasing the diameter of stenotic or occluded coronary arteries. A novel approach to myocardial revascularization involving laser technology is the creation of transmyocardial (epicardial to endocardial) channels for direct myocardial revascularization. This alternative revascularization method would clearly be of benefit to patients with diffuse coronary artery disease who are not candidates for conventional coronary artery bypass graft surgery or any of the currently available angioplasty modalities [120].

The creation of transmural left ventricular channels using a needle (so-called myocardial acupuncture) [121] was evaluated experimentally in the 1930s [122] and was used clinically to treat patients in 1960s. The technique was said to relieve ischemia by allowing blood to pass from the ventricle through the channels either directly into other vessels perforated by the channel or into myocardial sinusoids, which connect to the myocardial microcirculation [123]. In the reptilian heart, perfusion occurs via communicating channels between the left ventricle and the coronary arteries, and there is evidence for these communicating channels in the developing human embryo. The possibility of revascularizing the myocardium by creating transmyocardial channels with high-energy laser radiation was investigated initially by Mirhoseini [124]. He created 20–30 channels/cm^2 using 100 millisec pulses from a high power CO_2 laser in the left ventricular myocardium of dogs prior to LAD coronary artery ligation. Brisk bleeding from the sites of penetration resolved after several minutes of light pressure. Animals that had the channels created prior to LAD ligation acutely showed no evidence of ischemia or infarction in contrast to the control animals. The animals were sacrificed at intervals ranging from 4 weeks to 5 months. The laser-created channels could be demonstrated grossly and microscopically to be open and free of debris and scarring. Yano [125] created nontransmural myocardial channels (3 channels/cm^2) from the endocardial surface using a holmium:YAG laser (wavelength 2.14 μm) in six dogs acutely subjected to 90 min of LAD ligation followed by 6 hr of reperfusion. Two-dimensional echocardiography and segment length ultrasonic transducers documented preservation of myocardial contraction (shortening) in the ischemic region of four of the six laser-revascularized dogs. Despite these impressive acute results in a small group of dogs, Landreneau [126] found that regional myocardial blood flow estimated by radio-labeled microspheres and oxidative metabolism assessed by tissue pH measurements were severely depressed in the myocardial zone supplied by the occluded LAD despite the creation of multiple laser channels (25–30 channels, 3–5 mm apart). He also

reported that regional contractile dysfunction assessed by myocardial fiber shortening was no different in the lased region following LAD occlusion compared to a test LAD occlusion performed prior to creation of the laser channels. Whittaker [124] also could not demonstrate any immediate benefit to the ischemic myocardium in a canine model of coronary artery occlusion where myocardial laser channels were created using a holmium:YAG laser. Laser channels created 30 min into a 6-hr coronary artery occlusion failed to increase blood flow to the ischemic tissue, improve regional myocardial function, enhance washout of lactate, or decrease infarct size. Whittaker [124] also referenced several other recent studies that failed to demonstrate an acute benefit of laser-created transmyocardial channels for acute coronary artery occlusion. These data would suggest that the proposed connections between the transmyocardial channels and myocardial sinusoids either do not exist or are unable to supply sufficient blood flow acutely to compensate for epicardial coronary artery occlusion. However, the different results between the series of experiments using the canine LAD ligation model might possibly be explained by the greater number of channels created in the Mirhoseini experiments. Despite the discrepant results in acute animal investigations, it is possible that the creation of laser channels in the myocardium may promote long-term changes that could augment myocardial blood flow such as by inducing angiogenesis in the region of the lased (and thus damaged) myocardium. In support of this possibility, White [127] reported histologic evidence of probable new vessel formation adjacent to collagen-occluded transmyocardial channels.

Whittaker [128] evaluated the chronic response to direct myocardial revascularization in a rat model. Transmyocardial channels were made either using a holmium:YAG laser or a needle. Two months later, the rats were subjected to 90-min coronary artery occlusions. Prior to sacrifice, the heart was perfused with blue dye to detect collateral perfusion within the region of risk; the area of necrosis was determined by vital staining (tetrazolium). The area of necrosis as a percentage of the area at risk was reduced in the rats pretreated with needle channels but not in those pretreated with laser channels. Similarly, the number of blue dye containing vessels was increased in the rats treated with needle channels compared to the rats treated with laser channels or the control rats. Although laser revascularization did not demonstrate any chronic benefit in this model, the fact that needle-created channels had a chronic benefit in the face of acute arterial occlusion suggests the possibility that laser channels created either with different dosimetry or a different laser wavelength could be similarly beneficial. The greater lateral thermal damage of the holmium:YAG laser as compared to the CO_2 laser could account for acute or chronic differences in the response to laser-created transmyocardial channels.

Mirhoseini [29] reported the results of transmyocardial laser revascularization in a series of 12 patients in whom conventional bypass graft surgery would result in incomplete revascularization. Direct laser revascularization was performed in areas that were not suitable for insertion of a bypass graft with the creation of 10–12 channels using an 80-watt CO_2 laser. There were no operative deaths and clinical improvement was noted in all patients. A consistent finding in the follow-up studies was increased uptake of thallium isotope following thallium stress tests in the areas revascularized by laser, consistent with perfusion to these areas. Follow-up left ventriculography demonstrated patent channels in six of 10 patients, and an autopsy in one patient [130] revealed numerous patent and endothelialized vascular channels in the area revascularized by the laser.

Based on the animal and limited clinical data, a system for clinical laser transmycardial revascularization has been developed and is undergoing evaluation (The Heart Laser, PLC Systems). A phase I FDA protocol to study the safety of the procedure has been completed and a phase II protocol to study efficacy on 50 patients is ongoing. Typically, one 1 mm diameter channel is drilled per cm^2 of treatment area using a 35–50 msec pulse from a pulsed 850-watt CO_2 laser. This is a substantially reduced channel number and density compared to the earlier Mirhoseini dog experiments. The following preliminary results have been provided by PLC Systems. As of December 31, 1993, 46 patients with severe ischemic heart disease (66% with prior CABG) underwent transmyocardial laser revascularization using a left thoracotomy approach with an average of 21 channels being created during the procedure. Dedicated ECG electrodes were used to synchronize the pulsed CO_2 laser to the heart beat to minimize the risk of ventricular arrhythmias. Intraoperative transesophageal echocardiography was used in some patients to detect transmural

perforation by the appearance of echocardiographic density in the left ventricular cavity from steam due to the tissue vaporization. Perioperative mortality was 9%. In-hospital follow-up reported elimination of angina in 91% of treated patients and an increased activity level in 76% at the time of hospital discharge. Nuclear perfusion tests reportedly demonstrated increased perfusion at 3 and 6 months postoperatively. In five patients evaluated by positron emission tomography, metabolism increased in 27%, and perfusion increased in 20% of the lased areas. In the subset of patients evaluated at 3 months, 60–91% reported improvement in their anginal symptoms. One patient died following failed PTCA and emergency CABG performed 3 months after transmyocardial laser revascularization. Autopsy revealed multiple patent endothelial-lined laser channels with endocardial, and possibly intramyocardial, connections containing red blood cells. Based on these preliminary results, a critical evaluation of the potential role of transmyocardial laser revascularization for the treatment of patients with coronary artery disease appears indicated.

ANTIARRHYTHMIC LASER THERAPY
Ventricular Arrhythmias

Laser ablation has been investigated for several years as a means for treatment of ventricular and supraventricular arrhythmias. In vitro laser photoablation of pathological endocardium was demonstrated in 1984 by Isner [131] using a CO_2 argon laser. Subsequently, Saksena [132] and Isner [133] reported the use of the argon and CO_2 laser, respectively, to achieve superficial vaporization of endocardial tissue responsible for ventricular tachycardia in a small number of patients. Saksena [134] evaluated the safety and efficacy of intraoperative mapping-guided argon laser ablation alone, or in conjunction with standard surgical methods, in 20 consecutive patients with refractory sustained ventricular tachycardia or fibrillation. A mechanically chopped (1 sec pulses, 0.5 sec between pulses), 15-watt argon laser coupled to a 300-μm optical fiber was used for ventriculotomy and ventricular endocardial ablation. The area of laser endocardial ablation varied from 2 to 24 cm^2 (mean 9 cm^2). Thirty-eight VT morphologies were mapped and ablated with laser irradiation alone (82%), combined laser ablation and mechanical resection (13%), or mechanical resection alone (5%). Postoperative 30-day mortality was 5%, and only one patient required postoperative antiarrhythmic drug therapy. All survivors had suppression of inducible sustained VT at discharge, and no episodes of sudden death were reported at 1-year follow-up. These results compared favorably with the reported 25% need for additional antiarrhythmic therapy and 16% recurrence rate (over 27 months) following surgical subendocardial resection. Saksena reported a specifically improved success rate for inferior, septal, and posterior sites of VT origin using laser ablation compared to mechanical resection (46% vs. 55% in his series).

In contrast to the carbon dioxide and argon lasers that have been proposed for endocardial resection by tissue vaporization, the Nd:YAG laser has been proposed for antiarrhythmic therapy by in situ photocoagulation of the inciting focus without tissue vaporization. Svenson [135] reviewed the potential advantages of Nd:YAG laser photocoagulation for the treatment of ventricular tachycardia as compared to conventional surgical approaches. These benefits include the fact that the treated tissues are left intact preserving structural integrity of the myocardium. For example, mitral valve incompetence does not result from laser photocoagulation of the papillary muscles or the myocardium surrounding these structures [136]. Areas that are out of the reach of endocardial resection can be treated with improved access, and laser photocoagulation can be used in the absence of discrete areas of endocardial fibrosis. These benefits, however, are also shared by cryoablation. The major advantage compared to cryoablation is the fact that Nd:YAG laser photocoagulation can be performed on the normothermic beating heart during ventricular tachycardia at the time of surgery.

In contrast, cold cardioplegia is administered for effective cryoablation or for the performance of surgical endocardial resection. The ability to perform laser photocoagulation without cardioplegia enables improved assessment of efficacy during arrhythmia ablation. Upon rewarming the heart following cardioplegia, the inability to re-induce ventricular tachycardia could be secondary to a transient suppression from the cardioplegia as opposed to the surgical treatment. In contrast, using intraoperative mapping in the normothermic heart, the effects of laser irradiation can be monitored while the VT is ongoing; Nd:YAG irradiation can be delivered to the suspected site of origin until VT terminates and cannot be re-induced. Since the laser radiation can be applied to the epicardial surface of the heart, laser ablation is particularly useful for subepicardial in addition to subendocardial re-entry sites. Svenson, Selle, and Littman [135–138] reviewed their clinical experience with Nd:YAG laser ablation of ventricular tachycardia. A continuous wave Nd:YAG laser (wavelength 1.06 μm) coupled to a 600-μm diameter gas-cooled silica quart fiber was used to irradiate ~ 0.5^2 cm of tissue (spot size) at a power density of 70–150 watts/cm^2. The maximal depth of myocardial photocoagulation was estimated at 5–6 mm. In the largest series of 51 patients undergoing Nd:YAG laser photoablation, the number of intraoperative inducible forms of VT ranged from 0 to 6 (mean 2.5) per patient. In the five patients in whom intraoperative VT could not be induced, laser ablation was guided by the visible extent of endocardial fibrosis and by preoperative mapping data. Endocardial mapping and laser photoablation was performed through a ventriculotomy, whereas epicardial laser photocoagulation was performed directly. Electrophysiological recordings during laser irradiation demonstrated progressive prolongation of VT cycle length and then interruption of the presumed reentrant circuit. Sequential induction and laser ablation was performed until VT was finally no longer inducible. All 51 patients received endocardial laser applications ranging in surface area from 3 to 45 cm^2. Epicardial lasing was performed in 27 patients to surface areas ranging from 2 to 18 cm^2. Total time of lasing ranged from 3 to 25 min (mean 9.8). Nd:YAG laser photocoagulation was effective independent of the anatomic site of re-entry. Svenson [139] reported that 15% of the VT configurations induced intraoperatively required epicardial as opposed to endocardial photocoagulation for termination. At least one epicardial origin of VT was found in 1/3 of patients with either a right or left circumflex coronary artery related infarction without an aneurysm, suggesting that surgical endocardial resection alone would not be adequate therapy for this patient population.

Despite laser photocoagulation of myocardial foci, overall left ventricular function was not reduced in the operative survivors. Operative mortality in 12 patients with preoperative ejection fractions < 20% was 41%; in 39 patients with ejection fractions > 20% operative mortality was 8%, suggesting that ablative surgery should be targeted to this group of patients. Only one out of 25 patients had inducible sustained VT and only two had inducible nonsustained VT pre-discharge

[135]. Three of 34 patients had inducible VT on follow-up electrophysiologic study [137], and 88% of the 43 operative survivors were free of recurrent sustained VT at 1 year. There were no arrhythmic deaths in follow-up.

A significant potential of laser photocoagulation would be the development of catheter systems for percutaneous mapping and ablation. However, percutaneous laser antiarrhythmic therapy has been evaluated only in animal models. Lee [40] reported that endocardial lesions produced in vivo in a canine model by Nd:YAG laser radiation were comparable in gross morphology and size to those produced by DC electrical shock, but that transcatheter electrode shock produced significantly more ventricular tachycardia and wall motion abnormality. Although transcatheter laser photoablation could create controlled endocardial lesions with fewer dilaterious effects than transcatheter electrode DC shock for treatment of ventricular arrhythmias, the current clinical therapeutic approach uses percutaneous radiofrequency ablation, which is less damaging than DC shock [141].

Supraventricular Tachycardias

Laser treatment has been proposed as an alternative to surgical treatment of certain supraventricular tachycardias (SVT). Bypass pathway ablation for Wolff-Parkinson-White Syndrome, A-V node ablation for atrioventricular nodal re-entry tachycardia, sinus node ablation for automatic sinus tachycardia, and ablation, partition and/or isolation procedures for atrial reentrant tachycardia or fibrillation, are all potential procedures that may be performed more expeditiously and safely with laser radiation [137]. Atrioventricular node and sinus node ablation have been performed experimentally in dogs using argon or Nd:YAG laser radiation delivered through fiberoptic and angiographic catheters [142–144]. Narula [142] demonstrated PR interval prolongation following percutaneous argon laser irradiation of the A-V node. Additional radiation produced second- and eventually third-degree A-V nodal block. Persistence of A-V nodal delay was noted at re-study at 4 weeks. Curtis [143] reported two patterns of injury involved in conduction ablation: one was direct vaporization of tissue, and the other was formation of a hematoma and thermal necrosis without evidence of tissue vaporization. A single novel catheter with both bipolar electrodes for mapping of the A-V region and a 400-μm silica fiber for laser ablation

was developed for use in Curtis' study. Littmann [144] used an Nd:YAG laser to photocoagulate sinus node regions with long-lasting suppression of heart rate in dogs. Schuger [145] used a Spears Laser Balloon catheter inserted percutaneously into the coronary sinus in a canine model to produce a fibrotic lesion anatomically well-suited for left-sided accessory pathway ablation. Coagulation necrosis invading the atrioventricular groove and left atrial wall was demonstrated histologically at 6 weeks.

The effective prolongation of conduction following laser irradiation without acute or chronic complications suggests the potential application of this technique for management of supraventricular tachyarrhythmias. Saksena [146,147] treated seven patients with malignant SVT (4 Wolf-Parkinson-White Syndrome, 1 AV nodal re-entry, 1 atrial tachycardia, 1 atrial fibrillation) with intraoperative argon laser ablation. A 15-watt CW argon laser coupled to a 300-μm silica fiber was guided by electrophysiologic mapping to ablate the AV node or accessory pathway (combined with surgical dissection in the latter case). Spontaneous and inducible SVT was eliminated in all of the five patients with AV nodal reentry or WPW. AV nodal conduction was interrupted in the patient with atrial tachycardia and modified in the patient with atrial fibrillation. Excellent SVT control continued during follow-up of 1–16 months.

MYOCARDIAL ABLATION

Laser radiation may be effectively used for the ablation of myocardial tissue for the treatment of various cardiovascular disorders. Isner [148] demonstrated the feasibility of performing a myotomy-myectomy for idiopathic hypertrophic subaortic stenosis (IHSS) using laser radiation. In vitro investigations demonstrated that argon radiation could cut and vaporize the myocardium producing a myotomy-myectomy morphologically similar to that produced by the conventional blade technique. In vivo experiments confirmed that a laser myoplasty could be achieved in dogs by the use of an optical fiber inserted through a ventricular catheter. Laser myoplasty was successfully performed intraoperatively in a patient with hypertrophic cardiomyopathy using a 200-μm fiber coupled to a continuouswave argon laser. Dowling [149] performed a septal myectomy using a noncontact carbon dioxide laser, claiming the technique allowed improved visualization and cleaner resection of the septum compared to scalpel resection. In view of the feasibility of using laser therapy to create a myoplasty trough, a clinical trial of percutaneous laser myoplasty has been initiated using a newly developed catheter designed to orient an optical fiber against the septum. Two patients have been treated successfully with an acute reduction in their gradient and an improvement in their clinical status (J. Isner, pers. comm.). The major advantage of this laser procedure is the ability to perform percutaneously what otherwise would require a thoracotomy and open heart surgery.

The potential treatment of congenital heart defects using laser irradiation from an argon laser has been investigated in vitro [150] and in vivo in animal models [151,152]. Laser radiation was used in postmortem hearts to create an atrial septectomy and to relieve obstruction in valvular pulmonic and aortic stenosis, dysplastic pulmonary valve, pulmonary atresia, and coarctation of the aorta. CO_2 laser radiation has also been used for the laser debridement of calcified deposits from stenotic aortic valves in vitro. Atrial septostomies were able to be performed percutaneously in dogs using an argon laser coupled to flexible silica fibers [150,152] or a CO_2 laser coupled to silver halide infrared transmitting fibers [151]. Clinical application of laser irradiation for the treatment of congenital and valvular disease has been limited.

LASER DIAGNOSTICS
Arterial Laser-Induced Fluorescence Spectroscopy

Low-power laser radiation induces tissue fluorescence without tissue damage and can be used for diagnostic fluorescence spectroscopy. Fluorescent substances have long been identified in atherosclerotic plaques [153–155] and recent studies [156–159] have shown that normal and atherosclerotic arterial fluorescence differ. Laser-induced fluorescence spectroscopy of the arterial wall might therefore enable accurate detection of the presence of atheromatous plaque [160]. Accurate fluorescence imaging of the atherosclerotic vessel wall could detect early atherosclerotic changes, potentially identify atherosclerotic lesions at higher risk of complications, and guide laser or other ablative systems selectively and completely to ablate the obstructive atherosclerotic plaque.

The ability to differentiate atherosclerotic from normal tissue by fluorescence spectroscopy is suggested by differences in their composition, specifically differences in the quantity and character of fluorophores. Fluorophores have been reported to accumulate in the arterial wall as an atherosclerotic plaque develops, and these endogenous fluorescent substances, including carotenoids [155] and elastin derivatives [153], have been extracted from atheromatous plaques. Oraevsky [161] used fluorescence spectroscopy to detect peroxidized lipoproteins in atherosclerotic human plaques in vitro and in lesions in a hypercholesterolemic rabbit model in vivo. Since arterial fluorescence results from the contributions of several fluorophores, models have been proposed to determine the chemical composition of atherosclerotic plaques based on fluorescence characteristics [162]. Collagen and elastin are the major protein constituents of normal and atherosclerotic arteries [163]. However, the collagen to elastin ratio varies from 0.5 in normal arterial wall to 7.3 in atherosclerotic plaques, and this difference appears to account for much of the fluorescence difference between normal and atherosclerotic tissue [164].

Kitrell [156] demonstrated that fluorescence could be used to distinguish fibrous plaque from healthy arterial wall. Excitation at 480 nm resulted in distinct spectra for normal wall and atherosclerotic plaque. Normal samples displayed spectral peaks of approximately equal size at 550 and 600 nm. Atherosclerotic samples exhibited the same two peaks, but with the 600 nm peak smaller than the 550 nm peak. Sartori [157] found an inverse correlation between the fluorescence spectral intensity ratio and intimal thickness with argon laser-induced fluorescence spectroscopy of normal and atherosclerotic arteries.

Ultraviolet-induced arterial fluorescence has been studied by multiple investigators. Deckelbaum [158], using a nitrogen laser at a wavelength of 337 nm to induce fluorescence, reported not only the ability to distinguish between normal and atherosclerotic aorta, but also the ability to differentiate thin yellow fatty plaque from thick white atheromatous or fibrous plaque. Normal aortic specimens had maximal fluorescence intensity at 514 nm, white atheromatous plaque at 448 nm, and yellow fatty plaque at 530 nm. Anderson-Engels [159] also reported a difference in the nitrogen laser-induced fluorescence spectra of normal and atherosclerotic aorta and used fluorescence intensity ratios to classify arterial tissue as normal or as one of three different atherosclerotic histologic types. O'Brien [165] evaluated several discriminant algorithms for their ability to differentiate normal from atherosclerotic aorta, using helium cadmium (wavelength 325 nm), laser-induced fluorescence spectroscopy (Fig. 4) and reported that six of seven discriminant functions had classification accuracies greater than 90%. Gaffney et al. [166] reported that helium cadmium, laser-induced fluorescence spectra of atherosclerotic plaques correlated well with both fibrous plaque content and intimal thickness. Scott [167] developed a simplified LIF system using photomultiplier tubes and band pass filters to evaluate the ratio of arterial tissue fluorescence at 380–440 nm. Using a threshold fluorescence intensity ratio of 1.75, 41 of 44, or 93%, and of the normal specimens were correctly classified by ratios less than the threshold, whereas 50 of 57, or 88%, of the atherosclerotic specimens were correctly classified by ratios above this threshold. The classification accuracy increased at the extremes of intimal thickness. Specimens with an intimal thickness < 150 µm were correctly classified as normal in 22 of 22, or 100%, of the specimens. Thirty-six of 40, or 93%, of the atherosclerotic specimens with an intimal thickness of 500 µm or greater were correctly classified, whereas all 31, or 100%, of the specimens with an intimal thickness equal to or greater than 600 µm were correctly classified. The transition from normal to atherosclerotic ratios occurred at an intimal thickness of 200–300 µm. These observations are consistent with the previously reported 325 nm fluorescence sampling depth of 200 µm [168]. The use of ultraviolet radiation to induce fluorescence resulted in better normal and atherosclerotic tissue discrimination than achieved using visible radiation [169,170]. Leon [171] and Deckelbaum [172] have demonstrated the feasibility of in vivo fiberoptic ultraviolet-induced fluorescence spectroscopy by recording arterial fluorescence from patients undergoing vascular surgery or cardiac catheterization.

Since normal and atherosclerotic tissue have different fluorescence spectra, it may be possible to construct images of the arterial surface using fluorescence imaging [173–175]. Hoyt [173] performed laser spectroscopic imaging using laser-induced spectroscopic signals collected and transmitted via an array of optical fibers to produce a two-dimensional array of pixels ("picture elements") from which a map or image of the arterial wall was constructed. The catheter employed was composed of 19 optical fibers resulting in a 19-

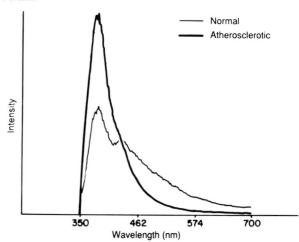

Fig. 4. Emission spectra. Representative helium-cadmium, laser-induced fluorescence spectra of normal and atherosclerotic aorta. The spectra are normalized to total intensity.

pixel image. With this imaging approach, more optical fibers could be added to enlarge the mapped area or to increase resolution. Anderson [174] suggested using one- and two-dimensional fluorescence imaging systems for atherosclerotic plaque demarcation. They used a computer-enhanced multicolor imaging system based on split-mirror, image-forming optics to obtain four individually filtered and congruent fluorescence spectral images simultaneously. Each image represented the fluorescence intensity at a given (filtered) wavelength. An arterial wall image could then be produced with the value of a discriminant function (e.g., a ratio of fluorescence intensity at different wavelengths derived from the different images) at each point to demarcate atherosclerotic from normal areas.

Clarke [176] studied laser Raman light scattering, laser-induced plasma photoemission, and electron paramagnetic resonance spectroscopy of arterial tissue. The Raman component of laser light that is scattered by tissue carries with it information about the chemical composition of the irradiated tissue. Laser Raman scattering was capable of detecting the presence of calcification in atherosclerotic coronary artery segments or degenerative aortic valve leaflets. The presence of tissue calcification could also be detected by calcium emission lines in the plasma emitted by cardiovascular tissue undergoing pulsed laser ablation [177]. Petit [178] was able to differentiate normal from atherosclerotic (calcified plaque) tissue by temporal differences in excimer laser pulses reflected from the arterial surface and suggested that dynamic reflectivity could be performed concurrently with excimer laser-induced fluorescence spectroscopy.

NADH Fluorimetry

The continuous monitoring of tissue NADH levels is an important means of monitoring tissue metabolism in terms of ischemia and viability. Renault [179] developed a laser fluorimeter designed for measurement of NADH levels in blood-perfused organs in an intact organism. A double-beam laser fluorimeter excited NADH fluorescence using light at a wavelength of 337 nm from a pulsed nitrogen laser. The NADH fluorescence emission at 480 nm was measured and compensation for blood circulation in the tissues was achieved by measuring the reflectance at 586 nm. Redox states could be assessed on-line as NAD does not fluorescence at these wavelengths; only the reduced form, NADH, fluoresces. Therefore, the NADH: NAD ratio would be proportional to the fluorescence emission at 480 nm. An increase in NADH fluorescence was demonstrated in isolated rat hearts rendered ischemic, [179,180] during skeletal muscle contraction in humans [181], and in a patient undergoing cardiac catheterization during contrast injection [182]. In the latter case, an optical fiber was inserted in a conventional catheter with the tip positioned on the left ventricular inferior wall endocardium. Injection of contrast medium into the right coronary artery provoked a marked transient increase in NADH fluorescence as a marker of the transient ischemia and/or anoxia induced by contrast injection. A prototype laser-fiberoptic based sensor for in situ NADH monitoring based on a compact Nd:YAG laser with associated harmonic generators has also been developed [183] with detection sensitivity of free NADH in the micromolar region. Immobilizing the enzyme lactate dehydrogenase on the fiber tip converts the monitoring channel into a lactate sensor. These studies suggest that laser fluorimetry might be a promising method of assessing and continuously monitoring regional myocardial ischemia and hypoxia in a clinical setting.

CONCLUSIONS

It is important to evaluate every new technology in terms of its cost and benefit. For a new interventional technology, one must consider the issues of whether the new technology can do something that conventional approaches cannot, or whether the new technology can do something cheaper than the conventional approaches. Developments in laser angioplasty, laser thrombolysis, transmyocardial laser revascularization, photochemotherapy, laser treatment of arrhythmias and/or laser diagnostics may improve upon conventional nonlaser approaches and provide new therapeutic or diagnostic options. As laser technology is further developed and its full potential in cardiovascular disease is realized, we may see an increasing application and acceptance of laser-based procedures in cardiology.

ACKNOWLEDGMENTS

The author acknowledges and thanks Ava Artaiz for her invaluable assistance with the preparation of this manuscript.

REFERENCES

1. McGuff PE, Bushnell D, Soroff HS, et al. Studies of the surgical applications of laser (light amplification by stimulated emission of radiation). Surg Forum 1963; 14: 143–145.
2. Choy DSJ, Stertzer RH, Myler RK, et al. Human coronary laser recanalization. Clin Cardiol 1984; 7:377–381.
3. Ginsburg R, Kim DS, Guthaner D, Tots J, Mitchell RES. Salvage of an ischemic limb by laser angioplasty: Description of a new technique. Clin Cardiol 1984; 7:54–58.
4. Lammer J, Karnel F. Percutaneous transluminal laser angioplasty with contact probes[1]. Radiology 1988; 168: 733–737.
5. Sanborn TA, Greenfield AJ, Guben JK, Menzoian JO, LoGerfo FW. Human percutaneous and intraoperative laser thermal angioplasty: Initial clinical results as an adjunct to balloon angioplasty. J Vasc Surg 1987; 5:83–90.
6. Belli AM, Cumberland DC, Procter AE, Welsh CL. Total peripheral artery occlusions: conventional versus laser thermal recanalization with a hybrid probe in percutaneous angioplasty—results of a randomized trial. Radiology 1991; 181:57–60.
7. Lammer J, Pilger E, Decrinis M, Quehenberger F, Klein GE, Stark G. Pulsed excimer laser versus continuous-wave Nd:YAG laser versus conventional angioplasty of peripheral arterial occlusions: Prospective, controlled, randomized trial. Lancet 1992; 340:1183–1188.
8. Cumberland DC, Oakley GDG, Smith GH, et al. Percutaneous laser assisted coronary angioplasty. Lancet 1986; 2:214.
9. Cumberland DC, Taylor DI, Welsh CL, et al. Percutaneous laser thermal angioplasty: Initial clinical results with a laser probe in total peripheral artery occlusions. Lancet 1986; 1:1457–1459.
10. Sanborn TA, Faxon DP, Kellett MA, et al. Percutaneous coronary laser thermal angioplasty with a metallic capped fiber. JACC 1987; 9(Suppl A):104A.

11. Cote G, Smith A, Andrus S, et al. Immediate results of percutaneous argon laser coronary angioplasty. Circulation 1989; 80(Suppl II):II–477.

12. Deckelbaum LI, Isner JM, Donaldson RF, et al. Reduction of laser-induced pathologic tissue injury using pulsed energy delivery. Am J Cardiol 1985; 56:662–666.

13. Linsker R, Srinivasan R, Wynne JJ, Alonso DR. Far-ultraviolet laser ablation of atherosclerotic lesions. Lasers Surg Med 1994; 4:201–206.

14. Grundfest WS, Litvack IF, Goldenberg T, et al. Pulsed ultraviolet lasers and the potential for safe laser angioplasty. Am J Surg 1985; 150:220–226.

15. Grundfest WS, Litvack F, Forrester JS, et al. Laser ablation of human atherosclerotic plaque without adjacent tissue injury. JACC 1985; 5:929–933.

16. Isner JM, Donaldson RF, Deckelbaum LI, et al. The excimer laser: Gross, light microscopic and ultrastructural analysis of potential advantages for use in laser therapy of cardiovascular disease. JACC 1985; 6:1102–1109.

17. Wollenek G, Laufer G, Grabenwoger F. Percutaneous transluminal excimer laser angioplasty in total peripheral artery occlusion in man. Lasers Surg Med 1988; 8:464–468.

18. Litvack F, Grundfest WS, Goldenberg T, et al. Percutaneous excimer laser angioplasty of aortocoronary saphenous vein grafts. JACC 1989; 14:803–808.

19. Geschwind HJ, Boussignac G, Dubois-Rande JL, Zelinsky R, Jea Tahk S. Laser angioplasty in peripheral arterial disease. Laser Med Surg 1991; 6:307.

20. Geschwind HJ, Dubois-Rande JL, Zelinsky R, et al. Percutaneous coronary mid-infrared laser angioplasty. Am Heart J 1991; 122:552–558.

21. Cook SL, Eigler NL, Shefer A, et al. Percutaneous excimer laser coronary angioplasty of lesions not ideal for balloon angioplasty. Circulation 1991; 84:632–643.

22. Bittl JA, Ryan TJ, Keaney JF, et al. Coronary artery perforation during excimer laser coronary angioplasty. JACC 1993; 21:1158–1165.

23. Werner G, Buchwald A, Unterberg C, et al. Excimer laser angioplasty in coronary artery disease. Eur Heart J 1991; 12:24–19.

24. Goodkind J, Coombs V, Golobic R. Excimer laser angioplasty. Heart Lung 1993; 22:26–35.

25. Isner JM, Rosenfield K, White CJ, et al. In vivo assessment of vascular pathology resulting from laser irradiation. Circulation 1992; 85:2185–2196.

26. Nakamura F, Kvasnicka J, Uchida Y, et al. Percutaneous angioscopic evaluation of luminal changes induced by excimer laser angioplasty. Am Heart J 1992; 124:1467–1472.

27. Larrazet FS, Dupouy PJ, Rande Dubois JL, Hirosaka A, Kvasnicka J, Geschwind HJ. Angioscopy after laser and balloon coronary angioplasty. JACC 1994; 23:(6)1321–1326.

28. Torre SR, Sanborn TA, Sharma SK, et al. Percutaneous coronary excimer laser angioplasty quantitative angiographic analysis demonstrates improved angioplasty results with larger laser catheters. Circulation 1990; 82(Suppl 3):III 671.

29. Margolis JR, Mehta S. Excimer laser coronary angioplasty. Am J Cardiol 92; 69:3F–11F.

30. Bittl JA, Sanborn TA. Excimer laser-facilitated coronary angioplasty. Circulation 1992; 86:71–80.

31. Hanet C, Wijns W, Michel X, et al. Influence of balloon size and stenosis morphology on immediate and delayed elastic recoil after percutaneous transluminal coronary angioplasty. JACC 1991; 18(2):506–511.

32. Isner JM, Rosenfield K, Losordo DW, et al. Combination balloon-ultrasound imaging catheter for percutaneous transluminal angioplasty. Circulation 1991; 84(2):739–754.

33. Rensing BJ, Hermans WR, Beatt KJ, et al. Quantitative angiographic assessment of elastic recoil after percutaneous transluminal coronary angioplasty. Am J Cardiol 1990; 66(15):1039–1044.

34. Safian RD, Freed M, Lichtenberg A, May MA, Juran N, Grines CL, O'Neill WW. Are residual stenoses after excimer laser angioplasty and coronary atherectomy due to inefficient or small devices? Comparison with balloon angioplasty. JACC 1993; 22(6):1628–1634.

35. Ellis SG, Vandeormael MG, Cowley MJ, et al. Coronary morphologic and clinical determinants of procedural outcome with angioplasty for multivessel coronary disease: Implications for patient selection. Circulation 1990; 82:1193–1202.

36. Ghazzal ZM, Hearn JA, Litvack F, et al. Morphological predictors of acute complications after percutaneous excimer laser coronary angioplasty. Circulation 1992; 86:820–827.

37. Holmes DR, Reeder GS, Ghazzal ZMB, Bresnahan JF, King III SB, Leon MB, Litvack F. Coronary perforation after excimer laser coronary angioplasty: The excimer laser coronary angioplasty registry experience. JACC 1994; 23(2):330–335.

38. Bittl JA, Sanborn TA, Tcheng JE, et al. Clinical success, complications and restenosis rates with excimer laser coronary angioplasty. Am J Cardiol 1992; 70:1553–1539.

39. Litvack F, Margolis J, Cummins F, et al. Excimer laser coronary registry: Report of the first consecutive 2080 patients. JACC 1992; 19:276A.

40. Litvack F, Eigler N, Margolis J, Rothbaum D, Bresnahan JF, Holmes D, Untereker W, Leon M, Kent K, Pichard A, King S, Ghazzal Z, Cummins F, Krauthamer D, Palacios I, Block P, Hartzler GO, O'Neill WO, Cowley M, Roubin G, Klein LLW, Frankel PS, Adams C, Goldenberg T, Laudenslager J, Grundfest WS, Forrester JS. Percutaneous excimer laser coronary angioplasty: Results in the first consecutive 3,000 patients. JACC 1994; 23(2):323–329.

41. Baumbach A, Haase K, Karsch KR. Usefulness of morphologic parameters in predicting the outcome of coronary excimer laser angioplasty. Am J Cardiol 1991; 68:1310–1315.

42. Safian RD, Freed M, Lichtenberg A, May MA, Strzelecki M, Grines CL, Pavlides G, Schreiber TL, O'Neill WW. Usefulness of percutaneous transluminal coronary angioplasty after new device coronary interventions. Am J Cardiol 1994; 73:642–646.

43. Knopf WD, Parr KL, Moses JW, et al. Multicenter registry report. Circulation 1992; 86(Suppl 1)I511.

44. Knopf W, Parr K, Moses J, et al. Holmium laser angioplasty in coronary arteries. JACC 1992; 19:352A.

45. de Marchena EJ, Mallon SM, Knopf WD, Parr K, Moses JW, Chutorian DM, Myerburg RJ. Effectiveness of holmium laser-assisted coronary angioplasty. Am J Cardiol 1994; 73:117–121.

46. Geschwind HJ, Nakamura F, Kvasnicka J, et al. Exci-

mer and holmium yttrium aluminum garnet laser coronary angioplasty. Am Heart J 1993; 125:510–522.

47. Estella P, Ryan TJ, Landzberg JS, et al. Excimer laser-assisted coronary angioplasty for lesions containing thrombus. JACC 1993; 21:1550–1556.

48. de Marchena E, Mallon S, Posada JD, et al. Direct holmium laser-assisted balloon angioplasty in acute myocardial infarction. Am J Cardiol 1993; 71:1223–1225.

49. Litvack F, Eigler NL, Forrester JS. In search of the optimized excimer laser angioplasty system. Circulation 1993; 87:1421–1422.

50. Baumbach A, Bittl JA, Fleck E, Geschwind HJ, Sanborn TA, Tcheng JE, Karsch KR. Acute complications of excimer laser coronary angioplasty: A detailed analysis of multicenter results. JACC 1994; 23(6):1305–1313.

51. Sanborn TA, Torre SR, Sharma SK, et al. Percutaneous coronary excimer laser-assisted balloon angioplasty. JACC 1991; 17:94–99.

52. Baumbach A, Haase KK, Voelker W., et al. Effects of intracoronary nitroglycerin on lumen diameter during early follow-up angiography after coronary excimer laser atherectomy. Eur Heart J 1991; 12:726–731.

53. Tenaglia AN, Tcheng JE, Kisslo KB, et al. Intracoronary ultrasound evaluation of excimer laser angioplasty. Circulation 1992; 86:I–516.

54. van Leeuwen TG, van Erven L, Meertens JH, et al. Origin of arterial wall dissections induced by pulsed excimer and mid-infrared laser ablation in the pig. JACC 1992; 19:1610–1618.

55. van Leeuwen TG, Meertens JH, Velema E., et al. Intraluminal vapor bubble induced by excimer laser pulse causes microsecond arterial dilation and invagination leading to extensive wall damage in the rabbit. Circulation 1993; 87:1258–1263.

56. Abela GS. Abrupt closure after pulsed laser angioplasty. J Interventional Cardio 1992; 5:259–262.

57. Isner JM, Pickering JG, Mosseri M. Laser-induced dissections. JACC 1992; 19:1619–1621.

58. Preisack MB, Voelker W, Haase KK, et al. Case Report: Formation of vessel aneurysm after stand alone coronary excimer laser angioplasty. Cathet Cardiovasc Diagn 1992; 27:122–124.

59. Feld MS, Kramer JR. Mutagenicity and the XeCl excimer laser. Am Heart J 1991; 6:1803–1806.

60. Buchwald AB, Werner GS, Unterberg C., et al. Restenosis after excimer laser angioplasty of coronary stenoses and chronic total occlusions. Am Heart J 1992; 123:878–885.

61. Kuntz RE, Gibson CM, Nobuyoski M, Baim DS. A generalized model of restenosis following conventional balloon angioplasty, stenting, and directional atherectomy. J Am Coll Cardiol 1993; 21:15–25.

62. Bittl JA, Kuntz RE, Estella P, Sanborn TA, Baim DS. Analysis of late lumen narrowing after excimer laser-facilitated coronary angioplasty. Am Coll Cardiol 1994; 23(6):1314–1320.

63. Holmes DR, Forrester JS, Litvack F, et al. Chronic total obstruction and short-term outcome: The excimer laser coronary angioplasty registry experience. Mayo Clin Proc 1993; 68:5–10.

64. Reeder GS, Bresnahan JF, Holmer DR, et al. Excimer laser coronary angioplasty. Cathet Cardiovasc Diagn 1992; 25:195–199.

65. Watson LE, Gantt S. Excimer laser coronary angioplasty for failed PTCA. Cathet Cardiovasc Diagn 1992; 26:285–290.

66. Waksman R, Carey D, Chazzal ZMB, King SB. Coronary excimer laser for unsuccessful angioplasty. J Invasive Card 1994; 6(1):21–24.

67. Grunkemeier JM, Gregory KW. Acoustic measurements of cavitation bubbles in blood, contrast and saline using an excimer laser. Circulation 1992; 86(Suppl 4):16.

68. Tcheng JE, Phillips HR, Wells LD, et al. A new technique for educing pressure pulse phenomena during coronary excimer laser angioplasty. JACC 1993; 21:386A.

69. Baumbach A, Haase KK, Rose C, Oberhoff M, Hanke H, Karsch KR. Formation of pressure waves during in vitro excimer laser irradiation in whole blood and the effect of dilution with contrast media and saline. Lasers Surg Med 1994; 14:3–6.

70. van Leeuwen TG, Jansen ED, Welch AJ, Borst C. Excimer laser induced bubble: Dimensions, theory and implications for laser angioplasty. Lasers Surg Med (in press).

71. Xie DY, Hassenstein S, Oberhoff M, et al. Preliminary evaluation of smooth excimer laser coronary angioplasty (SELCA) in vitro. Circulation 1992; 86(Suppl I): I–653.

72. Oberhoff M, Hassenstein S, Hanke H., et al. Smooth excimer laser coronary angioplasty (SELCA). Circulation 1992; 86(Suppl I):I–800.

73. Xie DY, Hassenstein S, Oberhoff M, Hanke H, Baumbach A, Hohla K, Haase KK, Karsch KR. In vitro evaluation of ablation parameters of normal and fibrous aorta using smooth excimer laser coronary angioplasty. Lasers Surg Med 1993; 13:618–624.

74. Henson KD, Leon MB, Pichard AD, et al. Successful directional excimer laser coronary angioplasty in unfavorable lesion morphologies. JACC 1993; 21:385A.

75. Ghazzal ZM, Leon MB, Shefer A, et al. The novel directional laser catheter. JACC 1993; 21:288A.

76. Garrand TJ, Stetz ML, O'Brien KM, et al. Design and evaluation of a fiberoptic fluorescence guided laser recanalization system. Lasers Surg Med 1991; 11:106–116.

77. Scott JJ, Desai SP, Deckelbaum LI. Optimization of laser angioplasty catheter position using arterial fluorescence feedback. Lasers Surg Med 1993; (Suppl 5):12.

78. Abela GS, Seeger JM, Barbieri E, Franzini D, Fenech A, Pepine CJ, Conti CR. Laser angioplasty with angioscopic guidance in humans. JACC 1986; 8(1):184–192.

79. Lee G, Ikeda R, Stobbe D, Ogata C, Theis J, Lui H, Mendizabal RC, Reis RL, Mason DT. Vaporization of human thrombus by laser treatment. Am Heart J 1993; 106(2):403–404.

80. Kaminow IP, Wiesenfeld JM, Choy SJ. Argon laser disintegration of thrombus and atherosclerotic plaque. Applied Optics 1984; 23(9):1301–1302.

81. Marco J, Silvernail PJ, Fournial G, Choy DS, Fajadet J, Case RB. Complete patency in thrombus-occluded arteries two weeks after laser recanalization. Lasers Surg Med 1985; 5:291–296.

82. LaMuraglia GM, Anderson RR, Parrish JA, Zhang D, Prince MR. Selective laser ablation of venous thrombus: Implications for a new approach in the treatment of pulmonary embolus. Lasers Surg Med 1988; (8):486–493.

83. Gregory KW, Block PC, Knopf WD, Buckley LA, Cates

CU. Laser thrombolysis in acute myocardial infarction. Lasers Surg Med 1993; (Suppl 5):13.

84. Topaz O, Rozenbaum EA, Battista S, Peterson C, Wysham DG. Laser facilitated angioplasty and thrombolysis in acute myocardial infarction complicated by prolonged or recurrent chest pain. Cathet Cardiovasc Diagn 1993; 28:7–16.

85. Pettit GH, Saidi IS, Tittel FK, Sauerbrey R, Cartwright J, Farrell R, Benedict CR. Thrombolysis by excimer laser photoablation. Lasers Life Sci 1993; 5:1–13.

86. Jenkins RD, Spears JR. Laser balloon angioplasty. Circulation 1990; 81(Suppl IV):IV–101–108.

87. Hiehle JF, Bourgelais JR. D, Shapsay S, Schoen FJ, Spears JR. Nd: YAG laser fusion of human atheromatous plaque arterial wall separations in vitro. Am J Cardiol 1985; 56:953–957.

88. Jenkins RD, Sinclair IN, Leonard BM, Sandor T, Schoen FJ, Spears JR. Laser balloon angioplasty versus balloon angioplasty in normal rabbit iliac arteries. Lasers Surg Med 1989; 9:237–247.

89. Alexopoulos D, Sanborn TA, Marmur JD, Badimon JJ, Badimon L, Dische R, Fuster V. Acute biological response to laser balloon angioplasty in the atherosclerotic rabbit. Lasers Surg Med 1994; 14:7–12.

90. Jenkins RD, Sinclair IN, McCall PE, Schoen FJ, Spears JR. Thermal sealing of arterial dissections and perforations in atherosclerotic rabbits with laser balloon angioplasty. Lasers Life Sci 1989; 3:13–30.

91. Ischinger T, Coppenrath K, Weber H, Enders S, Ruprecht L, Unsöld E, Hessel S. Laser balloon angioplasty: Technical realization and vascular tissue effects of a modified concept. Lasers Surg Med 1990; 10:112–123.

92. Sinclair IN, Jenkins RD, James LM, Sinefsky EL, Wagner MS, Sandor T, Schoen FJ, Spears JR. Effect of laser balloon angioplasty on normal dog coronary arteries in vivo. J Am Coll Cardiol 1988; 11(Suppl):108A (Abstract).

93. Spears JR, Reyes VP, Wynne J, Fromm BS, Sinofsky EL, Andrus S, Sinclair IN, Hopkins BE, Schwartz L, Aldridge HE, Plokker HWT, Mast EG, Rickards A, Knudtson ML, Sigwart U, Daer WE, Ferguson JJ, Angelini P, Leatherman LL, Safian RD, Jenkins RD, Douglas JS, King III SB. Percutaneous coronary laser balloon angioplasty: Initial results of a multicenter experience. J Am Coll Cardiol 1990; 16:293–303.

94. Jenkins RD, Sinclair IN, Anand RK, James LM, Spears JR. Laser balloon angioplasty: Effect of exposure duration on shear strength of welded layers of postmortem human aorta. Lasers Surg Med 1988; 8:392–396.

95. Schwartz L, Andrus S, Sinclair IN, Plokker T, Dear WE, Spears RJ. Restenosis following laser balloon coronary angioplasty: Results of a randomized pilot multicentre trial. Circulation 1991; 84(4):Suppl II:361.

96. Spears JR, Safian RD, Douglas JS, Plokker HWT, Sinclair IN, Jenkins RD, Reyes VP, Pichard AD, Ferguson JJ, Rickards AF, LBA Study Group. Multicenter acute and chronic results of laser balloon angioplasty for refractory abrupt closure after PTCA. Circulation 1991; 84(4)Suppl II:517.

97. McMath LP, Kundu SK, Spears RJ. Experimental application of bioprotective materials to injured arterial surfaces with laser balloon angioplasty. Circulation 1990; 82(4)Suppl III:72.

98. Fram DB, Gillam LD, Aretz TA, Tangco RV, Mitchel JF, Fisher JP, Sanzobrino BW, Kiernan FJ, Nikulasson S, Fieldman A, McKay RG. Low pressure radiofrequency balloon angioplasty: Evaluation in porcine peripheral arteries. J Am Coll Cardiol 1993; 21(6):1512–1521.

99. Yamashita K, Satake S, Ohira H, Ohtomo K. Radiofrequency thermal balloon coronary angioplasty: A new device for successful percutaneous transluminal coronary angioplasty. JACC 1994; 23(2):336–340.

100. Kessel D. Hematoporphyrin and HPD: Photophysics, photochemistry and phototherapy. Photochem Photobiol 1984; 39(6):851–859.

101. Spears RJ, Serur J, Shropshire D, Paulin S. Fluorescence of experimental atheromatous plaques with hematoporphyrin derivative. J Clin Invest 1983; 71:395–399.

102. Prevosti LG, Wynne JJ, Becker CG, Linsker R, Shires GT. Laser-induced fluorescence detection of atherosclerotic plaques with hematoporphyrin derivative used as an exogenous probe. J Vasc Surg 1988; 7:500–506.

103. Kessel D, Sykes E. Porphyrin accumulation by atheromatous plaques of the aorta. Photochemistry & Photobiology 1984; 40(1):59–61.

104. Spokojny AM, Serur JR, Skillman J, Spears RJ. Uptake of hematoporphyrin derivative by atheromatous plaques: Studies in human in vitro and rabbit in vivo. JACC 1986; 8:1387–1392.

105. Vever-Bizet C, L'Epine Y, Delettre E, Dellinger M, Peronneau P, Gaux JC, Brault D. Photofrin II uptake by atheroma in atherosclerotic rabbits. Fluorescence and high performance liquid chromatographic analysis on post-mortem aorta. Photochem Photobiol 1989; 49(6):731–737.

106. Litvack F, Grundfest WS, Forrester JS, Fishbein MC, Swan HJC, Corday E, Rider DM, McDermid IS, Pacala TJ, Laudenslager JB. Effects of hematoporphyrin derivative and photodynamic therapy on atherosclerotic rabbits. Am J Cardiol 1985; 56:667–671.

107. Neave V, Giannotta S, Hyman S, Schneider J. Hematoporphyrin uptake in atherosclerotic plaques: Therapeutic potentials. Neurosurgery 1988; 23:307–312.

108. Eton D, Colburn MD, Shim V, Panek W, Lee D, Moore WS, Ahn SS. Inhibition of intimal hyperplasia by photodynamic therapy using photofrin[1]. J Surg Res 1992; 53:558–562.

109. Mackie RW, Vincent GM, Fox J, Orme EC, Hammond MEH, Chang-Zong C, Johnson MD. In vivo canine coronary artery laser irradiation:photodynamic therapy using dihematoporphyrin ether and 632 nm laser: A safety and dose-response relationship study. Lasers Surg Med 1991; 11:535–544.

110. Dartsch PC, Ischinger T, Betz E. Differential effect of photofrin II on growth of human smooth muscle cells from nonatherosclerotic arteries and atheromatous plaques in vitro. Arteriosclerosis 1990; 10:616–624.

111. Dartsch PC, Ischinger T, Betz E. Responses of cultured smooth muscle cells from human nonatherosclerotic arteries and primary stenosing lesions after photoradiation: Implications for photodynamic therapy of vascular stenoses. JACC 1990; 15:1545–1550.

112. Morcos NC, Berns M, Henry WL. Phycocyanin: laser activation, cytotoxic effects, and uptake in human atherosclerotic plaque. Lasers Surg Med 1988; 8:10–17.

113. Ortu P, LaMuraglia GM, Roberts WG, Flotte TJ, Hasan

T. Photodynamic therapy of arteries: A novel approach for treatment of experimental intimal hyperplasia.

114. March KL, Patton BL, Wilensky RL, Hathway DR. 8-methoxypsoralen and longwave ultraviolet irradiation are a novel antiproliferative combination for vascular smooth muscle. Circulation 1993; 87:184–91.

115. Sumpio BE, Phan SM, Gasparro FP, Deckelbaum LI. Control of smooth muscle cell proliferation by psoralen photochemotherapy. J Vasc Surg 1993; 17:1010–1018.

116. Gregory KW, Buckley LA, Haw TE, Grunkemeier JM, Chasteney EA, Qu Z, Tuke-Bahlman D, Fahrenbach H, Block PC. Photochemotherapy of intimal hyperplasia using psoralen activated by ultra-violet light in a porcine model. Lasers Surg Med 1994; (Suppl 6):12 Abstract.

117. Sumpio BE, Li G, Deckelbaum LI, Gasparro FP. Selective inhibition of smooth muscle cell proliferation by visible light activated psoralen. (in press)

118. Gasparro FP, Gattolin P, Olack GA, Deckelbaum LI, Sumpio BE. The excitation of 8-methoxypsoralen with visible light: reversed phase HPLC quantitation of monoadducts and cross-links. Photochem Photobiol 1993; 57(6):1007–1010.

119. Spaedy TJ, March KL, Wilensky RL, Aita M, Gradus-Pizlo I, Hathway DR. The combination of 8-methoxypsoralen and ultraviolet A light in vivo inhibits smooth muscle proliferation after angioplasty. Circulation 1993; 88(4):1–81.

120. Mirhoseini M, Shelgikar S, Cayton MM. Transmyocardial laser revascularization: A review JCLMS 1993; 11(1):15–19.

121. Sen PK, Udwadia TE, Kinare SG, Parulkar GB. Transmyocardial acupuncture. A new approach to myocardial revascularization. J Thorac Cardiovasc Surg 1965; 50: 181–189.

122. Beck CS. The development of a new blood supply to the heart by operation. Ann Surg 1993; 102–801.

123. Whittaker P, Kloner RA, Przyklenk K. Laser-mediated transmural myocardial channels do not salvage acutely ischemic myocardium. JACC 1993; 22(1):302–309.

124. Mirhoseini M, Cayton MM. Revascularization of the heart by laser. J Microsurg 1981; 2:253–260.

125. Yano OJ, Bielefeld MR, Jeevanandam V, Treat MR, Marboe CC, Spotnitz HM, Smith CR. Prevention of acute regional ischemia with endocardial laser channels. Ann Thorac Surg 1993; 56:46–53.

126. Landreneau R, Nawarawong W, Laughlin H, Ripperger J, Brown O, McDaniel W, McKown D, Curtis J. Direct CO_2 laser "revascularization" of the myocardium. Lasers Surg Med 1991; 11:35–42.

127. White M, Hershey JE. Multiple transmyocardial puncture revascularization in refractory ventricular fibrillation due to myocardial ischemia. Ann Thorac Surg 1968; 6:557–563.

128. Whittaker P, Zheng S, Kloner RA (Heart Institute Good Samaritan Hospital & Univer Southern California, Los Angeles, CA (90017). Proceedings of the SPIE: O/E Lase 1992:1878–1828.

129. Mirhoseini M, Shelgikar S, Cayton MM. New concepts in revascularization of the myocardium. Ann Thorac Surg 1988; 45:415–420.

130. Mirhoseini M, Shelgikar S, Cayton M. Clinical and histological evaluation of laser myocardial revascularization. JCLMS 1990:73–78.

131. Isner JM, Michlewitz H, Clarke RH, Estes NAM, Donaldson RF, Salem DN, Bahn I, Payne DD, Cleveland RJ. Laser photoablation of pathological endocardium: In vitro findings suggesting a new approach to the surgical treatment of refractory arrhythmias and restrictive cardiomyopathy. Ann Thorac Surg 1985; 39(3):201–206.

132. Sakasena S, Hussain SM, Gielchinsky I, Gadhoke A, Pantopoulos D. Intraoperative mapping-guided argon laser ablation of malignant ventricular tachycardia. Am J Cardiol 1987; 59:78–83.

133. Isner JM, Estes NA, Payne DD, Rastegar H, Clarke RH, Cleveland RI. Laser-assisted endocardiectomy for refractory ventricular tachyarrhythmias: Preliminary operative experience. Clin Cardiol 1987; 10:201.

134. Saksena S, Gielchinsky I, Tullo NG. Argon laser ablation of malignant ventricular tachycardia associated with coronary artery disease. Am J Cardiol 1989; 64: 1298–1304.

135. Svenson RH. Neodymium: YAG laser ablation of ventricular tachycardia: A two-year experience. Arrhythmia Clinic 1987; 5(4):23–32.

136. Selle JG, Svenson RH, Gallagher JJ, Littmann L, Sealy WC, Robicsek F. Surgical treatment of ventricular tachycardia with Nd:YAG laser photocoagulation. PACE 1992; 15:1357–1361.

137. Selle JG, Svenson RH, Gallagher JJ, Littmann L, Sealy WC. Nd:YAG laser arrhythmia ablation. Cardiology 1989:72–78.

138. Littman L, Svenson RH, Gallagher JJ, Selle JG, Simmern SH, Fedor JM, Colavita PG. Functional role of the epicardium in postinfarction ventricular tachycardia. Circulation 1991; 83(5):1577–1591.

139. Svenson RH, Littmann L, Gallagher JJ, Selle JG, Zimmern SH, Fedor JM, Colavita PG. Termination of ventricular tachycardia with epicardial laser photocoagulation: A clinical comparison with patients undergoing successful endocardial photocoagulation alone. JACC 1990; 15(1):163–170.

140. Lee BI, Gottdiener JS, Fletcher RD, Rodriguez ER, Ferrans VJ. Transcatheter ablation: comparison between laser photoablation and electrode shock ablation in the dog. Circulation 1985; 72(3):579–86.

141. Gonska D, Brune S, Bethge KP, Kreuzer H. Radiofrequency catheter ablation in recurrent ventricular tachycardia. Eur Heart J 1991; 12:1257–1265.

142. Narula OS, Boveja BK, Cohen DM, Narula JT, Tarjan PP. Laser catheter-induced atrioventricular nodal delays and atrioventricular block in dogs: Acute and chronic observations. JACC 1985; 5(2):259–267.

143. Curtis AB, Abela GS, Griffin JC, Hill JA, Normann SJ. Transvascular argon laser ablation of atrioventricular conduction in dogs: Feasibility and morphological results. PACE 1989; 12:347–357.

144. Littmann L, Svenson RH, Gallagher JJ, Bharati S, Lev M, Linder KD, Tatsis GP, Nichelson C. Modification of sinus node function by epicardial laser irradiation in dogs. Circulation 1990; 81:350–359.

145. Schuger CD, McMath L, Abrams G, Zhan H, Spears JR, Steinman RT, Lehmann MH. Long-term effects of percutaneous laser balloon ablation from the canine coronary sinus. Circulation 1992; 86:947–954.

146. Saksena S, Munsif AN, Hussain SM, Gielchinsky I. Long term clinical results of intraoperative mapping-guided argon laser ablation of malignant supraventric-

ular and ventricular tachycardias. JADD 1988; 11(2): 178A (abstract).

147. Saksena S, Gielchinsky I. Argon laser ablation of modification of the atrioventricular conduction system in refractory supraventricular tachycardia. Am J Cardiol 1990; 66:767–770.

148. Isner JM, Clarke RH, Pandian NG, Donaldson RF, Salem DN, Konstam MA, Cleveland RJ. Laser myoplasty for hypertrophic cardiomyopathy. Am J Cardiol 1984; 53:1620–1625.

149. Dowling RD, Landreneau RJ, Gasior TA, Ziady GM, Armitage JM. Septal myectomy with a carbon dioxide laser for hypertrophic cardiomyopathy. Ann Thorac Surg 1993; 55:1558–1560.

150. Riemenschneider TA, Lee G, Ikeda RM, Bommer WJ, Stobbe D, Ogata C, Rebeck K, Reis RL, Mason DT. Laser irradiation of congenital heart disease: Potential for palliation and correction of intracardiac and intravascular defects. Am Heart J 1983; 106:1389.

151. Zeevi B, Gal D, Wolf N, Berant M, Abramovici A, Blieden LC, Katzir A. The use of carbon dioxide fiberoptic laser catheter for atrial septostomy. Am Heart J 1988; 116:117.

152. Bommer WJ, Lee G, Riemenschneider TA, Ikeda RM, Rebeck K, Stobbe D, Ogata C, Theis JH, Reis RL, Mason DT. Laser atrial septostomy. Am Heart J 1983:1152.

153. Banga I, Bihara-Varga M. Investigations of free and elastin bound fluorescent substances present in the atherosclerotic lipid and calcium plaques. Connect Tiss Res 1974; 2:237–241.

154. Blankenhorn DH, Braunstein H. Carotenoids in man, III. The microscopic pattern of fluorescence in atheromas, and its relation to their growth. J Clin Invest 1958; 37:160–165.

155. Prince MR, Deutsch TF, Matthews-Roth, et al. Preferential light absorption in atheromas in vitro. J Clin Invest 1986; 78:295–302.

156. Kittrell C, Willett Rl, de los Santos-Pancheo C, et al. Diagnosis of fibrous arterial atherosclerosis using fluorescence. Appl Opt 1985; 25:2280–2281.

157. Sartori M, Henry PD, Roberts R, et al. Estimation of arterial wall thickness and detection of atherosclerosis by laser-induced argon fluorescence. JACC 1986; 7:270A (Abstract).

158. Deckelbaum LI, Lam JK, Cabin HS, et al. Discrimination of normal and atherosclerotic aorta by laser-induced fluorescence. Laser Med Surg 1987; 7:330–335.

159. Andersson-Engels S, Gustafson A, Johnasson J, et al. Laser-induced fluorescence used in localizing atherosclerotic lesions. Laser Med Surg 1989; 4:171–181.

160. Deckelbaum LI. Fluorescence spectroscopy in cardiovascular disease: Fundamental concepts and clinical applications. Trends Cardiovasc Med 1991; 1:171–176.

161. Oraevsky AA, Jacques SL, Pettit GH, Sauerbrey RA, Tittel FK, Nguy JH, Henry PD. XeCl laser-induced fluorescence of atherosclerotic arteries. Circulation Res 1993; 72:84–90.

162. Richards-Kortum R, Rava RP, Cothren R, et al. A model for extraction of diagnostic information from laser-induced fluorescence spectra of human artery wall. Spectrochim Acta 1989; 45A:87–93.

163. Roskosova B, Rapp JH, Porter JM, et al. Composition and metabolism of symptomatic distal aortic plaque. J Vasc Surg 1986; 3:617–622.

164. Laufer G, Wollenek G, Rueckle B, et al. Characteristics of 308nm excimer laser activated arterial tissue photoemission under ablative and non-ablative conditions. Lasers Surg Med 1989; 9:556–571.

165. O'Brien K, Gmitro A, Gindi GR, Stetz ML, Cutruzzola FW, Laifer LI, Deckelbaum LI. Development and evaluation of spectral classification algorithms for fluorescence guided laser angioplasty. IEEE 1989; 36(4):424–431.

166. Gaffney EJ, Blarke RH, Lucas AR, et al. Correlation of fluorescence emission with the plaque content and intimal thickness of atherosclerotic coronary arteries. Lasers Surg Med 1989; 9:215–228.

167. Scott J, Stetz M, Imam K, Serafin J, Deckelbaum LI. A simplified laser-induced fluorescence spectroscopy system for coronary laser angioplasty guidance. Lasers Surg Med 1992; (Suppl IV):13.

168. Gmitro AF, Cutruzzola FW, Stetz ML, Deckelbaum LI. Measurement depth of laser-induced tissue fluorescence with application to laser angioplasty. Applied Optics 1988; 27(9):1844–1849.

169. Casale PH, Nishioka NS, Southern JF, et al. Improved criteria for detecting atherosclerotic plaque by fluorescence spectroscopy. Circulation 1987; 76(Suppl IV):2084 (Abstract).

170. Crilly RJ, Gunther S, Motamedei M, et al. Fluorescence spectra of normal and atherosclerotic human aorta: optimum discriminant analysis. SPIE 1989; 1067:110–115.

171. Leon MB, Prevosti LG, Smith PD, et al. In vivo laser-induced fluorescence plaque detection: Preliminary results in patients. Circulation 1987; 76(Suppl IV):1623 (Abstract).

172. Deckelbaum LI, Scott JJ, Rohls K, Desai S, Kim C, Cleman MW. Utility of arterial fluorescence feedback during excimer laser coronary angioplasty. Am Coll Card 43rd Annual Scientific Session 1993 (Abstract).

173. Hoyt CC, Richards-Kortum RR, Costello B, et al. Remote biomedical spectroscopic imaging of human artery wall. Lasers Surg Med 1988; 8:1–9.

174. Andersson PS, Montan S, Svanberg S. Multispectral systems for medical fluorescence imaging. IEEE J Quantum Electron 1987; QE-23:1798–1805.

175. Sartori M, Sauerbrey R, Kubodera S, Tittel FK, et al. Autofluorescence maps of atherosclerotic human arteries—A new tachnique in medical imaging. IEEE J QUantum Electron 1987-QE-23:1794–1797.

176. Clarke RH, Isner JM, Gauthier T, et al. Spectroscopic characterization of cardiovascular tissue. Lasers Surg Med 1988; 8:45–59.

177. Deckelbaum LI, Scott JJ, Stetz ML, et al. Detection of calcified atherosclerotic plaque by laser-induced plasma emission. Lasers Surg Med 1992; 12:18–24.

178. Pettit GH, Sauerbrey R, Tittel FK, Weilbacher D, Henry PD. Atherosclerotic tissue analysis by time-resolved XeCl excimer laser reflectometry. Lasers Surg Med 1993; 13:279–283.

179. Renault G, Raynal E, Sinet M, Muffat-Joly M, Berthier JP, Cornillault J, Godard B, Pocidalo JJ. In situ double-beam NADH laser fluorimetry: Choice of a reference wavelength. Am J Physiol 1984; 15:H491–H499.

180. Horvath KA, Torchiana DF, Daggett WM, Nishioka NS. Monitoring myocardial reperfusion injury with NADH fluorometry. 1992; 12:2–6.

181. Guezennec CY, Lienhard F, Louisy F, Renault G, Tusseau MH, Portero P, In situ NADH laser fluorimetry during muscle contraction in humans. Eur J Applied Physiol 1991; 63(1):36–42.

182. Duboc D, Toussaint M, Donsez D, Weber S, Guerin F, Degeorges M, Renault G, Polianski J, Pocidalo JJ. Detection of myocardial ischaemia by NADH laser fluorimetry during human left heart catheterization. Lancet 1986:522.

183. Orr CS, Arthurs SC. Tissue viability measurement by in situ fluorometry. ASAIO;1992; 38(3):M412–415.

Chapter 2

Lasers in Dentistry

Harvey A. Wigdor, DDS, MS, **Joseph T. Walsh, Jr.**, PhD,
John D.B. Featherstone, MSc, PhD, **Steven R. Visuri**, MS, **Daniel Fried**, PhD,
and **Joseph L. Waldvogel**, DDS

Ravenswood Hospital Medical Center, Wenske Laser Center, Chicago,
(H.A.W.); Biomedical Engineering Department, Northwestern University,
Evanston, (J.T.W., S.R.V.); Nobelpharma Industries, Chicago (J.L.W.);
Department of Oral Sciences, Eastman Dental Center, Rochester,
New York (J.D.B.F., D.F.)

INTRODUCTION

If asked what causes the most anxiety in the dental office, the typical patient undoubtedly would single out the drill (handpiece) as the most uncomfortable component in dental treatment. Many patients are so afraid of dental procedures that they frequently wait until the pain from infection is so great that they are willing to endure the perceived painful treatment to gain relief. Some dental patients are aware, mainly through the media, that a beam of light can cut metals and other hard objects. Why not, then, use this beam of light, instead of a drill, to cut into gingiva or teeth and make the visit to the dentist as easy as going for a haircut? The perception of the lay public seems to be that dental treatment can be made much easier if methods are developed to eliminate the use of the drill, and a laser may be just that method.

Almost immediately after the development of the ruby laser by Maiman in 1960, researchers postulated that it could apply to dental treatment. Stern and Sognnaes in 1964 [1] began looking at the possible uses of the ruby laser in dentistry. They were the first in a long list of investigators looking for a better way to treat dental patients with lasers. They began their laser studies on hard dental tissues by investigating the possible use of a ruby laser to reduce the subsurface demineralization [2–4]. Stern and Sognnaes found a reduction in permeability, to acid demineralization, of the exposed enamel. However, Adrian et al. [5] found that the ruby laser produced significant heat that caused damage to the pulp of the teeth. A number of other researchers looked at the effect lasers had on dental hard tissues [6–12]. Since these preliminary studies, research in this area has been sparse with but a few reports discussing the potential hard tissue uses. At present, the Food and Drug Administration has cleared laser soft tissue procedures with the CO_2, Nd:YAG, Ho:YAG, and Argon lasers. Also cleared is the use of lasers for the polymerization of light-activated restorative materials.

Our goal in this summary is to look at the past, present, and future of laser dentistry, trying to make some sense of recent claims and reports so that an understanding may begin to unfold. Summaries of published research papers form the core of this report, using them to establish the current knowledge in this ever-changing field. For reference, Dederich and Cheong et al. [13,14] have published summaries of the basic laser–tissue interaction.

We divide this article into sections based on application. Numerous reports have been directed toward both soft and hard dental tissue use. It seems appropriate that the bulk of this current work include these two major areas of accepted and possible future dental applications. Other possible applications also are discussed.

SOFT TISSUE

The interaction of laser radiation with various soft tissues of the human body has been reported in innumerable articles. Across a fairly broad spectrum of soft tissues, one can generalize the laser-tissue interactions. The general dentists, periodontists, endodontists, and oral and maxillofacial surgeons who were the pioneers in the use of lasers in dentistry faced a unique problem: there are teeth that pass through the soft tissue being treated. The ability of teeth to recover from traumatic injury is limited. Thus, during laser-based treatment of the soft tissue in the oral cavity, a practitioner must protect the teeth.

The effect of the CO_2 laser on soft tissue has been reported in several articles by Luomanen in 1987 [15–19]. In these articles the cellular and extracellular components of healing and repair of epithelium and connective tissue were evaluated following CO_2 laser incisions of rat mucosa and compared to scalpel incisions. A brief summary of these articles would suggest that there are differences in the tissue reactions seen when either the scalpel or the CO_2 laser are used to make the incision. The author suggests that these differences may be the cause of the effects seen clinically, i.e., slower healing and less scar formation when a CO_2 laser is used for surgery. The reader is encouraged to review these excellent articles on the basic histologic effect of the laser on oral mucosa. Walsh et al. [20–23] reported the use of CO_2 lasers for soft tissue ablation, directing attention to the ablation rate and thermal effects on various tissues. The authors showed that thermal damage could be controlled if the optimal parameters are used when cutting these tissues with either pulsed or continuous wave (CW) CO_2 lasers.

One of the early reports in 1968 of lasers in oral and maxillofacial surgery was by Goldman et al. [24]. They reported on the use of the CO_2 laser in preliminary investigative surgery. There was some concern by these early investigators about possible damage to the underlying bone around teeth. Clayman et al. [25] looked at the defects caused by the CO_2 laser to evaluate the effect of this laser on bone in both the short and long term. They reported in 1978 that the CO_2 laser does, in fact, cause minimal damage to the bone under the gingiva being treated, but the gingiva healed well, albeit over a longer period of time [25]. A pioneer in the area of clinical periodontal and oral surgery is Pick, who, along with colleagues in 1985 reported on the laser gingivectomy [26]. This procedure is usually limited to those lesions caused by drug-induced gingival overgrowth. The drug Dilantin® (phenytoin sodium, Parke-Davis, Morris Plains, NJ) has been implicated most often and has been reported to cause this problem in ~ 50% of patients receiving it. More recently, the drugs Sandimmune (cyclosporine, Sandoz, East Hanover, NJ), Procardia (nifedipinem Pratt Pharmaceuticals, New York City), and Cardizam (diltiazem hydochloride, Marrion Merrell Dow, Kansas City, MO) have been reported to cause gingival overgrowth.

Pick discussed the technique for removal of overgrown gingival tissue, paying close attention to and protecting the teeth and the surrounding bone. The advantages of using the CO_2 laser for this type of surgical procedure included dry and bloodless surgery, instant sterilization of the surgical site, and reduced bacteremia [27]. Further, there were reduced mechanical trauma, minimal postoperative swelling and scarring, and minimal postoperative pain. Some of the disadvantages included the cost of the laser for the dental practitioner, loss of tactile feedback since the CO_2 laser is used in the noncontact mode, and the special training needed for both the surgeon and assistant. Pick and Picaro [28], Abt et al. [29], and Frame [30] have all reported the successful use of the CO_2 laser for the treatment of oral pathologies.

The soft tissue applications have been restricted mostly to incising and excising masses from the mucosa and gingiva in the oral cavity. Only recently have reports suggested that the CO_2 laser may have a unique ability in periodontal surgery to impede the postoperative growth of oral epithelium. A major problem that occurs after surgery around teeth is that the epithelium grows faster then the healing connective tissues. The swiftly growing epithelium will progress down along the root surface of the tooth, causing a deep pocket to form next to the tooth. This pocket is a site for accumulation of bacteria and debris. The bacteria and debris are not cleansable in these deep pockets and can lead to a poor prognosis after periodontal surgery. Rossmann and Israel [31,32] have reported on a technique where the CO_2 laser was used to remove the epithelium from the connective tissue around the tooth. They have shown inhibition of epithelial in growth around the tooth [31,32]. More research needs to be performed in this area, but it seems as if the CO_2 laser may have the unique characteristic of being able to remove a thin layer of epithelium cleanly, unlike anything now available in dentistry.

A few examples of these dental procedures are presented in the following summaries of some experiences by one of the authors (H.A.W.) using the CO_2 laser as a surgical instrument in dental soft tissue applications. All the cases were performed by this author. The presented procedures represent a cross section of the types of surgeries presently performed by dentists with CO_2 lasers. It is not intended here to discuss the benefits of one laser over another for soft tissue procedures nor to specify the special techniques for a particular laser. Although other lasers have been cleared by the FDA, this author's experience has been only with the CO_2 laser; hence these cases were performed with this laser. Other cleared lasers could perform these procedures equally as well.

CASE EXPERIENCES

Patient 1. A 22-year-old black female presented to the Oral Diagnosis Department at the University of Illinois College of Dentistry for treatment of enlarged "gums." This patient had a

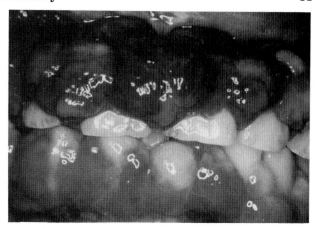

Fig. 1. Preoperative photograph of a patient with Dilantin-induced gingival overgrowth. Note the severe overgrowth of the gingiva.

history of seizure disorders and was taking Dilantin to control them. There were no other medical problems reported. She stated that she had been taking dilantin since she was very young and her gums had been enlarged for quite some time, but she was afraid of the surgery. At the presentation visit, the patient was given a prescription for Peridex® (chlorhexidine gluconate, Proctor and Gamble, Cincinnati, OH), an antibacterial rinse that reduces the inflammation causing the severe overgrowth seen in this patient. She was then rescheduled for surgery 2 weeks later. Figure 1 shows this patient before surgery and after 2 weeks of Peridex® therapy.

Prior to surgery, the patient was anesthetized with 2% lidocaine with 1:100,000 epinephrine. After suffcent anesthesia, the tissue was first debulked with a CO_2 laser (Pfizer, Irvine, CA) in the focused mode 10 watts CW. The teeth immediately adjacent to the surgical site were protected with a metal retractor. Figure 2 shows the retractor in place protecting the tooth below. After the lesion was significantly reduced, the laser was used in the defocused mode to contour the tissue. As stated earlier, the CO_2 laser procedure is noncontact, so the surgeon does not know when the laser has penetrated through the tissue. It is therefore essential that the tooth below the incision be protected.

The surgical objective was to create the contour of the normal gingiva. Once the bulk of the lesion was removed, the laser was used in the defocused mode to ablate thin layers of tissue to festoon the gingiva. Figure 3 shows the immediate postoperative results. There are some areas of

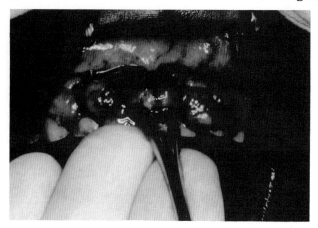

Fig. 2. Intraoperative photograph with retraction instrument in place to protect the tooth beneath.

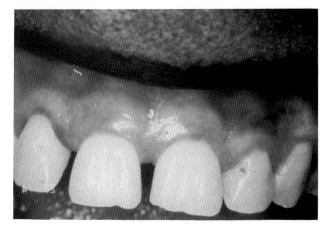

Fig. 4. Three-week postoperative view; appearance of the gingiva has normal contours.

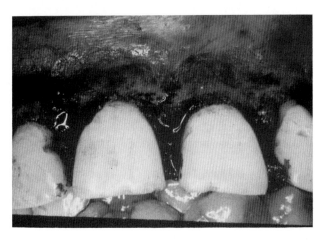

Fig. 3. Immediate postoperative photograph with minimal hemorrhage evident.

hemorrhagic tissue between the teeth. A sharp curette was used in these tissues to remove the hyperplastic tissue because of the close proximity of the teeth to each other. The laser could have damaged the teeth in this area if removal was attempted. The patient tolerated the procedure well, and there were no unusual postoperative complications. Figure 4 is a 3-week postoperative photograph showing good contour of the gingival tissue without any evidence of edema, inflammation, or ulceration. The patient denied any postoperative pain but had some mild discomfort controlled easily with acetaminophen.

The great benefit gained with this laser is the reduction of postoperative pain. The reduction of hemorrhage during the surgical procedure and after also makes the CO_2 laser an ideal treatment modality for these dental therapies. Time of surgery can also be reduced after the provider becomes experienced with laser surgical techniques.

Patient 2. A 53-year-old black female presented with the complaint of pain and bleeding beneath her existing lower full denture. An exam revealed a 2–3-cm-long epulis fissuratum in the buccal vestibule of her left ridge. Figure 5 indicates the lesion beneath the denture. These types of lesions are found frequently beneath ill-fitting dentures and can be a chronic source of infection and pain. Usually the treatment consists of surgical removal of the excess tissue and construction of a new denture to prevent the recurrence of the lesion. The patient was anesthetized with 2% lidocaine. The bulk of the lesion was removed with a CO_2 laser (Sharplan, Israel) in the focused mode using 7 watts CW. After debulking the lesion, the laser was defocused and used to festoon the tissue. Figure 6 is the immediate postoperative photograph showing the char that was created by the laser over the surgical site.

The patient experienced no postoperative discomfort, and Figure 7 shows the area 3 weeks after surgery. This patient had a similar procedure, done conventionally with a scalpel, a year prior to this surgery. The remarkable difference to her was that the postoperative pain was dramatically less after this laser surgery than with her prior surgical experience. This patient has been followed over the last 7 years; she still has no complaints and the lesion has not recurred.

Patient 3. Within the oral cavity are structures called frenula that attach the lips and tongue. Occasionally, such an attachment limits tongue movement or causes tension on gingival

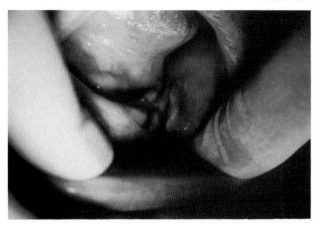

Fig. 5. Preoperative photograph of an epulis fissuratum.

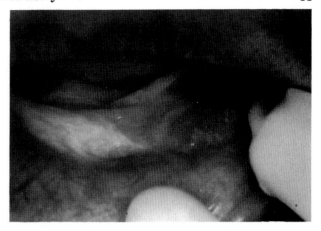

Fig. 7. Three-week postoperative result.

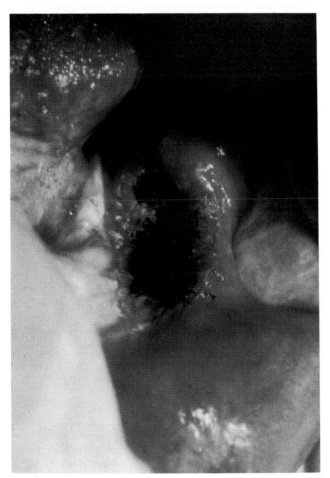

Fig. 6. Immediate postoperative photograph; note char covering operative site.

tissue, and thus gingival problems. A surgical treatment for such frenular problems can be curative.

A 12-year-old white female presented with a frenum that inhibited the movement of the tongue. Figure 8 shows the preoperative frenum. Note that it was attached to the total length of the tongue. For the procedure, 1–2 cm^3 of lidocaine were infiltrated into the base of the frenum. After sufficient anesthesia, the CO_2 laser (Luxar, Bothel, WA) emitting 5 watts CW was used to make a cut in the center of the frenum in a superior-to-inferior direction until the base of the tongue was reached. Because the base of the tongue can be very hemorrhagic if cut with a blade, the laser has the advantage of treatment without bleeding. Figure 9 is an immediate postoperative view of the sectioned frenum, and Figure 10 is a view 2 weeks later. The patient tolerated the procedure well and had no postoperative discomfort.

Patient 4. This patient (described below) had dental implants placed 6 months prior to the laser surgery. The principle of dental implants is to place them in bone as atraumatically as possible and allow them to heal in the bone covered by the gingiva for 6 months. After the 6-month healing period, an incision is made over the implants and a transmucosa cylinder (abutment) is placed on the implant. For this stage of the implant procedure, a CO_2 laser can be of value.

A 53-year-old white male presented for the placement of dental implants. Due to a severe gag reflex, he had been unable to wear full dentures and had been without teeth for many years. The implant placement surgery was uneventful; six implants were placed in the maxillary arch and five in the mandibular arch. Six months after the placement of dental implants, the patient presented for exposure of these implants and attach-

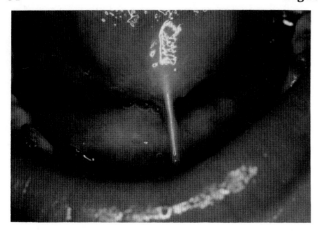

Fig. 8. Preoperative photograph of the tightly bound down tongue.

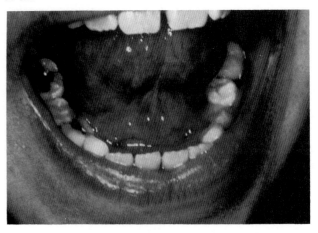

Fig. 10. Two-week postoperative view; note reduced limitation of movement of the tongue.

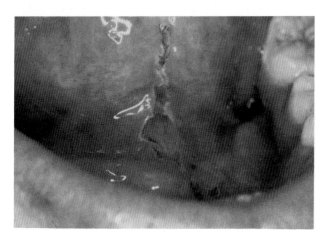

Fig. 9. Immediate postoperative photograph; no hemorrhage is evident.

ment of the abutments. The patient was anesthetized with lidocaine throughout the surgical sites.

Figure 11 shows the preoperative edentulous ridge. The implants are the dark bulges on the ridge. An incision was made with a CO_2 laser (Luxar, Bothel, WA) 7 watts CW with a spot size of ~ 800 µm on the crest of the alveolar ridge exposing the tops of the implant screws (see Fig. 12). After the incision was made with the laser, the implants were further exposed with a periosteal elevator. Both maxillary and mandibular implants were exposed and abutments placed. Figure 13 shows the abutments in place. Figure 14 shows the prosthesis in place and the postoperative result 6 weeks later. The patient tolerated the second procedure well and had no postoperative discomfort. For this procedure, the CO_2 laser allows for a better visualization of the implants because of the reduction of bleeding in the surgical site. Lasers also can be used in place of electrocautery because there is no electrical current with lasers that could be transmitted through the implant to the surrounding bone.

The CO_2 laser is the most frequently used laser in surgery; very few reports have been published discussing the use of the pulsed Nd:YAG, argon, and Ho:YAG lasers on oral soft tissues. White et al. [33] have discussed the use of the pulsed Nd:YAG laser on soft tissue lesions.

HARD TISSUES

The soft tissue interaction of different laser wavelengths is fairly well known, but hard dental tissue interaction is just beginning to be understood. Because light interacts much differently with hard tissues, an understanding of the optical properties of hard tissues must first be determined. The following is a brief summary of the optical properties of dental hard tissues.

Optical Properties

Background. For any procedures using lasers, the optical interactions between the laser and the tissue must be thoroughly understood to ensure safe and effective treatment. The laser-tissue interaction is controlled by the irradiation parameters, i.e., the wavelength, repetition rate, the pulse energy, spatial and temporal characteristics, and the optical properties of the tissue. Typically, the optical properties are characterized by the refractive index, and scattering (μ_s) and absorption coefficients (μ_a), and the scattering an-

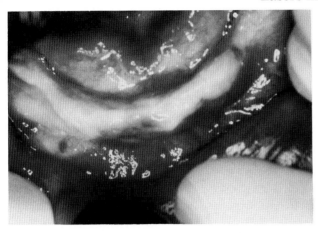

Fig. 11. Preoperative photograph of submerged dental implants. The bulges in the ridge are the location of the implants.

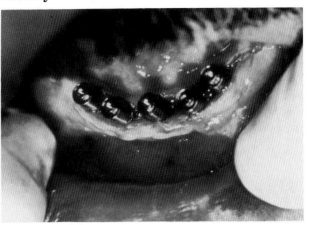

Fig. 13. Abutments in place on implants.

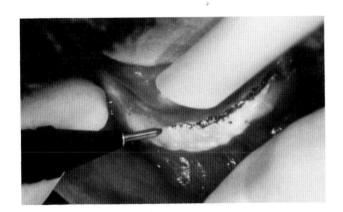

Fig. 12. Intraoperative photograph using the CO_2 laser to expose the implants.

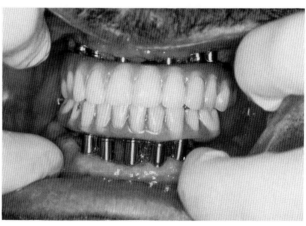

Fig. 14. Dental bridges in place with implants evident beneath the bridges.

isotropy. However, the ultimate effects of laser irradiation on tissue depend on the distribution of energy deposited inside the tissue. The concomitant temperature rise at each point in the exposed tissue is a result of this distribution and any heat conduction away from the source. The temperature rise is the fundamental effect determining the extent of changes in the morphology and chemical structure of the irradiated tissue.

For materials with high absorption, $\mu_a > 100$ cm^{-1}, the laser energy is absorbed within 100 μm of the surface and converted to heat. Energy transport into the tissue is primarily due to heat conduction away from this surface, and light scattering is insignificant. This condition is representative of the interaction between dental hard tissues and CO_2 lasers and perhaps also for the ArF excimer and Er:YAG lasers. In the visible and near IR, dentin and enamel only weakly absorb light, and light scattering plays a very important role in determining the deposited energy distribution in the tissue.

Dental enamel and dentin in the UV, visible, and near IR (weak absorption and strong scattering). An accurate knowledge of light transport in weakly and moderately absorbing tissues generally requires a complete characterization of the scattering and absorption properties of the tissue. Most current models that describe the propagation of laser light in highly scattering biological tissues are approximate solutions of the radiative transport equation [14,34–36]. These models require accurate knowledge of the absorption coefficient (μ_a), the scattering coefficient (μ_s), and the scattering phase function. For highly scattering tissues such as dentin

TABLE 1. Optical Properties of Dentin and Enamel Determined by Fried et al. [37,38] With Some Published Data for Comparison.*

λ	μ_s, cm^{-1}	μ_a, cm^{-1}	g	f	Previously published values
Enamel					
1053 nm	15 ± 5	<1.0	0.96 ± 0.02	35 ± 5 %	
632 nm	60 ± 18	<1.0	0.96 ± 0.02	35 ± 5 %	μ_s = 25 cm^{-1}, μ_a < 1.0 cm^{-1}, [39]
543 nm	105 ± 30	<1.0	0.96 ± 0.02	60 ± 10 %	μ_s = 45 cm^{-1}, μ_a < 1.0 cm^{-1}, [39]
Dentin					
1053 nm	260 ± 78	3–4	0.93 ± 0.02	0–2	
632 nm	280 ± 84	3–4	0.93 ± 0.02	0–2	μ_s = 130 cm^{-1}, μ_a = 4 cm^{-1}, [40]
					g = 0.4, [41]
543 nm	280 ± 84	3–4	0.93 ± 0.02	0–2	μ_s = 180 cm^{-1}, μ_a = 4 cm^{-1}, [40]

*Typical error for the scattering coefficients is ~30 % and is indicative of the sample variability.

and enamel, it is necessary to describe the directional nature, or anisotropy, of the scattering by a mathematical function called the scattering phase function. The exact form of the phase function is generally not known for each particular wavelength and tissue. In most cases involving biological tissue [14], the phase function is modeled by a function that contains a single parameter, the average cosine of the scattering angle, commonly referred to as g, (g = < cos θ >). For biological tissues, (g) is often close to one, g >0.9, which indicates highly forward directed scattering. Fried et al. [37,38] recently determined (see below) that g at 10.6 μm is close to one for dentin and enamel; consequently, transmitted and scattered light in the visible and near IR can penetrate deep into the interior of the tooth.

Enamel (μ_a and μ_s). Spitzer and ten Bosch [39] have measured the diffuse transmission and reflection values of thin enamel slabs in an integrating sphere and found that the absorption was very weak, (μ_a≤1 cm^{-1}) in the visible (400–700 nm) and moderate (μ_a≥10 cm^{-1}) in the ultraviolet, (240–300 nm). The reported scattering coefficients decreased exponentially between 240 and 700 nm from 400 cm^{-1} to 20 cm^{-1}. Fried et al. [37,38] have determined the scattering and absorption coefficients of fully index matched enamel samples at 543, 632, and 1053 nm. These values and the values reported by Spitzer and ten Bosch [39] are listed in Table 1. The implications of these data are that light in the visible (400–700 nm) and near infrared (1053 nm, Nd:YAG) is negligibly absorbed and moderately scattered by enamel.

Dentin (μ_a and μ_s). ten Bosch and Zijp [40,41,42] measured the scattering and absorption coefficients of 170-μm-thick sections of dentin between 400 and 700 nm. The absorption coefficient was essentially wavelength independent

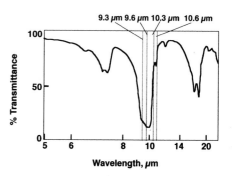

Fig. 15. The infrared spectrum of carbonated hydroxyapatite between 5 μm and 20 μm. The vertical dotted lines represent the wavelength of the center of the vibration-rotation bands of the CO_2 laser, 9.3, 9.6, 10.3, and 10.6 μm.

with a value of μ_a ~4 cm^{-1}. The scattering coefficient reported by ten Bosch and Zijp [40] varied from 30–200 cm^{-1} over the same wavelength range. Tissue sections with varying mineral content and tubule density showed a distinct dependence of the scattering coefficient on the tubule density. No dependence on the mineral content was found, suggesting that the scattering was largely a result of the dentinal tubules. The values of these coefficients measured by Fried et al. [37,38] for fully index matched dentin samples at 543, 632, and 1053 nm are comparable (Table 1). At 1053 nm, the absorption and scattering coefficients of dentin are considerably higher than those of enamel, and Seka et al. [44] have shown, using Monte Carlo simulations, that for 1,053 nm laser radiation, the higher absorption coefficient of dentin coupled with stronger scattering can lead to preferential energy deposition near the dentin-enamel interface. This deposition may cause subsurface heating, which may have negative consequences such as subsurface vaporization and cracking and pulpal necrosis.

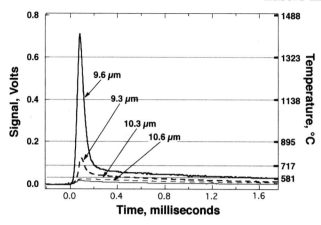

Fig. 16. The temporal evolution of the surface temperature profiles of bovine enamel irradiated by a single 100-μs-duration CO_2 laser pulse at $\lambda = 9.6$ (thick solid line), 9.3 (thick dashed line), 10.3 (thin dashed line), and 10.6 (thin solid line), and an absorbed fluence of 10 J/cm^2. The left axis represents the signal intensity as measured by the HCZT detector, and the right axis shows surface temperatures interpolated for the measured voltages [4,5].

TABLE 2. The Absorption Coefficients Calculated From Angularly Resolved Reflectance Measurements [46] and Measured Reflectance Values for Four CO_2 Wavelengths

Wavelength, μm	10.6	10.3	9.6	9.3
Reflectance, % [45]	13.8 ± 0.5	16.4 ± 1.0	48.7 ± 1.0	37.7 ± 2.0
Absorption, cm^{-1} [46]	5,200	6,500	31,300	18,500

Enamel and dentin scattering phase function. Fried et al. [37] determined the scattering anisotropy (g) and the scattering phase function for dental enamel and dentin at 543, 632, and 1,053 nm from angularly resolved scattering distributions of fully index matched samples of dentin and enamel and Monte Carlo simulations (Table 1). The scattering was best described by a complex phase function consisting of a linear combination of a Henyey Greenstein function [43] (g = 0.96 and 0.93 for enamel and dentin, respectively) and an isotropic phase function (35–60% for enamel and 0–2% for dentin) indicating highly forward directed scattering (deep penetration) in these tissues.

Dentin and enamel in the IR and UV (strong absorption). For materials with very high absorption coefficients, the laser energy is absorbed very close to the surface and light scattering is insignificant. The energy deposition within the sample can be adequately described by the absorption coefficient and the reflectance. The reflectance can be very high near a strong absorption band due to the increase in the imaginary component of the index of refraction, e.g., at 9.6 μm the reflectance of human dental enamel exceeds 50% [45,46].

The mineral of dental enamel is carbonated hydroxyapatite, which has strong absorption bands in the infrared region due to phosphate, carbonate, and hydroxyl groups in the crystal structure. The spectral output of the CO_2 laser overlaps the strong phosphate absorption bands of dental enamel apatite [47–49] (see Fig. 15); consequently, all the CO_2 laser radiation is absorbed in a very thin layer at the enamel surface (< 10 μm) [46]. Heat conduction is therefore the principle method of energy transport into the sample.

Duplain et al. [46] estimated absorption coefficients and optical constants for bovine enamel from polarization-dependent angular reflectance measurements at CO_2 wavelengths (Table 2). They found that both reflectance and absorption coefficients vary dramatically from $\lambda = 9.3$ to 10.6 μm [46]. Fried et al. [45] also measured the reflectance of human enamel at 9.3, 9.6, 10.3 and 10.6 μm, using an integrating sphere and report a similar trend in reflectance (Table 2).

The absorption coefficients of highly absorbing materials can also be estimated from time-resolved temperature measurements. Fried et al. [45] measured time-resolved surface temperatures of laser-irradiated bovine enamel at 9.3, 9.6, 10.3, and 10.6 μm (Fig. 16). The absorbed energy density at 9.6 μm was significantly higher than the other wavelengths for a given pulse duration, consequently resulting in much higher surface temperatures. The large relative differences in measured surface temperatures are consistent with previous SEM observations of wavelength-dependent surface morphologies [49] and the variance in the absorption coefficients calculated from reflectance data [46].

The erbium (~3.0 μm), HF (2.7–3.0 μm), and excimer lasers (193, 248, and 308 nm) are also strongly absorbed by dental hard tissues. Surface treatments employing the 193 nm wavelength for the ablation of dental hard tissues show that the 193 nm wavelength (ArF) of the excimer laser is efficiently absorbed by hard dental tissues [55,56]. Neev et al. [57–59] have also shown that the 308 nm wavelength is efficiently absorbed by dentin since it overlaps protein absorption ba

Erbium laser light is efficiently absorbed by the intrinsic H_2O and the OH^- in the apatite mineral of dental hard tissues [60,61]. The OH^- absorption band is centered at 2.8 μm, whereas the water absorption occurs over a very broad region that peaks near 3.0 μm. Altshuler [62] has suggested that the Er:YSGG laser [2.79 μm) may be absorbed more efficiently than the Er:YAG (2.94 μm) by the mineral in dental hard tissues because it overlaps the sharp peak of the OH^- band of hydroxyapatite. The HF laser emits in a similar wavelength range (tunable from 2.7–3.0 μm) and is strongly absorbed by calcified tissues [63].

Implications. Before the interactions of lasers with hard dental tissues can be well characterized and the optimum laser parameters for a particular application selected, the optical properties of these tissues must be known. As summarized above, some of these parameters are known, but there are still major gaps. Unfortunately, empirical and even clinical studies employing lasers are usually concluded before even a basic knowledge of the optical properties are acquired.

Lasers for Preventive Dentistry

Early studies of the effect of lasers on hard dental tissues were based simply on the empirical use of available lasers and an examination of the modified tissue by various techniques. Even though these studies were primitive, i.e., the optical properties of dental tissues at the respective laser wavelengths and the laser pulse shape and characteristics were not investigated, they suggested the potential uses of lasers in preventive dentistry. Studies by Stern et al. [1,64] utilizing a ruby laser ($\lambda = 693.4$ nm) demonstrated that the laser could be used to heat the surface of human enamel, consequently increasing enamel resistance to subsurface demineralization in vitro. Vahl [65] used electron microscopy and x-ray diffraction to study the effects of laser radiation on enamel. These studies clearly demonstrated ultrastructural and crystallographic changes in response to laser radiation. Later studies by Yamamoto et al. [66] showed the potential of a Nd:YAG laser ($\lambda = 1064$ nm) to fuse dental enamel at very high irradiation intensities (~ 1 GW/cm^2) and to make it highly resistant to subsequent dissolution.

The majority of the earliest studies were carried out using near IR and visible light lasers at wavelengths that are weakly absorbed by dental hard tissues. Often very high irradiation intensi-

ties ($>10^7$ W/cm^2) were used to generate the desired effects. Presumably the mechanism of coupling of the laser energy to the sample was by plasma formation at the high incident power densities applied. The high energies utilized as well as the high transmission of these tissues in the visible and near IR would be expected to result in subsurface damage to the pulp.

Similar studies utilizing carbon dioxide lasers were able to employ much lower energy density levels as a result of efficient transfer of energy from light to heat. Dental enamel, cementum, and dentin mineral are a carbonated apatite that has intense absorption bands in the 9.0–11.0 μm infrared region (Fig. 15); therefore, infrared radiation (IR) from the CO_2 laser is much more efficiently absorbed than radiation from the visible spectrum; see Fowler [67], Nelson and Featherstone [68], Nelson et al. [69], and Nelson and Williamson [70]. Meurman et al. [71] compared the effects of the Nd:YAG and CO_2 lasers on synthetic apatite and observed that only the CO_2 laser had an inhibitory effect on reactivity. There was no discernible effect on apatite after irradiation with the Nd:YAG laser. Launay et al. [72] compared the effects of the Nd:YAG, the continuous wave argon ion, and the continuous wave CO_2 lasers on dental enamel. They found that the pulsed Nd:YAG laser (200–2,000 J/cm^2) did not fuse the surface of enamel and that the light diffused to the pulp where overheating occurred. The argon ion laser (300–10,000 J/cm^2) produced irreproducible results due to the organic material on the surface that was absorbing the laser light. The continuous wave CO_2 laser (250–1,000 J/cm^2) melted the surface with some overheating of the pulp. Stern et al. [3], Kantola et al. [73], and Lenz et al. [74] carried out studies utilizing continuous wave CO_2 lasers and demonstrated ultrastructural crystallographic effects. Kuroda and Fowler [9] and Fowler and Kuroda [75] also reported structural and phase changes in surface enamel when treated with a continuous wave CO_2 laser.

Featherstone et al. [49] and Nelson et al. [69,76] measured the effects of low-energy pulsed laser radiation on human dental enamel and dentin for CO_2 laser wavelengths from 9.3 through 10.6 μm. SEM studies showed that the surface effects were highly wavelength-dependent in this region and that 9.3 μm and 9.6 μm wavelengths were highly efficient at heating the surface of enamel, much more so than even the 10.6 μm wavelength. All of these studies suggest that the carbon dioxide laser, preferably tuned to the highly absorbed 9.3 and 9.6 µm wavelengths, is the system of choice for preventive dental applications.

In most studies using the continuous wave CO_2 lasers, typical interaction times of 50 msec to 2 sec were used. These interaction times are much longer than the thermal relaxation time of enamel ($\sim$ 100 µs) [45]. For long interaction times, a large fraction of the absorbed laser energy is conducted away from the enamel surface into the interior of the tooth during the laser pulse, resulting in inefficient surface heating and possible pulpal damage. Ideally, the laser pulse duration should be on the order of the thermal relaxation time of the tissue. If the pulse duration is too short, the deposited power density may be too high, causing ablation of tissue instead of the desired heating and fusion. Pulsed lasers provide a way of increasing the peak power density while keeping the pulse energy density constant. This means that fusion, melting, and recrystallization of enamel crystals can be confined to a thin surface region without affecting the underlying dentin or pulp.

Featherstone et al. [49] and Nelson et al. [69,76] have measured the effect of low-energy pulsed CO_2 laser irradiation on human dental enamel and dentin in the infrared region from 9.3 through 10.6 µm. Multiple (100 at 1 Hz) short (100–200 ns) pulses at irradiation intensities of a MW/cm^2 per pulse were used. The pulsed laser melted the surface of enamel and dentin at much lower deposited energies than continuous wave CO_2 lasers. Recent studies [77] by the same group using a custom built CO_2 laser with the optimum pulse width of 100 µs (on the order of the relaxation time) and the optimum wavelengths of 9.3 and 9.6 µm, have shown that significantly lower irradiation intensities ($<$ 25 kW/cm^2) and fewer pulses can be used with a greater efficacy.

Mechanism of inhibition. Featherstone and Nelson [49] observed that the pulsed CO_2 laser produced a temperature rise ($>$1,000 °C) at the surface sufficient to fuse and melt enamel crystals, which are composed of carbonated apatite. This surface melt zone was no deeper than 5 µm, beneath which there was a region of interaction 10–40 µm deep, where the temperature rise was insufficient for the sintering process but sufficient for some compositional changes to the crystals. Subsequent infrared analysis [78] indicated that the carbonate content was dramatically reduced, and the surface phases were hydroxyapatite and tetracalcium diphosphate monoxide. Comparable

effects were reported after heat treatment or laser treatment of human enamel by Fowler and Kuroda [75]. Kuroda and Fowler [9] observed a reduction in the carbonate content (66%), the water content, and apatite hydroxide content (33%) of enamel after irradiation with a continuous wave CO_2 laser (10,000 J/cm^2, 20 W −1 second). Analysis of the irradiated product using powder x-ray diffraction and infrared analysis indicated a mixture of minor phases of α—$Ca_3(PO_4)_2$ and $Ca_4(PO_4)_2O$ and modified hydroxyapatite. Fowler and Kuroda [75] categorized the chemical and morphological changes in dental enamel observed during heating (in furnace) into three temperature zones: 100–650 °C, 650–1,100 °C, and > 1,100 °C. A summary (from ref. 9) follows of the structural and chemical changes that take place in each of these regions.

100–650 °C:
1. Loss of H_2O ($\sim$ 30%)
2. CO_3^{2-} loss ($\sim$ 66%) and rearrangement of carbonate to phosphate and OH^- positions
3. Acid phosphate HPO_4^{2-} condenses to form pyrophosphate P_2O_7
4. Decomposition and denaturation of proteins.
5. Contraction of a-axis lattice dimension at 250–300 °C.

650–1,100 °C:
1. Recrystallization, crystal growth of β—$Ca_3(PO_4)_2$ formed in tooth enamel.
2. Decrease in OH^-
3. Conversion of OH^- to O^{2-}
4. Loss of H_2O and CO_3^{2-}
5. Loss of trapped CO_2 + NCO^-

> 1,100 °
1. 1,450 °C disproportionates to α'— $Ca_3(PO_4)_2$ and $Ca_4(PO_4)_2O$ Melting at 1,280 °C
2. 1225 °C β—$Ca_3(PO_4)_2$ converted to α—$Ca_3(PO_4)_2$
3. α'—$Ca_3(PO_4)_2$ and $Ca_4(PO_4)_2O$ melts at 1600 °C Conversion of OH^- to O^{2-}

All of the observed processes above are dependent upon the rate and length of heating, which are of fundamental importance for the comparison of these observations with the effects of laser heating.

The reasons for the observed inhibition of lesion formation after laser modification are still not clear, although there are several possible explanations. It has been suggested by Stern et al. [64] and Lenz et al. [74] that the enamel surface is sealed by the laser and is less permeable for the subsequent diffusion of ions into and from the enamel. Oho and Morioka [79] treated the surface of enamel with an argon ion laser (surface coated with an absorbing ink to increase absorption) and analyzed the heated enamel with thermal analysis, infrared spectroscopy, polarized light spectroscopy, and x-ray diffraction. They identified the formation of microspaces in the lased enamel due to the removal of organics, water, and carbonate, which increased the permeability of enamel and may act as sites for deposition of ions released by an acid attack, thereby providing a possible mechanism of inhibition. Borggreven et al. [7] also suggested that laser irradiation increased the permeability of bovine dental enamel. In addition to permeability changes, the loss of organics and carbonate should dramatically increase the acid resistance of dental enamel [8].

Fowler and Kuroda [75] suggested that the laser treatment at temperatures < 650 °C may convert sufficient acid phosphate HPO_4^{2-} to P_2O_7 to inhibit demineralization. Christofferson and Christofferson [80] reported that P_2O_7 concentrates reduced the hydroxyapatite dissolution rate to zero.

Fox et al. [81] have proposed a model describing the mechanism of increased resistance of dental enamel to acid dissolution after laser irradiation. This model is based on studies of heat-treated and irradiated synthetic carbonated apatites. The authors describe a decrease in the apparent solubility of enamel after heat treatment to temperatures in excess of 1,200°C. This decrease in solubility is attributed to the change in the rate of the dissolution kinetics from the more accessible dissolution site of hydroxyapatite to control by the less reactive site of heat-treated apatite [82]. Fowler and Kuroda [75] hypothesize that heating to temperatures in excess of 1,200 °C may actually increase the susceptibility of dental enamel to acid dissolution because the α and β—$Ca_3(PO_4)_2$ and $Ca_4(PO_4)_2O$ phases formed at high temperature are more soluble then hydroxyapatite and dental enamel.

Oksuka et al. [83], Yu et al. [54], and Fox et al. [81] have shown that moderate heat treatment by CO_2 lasers (300–400 °C) reduced the solubility of dental enamel and synthetic carbonated apatite. Sato [84] found that the dissolution rate de-

creased after a 24-hour heat treatment at 350°C. This change in solubility after low temperature treatment can be attributed to the thermal decomposition of the more soluble carbonated hydroxyapatite into the less soluble hydroxyapatite.

At this time, the optimum temperature range for clinically applicable caries preventive treatments has not been determined. This is probably due to the complexity of the thermal decomposition of these materials. This complexity is compounded by several competing mechanisms that are optimized at different temperatures, e.g., high temperatures ($>1,100$ °C) may decrease the permeability of enamel; however, decomposition produces other phases that are more susceptible to acid dissolution. Lower temperature heat treatments (650°C) may increase the acid resistance by chemical changes (loss of organics and carbonate), even though the permeability has increased. In regard to subsurface enamel, we believe that the laser-induced compositional changes of the enamel surface reduce its solubility and that changes below the surface, not detected by methods utilized to date, will reduce the solubility beneath the surface.

Goodman and Kaufman [85], Yamamoto and Sato [8], and Kuroda and Fowler [9] observed that the combination of laser irradiation and subsequent topical fluoride application decreased the solubility of dental enamel more than either the fluoride treatment or the laser treatment alone. Tagomori and Morioka [86] treated dental enamel with acidulated phosphate fluoride (APF), then irradiated with a Nd:YAG laser (with ink applied to the surface to enhance absorption). They observed that the acid resistance was dramatically higher only if the sample was irradiated prior to APF application, indicating that the laser-modified enamel has an enhanced uptake of APF. Featherstone et al. [87] observed that irradiation of carious lesions in enamel with pulsed 9.3 μm CO_2 radiation, followed by subsequent treatment with APF, resulted in complete inhibition of lesion progression. Fox et al. [88] treated sound enamel with 10.6 μm continuous CO_2 radiation followed by treatments of fluoride, dodecylamine HCl (DAC), and ethane-1-hydroxyl-1,1-diphosphonic acid (EHDP), and considerable reduction was observed for all three agents, in combination with laser irradiation. The authors used calculations [89] to show that in the oral environment no dissolution is expected at a pH as low as 4.5 with as little as 0.01 moles/1 fluoride present. The authors hypothesized that there is a synergistic relationship between chemical inhibitors and heat treatment. The thermal treatment (laser) converts the carbonated hydroxyapatite mineral of tooth enamel to a less soluble mineral, and chemical inhibitors work by a common ion effect of the fluorapatitic surface, which is more effective on the less soluble laser-modified enamel.

Future of laser preventive treatment. Other lasers may have potential for preventive laser treatments on hard dental tissues. Frentzen et al. [56] have evaluated the potential uses of the excimer laser in dentistry and listed the areas of possible application. The principle wavelengths that are produced by excimer lasers are 193 nm, 248 nm, and 308 nm. The 308 nm laser should not work well on enamel because of weak absorption by hydroxyapatite at this wavelength and strong scattering [39]. It may, however, be well suited for dentin [90] due to the strong absorption by proteins and lipids [40]. The 248 nm wavelength is not desirable for use in the oral cavity because of the risk of mutagenic and carcinogenic effects [56]. These same arguments also apply to the 3rd and 4th harmonics of the Nd:YAG laser (266 and 355 nm). At 193 nm, there is strong absorption and minimal penetration reducing the mutagenic and carcinogenic risk. This wavelength is highly efficient at heating dental hard tissues with minimal heating of the pulp [56,55] and may be suitable for preventive treatments if lasers were developed with longer pulse durations in the microsecond range.

The Er:YAG laser (2.96 μm) can efficiently ablate hard tissue [61,62,91–93] and may be well suited for melting and cutting enamel and dentin due to the strong water and OH^- absorption of apatite. At this wavelength the strong absorption of water causes explosive vaporization of internal water, generating a porous surface with minimal fusion that may actually increase the permeability of enamel. Although the Er:YAG laser may be developed further for dentin and enamel removal and cutting, there have not been any dissolution studies to date to determine if this laser is suitable for caries preventive treatments.

It now appears possible for surface enamel, dentin, carious enamel, or carious dentin to be treated with specifically directed low-energy pulsed CO_2 laser light without biological damage to the inner tooth. A comprehensive analysis of the relative importance of all these various chemical and morphological changes on the mechanism of acid resistance has yet to be determined. However, it is now known that this treatment requires wavelength-specific laser irradiation for efficient conversion of laser energy into heat at the enamel surface and in the immediate subsurface, causing crystal transformation, loss of organics, and subsequent inhibition of subsurface lesion formation. For clinical applications, the optimal wavelength of laser radiation must be determined, together with the optimal energy density, optimal pulse shape, duration, and repetition rate. The fracture and wear resistance of laser modified enamel must also be thoroughly investigated before this treatment is acceptable for clinical use, because laser treatments may introduce stresses, cracking, and crazing that may reduce the structural integrity of dental enamel. The treatment of carious lesions, pits, and fissures [94], and occlusal surfaces, are all possibilities that could be explored in the future. If this laser technology that has been shown to be effective in the laboratory becomes available at a reasonable cost and the results hold up clinically, there will indeed be a future for the clinical application of lasers in preventive dentistry.

Hard tissue ablation

At a recent American Dental Association (ADA) meeting, a survey was conducted to evaluate dentists' perceptions of lasers and their interests in using lasers in their practices. Dentists stated that if the FDA cleared lasers for hard tissue surgery, > 75% of them would consider changing the method of treatment they presently use for hard tissue cutting [95]. It is fueled by the perception, still to be proven, that a laser that could cut hard dental tissues would be better accepted by dental patients. The dental handpiece (drill) presently used by dentists causes fear in many patients because of its sound and vibration. It would seem that a method that can accomplish the same effect without these stimuli would be less noxious to dental patients. An understanding of the basic tissue and material interaction of any laser must precede any treatment in humans. The preceding discussion of the spectroscopic analysis of dental tissues is just the beginning of the long story yet to be told of laser dental tissue interaction. The following discussion adds even more important information regarding these tissue interactions.

Some of the early researchers who looked at the possibility of using lasers to replace the dental drill found that the first lasers caused significant heat that led to severe irreversible damage to the dental pulp. Even though this damage was evident, there was enough interest for these early researchers to look at the interaction of lasers on dental hard tissues [2–11]. Melcer et al. [96,97] reported on the use of the CO_2 laser for the treatment of dental decay. A number of other investigators looked at the effect of the CO_2 laser on dental hard tissues and bone [45,49,96–105]. Other lasers have been investigated to determine their effects on dental hard tissues. Dederich et al. looked at the root canal wall after Nd:YAG laser radiation treatment [106]. Harris and Wigdor evaluated the effects of the Q-switched Nd:YAG laser on enamel and found that this method appeared to cause no thermal damage [107]. Bahcall et al. [108] investigated the use of the pulsed Nd:YAG laser to cleanse root canals. Their results showed that the Nd:YAG laser may cause harm to the bone and periodontal ligament [108]. Neev et al. [90,109] looked at the effect of the excimer laser on dental hard tissues. Pini et al. and Feuerstein et al. [55,110] also reported results of the use of excimer lasers on dental hard tissues.

Koort and Frentzen [111] reviewed the effects of pulsing a number of different lasers on dental hard tissues. They found cracking in dentin and enamel in teeth irradiated by lasers tested. Whether or not this finding has clinical significance is yet to be determined [111].

Altshuler et al. [112] evaluated the use of a model to determine the laser destruction of hard dental tissues. They also reported on the potential of the tooth as an optical device [113]. Zakariasen et al. [114] and Barron et al. [115] evaluated the use of laser scanned fluorescence in the detection of carious enamel.

At the present moment, as stated above, the lasers that show the most promise for hard tissue surgery are the Er:YAG and Er:YSGG lasers. Hibst and Keller [92,93,116] have performed the premier work in this area and have reported on the basic tissue interaction events with the Er:YAG on dental hard tissues. They showed that this laser can cut dental tissues and also remove dental materials. They studied the ablation efficiency of this laser and its effect on dental hard tissues under the scrutiny of light and SEM microscopy.

Lasers Under Study for Hard Tissue Applications

It is of great importance to understand that any laser that may be used by dentists must yield clinical effects at least similar to a dental handpiece. If a laser were to require much longer time, for instance, or cause more damage to achieve the same result as a drill, this laser would probably not be welcomed by the dental community in earnest. This concept must be understood by dental laser researchers for it is at the core of the acceptance of laser surgery by a significant number of dentists. The following is a summary of the lasers and techniques presently being studied for surgical hard tissue dental applications.

Er:YAG and Er:YSGG lasers. The Er:YAG ($\lambda = 2.94$ μm) and Er:YSGG ($\lambda = 2.79$ μm) lasers emit in the midinfrared near the IR peak of the water absorption curve and the OH^- absorption of hydroxyapatite. These lasers represent the best near-term hope for a laser that can effectively remove dental hard tissues. In brief, the radiation that these lasers emit is strongly absorbed by water. The absorbed energy induces a rapid rise in temperature and pressure, and the heated material is explosively removed. Although the amount of water in dentin or enamel (20% and 10%, respectively) is relatively low, there appears to be enough absorption to initiate the ablation process. Further, there is some evidence that carbonated hydroxyapatite, the mineral of dentin and enamel, also absorbs strongly in the midinfrared [69,70,76,78] because of the OH^- ions present in the structure.

The net result of this relatively high absorption is that the tissue is removed and little of the incident laser energy remains in the tissue to cause thermal damage. Hibst and Keller [92] measured the cutting rate for an Er:YAG laser. Using their 1.1-mm-diameter spot, a 50 J/cm^2 radiant exposure, and a 10 Hz pulse repetition rate, one would expect to be able to remove a 2.7 mm × 1 mm × 4 mm volume of enamel in ~ 30 seconds [92]. Such removal rates are adequate for crown preparation. Faster ablation rates have been reported for the removal of carious materials [117]. In brief, because decayed material has a lower ultimate tensile strength than the surrounding healthy enamel and dentin, such material is removed at lower laser-induced temperatures and pressures. Consequently, one can achieve higher ablation rates in carious material than in normal tissue. More importantly, it may be possible to selectively remove the decayed material and minimally affect the adjacent normal tissue.

Several problems remain to be solved before the erbium lasers can be used safely and effectively for the treatment of dental hard tissues. The first and most important issue is the temperature rise within the tooth. The rise induced by a single erbium laser pulse is several hundred degrees at the site of absorption, but only a few hundred μm from the ablation site, the temperature rise is but a few degrees. The temperature rise distant from the absorption site is, however, minimal only for a single pulse. It has been shown that multiple pulses induce a temperature increase that can be > 30°C throughout the entire tooth [118]. Such a temperature rise likely does not damage the dentin or enamel immediately adjacent to the ablation site. Thus histologic examination of ablated teeth that were fixed immediately following laser irradiation fail to show changes induced by such minimal temperature rises. Nonetheless, it is recognized that temperature rises of 5°C or greater in the pulp for >~1 minute can necrose the pulp cavity [119].

The solution to the temperature increase is to cool the tooth surface with water [139,141]. Recent data indicate that the water flow rate can be relatively slow (e.g., 5 ml/min) to limit effectively the temperature rise to < 3°C even during prolonged ablation at 10 Hz [141]. Such water flow rates do inhibit the ablation but only minimally when compared with ablation in the absence of water flow. The ablation of tissue with an erbium laser through a layer of water seems contradictory when one considers that water strongly absorbs the incident laser radiation. However, it is clear that first segment of the incident laser pulse induces a cavity within the water layer through which the remainder of the pulse can propagate to the tissue surface. The challenge that remains is to incorporate the water spray mechanism into an ergonomic handpiece that can effectively deliver laser radiation.

The other major problem that erbium laser radiation can cause is cracking of the teeth [111,118]. Such cracking has been noted but mainly at higher radiant exposures. It appears that these cracks are produced by shock waves that propagate into the teeth following ablation. Such shock waves are an unavoidable aspect of the ablation process. Basically, to achieve ablation of a dental hard material, one needs to induce a pressure rise sufficient to explode the material away from the site of absorption. The challenge is to select a radiant exposure that achieves the desired ablation yet minimizes the unwanted side effect.

As mentioned above, one would hope that a laser capable of removing dental hard tissue could also be used to remove restorative materials such as composites, amalgams, and cements. Limited studies using an Er:YAG laser indicate that the ablation of various composites and cements is readily achieved. Ablation of amalgam is possible, although the process is less efficient [120]. The question of toxicity of the ablation products, which leave the ablation site at high temperature and with considerable velocity (e.g., greater than Mach 1), remains a problem that must be addressed in light of current knowledge of the toxicity of particles produced using the traditional dental drill.

Finally, this section groups the Er:YAG and Er:YSGG lasers into a single discussion. Based upon the low-intensity water absorption curve, one would expect that the 2.5-fold greater absorption by water at 2.94 μm when compared with that at 2.79 μm would result in a significant difference in the effects of the two lasers. However, the absorption coefficient of water is strongly temperature-dependent; the absorption shifts during the erbium laser pulse. Consequently, the incident laser radiation penetrates much farther into any treated tissue than might be expected. For example, Er:YAG laser radiation actually penetrates as much as 100 μm into the tissue, whereas the water absorption curve would predict only 1–2 μm of penetration. In fact, the Er:YAG laser radiation penetrates farther into the tissue than the Er:YSGG laser radiation. An opposite prediction follows from the low-intensity water absorption curve. The bottom line is that there is relatively little difference between the penetration of Er:YAG and Er:YSGG laser radiation, and such differences are likely to be inconsequential to the ablation of dental hard tissues. The determination of which laser to use (Er:YAG vs. Er:YSGG) will likely be based more upon engineering considerations (e.g., which medium yields the most efficient laser and which wavelength is easier to deliver) than tissue considerations.

Carbon dioxide (CO_2) lasers. These were among the first to be used experimentally for the ablation of dental hard tissues [3,6]. It has become quite clear that a continuous wave (cw) CO_2 laser does not deliver the irradiance necessary to explosively remove tooth materials. Instead, the cw CO_2 laser only chars a tooth surface and overheats the pulpal chamber [105,121].

Short-pulsed CO_2 lasers, however, can effectively ablate hard biological materials [45,54,74]. The most efficient CO_2 laser for hard tissue ablation is the transversely excited, atmospheric pressure, or TEA, CO_2 laser, which emits 0.1–2.0 μsec-long pulses of typically 10.6 μm radiation. The infrared radiation is fairly strongly absorbed by the water within the tooth and more strongly by the carbonated hydroxyapatite mineral of the tooth. As a result of absorption of the 10.6 μm radiation, there is a rapid pressure rise at the absorption site, which causes ablation. This induced pressure has been shown to selectively ablate carious material preferentially over normal dentin, a result that is likely related to the higher tensile strength of the normal dentin [122].

As with other lasers used for the ablation of dental hard tissues, the best results appear to be obtained when the tissue is simultaneously cooled with a water spray [123]. The TEA CO_2 appears to induce a larger plasma than other infrared lasers. The plasma is a problem in two respects: (1) the plasma absorbs incident laser radiation before it reaches the tooth surface, thus diminishing the ablation efficiency, and (2) the shock wave that results from the plasma can be damaging. Thus the problems that need to be addressed include diminution of the induced plasma, minimization of the shock wave induced damage to unablated tooth material, characterization and control of the potential shock wave induced damage to the inner ear structures in the practitioner or the patient, and elimination of the overheating of the tooth structures [123]. The latter problem can likely be solved with an appropriate water spray system. The former problems require the judicious selection of laser irradiation parameters. It is not clear that such a parameter range can be appropriately designed into a TEA CO_2 laser system; thus work on such systems remains limited.

Optical parametric oscillators (OPO). These oscillators have not yet been used in dentistry, but one can speculate that such devices have potential. An OPO system consists of a pump laser (e.g., a 1.06 μm Nd:YAG laser) and a crystal (e.g., KTA) [124]. The pump beam is used to excite the crystal, which then emits two new beams of light, both at a longer wavelength than the pump wavelength. These new wavelengths can be varied by rotating the crystal. The OPOs currently being developed emit radiation near the 2- and 3-μm absorption bands of water and in the 4–5 μm region. For further details, the reader is referred to more technical sources [125], but it should be noted that it is now possible to use a diode laser to pump Nd ions embedded in an OPO crystal, thus emitting tunable radiation in the IR. Such a system can be low cost, lightweight, and portable. Further, the output from an OPO can be fairly powerful, e.g., 10 W or more [126]. Currently, the OPOs are limited by the ability of the crystals to handle high peak power. Such a limi-

tation will continue to decrease as crystal growers become more proficient at eliminating impurities.

Dye enhanced laser ablation. As noted above, the infrared lasers that have shown the most promise for hard tissue removal take advantage of the absorption peaks of water and hydroxyapatite that are present in dentin and enamel. An alternative that is being explored is to increase the absorption of the incident laser radiation by the addition of an exogenous dye [127,128]. This technique, termed dye-assisted or dye-enhanced laser ablation, uses microdrops of dye deposited on the surface of the tissue to increase the absorption of a particular laser. Energy that would normally be reflected or scattered is now coupled into the dye-tissue interface. The lasers currently being utilized are either a diode ($\lambda = 805$ nm) or a tunable Alexanderite ($\lambda = 700$–825 nm) laser. Microliters of indocyanine green dye are precisely deposited, using ink-jet technology, onto the tooth surface prior to irradiation. The laser is pulsed and the procedure repeated. Early results show that the process is fairly efficient, removing ~ 50–75 μm of material per laser pulse of 1 Joule [128]. Light and electron microscopy of ablation craters is also encouraging. Irradiated enamel shows no cracking or fissuring but only smooth walls [127,128]. The major drawback to overcome is the slow rate at which the process occurs. Because the dye is essentially removed with each laser pulse, it has to be redeposited prior to the next pulse. Presently only very slow repetition rates are obtainable. Thermal studies also need to be performed to determine the extent of heat that is deposited in the tissue during the procedure. This will, of course, become a larger issue as the repetition rates are increased to practical levels.

Excimer. The ultraviolet (UV) wavelengths of excimer lasers are relatively efficient in the removal of bone and thus are good candidates for dentistry as well [63,129]. In the past, excimer lasers were thought to interact with biological tissue through a photochemical process, ablation being the result of breaking bonds within the tissue [130]. Thus excimer lasers are often thought of as nonthermal lasers despite the fact that they do produce heat in the target material. More recently some of the researchers have found evidence that the excimer ablation is a thermal process [59].

The two most prevalent excimer lasers are the ArF (193 nm) and the XeCl (308 nm). However, there are other excimers as well as frequency multiplied lasers that emit in the UV. Although the fluences and resulting ablation rates are generally much lower than with erbium lasers, the latter are capable of much higher pulse repetition rates. Limited data exist on the temperatures induced within the teeth during UV ablation of teeth. However, there is a moderate amount of data on the surface temperatures [57,58,90,131]. Not surprisingly, the temperature rises produced are largely parameter-dependent; the temperature is mostly dependent on the repetition rate and less dependent on the fluence and spot size [58]. Even with low fluence settings and a low repetition rate, which should have yielded small temperature increases, SEM analysis showed a melted layer of dentin surrounding the ablation craters [58]. Depending on the parameters chosen, the surface temperatures can be as little as 40°C to several hundred degrees [58,131]. It is interesting to point out that the XeCl laser evidently produces considerably higher temperatures compared to the ArF laser [131]. More importantly, studies need to determine the thermal effects to the temperature sensitive pulp chamber.

There are two potential advantages to using excimer wavelengths besides the issue of thermal damage. There is less absorption by water in the UV than in the IR, which allows for water cooling while drilling single spots. It has been seen by S.R. Visuri (unpub. data) that there is a limit to the depth one can achieve while drilling a single channel into a tooth with a combination of an Er: YAG laser and a cooling water spray. As the channel gets deeper, water flows into it and has no means of escaping, eventually preventing further ablation. With the excimer, it is likely that ablation can be continued through a greater water thickness, allowing for deeper drilling of small channels. This problem is not an issue for drilling of larger areas where the water has a path out of the ablation site. The second advantage excimer lasers may have is that they may be more caries selective. The UV wavelengths appear to have an affinity to caries ablation in both dentin and enamel [117,132,133]. At a wavelength of 377 nm, the threshold for ablation of healthy dentin is four times higher than the threshold for carious dentin [117]. Because of the minimal relative time a dentist spends removing decay (more time is spent removing old restorations and preparing healthy dentin and enamel), it is questionable whether the selective ablation will be an important action of this laser in the clinical setting.

Holmium. There has been some interest in using the holmium laser for removal of hard dental tissue. Having stronger absorption than Nd:YAG laser radiation in teeth, the holmium laser causes less thermal damage, yielding necrosis zones on the order of 50 μm [134]. The holmium laser is less efficient at removing dental material for a given radiant exposure than either the erbium or the excimer [134], leading one to speculate that the holmium laser will cause a larger temperature increase in the tooth subsequent to ablation. The erbium laser wavelengths cause the least thermal damage of the infrared lasers and would be the preferred wavelength if that were the only consideration. The advantage that the holmium laser has over the erbium laser is that 2.1 μm radiation travels down optical fibers without significant energy losses. The ease of a fiber delivery system may be a considerable advantage when working in the confined spaces of the oral cavity. A second advantage of a holmium laser system is that the ratio of the radiant exposure needed to induce cracks in a tooth to that needed to initiate ablation is fairly large when compared with an erbium laser [135]. In effect, when using a holmium laser there is a wider range of laser energies prior to the onset of mechanical damage. It remains to be seen whether this increased permissible range of operation is a significant advantage. Although the potential cracking of teeth is an issue, the major challenges that remain in the development of a holmium laser for the ablation of dental hard tissues is the limiting of thermal damage to the pulp chamber and the minimization of thermal damage at the ablation crater edge such that there can be adequate bonding of restorative materials.

Laser Ablation Research

Research reported by Wigdor et al. [136] investigated the effects of two lasers (CO_2 $\lambda = 10.6$ and Er:YAG $\lambda = 2.94$) on dental hard tissue. This research attempted to compare lasers after they created a hole in a canine tooth that was similar to one created by a dental drill. The SEM photograph in Figure 17 shows a low power view of the defect caused by a CO_2 laser. Note that the dentinal tubules are not evident. There is also a significant amount of cracking in the dentin. SEM views of an Er:YAG laser cut (Fig. 18) show good definition of the dentin. Figure 19, a SEM photograph, shows the effects of a slow-speed dental handpiece as a control. Note the similarities of the dentinal tubules to the Er:YAG laser photograph.

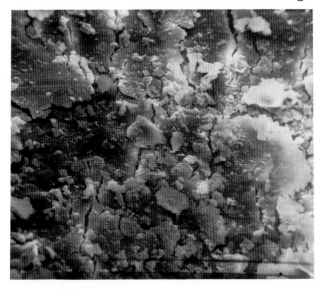

Fig. 17. SEM photograph of dentin irradiated with a CO_2 laser ($\times$ 1,000).

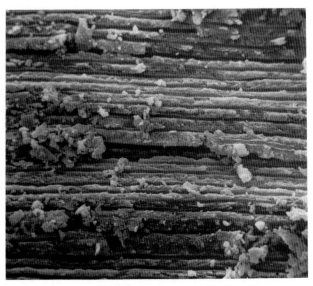

Fig. 19. SEM photograph of dentin treated with a slow speed dental drill ($\times$ 1,000).

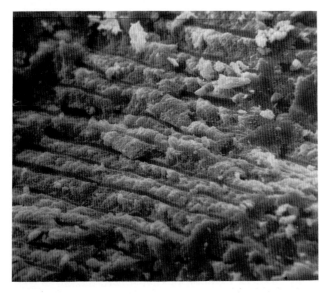

Fig. 18. SEM photograph of dentin irradiated with an Er: YAG laser ($\times$ 1,000).

The CO_2 laser-treated teeth investigated under light microscopy four days after laser exposure showed several pupal responses close to the irradiated surface. These included loss of the odontoblastic cell layer, an absence of the predentin layer, and congestion of the blood vessels without extravasation (Fig. 20). The CO_2 laser photomicrograph shows that the laser defect came very close to the pulpal tissue ($\sim$ 50 μm). The pulpal response is minimal considering the depth of the

laser defect. There is also a lack of a noticeable inflammatory cell infiltrate.

The Er:YAG laser-treated teeth also investigated under light microscopy four days after laser exposure have retained a normal architecture of the odontoblastic cell layer and the predentinal layer (Fig. 21). The vascularity and cellularity of the connective tissue appeared similar to that of the untreated control specimens (Fig. 22). There was no inflammatory cell infiltrate evident. On some of the Er:YAG laser-treated specimens, there was a loss of the odontoblastic layer in the area of laser treatment. However, no other changes of the pulp were noted even on higher power (Fig. 23).

A finding of great interest was noticed upon examining the various histologic sections. This finding can be seen in Figure 24, which shows a tooth irradiated with an Er:YAG laser. There is reparative dentin formation immediately adjacent to the laser defect. The great interest in this finding stems from the fact that the thickened dentin is just adjacent to the laser defect and it occurred in just 4 days. What accounts for this change in the dentin is unknown. The separation of the pulpal tissue from the dentin is probably a histologic artifact.

A change was seen on another canine tooth after Er:YAG laser ablation. The teeth were removed and fixed with 10% formalin and decalcified. Figure 25 is a photomicrograph of the pulp cavity with the Er:YAG laser hole just above

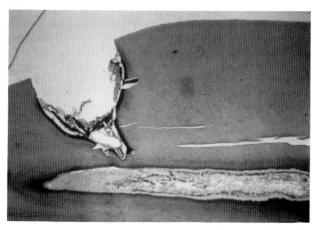

Fig. 20. Light photomicrograph showing tooth and pulpal tissue, of a CO_2 laser defect in a canine tooth. H&E ($\times 100$).

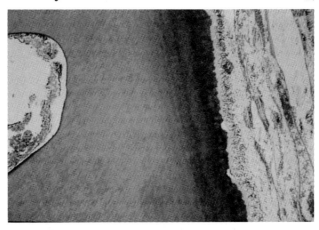

Fig. 21. Light photomicrograph showing tooth and pulpal tissue of an Er:YAG laser defect in a canine tooth. H&E ($\times 100$). See insert for color representation.

the pulp. Figure 26 shows the normal predentin, which is distant from the Er:YAG laser-created hole; note the lack of any inclusions in the lighter predentin layer. Figure 27 is a view of the predentin just below the laser hole; note the dark inclusions in the predentin layer. Some event occurred that forced these dark objects into the predentin layer, but it is not known at this time what could have caused this change.

To understand the basic tissue interaction and to develop parameters of safe laser action on hard dental tissues, basic laser tissue and material interaction studies must be performed. The following is a summary of some projects that shed light on this interaction.

Wigdor et al. and Visuri et al. [137–140] evaluated the effects of the Er:YAG laser on dental hard tissues and dental materials and the effects of a water spray. Because of the high absorption of the Er:YAG laser radiation in water, there has been some concern that water, when used to cool the ablation of dental tissues and materials, would inhibit the ablation significantly. Reports suggest that the water only minimally reduces the ablation efficiency. The thermal effect of the Er:YAG laser was also studied to substantiate the need for a water coolant. Figure 28 shows the plume created by the Er:YAG laser on dentin.

Sections of dental composite material were placed so that one side of the sample was in front of the laser beam. On the opposite side, a thermocouple was placed to detect temperature changes. A water stream was directed at varying flow rates to the spot of laser impact (Fig. 29).

There is a significant increase in the temper-

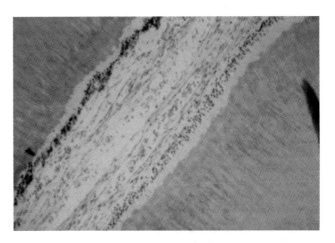

Fig. 22. Light photomicrograph showing tooth and pulpal tissue of a tooth with a defect created by a slow speed handpiece. H&E ($\times 100$). See insert for color representation.

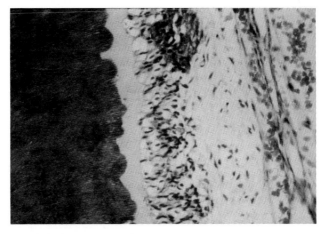

Fig. 23. Light photomicrograph of higher power view of the pulp in the tooth treated with the Er:YAG laser. H&E ($\times 400$). See insert for color representation.

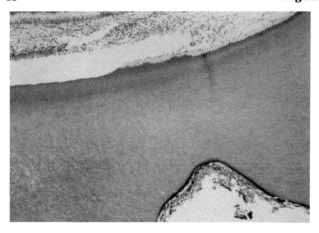

Fig. 24. Light photomicrograph of the area of the predentin layer just beneath the Er:YAG laser defect. H&E (×100).

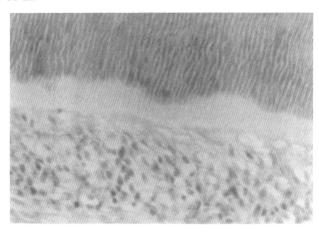

Fig. 26. Light photomicrograph of the predentin and pulpal tissue in an area normal pulpal tissue. H&E (×400).

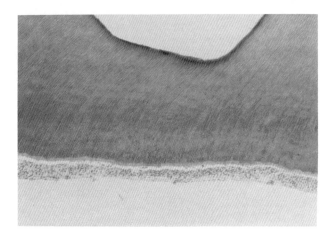

Fig. 25. Light photomicrograph of the dentin and pulpal tissue just beneath an Er:YAG laser defect. H&E (×100).

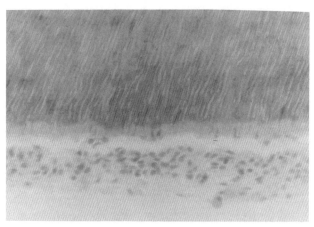

Fig. 27. Light photomicrograph of the predentin and pulpal tissue just beneath the laser ablation defect. H&E (×400).

ature of the dental materials when no water is used. The graph in Figure 30 indicates changes in the temperature with and without water when composite material was ablated and also represents the dental hard tissue values since they were almost the same as the composite values. The water controlled the temperature so that the increase was just about 1°C above the baseline temperature. There was a significant increase in temperature when water was not used.

The graph in Figure 31 shows the ablation rate of the composite material. The fluence and water were varied and the ablation per pulse was calculated. Figure 32 is a photograph of the ablation plume of an Er:YAG laser impact on composite material. The ablation rate was about the same with and without water at each fluence. Figure 33 shows the ablation holes created by the Er:YAG laser with and without waterspray. There is an obvious area of char in and around the hole created without water (Fig. 33, left).

To summarize, it seems that when the Er:YAG laser is used for the ablation of either dental hard tissues or dental materials, water will be necessary for cooling. The water may also reduce the shock wave effect, which possibly causes the cracks reported by Koort and Frentzen [111]. Dentists are presently using water for cooling with dental handpieces so the addition of water with a laser should be an easy transition. Both the histologic and SEM results presented here appear promising. Of note is that these results were created without waterspray. It would be of great interest to evaluate the effects of these laser conditions with water. Of great concern when ablating dental materials are the products being pro-

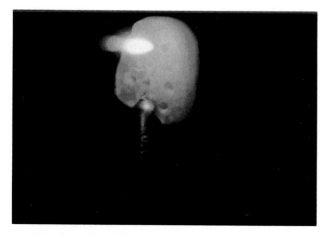

Fig. 28. Laser plume from a Er:YAG laser impact on tooth. See insert for color representation.

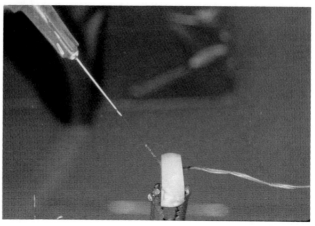

Fig. 29. Photograph of the scientific setup with the laser beam coming from the left. See insert for color representation.

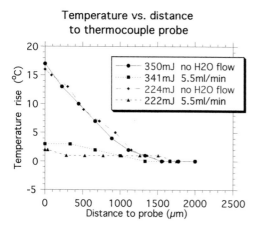

Fig. 30. Graph of the temperature changes from the Er:YAG laser impacted on dental composite.

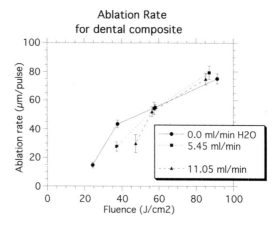

Fig. 31. Graph of the ablation efficiency of the Er:YAG laser on composite materials without waterspray and at varying rates of water flow.

duced by the laser. It seems likely that the water may reduce the plume size and possibly the amount of air-borne products that are created, but first an understanding of how this laser affects common dental materials must be studied.

Laser Composite Curing

Another use of light in dentistry began with the advent of photopolymerized dental composite materials. The first materials introduced in the late 1970s were cured with a light in the ultraviolet wavelength [141,142]. Due to the concern about UV light in the mouth, composites that polymerize in the visible light spectrum were developed [143–145]. These composites were used for anterior esthetic dental restorations and also for sealing the occlusal pits and fissures in posterior teeth to reduce decay. Powell et al. [146] showed that an argon laser requires shorter curing times and that the materials-dentin bond strength were considerably stronger when cured with the laser. Kelsey et al. [147,148] reported that the argon laser also decreased curing time and further stated that all physical properties were enhanced when compared with conventional light curing units. The variables that control the depth and extent of cure include time of exposure, composite material, wavelength and intensity of the light, and particle size of the filler. Because laser light is intense, monochromatic, coherent, and collimated, it was thought that it may be a superior light source for photopolymerization of dental composite materials. Blankenau [149] showed that if the testing time after laser polymerization

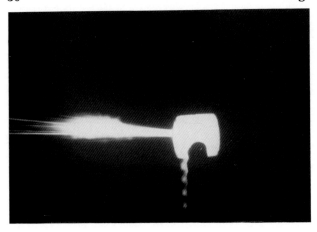

Fig. 32. Photograph of the ablation plume created by an Er:YAG laser on dental composite material.

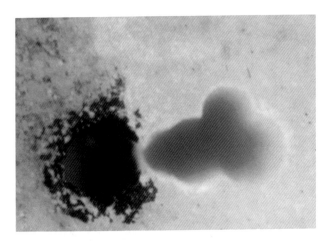

Fig. 33. Magnified view of the holes created by the Er:YAG laser. Left is without waterspray; right is with waterspray.

varied, there were considerable differences in results taken during the first 20 days postpolymerization.

Wigdor [150] looked at the cure depth of composite materials using two lasers (HeCad $\lambda = 443$ nm and Argon $\lambda = 488$ nm). Using a 50 mw laser, the amount of cure depth was about the same with the laser as the conventional xenon light source used by dentists presently for composite curing filtered to 460 nm. From the results reported, the argon and HeCd lasers appear to be similar to present methods of curing dental composite resins. The use of a more powerful laser may have cured the material faster and deeper. Since the physical properties of the composites postlaser irradiation were not determined, no

judgment can be made regarding improved results with the laser.

LASER ETCHING

A relevant topic is the use of the laser to etch tooth surfaces to increase bond strength. Presently, a 10% phosphoric acid is used to remove the organic component of enamel, which causes deep microscopic grooves to increase bonded surface area. Liberman et al. and Cooper et al. [151,152] used a CO_2 laser and compared the bonding strength with phosphoric acid etching. These studies showed similar etch strengths when either method was used with enamel. In dentin, however, Cooper et al. [152] reported a 300% increase in bond strength when the dentin was laser treated prior to bonding. Roberts-Harry [153] used the Nd:YAG laser for enamel etching and found that bond strength was less than that obtained with 10% phosphoric acid. Dederich and Tulip [154] investigated the use of the Nd:YAG laser on dentin as a pretreatment for bonding efficiency. They found that the bond strength was less with the laser than without.

Laser Welding of Dental Bridges

With the development of dental implants, there is need for more precise methods for creating dental bridges that adapt to these implants. Inherent in the casting technology presently used for most crowns and bridges is a very slight shrinkage of the metal. In traditional bridgework, this shrinkage is not significant enough to cause a problem with bridges adapting properly. Bridges that are created to adapt to implants are much more precise, and this shrinkage can cause these bridges to fit improperly. Because of the need for a more precise method for creating implant bridges, a stereo laser welding system was developed in the PROCERA® (Nobelpharma, Westmont, IL) manufacturing process for implant and conventional precision prosthetics. In this process, the stereo laser welder is used to weld together the premachined commercially pure grade II titanium bridge elements in the fabrication of implant-supported prosthetic frameworks [156].

The laser system is a flashlamp pumped Nd:YAG laser. Figure 34 is the laser welding the titanium bridge. Because of the characteristics of the titanium to develop an oxide layer, the welding must take place under an atmosphere of argon gas. This atmosphere assures that the weld joint is oxide free and of maximum strength. With the

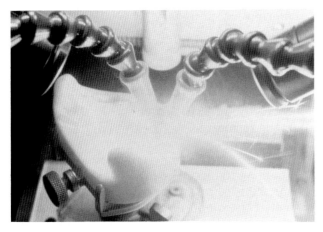

Fig. 34. Laser weld of titanium bridge.

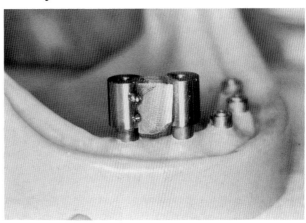

Fig. 35. Titanium welded joint is on the left, two welds are obvious.

lens system and mirror focal point, a weld of 600–800 μm deep is generated at the joint. The energy provided from the laser melts each piece of titanium on either side of the joint. As the metal cools, the two pieces of titanium join together. Figure 35 notes the appearance of the weld on the left joint. This method is different from the soldering methods presently used because with the laser similar metals are welded, whereas in soldering impurities (flux) and dissimilar metals are soldered, which can lead to a weaker joint.

Another important aspect of this technique is the use of the stereo laser weld. Welds are made at exactly the same time with two different beams of the laser on either side of the joined metals. If the welds are done at different times, there is differential shrinking, which leads to distortion. The simultaneous welding of the titanium pieces contributes significantly to the precise adaptation of these implant bridges to the underlying implants. Figure 36 is the completed welded bridge.

LASER SAFETY

The status of dental lasers and their safe use is based on a number of issues, including good controlled research, unbiased education of the practitioners using the lasers, continuing education requirements, and possible periodic examination leading to a method of credentialing of dental laser users. These actions are necessary because of the way dental care is provided to patients. Most dentists are independent practitioners and do not have any governing body reviewing their care of patients. This is quite different from hos-

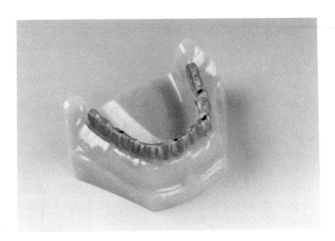

Fig. 36. A finished titanium bridge welded together.

pitals where departments of surgery review credentials of laser users.

What seems to be an important quest of all laser researchers, manufacturers, and dentists is to find a laser that can replace the dental handpiece (drill) to remove decay in a more acceptable way. To date, however, no laser has been cleared by the FDA for dental hard tissue treatment or removal. Clearance has not been granted because research to date has not shown that lasers are safe and effective. The lack of sufficient controlled research is also why lasers have not been embraced by the dental community as a new method of treatment. In addition, the lack of research is the fundamental reason why dental lasers are in the precarious place they find themselves today.

All of which leads to another problem, which is the educational process presently used to train dentists. It is essential that any education in laser training be unbiased and have as a goal to educate dentists in general laser use and safety. The intent of a good educational process is to give the users basic information so that they can decide which laser would be best for a certain indication.

Following are the authors' suggested actions that could lead to the desired goal: the efficient, safe, and effective use of lasers in dentistry.

Research

Laser treatment in humans must be based on research that has proven the treatment to be safe and effective. Indicated methods must not be based on financial gain and/or improved reputation of the user. The use of the scientific method should not be ignored by laser researchers and practitioners, and all research must be scrutinized for its scientific merit. An additional intent of this research is to review the parameters of a specific laser for optimal use of a specific condition. The FDA has established guidelines to protect patients, and these rules must be followed. Changes in the FDA's stated guidelines will be based on controlled research proving that lasers are of value by the results of research.

There is a great need at present for an educational process that will inform dental practitioners of accepted and potential laser uses. This education initially should only be didactic in nature, covering basic laser physics and safety and tissue effects of lasers without "hands-on" training. This didactic training is essential so that practitioners can acquire a firm knowledge of the physics and tissue interaction of lasers before training in their surgical techniques. It should also be understood that a specific treatment may not be restricted to one wavelength. Changing parameters of different wavelengths may have similar effects on tissues.

Credentialing of Use

Establishing standards. To establish a uniform understanding of the guidelines that will regulate laser use in dentistry, standards must be developed. As knowledge expands in this field, there must be flexibility to incorporate new technology. Three general areas must be considered:

1. Governing agency. To insure the safe use of lasers, a private or governmental group must be developed. The intent of this agency should be to provide state licensing boards with the information necessary to regulate safe laser usage.
2. Education standards. Education of laser users must be uniform, with the main intent to provide unbiased training. The training should be divided into didactic and clinical components where the practitioner must show proficiency in the former before progressing to the latter training.
3. Continuing education standards. All laser users must be required to attend continuing education courses. With this area of clinical dentistry expanding at such a fast pace, it is imperative that users maintain their proficiency on a regular basis.

All practitioners that use lasers for surgery must keep abreast of new advances in laser research, use lasers only in FDA-cleared applications, and keep the interest of their patients in mind. Only when there is a concerted effort by dental researchers and practitioners to understand lasers and their potential use can patients be assured of safe and effective treatment.

FDA and Regulations

The three agencies that have regulatory control or have developed safety standards are the Food and Drug Administration (FDA), the Occupational Health and Safety Administration (OSHA), and the American National Standards Institute (ANSI). The Laser Institute of America has approved Z136.1 and Z136.3 laser safety standards for operators of lasers and for patients. Because of the impact that the three agencies now have and their potential for increased future influence, information concerning their actions is included here.

The FDA has developed a system, only recently applied to dentistry, to evaluate new technologies to treat patients in the United States. Lasers for dentistry are being scrutinized by the FDA, and they come under the purview of the Center for Devices and Radiologic Health (CDRH). The CDRH was developed in 1982 to develop and implement national programs to protect the public wellbeing in the fields of medical devices and radiological health. The "programs are intended to assure the safety, effectiveness, and proper labeling of medical devices, to control unnecessary human exposure to potentially hazardous ionizing and nonionizing radiation, and to insure the safe, efficacious use of such radiation" [156].

The Medical Device Amendments were formally initiated in 1976 to guide the medical device industry. Section 201(h) of the Federal Food, Drug and Cosmetic Act defines "device" as: "an instrument, apparatus, implement, machine, contrivance, implant, in vitro reagent, or other similar or related article, including any component part, or accessory, which is

- recognized in the National Formulary, or the United States Pharmacopoeia, or any supplement to them,
- intended for use in the diagnosis of disease or other condition, or in the cure, mitigation, treatment, or prevention of disease, in man or other animals, or
- intended to affect the structure or any function of the body, of man or other animal, and

which does not achieve its primary intended purposes through chemical action within or on the body of man or other animals and which is not dependent upon being metabolized for the achievement of its principal intended purposes."

The act and amendments are intended to affect manufacturers and other persons marketing medical devices, not practitioners. The three components that have an affect on dentistry are 510K, investigational device exemption (IDE), and premarket approval application (PMA).

A progression of events must occur that may ultimately lead to FDA clearance of a device. This progression starts with the determination of whether a new device is substantially equivalent to one on the market before May 28, 1976, or currently legal on the U.S. market. On that date, the amendments became law, giving the FDA jurisdiction over devices used to treat patients. If a new product caused an effect similar to the effect by a product already in use, a clearance could be given for the new product by the FDA under the 510K provision. Manufacturers desiring an 510K clearance by the FDA had to show that their device, by application, was substantially equivalent to a device in existence before May 28, 1976. Such devices were "grandfathered" because of their equivalency. Under the Safe Medical Device Act of 1990, devices may be found substantially equivalent to other legally marketed devices.

The clearance given to all the "dental" lasers, to date, is for soft tissue surgery only and comes under the 510K section, which states that these lasers affect oral soft tissues in a way similar to lasers in use for other tissues before the May 1976 date or are currently on the U.S. market. Equivalency does not have to be in oral soft tissue only; any soft tissue laser surgery can be used for 510K clearance. The only nonsoft tissue application, for the oral cavity, cleared by the FDA is for composite curing with the Argon laser. Since CO_2 lasers were used for surgery on oral tissues and other soft tissues prior to the 1976 date, manufacturers of dental lasers needed only to prove substantial equivalency to these CO_2 lasers to market them for oral soft tissue surgery. The application for Premarket Notification [510(K)] just needs to prove equivalency and does not need the extensive research necessary to prove safety and efficacy for a new device.

When the intent is to use a laser for a new dental application, such as hard tissue surgery, a premarket approval application (PMA) is required. Since at the time of writing there are no lasers with clearance to do surgery on dental hard tissue, any laser manufacturer wishing to market their laser for that purpose must apply for a PMA. The FDA suggests that a PMA application include multicenter research first evaluating the effect of the specific laser on dental hard tissue in vitro. Only after a sufficient amount of basic research can the manufacturer apply for an Investigational Device Exemption (IDE). The research must address the questions of safety and potential harm to patients. The IDE allows a clinician to treat patients in a very limited scope after proving that the intended treatment method is safe. An IDE must be granted for a new device to be used in human trials and shipped in interstate commerce.

The transition from the laboratory to the clinic where the device will be used on human subjects is not well defined. It is left to the FDA to decide whether enough basic research has been completed to allow clinical studies to begin.

The FDA states that PMA requirements must apply to the first four units that have the same wavelength and treatment parameters. A device that is brought to the market after the first four PMAs can apply for clearance under substantial equivalence (510K).

An important part of the FDA monitoring policy is that any manufacturer who develops a device must maintain an inventory of incidences that occur with the product. Through this inventory and reports from practitioners who use the product, the FDA can determine if the device has the potential for causing harm to patients.

ANSI Z136.3 and OSHA Standards

Two agencies have a special interest in the safe and effective use of lasers on the American public. The American National Standards Institute (ANSI) has approved the Z136.3 standard ("For the Safe Use of Lasers in Health Care Facilities"), with the Laser Institute of America (LIA) as secretariat. The LIA is responsible for the development and publication of these standards, recommending basic laser safety parameters in general and for specific applications.

The basic standard "provides guidance for the safe use of lasers and laser systems for diagnostic and therapeutic uses in health care facilities. It is intended for use by all persons associated with the installation, operation, maintenance, and service of Health Care Laser Systems (HCLS). This standard covers engineering, procedural, and administrative controls necessary for the safety of patients and health care professionals. These controls are based upon: evaluation of potential hazards from laser radiation; unique problems related to operating rooms, outpatient clinics, private medical, and dental offices; and exposure risks to patients and professional staff. Included are engineering and administrative controls, personal protective equipment and laser safety training" [157].

The specific standards for safe use of lasers in general, and specifically in dentistry, are available through the LIA. A summary of the dental standards are included here. These standards are continually being updated to include new lasers and applications. Note the following from the American National Standard *For the Safe Use of Lasers in Health Care Facilities,* ANSI Z136.3-1988 [158].

When the laser is not in use, it should be placed in the stand-by mode to reduce the chance of inadvertent laser burns. Only instruments that have a low reflectivity should be used.

Great concern must be directed to fire protection of the surgical area and surrounding environment. All flammable material must be protected from the laser beam. Eye protection is essential and achieved by using barrier lenses specific to the laser wavelength and are to be worn by all personnel within the laser treatment zone.

If general anesthesia is used, great care must be taken to protect the endotrachial tube. Because this tube is in close proximity to the tissue being treated, it can be impacted by the laser beam. If the laser beam burns through the tube, the gases can be ignited causing a fire in the patient's lungs.

All oral tissues not being treated must be protected from the laser. Enamel, dentin, and bone can be burned by the laser, causing damage to these tissues. Retractors should be placed between the treated tissues and the underlying hard tissues.

During laser ablation of any tissues, plumes are created that may have toxic materials within them. Effective evacuation is essential to remove these plumes from the surgical area to protect personnel.

The Occupational Safety and Health Administration (OSHA) has established safety guidelines using the ANSI Z136.3 standards as a guide. The object of the guidelines is "to provide a general overview to lasers, laser uses, laser hazards and hazard analysis that are required to provide appropriate background for understanding the applicable industry standards and regulatory requirements" [158]. The two documents listed above (ANSI Z136.3 and OSHA) in combination give the dental practitioner all the relevant information and regulations on the safe and effective use of lasers in dentistry.

It is the intent of these regulations to protect both the patient and dental personnel. These regulations have at their core the basic research that has been performed with lasers since their development in the early 1960s. Understanding the effect of lasers on tissue, especially dental hard tissues, has to be a prerequisite before additional standards can be developed.

SUMMARY AND THE FUTURE

As can be seen, there has been much progress in the area of lasers in dentistry since the early report by Stern and Sognnaes [1]. These early researchers and those who followed wished to develop clinical uses for lasers with the aim of bringing the laser to the dental practitioner to improve dental care. The progression has been slow, and some of the ambitions of the early researchers have yet to be realized.

To date, soft tissue applications have constituted the primary area for the clinical use of lasers in dentistry. Clinicians and patients alike have great interest in the development of lasers for dental use. In order to expand future applications in dentistry, developments must be based on understanding the effects of various wavelengths and other parameters on laser/tissue interactions in the oral cavity. With this understanding, lasers can be developed to treat specific conditions or for specific purposes in the mouth.

Research has shown that pretreatment of dental enamel with carbon dioxide laser light within certain parameters can markedly reduce subsequent acid dissolution of the enamel. Since dental decay is a demineralization process, such laser treatment is expected to be useful for inhibition of decay in the mouth. Understanding the effects of the parameters involved will allow for optimum conditions to be chosen for clinical inhibition of caries progression. The potential is good for this concept to be expanded for: (1) treatment of early enamel lesions to inhibit progression, (2) treatment of occlusal surfaces, (3) prevention of root caries' susceptible sites, and (4) treatment of early root caries to inhibit progression.

There are numerous other potential applications. Following is a list of possible uses of lasers in dentistry.

Lasers can be beneficial for selective removal of malignant tissue with the aid of porphorin compounds. These compounds are selectively absorbed by malignant cells and when combined with specific wavelength laser light, malignant tissue is destroyed. Some of the bacteria implicated in periodontal disease have porphorin compounds in their cell walls. Lasers may be used selectively to kill these bacteria, leaving other nonpathogenic bacteria intact. This action may also be expedited by using compounds similar to the porphorins that are painted in the gingiva before laser treatment.

Laser welding of bridges in vitro is progressing into the clinic; however, the potential to replace missing teeth by welding to natural teeth with lasers seems promising. This would reduce the need for abutment teeth in dental bridge fabrication.

The use of lasers to create holograms of dental models is now a reality. These holograms can be used by dentists and orthodontists who store models of their patients. Holograms can be kept in patients' records, eliminating many storage problems in the typical dental and orthodontic practice. Similar measurements made with the dental models can be made on these holograms. Later, holograms can also be superimposed over earlier ones for posttreatment assessment.

One of the most obvious applications of lasers is for the controlled removal of dental enamel, dentin, bone, or cementum. Using lasers to ablate hard dental tissue for bonding pretreatment, dental decay removal, and tooth preparation has recieved considerable attention by researchers. This worthy goal can be achieved only after more information is available on tissue/laser interactions and technology can be developed to make use of this knowledge. Replacement or supplementation of the dental drill is a real possibility for the future.

The laser of the future will probably have the ability to produce a multitude of wavelengths and pulsewidths, each specific to a particular application. When the knowledge of what parameters are necessary for ideal treatment is a reality, lasers can be developed that can provide dentists with the ability to care for patients with improved techniques and equipment. This must be the goal of laser dentistry.

ACKNOWLEDGMENTS

J.D.B.F. and D.F. were supported by NIH/NIDR grant RO1 DE 09958. H.W., J.W., and S.V. were supported by a grant from the Luxar Corporation. J.W. and S.V. were supported by NSF grant BCS-9257492.

REFERENCES

1. Stern RH, Sognnaes RF. Laser beam effect on dental hard tissues. J Dent Res 1964; 43 (Suppl.):873 (Abs 307).
2. Stern R, Renger HL, Howell FV. Laser effects on vital dental pulps. Br Dent J 1969; 26–28.
3. Stern RH, Vahl J, Sognnaes RF. Laser enamel: Ultrastructural observations of pulsed carbon dioxide laser effects. J Dent Res 1972; 51:455–460.
4. Stern RH, Renger HL, Howell FV. Laser effects on vital dental pulps. Br Dent J 1969; 26–28.
5. Adrian JC, Bernier JL, Sprague WG. Laser and the dental pulp. JADA 1971; 83:113–117.
6. Lobene RR, Bhussry BR, Fine S. Interaction of carbon dioxide laser radiation with enamel and dentin. J Dent Res 1968; 47:311–317.
7. Borggreven JMPM, van Dijk JWE, Driessens FCM. Effect of laser irradiation on permeability of bovine dental enamel. Arch Oral Biol 1980; 25:831–832.
8. Yamamoto H, Sato K. Prevention of dental caries by acousto-optically Q-switched Nd:YAG laser irradiation. J Dent Res 1980; 59(2):137.
9. Kuroda S, Fowler BO. Compositional, structural, and phase changes in vitro laser irradiated human tooth enamel. Calcif Tissue Int 1984; 36:361–369.
10. Goldman L, Hornby P, Meyer R, Goldman B. Impact of the laser on dental caries. Nature 1964; 203:417.
11. Lobine RR, Fine SF. Interaction of laser radiation with oral hard tissues. J Prosth Den 1966; 16:589–597.
12. Taylor R, Shklar G, Roeber F. The effects of laser radiation on teeth, dental pulp and oral mucosa of experimental animals. Oral Surg 1965; 19:786–795.
13. Dederich DN. Laser/tissue interaction. Alpha Omega Dental Fraternity 1991; 84:4, 33–36.

14. Cheong W, Prahl SA, Welch AJ. A review of the optical properties of biological tissues. IEEE J Quantum Electron 1990; 26:2166–2185.

15. Luomanen M, Virtaen I. Fibronectins in healing incision, excision and laser wounds. J Oral Pathol Med 1991; 20:133–138.

16. Luomanen M, Meurman JH, Letho V-P. Extracellular matrix in healing CO2 laser incision wound. J Oral Pathol 1987; 16:322–331.

17. Luomanen M, Virtanen I. Healing of laser and scalpel incision wounds of rat tongue mucosa as studied with cytokeratin antibodies. J Oral Pathol 1987; 16:139–144.

18. Luomanen M. Oral focal epithelial hyperplasia removed with CO_2 laser. Int J Oral Maxillofac Surg 1990; 19: 205–207.

19. Luomanen M. Experience with a carbon dioxide laser for removal of benign oral soft-tissue lesions. Proc Finn Dent Soc 1992; 88:49–55.

20. Walsh JT, Flotte TJ, Anderson RR, Deutsch TF. Pulsed CO_2 laser tissue ablation: Effect of tissue type and pulse duration on thermal damage. Lasers Surg Med 1988; 8:108–118.

21. Walsh JT, Deutsch TF. Pulsed CO_2 laser tissue ablation: Measurement and modeling of ablation rates. Lasers Surg Med 1988; 8:264–275.

22. Walsh JT, Deutsch TF. Pulsed CO_2 laser ablation of tissue: Effect of mechanical properties. IEEE Trans Biomed Eng 1989; 36:1195–1201.

23. Schomaker KT, Walsh JT, Flotte JT, Deutsch TF. Thermal damage produced by high irradiance CW CO_2 laser cutting tissue. Lasers Surg Med 1990; 10:74–84.

24. Goldman L, Shumrick DA, Rockwell RJ, Meyer R. The laser in maxillofacial surgery. Arch Surg 1968; 96:397–400.

25. Clayman L, Fuller T, Beckman H. Healing of continuous-wave and rapid superpulsed, carbon dioxide, laser induced bone defects. J Oral Surg 1978; 36:932–937.

26. Pick RM, Picaro BC, Silverman CJ. The laser gingivectomy: The use of the CO_2 laser for the removal of phenytoin hyperplasia. J Periodontol 1985; 56(8):492–496.

27. Pecaro BC, Garehime WJ. The CO_2 laser in oral and maxillofacial surgery. J Oral Maxillofac Surg 1983; 41: 725.

28. Pick RM, Becaro BC. Use of the CO_2 laser in soft tissue dental surgery. Lasers Surg Med 1987; 7:207–213.

29. Abt E, Wigdor HA, Lobraico R, Carlson B, Harris D, Pyrcz R. Removal of benign intraoral masses using the CO_2 laser. JADA 1986; 115(11):729–731.

30. Frame JW. Removal of oral soft tissue pathology with the CO_2 laser. J Oral Maxillofac Surg 1985; 43:850–855.

31. Rossmann JA. Current research using the CO_2 laser in guided tissue regeneration: Animal studies. Proceedings Second Annual Advanced Application Seminar, Luxar Corp., 1993.

32. Israel M. Current research using the CO_2 laser in guided tissue regeneration: Clinical studies. Proceedings Second Annual Advanced Application Seminar, Luxar Corp., 1993.

33. White JM, Goodis HE, Rose CL. Use of the pulsed Nd: YAG laser for intraoral soft tissue surgery. Lasers Surg Med 1991; 11:455–461.

34. Graaff R, Aarnoudse JG, de Mul FFM, Jentink HW. Light propagation parameters for anisotropically scattering media based on rigorous solution of the transport equation. Appl Optics 1989; 28:2273–2279.

35. Ishimaru A. "Wave Propagation and Scattering in Random Media." New York: Academic Press, 1978.

36. Wilson BC, Jacques SL. Optical reflectance and transmittance of tissues: Principles and applications. IEEE J Quantum Electron 1990; 26:2186–2191.

37. Fried D, Featherstone JDB, Glena RE, Seka W. The nature of light scattering in dental enamel and dentin at visible and near-IR wavelengths. Appl Optics (in press).

38. Fried D, Featherstone JDB, Glena RE, Bordyn B, Seka W. The light scattering properties of dentin and enamel at 543, 632, and 1053 nm. In: "Lasers in Orthopedic, Dental, and Veterinary Medicine II." Bellingham, WA: SPIE 1993, pp 240–245.

39. Spitzer D, ten Bosch JJ. The absorption and scattering of light in bovine and human dental enamel. Calcif Tiss Res 1975; 17:129–137.

40. ten Bosch JJ, Zijp JR. Optical properties of dentin. In: Thylstrup, A, ed. "Dentine and Dentine Research in the Oral Cavity." Oxford: IRL Press, 1987, pp 59–65.

41. Zijp JR, ten Bosch JJ. Theoretical model for the scattering of light by dentin and comparison with measurements. Appl Optics 1993; 32:411–415.

42. Zijp JR, ten Bosch JJ. Angular dependence of HeNe laser light scattering by bovine and human dentine. Arch Oral Biol 1991; 36:283–289.

43. Henyey IG, Greenstein JL. Diffuse radiation in the galaxy. Astrophys J 1941; 93:70–83.

44. Seka W, Fried D, Glena RE, Featherstone JDB. Laser energy deposition in dental hard tissue. J Dent Res 1994; 73:340.

45. Fried D, Borzillary SF, McCormack SM, Glena RE, Featherstone JDB, Seka W. The thermal effects on CO_2 Laser irradiated dental enamel at 9.3, 9.6, 10.3, and 10.6 μm. In "Laser Surgery: Advanced Characterization, Therapeutics, and Systems IV." Bellingham, WA: SPIE 1994, pp 319–328.

46. Duplain G, Boulay R, Belanger PA. Complex index of refraction of dental enamel at CO_2 wavelengths. Appl Optics 1987; 26:4447–4451.

47. Fowler BO, Moreno EC, Brown WE. Infra-red spectra of hydroxyapatite, octacalcium phosphate and pyrolysed octacalcium phosphate. Arch Oral Biol 1966; 11:477–492.

48. Fowler BO. Infrared studies of apatites. II. Preparation of normal and isotopically substituted calcium, strontium, and barium hydroxyapatites and spectra-structure-composition correlations. Inorg Chem 1973; 13:207.

49. Featherstone JDB, Nelson DGA. Laser effects on dental hard tissue. Adv Dent Res 1987; 1:21–26.

50. Boehm RF, Chen M, Blair CK. Temperature in human teeth due to laser heating. ASME Paper No. 75-WA/Bio-8, 1975.

51. Laufer G, Haber S. Numerical analysis of the thermochemical tooth damage induced by laser radiation. J Biomech Eng 1985; 107:234–239.

52. Sagi A, Segal T, Dagan J. A numerical model for temperature distribution and thermal damage calculations in teeth exposed to a CO_2 laser. Mathematical Biosci 1984; 71:1–17.

53. Sagi A, Shitzer A, Katzir A, Akselrod S. Heating of biological tissue by laser irradiation: theoretical model. Opt Eng 1992; 31:1417–1424.

54. Yu D, Fox JI, Hsu J, Powell GL, Higuchi WI. Computer simulation of surface temperature profiles during CO_2 laser irradiation of human enamel. Opt Eng 1993; 32: 298–305.

55. Feuerstein O, Palanker D, Fuxbrunner A, Lewis A, Deutsch D. Effect of the ArF excimer laser on human enamel. Lasers Surg Med 1992; 12:471–477.

56. Frentzen M, Koort HJ, Thiensiri I. Excimer lasers in dentistry: Future possibilities with advanced technology. Quintessence Int 1992; 23:117–133.

57. Neev J, Liaw LL, Raney DV, Fujishige JT, Ho PD, Berns MW. Selectivity, efficiency and surface characteristics of hard dental tissues ablated with ArF pulsed excimer lasers. Lasers Surg Med 1991; 11:499–510.

58. Neev J, Liaw LL, Stabholtz A, Torabinejad JT, Fujishige JT, Berns MW. Tissue alteration and thermal characteristics of excimer laser interaction with dentin. SPIE Proceedings 1992; 1643:386–397.

59. Neev J, Stabholtz A, Liaw LL, Torabinejad JT, Fujishige, Ho PD, Berns MW. Scanning electron microscopy and thermal characteristics of dentin ablated by a short pulsed XeCl excimer laser. Laser Surg Med 1993; 12: 353–361.

60. Walsh JT Jr, Deutsch TF. Measurement of Er:YAG laser ablation plume dynamics. Appl Phys B 1991; 52: 217–224.

61. Wigdor HA, Walsh JT, Visuri S. Effect of water on hard dental tissue ablation of the Er:YAG laser. SPIE 1994 (in press).

62. Altshuler GB, Belikov AV, Erofeev AV. Laser treatment of enamel and dentin by different Er-lasers. SPIE 1994 (in press).

63. Izatt JA, Sankey ND, Partovi F, Fitzmaurice M, Rava RP, Iyzkan I, Feld MS. Ablation of calcified biological tissue using pulsed hydrogen fluoride laser radiation. IEEE J Quant Electron 1990; 26:2261–2270.

64. Stern RH, Sognnaes RF, Goodman F. Laser effect on in vitro enamel permeability and solubility. J Am Dent Assoc 1966; 78:838–843.

65. Vahl J. Electron microscopical and X-ray crystallographic investigations of teeth exposed to laser rays. Caries Res 1968; 28:10–18.

66. Yamamoto H, Ooya K. Potential of yttrium-aluminium-garnet laser in caries prevention. J Oral Pathol 1974; 38:7–15.

67. Fowler BO. Infrared studies of apatites. I. Vibrational assignments for calcium, strontium, and barium hydroxyapatites utilizing isotopic substitution. 1974; 13: 194–206.

68. Nelson DGA, Featherstone JDB. Preparation, analysis, and characterization of carbonated apatites. Calcif Tissue Int 1982; 34:S69–S81.

69. Nelson DGA, Shariati M, Glena R, Shields CP, Featherstone JDB. Effect of pulsed low energy infrared laser irradiation in artificial caries-like lesion formation. Caries Res 1986; 20:289–299.

70. Nelson DGA, Williamson BE. Low-temperature laser Raman spectroscopy of synthetic carbonated apatites and dental enamel. Aust J Chem 1982; 3S:715–727.

71. Meurman JH, Voegel JC, Rauhamaa-Makinen R, Gasser P, Thomann JM, Hemmerle J, Luomanen M, Paunio I, Frank RM. Effects of carbon dioxide, Nd:YAG and carbon dioxide-Nd:YAG combination lasers at high energy densities on synthetic hydroxyapatite. Caries Res 1992; 26:77–83.

72. Launay L, Mordon S, Cornil A, Brunetaud JM, Moschetto Y. Thermal effects of lasers on dental tissues. Lasers Surg Med 1987; 7:473–477.

73. Kantola S, Laine E, Tarna T. Laser-induced effects on tooth structure: VI. X-ray diffraction study of dental enamel exposed to a CO_2 laser. Acta Odontol Scand 1973; 31:369–379.

74. Lenz P, Glide H, Walz R. Studies on enamel sealing with the CO_2 laser. Dtsch Zahnarztl Z 1982; 37:469–478.

75. Fowler BO, Kuroda S. Changes in heated and in laser-irradiated human tooth enamel and their probable effects on solubility. Calcif Tissue Int 1986; 38:197–208.

76. Nelson DGA, Jongebloed WL, Featherstone JDB. Laser irradiation of human dental enamel. NZ Dent J 1986; 82:74–77.

77. Featherstone JDB, Fried D, Kantorowitz Z, Barrett-Vespone NA, Seka W. CO_2 laser inhibition of artificial caries-like lesion progression in dental enamel. J Dent Res (in press).

78. Nelson DGA, Wefel JS, Jongebloed WL, Featherstone JDB. Morphology, histology and crystallography of human dental enamel treated with pulsed low energy IR laser radiation. Caries Res 1987; 21:411–426.

79. Oho T, Morioka T. A possible mechanism of acquired acid resistance of human dental enamel by laser irradiation. Caries Res 1990; 24:86–92.

80. Christofferson J, Christofferson MR. Kinetics of dissolution of calcium hydroxyapatite: IV. The effect of some biologically important inhibitors. J Crystal Growth 1981; 53:42–54.

81. Fox JL, Yu D, Otsuka M, Higuchi WI, Wong J, Powell GL. Initial dissolution rate studies on dental enamel after CO_2 laser irradiation. J Dent Res 1992; 71:1389–1397.

82. Fox JL, Higuchi WI, Fawzi MB, Wu MS. A new two-site model for hydroxyapatite dissolution in acidic media. J Colloid Interface Sci 1978; 67:312–330.

83. Otsuka M, Wong J, Higuchi WI, Fox JL. Effects of laser irradiation on the dissolution kinetics of hydroxyapatite preparations. J Pharm Sci 1990; 79:510–515.

84. Sato K. Relation between acid dissolution and histological alteration of heated tooth enamel. Caries Res 1983; 17:490–495.

85. Goodman BD, Kaufman HW. Effects of an argon laser on the crystalline properties and rate of dissolution in acid of tooth enamel in the presence of sodium fluoride. J Dent Res 1977; 56:1201–1207.

86. Tagomori S, Morioka T. Combined effects of laser and fluoride on acid resistance of human dental enamel. Caries Res 1989; 23:225–231.

87. Featherstone JDB, Zhang SH, Shariati M, McCormack SM. Carbon dioxide laser effects on caries-like lesions of dental enamel. SPIE 1991; 1424:145–149.

88. Fox JL, Yu D, Otsuka M, Higuchi WI, Wong J, Powell GL. The combined effects of laser irradiation and chemical inhibitors on the dissolution of dental enamel. Caries Res 1992; 26:333–339.

89. Fox JL, Wong J, Yu D, Otsuka M, Higuchi WI, Hsu J, Powell GL. Carbonate apatite as a model for the effect of laser irradiation on human dental enamel. J Dent Res 1994 (in press).

90. Neev J, Stabholtz A, Liaw LL, Torabinejad M, Fujishige

JT, Ho PD, Berns MW. Scanning electron microscopy and thermal characteristics of dentin ablated by a short-pulse XeCl excimer laser. Lasers Surg Med 1993; 12: 353–361.

91. Walsh JT, Deutsch TF. Er:YAG ablation of tissue: Measurement of ablation rates. Lasers Surg Med 1989; 9:327–337.

92. Hibst R, Keller U. Experimental studies of the application of the Er:YAG laser on dental hard substances: I. Measurement of the ablation rate. Lasers Surg Med 1989; 9:338–344.

93. Hibst R, Keller U. Experimental studies of the application of the Er:YAG laser on dental hard substances: II. Light microscopic and SEM investigations. Lasers Surg Med 1989; 9:345–351.

94. Stewart L, Powell GL, Wright S. Hydroxyapatite attached by laser: A potential-sealant for pits and fissures. Operat Dent 1985; 10:2–5.

95. Trends in Dentistry, Dental Products Report, MEDEC Dental Communications, Northfield, IL, 1993, p 38.

96. Melcer J, Chaumette MT, Melcer F, Dejardin J, Hasson R, Merard R, Pinaudeau Y, Weill R. Treatment of dental decay by CO_2 laser beam: Preliminary results. Lasers Surg Med 1984; 4:311–321.

97. Melcer J. Latest treatment in dentistry by means of the CO_2 laser beam. Lasers Surg Med 1986; 6:396–398.

98. Zachariasen K, Barron J, Boran T. Carbon dioxide laser effects on dental hard tissues. Laser Institute of America Proceedings (ICALEO) 1988; 64:163–169.

99. Wigdor HA, Lobraico R, Abt E, Carlson B, Harris D, Pyrcz R. The use of the CO_2 laser to remove dental decay. Laser Institute of America Proceedings (ICALEO), 1988; 64:153–162.

100. Miserendino LJ. The laser apicoectomy: Endodontic application of the CO_2 laser for periapical surgery. Oral Surg 1988; 66(5):615–619.

101. Miserendino LJ, Abt E, Wigdor HA, Miserendino CA. Evaluation of thermal cooling mechanisms for laser application to teeth. Lasers Surg Med 1993; 13:83–88.

102. McKee MD. Effects of CO_2 laser irradiation in vivo on rat alveolar bone and incisor enamel, dentin and pulp. J Dent Res 1993; 73:1406–1417.

103. Jeffrey IWM, Lawrenson B, Longbottom C, Saunders EM. CO_2 laser application to the mineralized dental tissues—the possibility of iatrogenic sequelae. J Dent 1990; 18:24–30.

104. Shoji S, Nakamura M, Horoshi H. Histopathological changes in dental pulps irradiated by CO_2 laser: A preliminary report on laser pulpotomy. J Endodontics 1985; 11:379–384.

105. Pogrel MA, Chung KY, Taylor RC. Thermographic evaluation of the temperatures achieved by carbon dioxide laser on soft tissues and teeth. Thermology 1988; 3:50–52.

106. Dederich DN, Zakariasen KL, Tulip J. Scanning electron microscopic analysis of canal wall dentin following Nd:YAG laser irradiation. J Endodontics 1984; 10(9):428–431.

107. Harris D, Wigdor HA. The Q-switched Nd:YAG as a dental drill. Newsletter, Midwest Bio-Laser Institute, 1987.

108. Bahcall J, Howard P, Miserendino L, Walia H. Preliminary investigation of the histological effects of laser endodontic treatment of the periradicular tissues in dogs. J Endodontics 1992; 18(2):47–51.

109. Neev J, Liaw LL, Raney Dv, Fujishige JT, Ho PD, Berns MW. Selectivity, efficiency and surface characteristics of hard dental tissues ablated with ArF pulsed excimer lasers. Lasers Surg Med 1991; 11:499–510.

110. Pini R, Salimbeni R, Vannini M, Barone R. Laser dentistry: A new application of excimer laser in root canal therapy. Lasers Surg Med 1989; 9:352–357.

111. Koort HJ, Frentzen M. Pulsed laser in dentistry—Sense of Nonsense? SPIE Proceedings 1991; 1424:87–98.

112. Altschuler GB, Belikov AV, Erofeev AV, Egorov VL. Simulation of laser destruction of hard tooth tissues. Proceedings of Dental Applications of Lasers, SPIE 1993; 2080:10–19.

113. Altshuler GB, Belikov AV, Erofeev AV, Vitiaz IV. Optical model of human tooth. International Society of Laser Dentistry Proceedings 1992; 247–248.

114. Zakariasen K, Barron J, Paton B. Laser scanned fluorescence of non-lased/normal, lased/normal, non-lased/carious and laser/carious enamel. SPIE Proceedings 1992; 1643:493–502.

115. Barron J, Paton B, Zakariasen K. Micro-analysis of dental caries using laser scanned fluorescence. SPIE Proceedings 1992; 1643:503–509.

116. Keller U, Hibst R. Tooth pulp reaction following Er:YAG laser application. SPIE Proceedings 1991; 1424:127–133.

117. Rechmann P, Hennig T, von den Hoff U, Kaufmann R. Caries selective ablation: Wavelengths 377 nm versus 2.9 μm. SPIE 1993; 1880:235–239.

118. Burkes EJ, Hoke J, Gomes E, Wolbarsht M. Wet versus dry enamel ablation by Er:YAG laser. J Prothetic Dentistry 1992; 67:847–851.

119. Zach L, Cohen G. Pulp response to externally applied heat. Oral Surg Oral Med Oral Surg 1965; 19 (4):515–530.

120. Hibst R, Keller U. Removal of dental filling materials by Er:YAG laser radiation. SPIE 1991; 1424:120–126.

121. Miserendino LJ, Neiburger EJ, Walia H, Luebke N, Brantly W. Thermal effects of continuous wave CO2 laser exposure on human teeth: An in vitro study. J Endodontics 1989; 15:302–305.

122. Meese G, Zuhrt R. Therapy of deep caries by transverse excited atmosphere pressure carbon dioxide laser: an in vitro investigation. SPIE 1993; 1880:193–198.

123. Ertl T, Muller G. Hard tissue ablation with pulsed CO2 lasers. SPIE 1993; 1880:176–181.

124. Yariv A. "Optical Electronics." New York: Holt, Rinehart and Winston, 1985.

125. "Advanced Solid-State Lasers Technical Digest, 1992," Washington, DC: Optical Society of America, 1992.

126. Chadra S, Ferry MJ, Daunt G. 115mJ, 2-micron Pulses by OPO in KTP. In: "Advanced Solid-State Lasers Technical Digest, 1992." Washington, DC: Optical Society of America, 1992, pp 271–273.

127. Arcoria CJ, Fredrickson CJ, Hayes DJ, Wallace DB, Judy MM. Dye microdrop assisted laser for dentistry. Lasers Surg Med 1993; Suppl 5:17.

128. Jennett E, Motamedi M, Rastegar S, Arcoria C, Fredrickson C. Dye enhanced Alexanderite laser for ablation of dental tissue. Lasers Surg Med 1994; Suppl 6:15.

129. Izatt JA, Albagi D, Britton M, Jubas JM, Itzkan I, Feld

MS. Wavelength dependence of pulsed laser ablation of calcified tissue. Lasers Surg Med 1991; 11:238–249.

130. Srinivasan R. Ablation of polymers and biological tissue by ultraviolet lasers. Science 1986; 234:550–565.

131. Arima M, Matsumoto K. Effects of ArF:excimer laser irradiation on human enamel and dentin. Lasers Surg Med 1993; 13:97–105.

132. Henning T, Techmann P, Jeitner P, Kaufmann R. Caries selective ablation: The second threshold. SPIE 1993; 1880:117–124.

133. Henning T, Rechmann P, Pilgrim C, Schwartzmaier HJ, Kaufmann R. Caries selective ablation by pulsed lasers. SPIE 1991; 1424:99–105.

134. Altshular G, Belikov A, Erofeev A. Human tooth enamel and dentin damage by holmium laser radiation. SPIE 1992; 1643:454–463.

135. Altshuler GB, Belikov AV, Erofeev AV, Sam RC. Optimum regimes of laser destruction of human tooth enamel and dentin. SPIE 1993; 1880:101–107.

136. Wigdor HA, Abt E, Ashrafi S, Walsh JT. The effects of lasers on dental hard tissues. JADA 1993; 124:65–70.

137. Wigdor HA, Walsh JT, Cummings JP. New method for determination of ablation of hard tissues with the Er:YAG laser. SPIE Proceedings 1993; 1880:142–148.

138. Wigdor HA, Walsh JT, Visuri S. Thermal effect of Er:YAG laser radiation on dental hard tissues. SPIE Proceedings 1993; 2080:26–32.

139. Wigdor HA, Visuri SR, Walsh JT. Effect of water on dental material ablation of the Er:YAG laser. SPIE Proceedings 1994 (in press).

140. Visuri SR, Walsh JT, Wigdor HA. Erbium laser ablation of hard tissue: Modeling and control of the thermal load. SPIE Proceedings 1994 (in press).

141. Cook WD. Factors affecting the depth of cure of UV-polymerized composites. J Dent Res 1980; 59(5):800–808.

142. Salako NO, Cruickshanks-Boyd DW. Curing depths of materials polymerized by ultra-violet light. Brit Dent J 1979; 146(12):375–379.

143. Swartz ML, Phillips RW, Rhodes B. Visible light-activated resins depth of cure. JADA 1983; 106:634–637.

144. Yearn JA. Factors affecting cure of visible light activated composites. Int Dent J 1985; 35:218–225.

145. Tittha R, Fan PL, Dennison JB, Powers JM. In vitro depth of cure of photo-activated composites. J Dent Res 1982; 61(10):1184–1187.

146. Powell GL, Kelsey WP, Blankenau RJ, Barkmeier WW. The use of an argon laser for polymerization of composite resin. Esthetic Dentistry 1989.

147. Kelsey WP, Blankenau RJ, Powell GL, Barkmeier WW, Cavel WT, Whisenant BK. Enhancement of physical properties of resin materials by laser polymerization. Lasers Surg Med 1989; 9:623–627.

148. Kelsey WP, Blankenau RJ, Powell GL. Application of the argon laser dentistry. Lasers Surg Med 1991; 11:495–498.

149. Blankenau RJ, Powell Gl, Kelsey WP, Barkmeier WW. Post polymerization strength values of argon laser cured resin. Lasers Surg Med 1991; 11:471–474.

150. Wigdor HA. The use of the HeCd and argon lasers to cure dental composites when compared with white light sources. SPIE Proceedings 1990; 1200:372–378.

151. Liberman R, Segal TH, Nordenberg D, Serebro LI. Adhesion of composite materials to enamel: Comparison between the use of acids and lasing as pretreatment. Lasers Surg Med 1984; 4:232–327.

152. Cooper LF, Myers ML, Nelson DGA, Mowery AS. Shear strength of composite bonded to laser-pretreated dentin. J Prosth Dent 1988; 60:45–49.

153. Roberts-Harry DP. Laser etching of teeth for orthodontic bracket placement: A preliminary clinical study. Lasers Surg Med 1992; 12:467–470.

154. Dederich DN, Tulip J. The effect of Nd:YAG laser on dentinal bond strength. SPIE Proceedings 1991; 1424:134–137.

155. Jemt T, Linden B. Fixed implant-supported prostheses with welded titanium frameworks. Int J Periodontics Restorative Dent 1992; 12:177–183.

156. U.S. Department of Health and Human Services Public Health Service, Food and Drug Administration, Center for Device and Radiological Health. Everything You Always Wanted to Know About the Medical Device Amendments . . . and Weren't Afraid to Ask, 3rd ed, August 1990. HHS Publication FDA 90-4173.

157. For Safe Use of Lasers in Health Care Facilities, American National Standards Institute ANSI Z136.3-1988.

158. OSHA Guidelines on Laser Devices, Rockwell Laser Industries, Cincinnati, OH, February 15, 1990.

Chapter 3

Clinical Uses of Lasers in Dermatology

Ronald G. Wheeland, MD

Department of Dermatology, University of New Mexico, Albuquerque

INTRODUCTION

Lasers were introduced in the specialty of dermatology in the mid-1960s. Since then, their wide acceptance and use provide striking evidence of their extraordinary ability to treat, precisely and effectively, a number of skin diseases that were previously incapable of being managed by other medical or surgical methods. Continued evolutionary changes in both the laser technology and the understanding of the mechanisms involved in the laser–tissue interaction have improved the precision with which cutaneous laser surgery can be performed and have also increased the indications for it.

HISTORICAL ASPECTS OF LASER SURGERY

The concepts and principles necessary to create a functional laser system were developed in 1916 [1] by Albert Einstein as part of his quantum theory. However, the first device to utilize these concepts was not developed until 1954 when Townes and Gordon produced an ammonia gas MASER (Microwave Amplification for the Stimulated Emission of Radiation) [2], and the first functional laser system, utilizing a ruby crystal, was not developed until the following year by Maiman [3]. Since then, a rapid proliferation of laser systems has markedly improved the specificity and precision of treatment for vascular, pigmented, and neoplastic disorders by providing ad-

TABLE 1 Dermatologic Laser Systems

Emission	Laser system	Wavelength (nm)	Mode of output	Absorption characteristics
Visible (400–700 nm)				
	Argon (blue-green)	488–514	CW	Hemoglobin, melanin
	Dye (pigment)	510	Pulsed	Melanin
	Krypton (green)	521, 530	CW	Hemoglobin, melanin
	Frequency doubled:YAG (green)	532	Q-switched	Melanin, tattoos (red), Hemoglobin
	Copper (green)	511	Pulsed	Hemoglobin, melanin
	Krypton (yellow)	568	CW	Hemoglobin
	Copper (yellow)	578	Pulsed	Hemoglobin
	Dye (vascular)	577, 585	CW, Pulsed	Hemoglobin
	Ruby	694	Q-switch	Melanin, tattoos
	Alexandrite	755	Q-switch	Tattoos, melanin
Infrared (700–100,000 nm)				
	Nd:YAG	1,064	CW, Q-switch	Protein, tattoos
	CO_2	10,600	CW, SP	H_2O

ditional wavelengths, different delivery systems, and shorter pulse durations. Despite the relatively large number of laser systems currently available for medical use, they span only a narrow portion of the electromagnetic spectrum (Table I).

LASER–TISSUE INTERACTION

In addition to wavelength, a number of other factors, including irradiance, energy fluence, spot size, pulse duration, and the optical characteristics of the tissue, can influence the specificity of the laser-tissue interaction. Our understanding of this interaction has been improved by one of the more important recent conceptual advances, known as selective photothermolysis, which has helped to explain the effects that the duration of the laser pulse can have on the vascular or pigmented components of the skin. The first concept required to understand the mechanism of selective photothermolysis is thermal relaxation time (Tr). This is defined as the time required for an object to cool to 50% of the temperature achieved immediately following laser exposure without conducting heat to the surrounding tissue [4]. In order selectively to damage only one component of the skin, it is necessary for the exposure time to be shorter than the Tr. Otherwise, energy will be conducted to adjacent structures and result in nonspecific thermal damage. In the treatment of portwine stains, where the microvessels have a thermal relaxation time of 0.05–1.2 msec, it is possible to damage selectively only the vasculature by using a short-pulsed system, like the flashlamp-pumped pulsed dye laser, to effectively removal these types of birthmarks [4,5].

Q-Switching

The same concept of selective photothermolysis has also been employed to treat structures in the skin that are smaller than microvessels, like subcellular melanosomes or tattoo pigments, by using even shorter laser pulses generated by Q-switching. The Q-switched lasers confine the photons in the optical cavity until high peak powers have been reached and then dump the energy as a single short, 5–10 nsec pulse of very high intensity. These pulses generate both a mechanical acoustic wave in tissue as well as produce thermal effects, but the result is precise injury produced by selective photothermolysis.

Optical Properties

The optical properties of skin are an exceedingly important determinant of the selectivity by which lasers interact with tissue. The goal in performing laser surgery is to use a wavelength of light that is maximally absorbed by the component of skin that is to be treated [6]. When the absorptive characteristics of the targeted tissue are precisely matched with the most ideal wavelengths, maximal specificity of the laser-tissue interaction will occur [7]. An understanding of the spectral properties and relative concentration of the various chromophores in the target is also a prerequisite for maximizing the precision of the laser-tissue interaction. Fortunately, there are only two primary chromophores in the skin: oxygenated hemoglobin with three main absorption peaks at 418, 542, and 577 nm, and melanin, which has a very broad range of absorption. Although not representing a true chromophore, intracellular and extracellular water is another component of skin that can determine the specificity of laser-tissue interaction, especially for the infrared lasers [8]. The water content influences the quality of the thermal effect produced by some lasers, which can range from protein denaturation at temperatures of 40°C, to coagulation at temperatures of 60°C, vaporization at 100°C, and carbonization at 300°C.

INFRARED LASERS
Carbon Dioxide Laser

Over their years of development, infrared lasers have found numerous applications in dermatology, so much so that even though the carbon dioxide laser was developed back in 1964, it is still the most commonly used system in medicine today. This is largely a function of the precision of the laser-tissue interaction that occurs between infrared light and the intracellular and extracellular water content of the soft tissues found in the skin. This interaction results in the instantaneous conversion by thermal energy of water in a liquid state to a gaseous state consisting of steam and smoke [9]. This conversion occurs so quickly that there is minimal thermal conduction to the adjacent tissues, and the zone of thermal injury in soft tissue is only 0.1 mm thick. As a consequence, the carbon dioxide laser has become the preferred treatment for many dermatologic conditions and, in select cases, may represent the only available form of treatment [8,10].

Excisional surgery. Additional versatility for using the carbon dioxide laser in dermatology comes from its ability to function both as a precise cutting instrument to perform excisional surgery and to ablate superficially thin layers of soft tissue [11]. In order to perform excisions using the carbon dioxide laser, a small, focused beam of 0.1–0.2 mm in diameter and high power of 15–25 watts are used to produce an irradiance of 50,000–100,000 W/cm^2. This permits bloodless incisions to be made in most soft tissues as blood vessels up to 0.5 mm in diameter are immediately sealed by the laser [12]. Although the quality of hemostasis provided during CO_2 laser excision is usually excellent in most cases, an electrosurgical device should also be available in order to control any bleeding that may occur from large or high

flow vessels. Lymphatic vessels are also sealed by the laser as the incision is made and may help prevent dissemination of certain types of tumor cells that might otherwise occur by manipulation of malignant tumors during their surgical removal [13].

Several safety precautions must be taken when performing carbon dioxide laser excisional surgery to reduce the risk of injury to the patient, the surgeon, and operating room personnel [14]. As with all laser procedures, appropriate eyewear must be worn by all individuals in the operating room. Flammable surgical skin preparation agents, dry surgical drapes, and certain types of anesthetic gases must not be used in the laser operating room to avoid the possible hazard of combustion through inadvertent contact with the laser beam. A laser smoke evacuator must always be employed to remove potentially infectious particulates that are released into the air as a plume. It has now been established that papilloma viral DNA fragments can be recovered from the CO_2 laser plume during the treatment of warts [15], which is also true for electrosurgical plumes [16]. It has also been shown that bacterial spores can survive CO_2 laser vaporization [17,18]. The potential risk of transmission of other viral infections, including human immunodeficiency virus (HIV), by laser surgical plumes has not yet been determined. However, no viable simian immunodeficiency virus (SIV) was recovered from the carbon dioxide laser plumes generated under experimental conditions using different irradiances [19].

One side effect seen when using the carbon dioxide laser for excisional procedures is an apparent delay in the rate of development of wound tensile strength. Possibly as a result of the high degree of hemostasis and the consequent inhibition of fibrin clot formation, it appears that both wound contraction and re-epithelialization of carbon dioxide laser wounds are delayed compared to scalpel-incised wounds [20,21]. However, at least one contradictory study has also been published [22]. In spite of this, patients who undergo laser excision are generally managed postoperatively in an identical fashion to those treated with the standard nonlaser surgical technique.

The hemostatic ability of the CO_2 laser in its excisional mode of operation allows it to be successfully used in treating lesions in vascular anatomic locations (Table 2), like the scalp [23], or in the treatment of anticoagulated patients. The precision of the excisional mode of the carbon dioxide laser has also demonstrated usefulness in

TABLE 2. Indications for CO₂ Laser Excision

Medical conditions
  Anticoagulation
  Cardiac pacemaker
  Cardiac monitoring
High vascularity
  Vascular tumors
  Vascular anatomic locations
  Nail surgery
Stromal-independent tumors
  Melanoma
  Squamous cell carcinoma
Cosmetic conditions
  Keloids
  Rhinophyma
  Blepharoplasty

TABLE 3. Indications for CO₂ Laser Vaporization

Benign tumors
  Adenoma sebaceum (angiofibroma)
  Lymphangioma circumscriptum
  Tricholemmoma
  Neurofibroma
  Syringoma
  Trichoepithelioma
Cosmetic conditions
  Rhinophyma
  Acne scars (pitted)
  Epidermal nevus
  Lentigines
  Xanthelasma
  Tattoo
Premalignant conditions
  Actinic cheilitis
Malignant conditions
  Basal cell carcinoma (superficial variant)
  Erythroplasia of Queyrat
Inflammatory conditions
  Chondrodermatitis nodularis helicis
  Granuloma faciale
Cysts
  Digital mucous cyst
  Steatocystoma
  Vellus hair cyst
  Apocrine hidrocystoma
Infectious lesions
  Verrucae in immunosuppressed individuals
  Massive or refractory condyloma
  Recurrent periungual warts
  Refractory plantar warts
  Cutaneous deep fungal infections
Vascular lesions
  Pyogenic granuloma
  Angiokeratoma
  Lymphangioma circumscriptum
  Nodular portwine stains in adults
Miscellaneous conditions
  Porokeratosis
  Balanitis xerotica obliterans
  Nail matricectomy
  Nodular amyloidosis

performing certain types of cosmetic surgical procedures, such as removal of rhinophyma [24,25], blepharoplasty [26–28], and excision of keloids [29–31] removal from the earlobes [29] (see Fig. 6) and scalp [30,31].

Vaporization surgery. The carbon dioxide laser can also be used precisely and reproducibly to vaporize thin layers of soft tissue since its absorption by intracellular and extracellular water limits the depth of penetration [32]. This feature allows it to treat precisely a number of unrelated dermatologic conditions [10,18,33]. In these clinical situations, the carbon dioxide laser is used with relatively low irradiances of 200–600 W/cm^2, which is produced using a defocused beam with a diameter of 1–3 mm and low power settings of 4–10 watts. Using these parameters, a number of vascular [34], infectious [35,36], and inflammatory conditions [37–40], as well as cysts [41–43], deposition products [44], premalignancies [45–47], benign tumors [48–56], tattoos [57–59] (Figs. 1 and 2), certain types of cosmetic problems [60], malignancies [61,62], pigmentary conditions [63–65], and conditions involving the nails [66,67] and ears [68] have all been successfully treated using the defocused carbon dioxide laser in its vaporizational mode of operation (Table 3).

In each of these procedures, a thin layer of soft tissue is precisely vaporized as the beam passes over the treatment area. The resulting surface char is always removed by lightly scrubbing the surface with either sterile saline or 3% hydrogen peroxide to avoid thermal buildup. This process is repeated layer-by-layer using the same laser parameters until all remaining abnormal tissue has been grossly removed. The wound heals by second intention over a period of 7–10 days with minimal postoperative discomfort.

Superpulsed mode. The carbon dioxide laser also can be utilized as a chain of rapid, short, 200–400 μsec pulses with high peak power, which reduce collateral thermal damage by minimizing heat conduction from the treatment site to the surrounding tissues. This concept takes advantage of the known thermal relaxation time of soft tissue [69]. The individual pulses are separated from one another by brief pauses so that the duty cycle is only 5–15% and the average power delivered is only 30% of a continuous discharge system.

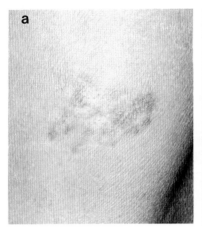
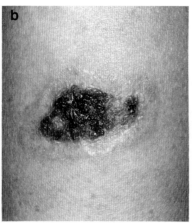
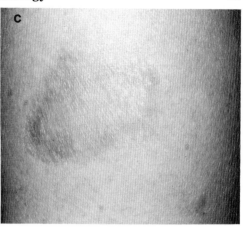

Fig. 1. (**a**) Preoperative appearance of an amateur tattoo. (**b**) Early wound contraction and persistent central crusting are seen three weeks following carbon dioxide laser vaporization. (**c**) An acceptable, flat textural scar is present 6 months later.

The superpulsed carbon dioxide lasers are capable of such precise ablation that they can be used in cosmetically sensitive areas like the nose [70], face [71], and lips [72] with minimal thermal damage [73] and excellent results. Although the precise clinical role for the superpulsed carbon dioxide laser has yet to be accurately defined, the potential benefits offered by its use appears to be substantial.

NEODYMIUM:YTTRIUM-ALUMINUM-GARNET (Nd:YAG) LASER

A second infrared laser, the Nd:YAG, has also been used by dermatologists in the management of a select group of skin diseases. This laser produces near-infrared light at a wavelength of 1,064 nm in a continuous fashion or it can be electronically gated into shorter pulses, Q-switched into very short pulses, or frequency-doubled to produce green light. Originally, this laser was primarily used to photocoagulate large caliber blood vessels [74] commonly found in hemangiomas and nodular port wine stains of adults [75,76]. However, because of deep penetration and poor absorption by the two chromophores of skin when used in the continuous output, noncontact mode of operation, this laser produces a wide zone of thermal destruction, which limits its use in treating many dermatologic disorders. However, more recently, synthetic sapphire tips have been developed that focus the Nd:YAG laser energy to a precise point and allow it to perform bloodless incisional surgery [77], much like the focused carbon dioxide laser [23,27].

This laser can be Q-switched to yield high-intensity, short pulses and frequency-doubled to produce green light. The Q-switched laser are presented in greater detail later in the tattoo removal discussion. However, frequency-doubling is possible when the near-infrared energy is passed through an optical crystal that doubles the frequency and halves the wavelength. This produces green light with a wavelength of 532 nm. Because this wavelength overlaps the absorption spectrum for oxyhemoglobin and melanin, the frequency-doubled Nd:YAG laser can be used to treat both vascular lesions [78] and benign pigmented lesions [79].

VISIBLE LIGHT LASERS

The extraordinary opportunities provided by the visible light lasers in the treatment of cutaneous vascular (Table 4) and pigmented lesions (Table 5), such as port wine stains, hemangiomas, lentigines, nevus of Ota, and tattoos, have yielded many emotionally rewarding experiences for both dermatologists and their patients because of the significant clinical improvement in these conditions that has been made possible by these devices.

Vascular Lesions—Port Wine Stain

One vascular condition for which no satisfactory form of treatment previously existed before the development of the visible light lasers is the port wine stain. Despite this fact, treatment has always been exceedingly important for this congenital birthmark since it may be associated even early in life with many serious psychological

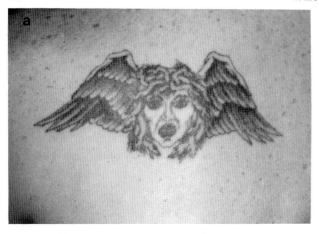
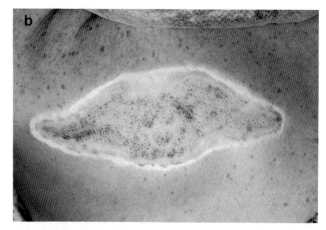
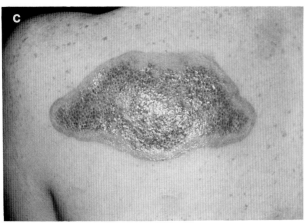
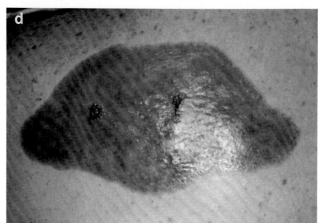

Fig. 2. **(a)** A large professional tattoo is seen preoperatively. **(b)** Appearance immediately following carbon dioxide laser vaporization with complete removal of all tattoo pigment. **(c)** After 4 week, the wound base has filled in with healthy granulation tissue. **(d)** The wound has nearly completely re-epithelialized after 3 months of daily wound care.

[80,81], medical, and social problems that can adversely influence the ability of the affected individual to function. In addition, some of the difficulties, such as progressive ectasia of blood vessels, which create multiple small, elevated, fragile, aneurysmal dilatations and surface irregularities, known as blebs, or soft tissue hypertrophy, which results in asymmetry and distortion of the lips or eyelids [82,83], may not develop until later in life [84]. Laser photocoagulation using a variety of different techniques and devices can typically treat this condition and their associated complications while simultaneously improving the appearance, function, and psychological status of the patient.

Argon laser. Although many different lasers and surgical techniques have been used over the years to treat port wine stains, there currently is no uniformity in the clinical management of this condition. As an example, the argon laser was historically the first laser to be effectively used in the management of port wine stains [85–87]. The blue-green light produced by this laser system at wavelengths of 488 and 514 nm could produce much more selective injury to blood vessels than was possible with other older, nonlaser techniques [88]. However, even though these wavelengths overlapped the oxyhemoglobin absorption spectrum [6], they occurred at a trough in this curve, which reduced the precision of the interaction since the thermal injury was not confined to the vasculature and heat was conducted throughout the dermis. As a result, the argon laser caused inadvertent thermal injury to the adjacent nonvascular tissues, which increased the risk of scarring [89] and textural changes [90]. In addition, epidermal injury also resulted from the competitive absorption of the blue-green argon laser light by melanin found in the epidermis. This represented a serious problem since epidermal

TABLE 4. Indications for Visible Light Lasers—Vascular Lesions

Telangiectasia
  Acne rosacea
  Essential
  Collagen vascular disorders
  Solar-induced
  Poikiloderma of Civatte
  Hereditary hemorrhagic telangiectasia
  Postrhinoplasty red nose
  Spider (nevus araneus)

Benign appendigeal tumors
  Adenoma sebaceum (angiofibroma)
  Glomus tumor

Congenital vascular lesions
  Portwine stain
  Angioma serpiginosa
  Blue rubber bleb syndrome
  Capillary hemangioma
  Cavernous hemangioma
  Angiokeratoma

Acquired vascular lesions
  Angiolymphoid hyperplasia
  Cherry angioma
  Venous lake
  Kaposi's sarcoma
  Pyogenic granuloma

TABLE 5. Indications for Visible Light Lasers—Pigmented Lesions

Congenital pigmented lesions
  Epidermal nevus
  Nevocellular nevus
  Nevus of Ito
  Nevus of Ota
  Cafe-au-lait macule
  Peutz-Jegher's spot

Acquired pigmented lesions
  Ephelides
  Lentigo benigna
  Melasma
  Postinflammatory hyperpigmentation
  Seborrheic keratosis

Tattoos
  Traumatic
  Decorative
  Medical
  Cosmetic

Premalignant lesions
  Lentigo maligna

Malignant lesions
  Basal cell carcinoma (pigmented type)

damage occurred as the light traversed the epidermis on its way to the dermal vasculature and resulted in vesiculation and crusting [91]. In addition, absorption within the epidermis reduced the amount of energy that reached the dermal blood vessels and higher energies were required to achieve photocoagulation. Because of these characteristics of the laser–tissue interaction with the argon laser, a number of complications such as scars, textural changes, and permanent hypopigmentation (Fig. 3) were recognized that limited the potential usefulness of this laser system [91].

A number of different techniques were employed in an attempt to improve the response of the argon laser treatment of port wine stains. One of these modifications recommended performing a series of small test exposures at different settings to a representative portion of the birthmark and then waiting 6–12 weeks to see the response before choosing the actual treatment parameters for the remainder of the lesion [88,92]. Also, the use of stripes [93] or polka dot [94] treatment patterns was recommended to reduce the potential for complications from excessive thermal damage. Despite the use of these innovative techniques, the development of permanent hypopigmentation [95] and an unacceptably high risk of hypertrophic scars and textural changes made impossible the treatment of children [96] and certain anatomic locations that are prone to scarring [97,98]. Newer, more precise lasers have largely supplanted the argon laser from consideration in the treatment of children with port wine stains, but select adult patients with small, thick, blue, or nodular port wine stains at anatomic locations with a low potential for scarring can still be effectively treated with the argon laser.

Yellow light lasers. Recognition of the limitations of the argon laser [91] in the treatment of portwine stains led to the development of a number of new systems that provided greater specificity in the laser–tissue interaction. One of these developments took advantage of the absorption peak for oxyhemoglobin that occurs at 577 nm [99,100]. Yellow light, which is emitted at this wavelength, penetrates deeper into the dermis than blue or green light and also is less well absorbed by melanin [101]. By taking advantage of these two features, the precision of the laser–tissue interaction in the treatment of most cutaneous vascular lesions, including port wine stains, was greatly improved by the use of yellow light. As a result, a number of different laser systems that produce yellow light have been developed, including the argon-pumped tunable dye, copper vapor, copper bromide, and krypton lasers.

Argon-pumped tunable dye laser. The ar-

Fig. 3. Patchwork hypopigmentation remains at the site of a large port wine stain following treatment with the argon laser. See insert for color representation.

Fig. 4. **(a)** Diffuse telangiectases are present on the cheek prior to treatment. **(b)** Nearly complete resolution without textural or pigmentary changes or scarring is seen 6 weeks after laser photocoagulation. See insert for color representation.

Fig. 5. **(a)** Large channel, high flow telangiectases are present on the nasal ala prior to laser treatment. **(b)** Excellent, but incomplete lightening is seen 6 weeks after laser photocoagulation performed at intervals along the length of each individual blood vessel. See insert for color representation.

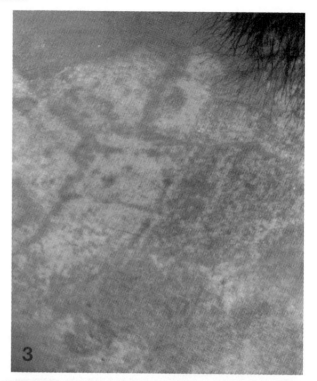

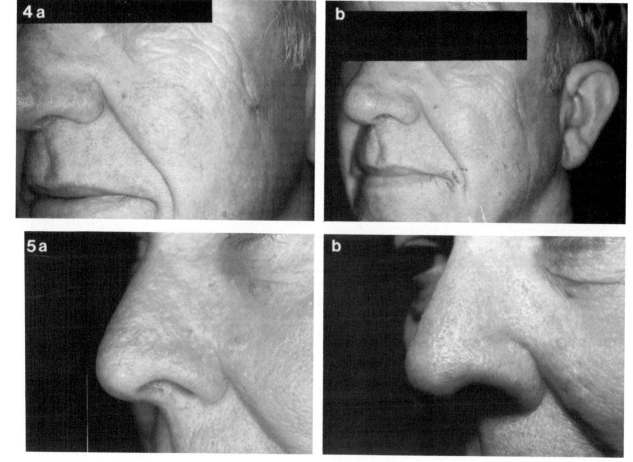

gon-pumped tunable dye laser was the first of the new yellow light lasers to be approved for the treatment of cutaneous vascular lesions. In these laser systems, an argon laser pumps an organic dye solution to stimulate the production of an adjustable band of wavelengths ranging from 488 nm to 638 nm. Light is produced in continuous fashion, but can be mechanically or electronically shuttered to yield shorter pulses of light. To treat vascular lesions, including port wine stains, the argon-pumped tunable dye laser is most often used at wavelength of 577 or 585 nm.

In addition to the pointillistic or polkadot technique originally described for use with the argon laser, the argon-pumped tunable dye laser can also be to treat port wine stains with a low power, tracing technique [102,103]. In this procedure, using magnified vision and a 50–100 μm laser beam with low power, individual blood vessels can be traced out and photocoagulated with minimal injury to the surrounding skin. Also, a computer-controlled, robotic optical scanning device can be coupled with the argon-pumped tunable dye laser system to treat large areas using geometric patterns created by individual pulses that are temporally separated from one another so that thermal damage can be minimalized.

These robotic optical scanning devices and automated handpieces can improve upon the effectiveness of the older free-hand polkadot or tracing techniques by providing greater consistency in the treatment of port wine stains while also reducing both the time required to treat large areas and the tedium associated with these other techniques [104–106]. The fiber optics from these devices can be easily attached with simple couplers to many different types of laser systems, including the argon and argon-pumped tunable dye lasers. The computer-controlled programs are designed automatically to deliver uniform pulses of light in precise geometric patterns. This reduces the risk of error that could adversely influence the outcome. Currently, there are two types of robotic scanners, Scanall™ and Multiscan™, and two types of automated handpieces, Hexascan™, CC-Scan™, available [107]. These systems most commonly have an adjustable pulse duration that varies from 30–990 msec and a pause interval of 50 msec. They deliver a 1 mm beam of light in geometric grids that vary in size from 1–13 mm in diameter.

The biggest advantages offered by the argon-pumped tunable dye laser are a function of the improved precision of the laser–tissue interaction made possible by the use of yellow light. This allows rapid clearing of the treated blood vessels with reduced epithelial damage and minimal postoperative care. These features allow effective treatment of children [103] without a significant risk of scarring, textural changes, or hypopigmentation.

Flashlamp-pumped pulsed dye laser. The flashlamp-pumped pulsed dye laser was the first laser system designed around the concept of selective photothermolysis [4,5,108,109]. This system is characterized by the production of short, 450 μsec, pulses of light that precisely match the thermal relaxation time for the microvessels of port wine stains and reduce the conduction of heat to the adjacent tissues [110]. Like the argon-pumped tunable dye lasers, this system also utilizes a solution containing an organic dye that, when pumped by a flashlamp, produced a 5 mm beam of yellow light at a wavelength of 577 or 585 nm [111].

The biggest advantage from use of the pulsed dye laser is a direct result of the precision of the laser-tissue interaction, which spatially confines the thermal effects to just the microvessels [112]. This feature permits the effective treatment of infants [113,114], children [113], and anatomic locations at high risk for scar formation [115–117] without a significant risk of complications. In addition, the large spot size produced by the flashlamp-pumped pulsed dye laser, in contrast to the small beam diameters produced by both the argon and argon-pumped tunable dye lasers, allows the treatment of even large areas of involvement in a relatively short treatment session without significant difficulty. The biggest disadvantages of the flashlamp-pumped pulsed dye laser are the purpura that develops shortly after treatment and persists for 10–14 days and the common need for multiple retreatments in order to obtain maximal resolution of the blood vessels.

Copper vapor and copper bromide lasers. The two different copper laser systems both produce yellow light at a wavelength of 578 nm by heating elemental copper or copper salts in the optical cavity. The energy is released as a chain of short, 20–40 nsec pulses [118] at a frequency of 10–15 kHz. This chain can be electronically broken into short series of pulses of 0.075–0.3 sec in duration and used to treat port wine stains with the previously mentioned overlapping polkadot technique, the low-power, small-beam tracing technique, or even attached to an optical scanner to treat larger geometric shapes with precise and reproducible control. These devices share many similarities with the argon-dye laser in both their indications [119,120] and response to treatment [121–123].

Krypton laser. Also capable of producing yellow light lasers is the gas-medium, krypton laser. This light energy is emitted at 568 nm and can be used in much the same way as the argon-dye and copper lasers to treat port wine stains. A significant benefit provided by the krypton laser over the two types of dye lasers is that potential toxic exposure to solvents or dyes is completely eliminated due to nature of its gas medium.

Nd:YAG laser. Although not a source of yellow light, the Q-switched Nd:YAG laser has recently been approved for the treatment of vascular lesions, including port wine stains. Traditionally, the conventional Nd:YAG laser is a source of near-infrared light having a wavelength of 1,064 nm. However, since this wavelength is poorly absorbed by either of the two primarily chromophores in skin [74], it produces a diffuse zone of thermal injury following exposure, which results in significant scarring. Because of this, until recently this device was not considered to be significantly useful in the treatment of skin disorders except in unusual patients with soft tissue hypertrophy secondary to long-standing port wine stains [76]. However, a modification of this laser allows the Nd:YAG laser to be used in the treatment of port wine stains. This modification consists of passing the 1,064 nm infrared light through an optical crystal composed of potassium titanyl phosphate (KTP), which serves to double the frequency and halve the wavelength to 532 nm, which is green in color [78]. This wavelength, coupled with the extremely short pulses and high peak energies provided by a Q-switch, allows these lasers to treat vascular lesions with minimal collateral thermal damage [79].

Vascular Lesions—Telangiectasia

Green light lasers. Despite the fact that there was a significant risk of complications when the green light lasers were used to treat some types of port wine stains, these systems remain very useful in the management of other types of cutaneous vascular lesions, including facial telangiectases (Fig. 4) [124–126]. It appears that the immediate edema, which forms in a perivascular distribution as a result of the imprecision of the interaction between green light and oxyhemoglobin, serves to reduce the blood flow rate and allows the subsequent laser impacts to seal even relatively large vascular channels, especially those with high flow rates like on the nasal alae, with a high degree of success.

Green light is produced by a number of different systems, including the argon [87,90], argon-pumped tunable dye, copper vapor [119,127], copper bromide, krypton, and frequency-doubled Nd:YAG lasers [79]. The results obtained in the treatment of most vascular lesions with each of the green light lasers systems are generally indistinguishable from one another. The commonest technique used to treat isolated, nonconfluent, linear telangiectases delivers pulses of 0.1–0.2 sec in duration with a 1 mm beam to photocoagulate the vessel at spaced intervals along its length. With this interrupted approach, the least amount of energy necessary is delivered to cause photocoagulation, which reduces inadvertent injury and minimizes the risk of scarring. When isolated, individual blood vessels are present over larger areas, as with rosacea or severe solar damage, use of one of the robotic scanners may be particularly helpful [104,106].

Yellow light lasers. In those cases where there is a mixture of both large and small caliber blood vessels in the same treatment field, it is generally best to try and minimize the risk of scarring or textural changes by treating the larger vessels (Fig. 5), first with green laser light and then using yellow laser light to remove the finer blood vessels, perhaps at the same or subsequent treatment session. If complete resolution does not occur following one treatment, retreatment can be considered in 6–12 weeks.

When fine telangiectases involve very large areas, as with poikiloderma of Civatte [128] or severe acne rosacea [129], the flashlamp-pumped pulsed dye laser may be required to satisfactorily manage the patient in a timely fashion. This is a result of the large beam of light produced by this system and the established parameters that allow it to successfully treat small caliber, low-flow vasculature [130].

Lower extremity telangiectasia. Many patients with lower extremity telangiectasia will often request laser surgery to eradicate these types of blood vessels. However, a generally poor response is obtained with all of the currently available lasers when red vessels of 0.2 mm or larger are treated on the legs. This is presumably due to greater difficulty in permanently sealing these vessels with laser photocoagulation due to the higher hydrostatic pressures found on the lower extremity compared with similar blood vessels found on the face. About the only clinical situation where lasers appear to be beneficial on the lower extremity is with the use of the flashlamp-pumped pulse dye laser to treat small matlike telangiectases that occasionally form following traditional injection sclerotherapy [131].

Tattoos

Dermatologists use a number of surgical procedures and techniques to remove tattoos, including lasers. These have included a number of ablative procedures such as salabrasion [132], dermabrasion [133], split-thickness excision [134], chemical scarification [135], excision [136], infrared coagulation [137], and argon [90,138] and carbon dioxide laser photocoagulation [139,140]. However, none of these techniques could completely remove all tattoo pigment in one procedure without also producing scars, hypopigmentation, or textural changes. In many cases, an 18–24-month interval was typically required to achieve the final cosmetic result. Most of these difficulties with treatment were largely solved with the introduction of the short-pulsed, high-intensity, Q-switched lasers for the removal of decorative, cosmetic, traumatic, and medical tattoos.

Ruby laser. Through Q-switching, the ruby laser produces high-intensity red light at a wavelength of 694 nm in extremely short pulses of only 20–40 nsec. This light is well absorbed by the carbon particles found in most amateur, traumatic, and many professional tattoos. It is also moderately well absorbed by melanin [141,142]. The tattoo pigments can be selectively targeted by the ruby laser, as a result of selective photothermolysis [4] from the mechanoacoustic shock wave that is generated in skin by the pulse of light [143–145]. The tattoo pigment granules are altered both in their size and shape following Q-switched laser exposure and are then phagocytosed by macrophages and slowly removed from the skin. This probably is a result of fragmentation of the pigment granules by cavitation, which markedly reduces the average size of the tattoo pigment clusters from 147–180 μm in diameter prior to ruby laser treatment into much smaller particles.

The ruby laser technique for treating tattoos was first developed in the early 1960s [146,147]. Today, the technique most commonly employed with the ruby laser uses slightly overlapping pulses at energy fluences of 4–8 J/cm^2, which are delivered in most cases without use of local anesthesia [148–152]. With this technique, the skin appears white in color for 15–20 min as a result of steam generated within the dermis by the photoacoustic wave.

Several weeks are necessary before substantial lightening of the tattoo is seen, but retreatment is usually not performed until 6–12 weeks later in order for fading to occur by phagocytosis of the fragmented particles. The response in tattoos treated with the Q-switched ruby laser is extremely variable and impossible to predict. In general, the response can be influenced by the nature of the tattoo, its age, color, size, and anatomic location (Table 6). The best results are obtained with amateur, traumatic, and black professional tattoos. However, an average of four retreatments may still be required to obtain maximal fading in amateur tattoos, whereas only 2–3 treatments are typically necessary for traumatic tattoos, and 6–8 treatments may be required for professional multicolored tattoos. In addition, certain colors, such as green, red, and yellow, either may fade very slowly or not at all. This is probably a result of greater pigment density in professional tattoos, larger particle size, and variable energy absorption by the different metals used to produce the different colors. Older tattoos that have been present for 10 years or more will usually respond more quickly to treatment with the Q-switched laser than newer tattoos since the particles may have already been partially phagocytosed or are more amenable to fragmentation [153]. Tattoos applied for cosmetic enhancement of the eyebrows, eyelids, or lips also can be treated with the ruby laser. However, these tattoo pigments may be oxidized by the laser pulse from the red-colored ferric oxide to the black-colored ferrous oxide [154]. This black discoloration may be very resistant to subsequent treatment and can be permanent.

Allergic granulomas. Some tattoo pigments can produce localized allergic reactions within the tattoo and cause pruritus and chronic eczematous changes as well as systemic symptoms and lymphadenopathy [155]. These reactions have been reported in association with mercury, which is used to make red colors [156–158], manganese to make purple colors [159,160], chromium to make green colors, cobalt to make blue colors, and cadmium to make yellow color. Because of the risk of producing a generalized allergic reaction or even anaphylaxis by fragmenting the various tattoo pigments found in allergic granulomas with

TABLE 6. Factors Influencing Outcome of Tattoo Treatment

Size
Desired postoperative appearance
Anticipated cost
Pigment density
Pigment depth
Age of tattoo
Patient deadlines
Tattoo type
   Amateur
   Professional
     single color
      multicolored
   Traumatic
   Cosmetic
History of adverse scarring
Skin type
Anatomic location
Presence of allergic granulomas

Q-switched laser pulses, the best approach to tattoo granulomas should be to remove them with curettage, excision, or carbon dioxide laser vaporization [157,161].

Skin type. The patient's skin type can also influence the outcome of laser treatment for type IV, V, and VI patients will obtain less fading of their tattoo following ruby laser treatment than light-skin types as a result of melanin absorption. For the same reason, this group of patients will also develop transient hypopigmentation that may last 4–6 months in some cases.

Nd:YAG laser. As previously discussed [74–77], the Nd:YAG laser is an invisible, near-infrared light source with a wavelength of 1,064 nm. The conventional Nd:YAG laser can be Q-switched to produce high peak energies and short pulse durations (10 nsec) similar to the ruby laser. A further modification of the Nd:YAG laser passes the near-infrared light through an optical crystal composed of potassium titanyl phosphate (KTP) doubling the frequency and halving the wavelength. This converts the invisible infrared energy to green light having a wavelength of 532 nm [78]. Each of the two wavelengths from the Nd:YAG laser can be used to treat tattoos, with the infrared wavelength used for removing the black (Fig. 6), yellow and blue colors, and the green wavelength for removing the red color (Fig. 7) [162–164]. The mechanism of action for the Nd:YAG laser treatment of tattoos is probably identical to that seen with the Q-switched ruby laser. The biggest difference comes from the fact that the 1,064 nm light is poorly absorbed by melanin so there is less absorptive interference by the epidermis compared with the ruby laser, and this longer wavelength of light also penetrates deeper into tissue. Furthermore, use of the frequency doubled Nd:YAG laser at a wavelength of 532 nm will often produce a favorable response in orange and red colored tattoos. However, capillary bleeding usually develops following with the Nd:YAG laser at 1,064 nm (Fig. 8) and the incidence of hypopigmentation is less than with the ruby laser.

Alexandrite laser. The latest Q-switched laser to be approved for the treatment of amateur and professional tattoos is the alexandrite laser [165,166]. This laser produces red light at a wavelength of 755 nm in a pulse of 100 nsec [116,117]. Its effectiveness is much like the other Q-switched lasers, with benefits, results, and complications that are most similar to the ruby laser.

Pigmented Lesions

Based on the principle of selective photothermolysis, a number of benign pigmented lesions [167] have been successfully treated (Table 5) with the Q-switched and short-pulsed lasers.

Ruby laser. The ruby laser can effectively target pigmented lesions because the pulse duration is shorter than the thermal relaxation time for melanocytes and melanosomes [168]. In addition, since melanin has such a broad absorption spectrum, it overlaps the emission of the ruby laser [169]. As a result, the melanosomes can be targeted for selective photothermolysis [170,171] by the short pulses of ruby light causing microscopic photodisruption [172].

As a function of the specificity of the laser–tissue interaction, the ruby laser can be used to treat Peutz-Jegher's spots [172], lentigines [173], ephelides, cafe-au-lait macules, Becker's nevus [174], melasma, nevus of Ota [175,176], and postinflammatory hyperpigmentation. The technique is similar to that used for tattoos except the number of treatments required for obtaining improvement is typically less than for tattoos and the energy fluences used are typically lower. The best results are generally seen with lentigines and nevus of Ota, but good results are also common with Becker's nevus. Cafe au lait macules, melasma, and postinflammatory hyperpigmentation are much more variable in their response and may even hyperpigment following treatment [174].

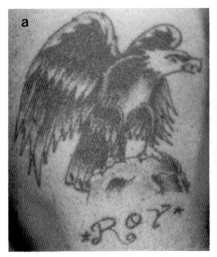 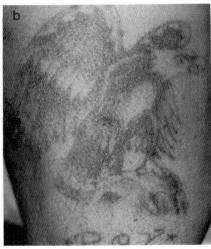 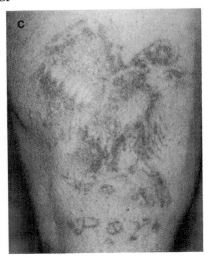

Fig. 6. (a) Preoperative appearance of a professional tattoo. (b) Marked lightening is seen 6 weeks after one treatment with the Q-switched Nd:YAG laser. (c) Additional lightening without textural changes or scarring has been obtained after two additional Nd:YAG laser treatments.

Frequency-doubled Nd:YAG laser. The Q-switched Nd:YAG laser can also be very effective in the treatment of benign pigmented lesions. For most superficial lesions, like lentigines, the green wavelength at 532 nm, produced by frequency-doubling, is used. However, the treatment of pigmented lesions that which are found deeper in the dermis, such as nevus of Ota, the invisible, near-infrared Nd:YAG laser light at 1,064 nm is used since in will penetrate farther into the skin than the visible green wavelength.

Copper vapor and copper bromide lasers. Some superficial benign pigmented lesions, such as lentigines and ephelides, can be effectively treated using the 511 nm green band from either of the copper lasers [119,122]. This light is delivered in a similar fashion to that used for the treatment of vascular lesions, in short pulses of 0.1–0.2 sec, but robotic scanners can also be used for this purpose. Hyperpigmentation that forms after injection sclerotherapy on the lower extremity as a result of hemosiderin deposition in the superficial dermis can be substantially lightened in a majority of patients by treatment with the copper laser [177].

Pulsed dye laser for pigmented lesions. Another flashlamp-pumped pulsed dye laser is currently available for the treatment of pigmented lesions [178]. This laser differs from the original system used to treat vascular lesions in that it produces green light at a wavelength of 510 nm in short pulses of 300 nsec. Since the green wavelength is selectively absorbed by melanin, benign pigmented lesions respond to selective photothermolysis. Like the other green light lasers, this system can be used to treat a number of different pigmented lesions such as lentigines, ephelides, melasma, nevus spilus, nevus of Ota, postinflammatory hyperpigmentation, seborrheic keratoses, and cafe-au-lait macules. Patients who develop temporary hyperpigmentation as a result of hemosiderin deposition from extravasated red blood cells following sclerotherapy will typically show substantial lightening with the pulsed dye laser [179].

Krypton laser. Like the copper lasers, the krypton laser also produces both yellow light to treat vascular lesions and two bands of green light, at wavelengths of 521 nm and 530 nm, which can be used to treat pigmented lesions. Since this laser can produce only relatively long pulses of light, there is a potentially greater risk of causing inadvertent thermal damage and scarring than with the shorter Q-switched laser. As a result, the krypton laser is most typically used to treat smaller pigmented lesions, such as lentigines, where excellent results can be readily achieved.

Alexandrite laser. Although only preliminary results are currently available as to the effectiveness of the new Q-switched alexandrite laser in the treatment of benign pigmented lesions, it is anticipated that the red light from this system will provide results that are comparable with

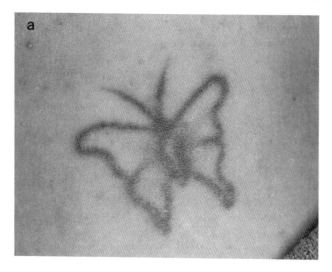

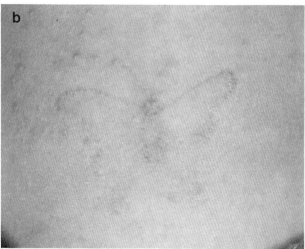

Fig. 7. (a) Preoperative appearance of a small mostly black professional tattoo with focal areas of red pigment. (b) Almost complete clearing has been achieved following two treatments with 1,064 nm infrared Nd:YAG light to the black portions of the tattoo and 532 nm frequency doubled green Nd:YAG laser light to the red portions of the tattoo.

the ruby laser. Obviously, further clinical investigation is required before the benefits of using this laser are firmly established.

Miscellaneous Lesions

Capillary hemangioma. Capillary hemangiomas represent a relatively common congenital vascular lesion [180] that can be effectively treated with several of the visible light lasers. Use of the flashlamp-pumped pulsed dye laser to treat capillary hemangiomas has shown great efficacy, particularly when the lesion is complicated by ulceration, bleeding, infection, or functional problems. In these situations, it appears that the pulsed dye laser can stimulate involution, especially if performed during the early proliferative phase [181–184]. Treatment with the pulsed dye laser should also be considered when the hemangioma interferes with normal function, such as with involvement of the hands or feet or around the eyes and mouth. Further, when large areas of involvement are affected that may cause disfigurement or be subject to secondary infection, bleeding, or trauma, the pulsed dye laser may also promote involution or prevent further capillary proliferation, even in rapidly enlarging lesions [184].

Pyogenic granuloma. Another vascular lesion that can be successfully managed with various laser systems is the pyogenic granuloma [185]. One laser system that has been reported to provide excellent results is the flashlamp-pumped pulse dye laser. Although only one treatment may be required to produce complete clearing, an accurate prediction of the outcome in each individual situation cannot be given.

Venous lakes Venous lakes represent large dilated vascular ectasia that most commonly form on the lips and ears following chronic sun exposure or minor trauma. These lesions can be effectively photocoagulated with many of the visible green and yellow light lasers (Fig. 9). Increased effectiveness is often seen if the elevated portion of the lesion is first compressed using plastic or glass to reduce the total thickness of the channel and then firing the laser through it.

Kaposi's sarcoma. A proliferative vascular tumor that is seen most commonly today in association with human immunodeficiency viral (HIV) infection is Kaposi's sarcoma. Since penetration by visible light is generally limited to ~ 1 mm, the small, flat Kaposi's lesions are amenable to treatment with either the flashlamp-pumped pulsed dye or argon lasers [187].

Lymphangioma circumscriptum. The flashlamp-pumped pulsed dye laser has been used to effectively treat lymphangioma circumscriptum when there is a significant vascular component present [187]. However, little response can be anticipated when only limited numbers of red blood cells are present.

EXPERIMENTAL LASER SYSTEMS AND SURGICAL TECHNIQUES
Low-Energy Lasers

Like the helium-neon and gallium-arsenide, low-energy lasers are a controversial area of laser

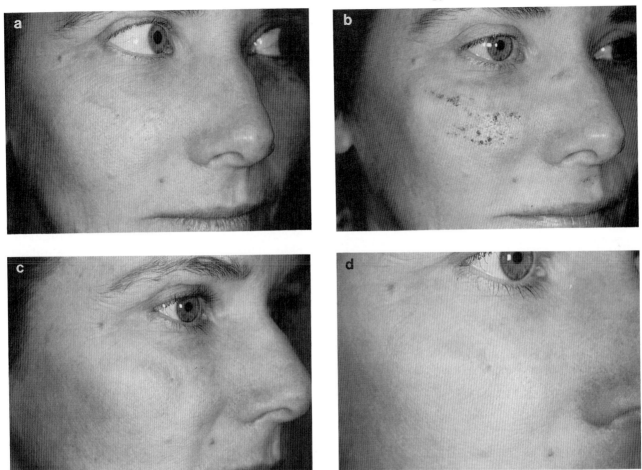

Fig. 8. (a) Diffuse blue-black discoloration is present on the cheek from a traumatic tattoo prior to treatment. (b) Capillary bleeding has occurred immediately following treatment with the Q-switched Nd:YAG laser at 1,064 nm. (c) Marked lightening is seen after the first treatment. (d) Additional lightening with nearly complete resolution has occurred following a second Nd:YAG laser treatment.

application in dermatology. These devices produce little or no temperature elevation following exposure. Since the generation of heat does not occur, it is felt that any effects seen are due directly to the laser radiation. One of the areas in which these systems have been employed is in an attempt to influence various aspects of wound healing [189–197].

Laboratory techniques have shown that low energy laser radiation increases the rate of DNA and RNA synthesis [198,199], fibroblast proliferation [200], and collagen synthesis [201]. Although the mechanism for these effects remains unclear, it may be due to photoactivation of a porphyrin-containing enzyme, which stimulates the mitochondrial synthesis of ATP [202]. An intriguing apparently contradictory effect has also been seen with low energy from a Nd:YAG laser in which fibroblast DNA replication and procollagen synthesis are inhibited [203,204]. Stimulatory effects on keratinocyte activity in culture by low energy lasers have also been reported [205] along with positive effects on the rate of second intention wound healing [206].

Photodynamic therapy (PDT). Photodynamic therapy utilizes low levels of laser energy to activate a photosensitizer that has accumulated in neoplastic cells following intravenous [210–215] or topical application [216]. Most of the currently experimental photosensitizers are based on the molecular structure of porphyrin. They can be activated by many wavelengths of light, but red is often chosen due to its greater depth of penetration. Exposure to laser light produces a photochemical reaction that releases singlet oxygen and superoxide radicals [217] that damage cell mem-

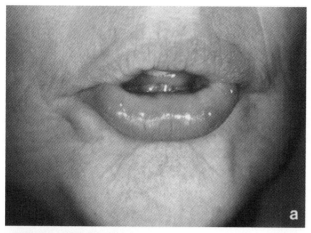

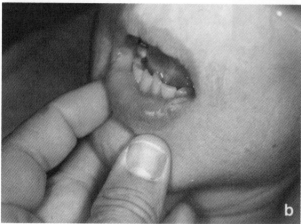

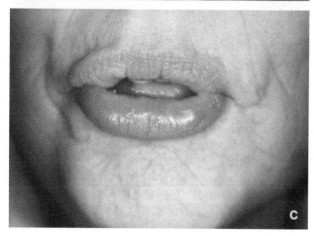

Fig. 9. (a) Two venous lakes are present on the lower lip prior to treatment. (b) Immediate whitening has occurred following photocoagulation with green laser light. (c) Complete disappearance of both lesions has occurred 6 weeks after one treatment without scarring or textural changes. See insert for color representation.

branes, subcellular organelles, and the endothelium of the blood vessels that supply the tumor [218].

Titanium:sapphire laser. The titanium:sapphire laser is an experimental solid-state system that employs titanium-doped sapphire (Al_2O_3) as its laser medium [219,220]. This pulsed laser system is most commonly operated at 800 nm where it produces peak intensities of 10 terrawatts (10^{12}) in very short pulses that are less than 120 femtoseconds (10^{-15}) in duration. This laser is capable of precisely ablating tissue without creating any thermal injury through a process known as ablative photodecomposition [219]. This process results in the creation of a "plasma" [221], which forms as high-energy photons from the laser break molecular bonds through the production of photoacoustic shock waves [222] and cavitation bubbles. This produces fragments from the impact site to be ejected without thermal injury. With this system, it is possible to produce precise ablation only of the epidermis by controlling the number and energy of pulses delivered. Nonthermal, collateral damage is minimal and ranges from 0–30 μm [220].

Diode Lasers

High-powered semiconductor diode lasers have recently been developed that emit energy at a wavelength of 805 nm in continuous or pulsed fashion [223]. Light from this laser can be transmitted by fiberoptics and delivered using synthetic sapphire tips in a contact mode to incise or vaporize soft tissue.

Laser welding. Several laser systems have been used to thermally weld skin incisions together by creating a protein coagulum [207–209]. Standardization of this technique must be completed before this procedure will achieve wide clinical acceptance.

CONCLUSION

Lasers have become an essential tool to the dermatologist in the management of many common cutaneous disorders that were simply not effectively managed previously. Lasers have been incorporated into most clinical dermatology practices because of the numerous benefits they can provide. Our understanding of the complex nature of the laser–tissue interaction has allowed these devices to be used in many innovative and beneficial ways. The anticipated continued evolutionary changes that are likely to occur in the future will certainly increase the already important position these devices hold in the specialty of dermatology.

REFERENCES

1. Einstein A. Zur quantentheorie der strahlung. Physiol Z 1917; 18:121–128.
2. Bromberg JL. "The Laser in America, 1950–1970." Cambridge: MIT Press, 1991; 19–23.
3. Maiman TH. Stimulated optical radiation in ruby. Nature 1960; 187:493–494.
4. Anderson R, Parrish J. Selective photothermolysis: Precise microsurgery by selective absorption of pulsed radiation. Science 1983; 220:524–527.
5. Parrish J, Anderson R, Harris T, et al. Selective thermal effects with pulsed irradiation from organ to organelle. J Invest Dermatol 1983; 80:75–80.
6. Anderson R, Parrish J. The optics of human skin. J Invest Dermatol 1981; 77:13–19.
7. Adams S, Swain C, Mills T, et al. The effect of wavelength, power and treatment pattern on the outcome of laser treatment of portwine stains. Br J Dermatol 1987; 117:487–494.
8. Wheeland RG, Walker NPJ. Lasers—25 Years Later. Int J Dermatol 1986; 25:209–216.
9. Sliney DH. Laser-tissue interactions. Clin Chest Med 1985; 6:203–208.
10. Garden JM, Geronemus RG. Dermatologic laser surgery. J Dermatol Surg Oncol 1990; 16:156–168.
11. Polanyi TG. Physics of surgery with lasers. Clin Chest Med 1985; 6:179–202.
12. Slutzki S, Shafir R, Bornstein LA. Use of the carbon dioxide laser for large excisions with minimal blood loss. Plast Reconstr Surg 1977; 60:250–255.
13. Lanzafame RJ, Rogers DW, Naim JO, et al. Reduction of local tumor recurrence by excision with the CO_2 laser. Lasers Surg Med 1986; 6:439–441.
14. Olbricht SM, Stern RS, Tang SV, et al. Complications of cutaneous laser surgery: A survey. Arch Dermatol 1987; 123:345–349.
15. Garden JM, O'Banion MK, Schelnitz LS, et al. Papillomavirus in the vapor of carbon dioxide laser-treated verrucae. JAMA 1988; 259:1199–1202.
16. Sawchuk WS, Weber PJ, Lowy DR, et al. Infectious papillomavirus in the vapor of warts treated with carbon dioxide laser or electrocoagulation: Detection and protection. J Am Acad Dermatol 1989; 21:41–49.
17. Mullarky MB, Norris CW, Goldberg ID. The efficacy of the CO_2 laser in the sterilization of skin seeded with bacteria: Survival at the skin surface and in the plume emissions. Laryngoscope 1985; 95:186–187.
18. Walker NPJ, Matthews J, Newsom SWB. Possible hazards from irradiation with the carbon dioxide laser. Lasers Surg Med 1986; 6:84–86.
19. Starr JC, Kilmer SL, Wheeland RG. Analysis of the carbon dioxide laser plume for simian immunodeficiency virus. J Dermatol Surg Oncol 1992; 18:297–300.
20. Buell BR, Schuller DE. Comparison of tensile strength in CO_2 laser and scalpel skin incisions. Arch Otolaryngol 1983; 109:465–467.
21. Jarmuske M, Stranc M, Stranc L. The effect of carbon dioxide laser on wound contraction epithelia regeneration in rabbits. Br J Plast Surg 1990; 43:40–46.
22. Finsterbush A, Rousso M, Ashur H. Healing and tensile strength of CO_2 laser incisions and scalpel wounds in rabbits. Plast Reconstr Surg 1982; 70:360–362.
23. Wheeland RG, Bailin PL. Scalp reduction surgery with the carbon dioxide CO_2 alser. J Dermatol Surg Oncol 1984; 10:565–569.
24. Wheeland RG, Bailin PL, Ratz JL. Combined carbon dioxide laser excision and vaporization in the treatment of rhinophyma. J Dermatol Surg Oncol 1987; 13:172–177.
25. Haas A, Wheeland R. Treatment of massive rhinophyma with the carbon dioxide laser. J Dermatol Surg Oncol 1990; 16:645–649.
26. Baker S, Muenzler WS, Small RG, et al. Carbon dioxide laser blepharoplasty. Ophthalmol 1984; 91:238–243.
27. David L, Sanders G. CO_2 laser blepharoplasty: A comparison to cold steel and electrocautery. J Dermatol Surg Oncol 1987; 13:110–114.
28. Morrow DM, Morrow LB. CO_2 laser blepharoplasty: A comparison with cold-steel surgery. J Dermatol Surg Oncol 1992; 18:307–313.
29. Kantor GR, Wheeland RG, Bailin PL, et al. Treatment of earlobe keloids with carbon dioxide laser excision. J Dermatol Surg Oncol 1985; 11:1063–1067.
30. Glass F, Berman B, Laub D. Treatment of perifolliculitis capitis abscedens et suffodiens with the carbon dioxide laser. J Dermatol Surg Oncol 1989; 15:673–676.
31. Kantor GR, Ratz JL, Wheeland RG. Treatment of acne keloidalis nuchae with carbon dioxide laser. J Am Acad Dermatol 1986; 14:263–267.
32. Fitzpatrick RE, Ruiz-Esparza J, Goldman MP. The depth of thermal necrosis using the CO_2 laser: A comparison of the superpulsed mode and conventional mode. J Dermatol Surg Oncol 1991; 17:340–344.
33. Arndt KA, Noe JM, Northam DBC, Itzkan I. Laser therapy basic concepts and nomenclature. J Am Acad Dermatol 1981; 5:649–654.
34. Ratz JL, Bailin PL. The case for use of the carbon dioxide laser in the treatment of port-wine stains. Arch Dermatol 1987; 123:74–75.
35. McBurney EL, Rosen DA. Carbon dioxide laser treatment of verrucae vulgares. J Dermatol Surg Oncol 1984; 10:45–48.
36. Ferenczy A, Mitas M, Nigai N, et al. Latent papilloma virus and recurring genital warts. N Engl J Med 1985; 313:784–788.
37. Wheeland RG, Ashley JA, Smith DA, et al. Carbon dioxide CO_2 laser treatment of granuloma faciale. J Dermatol Surg Oncol 1984; 10:730–733.
38. Dinehart S, Gross D, Davis C. Granuloma faciale: Comparison of different treatment modalities. Arch Otolaryngol 1990; 116:849–851.
39. Don P, Carney P, Lynch W, et al. Carbon dioxide laser-abrasion: A new approach to management of familial benign chronic pemphigus (Hailey-Hailey Disease). J Dermatol Surg Oncol 1987; 13:1187–1194.
40. Baldwin H, Geronemus R. Carbon dioxide laser vaporization of Zoon's balanitis: A case report. J Dermatol Surg Oncol 1989; 15:419–494.
41. Huerter C, Wheeland R. Multiple eruptive vellus hair cysts treated with carbon dioxide vaporization. J Dermatol Surg Oncol 1987; 13:260–263.
42. Huerter CJ, Wheeland RG, Bailin PL, et al. Treatment of digital myxoid cysts with carbon dioxide laser vaporization. J Dermatol Surg Oncol 1987; 13:723–727.
43. Bickley L, Goldberg D, Imaeda S, et al. Treatment of multiple apocrine hidrocystomas with the carbon dioxide laser. J Dermatol Surg Oncol 1989; 15:599–602.

44. Apfelberg D, Maser M, Lash H, et al. Treatment of xanthelasma palpebrarum with the carbon dioxide laser. J Dermatol Surg Oncol 1987; 13:149–151.

45. David LM. Laser vermilion ablation for actinic cheilitis. J Dermatol Surg Oncol 1985; 11:209–212.

46. Whitaker DC. Microscopically proven cure of actinic cheilitis by CO_2 laser. Lasers Surg Med 1987; 7:520–523.

47. Stanley RJ, Roenigk RK. Actinic cheilitis: Treatment with the carbon dioxide laser. Mayo Clin Proc 1988; 63: 230–235.

48. Wheeland RG, Bailin PL, Kronberg E. Carbon dioxide (CO_2) laser vaporization for the treatment of trichoepitheliomata. J Dermatol Surg Oncol 1984; 10:470–475.

49. Wheeland RG, Bailin PL, Reynolds OD, Ratz JL. Carbon dioxide (CO_2) laser vaporization of multiple facial syringomas. J Dermatol Surg Oncol 1986; 12:225–228.

50. Roenigk RK, Ratz JL. CO_2 laser treatment of cutaneous neurofibromas. J Dermatol Surg Oncol 1987; 13:187–190.

51. Wheeland RG, Bailin PL, Kantor GR, et al. Treatment of adenoma sebaceum with carbon dioxide laser vaporization. J Dermatol Surg Oncol 1985; 11:861–864.

52. Janniger C, Goldberg D. Angiofibromas in tuberous sclerosis: Comparison of treatment by carbon dioxide and argon laser. J Dermatol Surg Oncol 1990; 16:317–320.

53. Becker D. Use of the carbon dioxide laser in treating multiple cutaneous neurofibromas. Ann Plast Surg 1991; 26:582–588.

54. Hunziker T, Bayard W. Carbon dioxide laser in the treatment of porokeratosis. J Am Acad Dermatol 1987; 16:625.

55. Bailin PL, Kantor GR, Wheeland RG. Carbon dioxide laser vaporization of lymphangioma circumscriptum. J Am Acad Dermatol 1986; 14:257–262.

56. Eliezri Y, Sklar J. Lymphangioma circumscriptum: Review and evaluation of carbon dioxide vaporization. J Dermatol Surg Oncol 1988; 14:357–364.

57. Reid R, Muller S. Tattoo removal of CO_2 laser dermabrasion. Plast Reconstr Surg 1980; 65:717–728.

58. Levine H, Bailin P. Carbon dioxide laser treatment of cutaneous hemangiomas and tattoos. Arch Otolaryngol 1982; 108:236–238.

59. Apfelberg DB, Maser MR, Lash H, et al. Comparison of argon and carbon dioxide laser treatment of decorative tatoos: A preliminary report. Ann Plast Surg 1985; 14: 6–15.

60. Garrett A, Dufresne R, Ratz J, et al. Carbon dioxide laser treatment of pitted acne scarring. J Dermatol Surg Oncol 1990; 16:737–740.

61. Wheeland RG, Bailin PL, Ratz JL, et al. Carbon dioxide laser vaporization and curettage in the treatment of large or multiple superficial basal cell carcinomas. J Dermatol Surg Oncol 1987; 13:119–125.

62. Greenbaum S, Glogau R, Stegman S, Tromovitch T. Carbon dioxide laser treatment of erythroplasia of Queyrat. J Dermatol Surg Oncol 1989; 15:747–754.

63. Dover J, Smoller B, Stern R, et al. Low-fluence carbon dioxide alser irradiation of lentigines. Arch Dermatol 1988; 124:1219–1224.

64. Benedict LM, Cohen B. Treatment of Peutz-Jeghers lentigines with the carbon dioxide laser. J Dermatol Surg Oncol 1991; 17:954–955.

65. Ratz JL, Bailin PL, Wheeland RG. CO_2 laser treatment of epidermal nevi. J Dermatol Surg Oncol 1986; 12:567–570.

66. Leshin B, Whitaker DL. Carbon dioxide laser matriectomy. J Dermatol Surg Oncol 1988; 14:608–611.

67. Geronemus RG. Laser surgery of the nail unit. J Dermatol Surg Oncol 1992; 18:735–743.

68. Taylor MB. Chondrodermatitis nodularis chronica helicis: Successful treatment with the carbon dioxide laser. J Dermatol Surg Oncol 1991; 17:862–864.

69. Hobbs ER, Bailin PL, Wheeland RG, et al. Superpulsed lasers: Minimizing thermal damage with short duration, high irradiance pulses. J Dermatol Surg Oncol 1987; 13:955–964.

70. Wheeland RG, McGillis ST. Cowden's disease—Treatment of cutaneous lesions using carbon dioxide laser vaporization: A comparison of conventional and superpulsed techniques. J Dermatol Surg Oncol 1989; 15: 1055–1059.

71. Apfelberg DB, Maser MR, Lash H, et al. Superpulse CO_2 laser treatment of facial syringomata. Lasers Surg Med 1987; 7:533–537.

72. Fitzpatrick RE, Goldman MP, Ruiz-Esparza J. Clinical advantage of the CO_2 laser superpulsed mode. J Dermatol Surg Oncol 1994; 20:449–455.

73. Walsh JT, Deutsch TF. Pulsed CO_2 laser ablation: Measurement of the ablation rate. Lasers Surg Med 1988; 8:264–275.

74. Landthaler M, Haina D, Brunner R, et al. Neodymium-YAG laser therapy for vascular lesions. J Am Acad Dermatol 14:107–117.

75. Apfelberg DB, Smith T, Lash H, et al. Preliminary report on use of the neodymium-YAG laser in plastic surgery. Lasers Surg Med 1987; 7:189–198.

76. Dixon JA, Gilbertson JJ. Argon and neodymium YAG laser therapy of dark nodular port wine stains in older patients. Lasers Surg Med 1986; 6:5–11.

77. Hukki J, Krogerus L, Castren M, et al. Effects of different contact laser scalpels on skin and subcutaneous fat. Lasers Surg Med 1988; 8:276–282.

78. Apfelberg DB, Bailin PL, Rosenberg H. Preliminary investigation of KTP/532 laser light in the treatment of hemangiomas and tattoos. Lasers Surg Med 1986; 6:38–42.

79. Lanzafame RJ, Naim JO, Blackman JR. Preliminary assessment of the Con-Bio laser in vivo. J Clin Laser Med Surg 1994; 12:147–151.

80. Malm M, Calberg M. Port-wine stain—A surgical and psychological problem. Ann Plast Surg 1988; 20:512–516.

81. Lanigan SW, Cotterill JA. Psychological disabilities amongst patients with port wine stains. Br J Dermatol 1989; 121:209–215.

82. Wagner K, Wagner R. The necessity for treatment of childhood portwine stains. Cutis 1990; 5:317–318.

83. Geronemus RG, Ashinoff R. The medical necessity of evaluation and treatment of port-wine stains. J Dermatol Surg Oncol 1991; 17:76–79.

84. Barsky SH, Rosen S, Geer D, Noe JM. The nature and evaluation of port wine stains: A computer-assisted study. J Invest Dermatol 1980; 74:154–157.

85. Goldman L. The argon laser and the port wine stain. Plast Reconstr Surg 1980; 65:137–139.

86. Cosman B. Experience in the argon laser therapy of port wine stains. Plast Reconstr Surg 1980; 65:119–129.

87. Apfelberg DB, Maser MR, Lash H, et al. The argon laser for cutaneous lesions. JAMA 1981; 245:2073–2075.

88. Noe JM, Barsky SH, Geer DE, et al. Port-wine stains and the response to argon laser therapy: Successful treatment and the predictive role of color, age, and biopsy. Plast Reconstr Surg 1980; 65:130–136.

89. Dixon JA, Huether S, Rotering R. Hypertrophic scarring in argon laser treatment of port wine stains. Plast Reconstr Surg 1984; 73:771–777.

90. Dixon JA, Rotering RH, Huether SE. Patients' evaluation of argon laser therapy of port-wine stain, decorative tattoo, and essential telangiectasia. Lasers Surg Med 1984; 4:181–190.

91. Yanai A, Fukuda O, Soyano S, et al. Argon laser therapy of portwine stains: Effects and limitations. Plast Reconstr Surg 1985; 75:520–525.

92. Brauner GJ, Schliftman A. Laser surgery for children. J Dermatol Surg Oncol 1987; 13:178–186.

93. Apfelberg DB, Flores JT, Maser MR, et al. Analysis of complications of argon laser treatment of port wine hemangiomas with reference to the striped technique. Lasers Surg Med 1983; 2:357–371.

94. Apfelberg DB, Smith T, Maser MR, et al. Dot or point-illistic method for improvement in results of hypertrophic scarring in the argon laser treatment of portwine hemangiomas. Lasers Surg Med 1987; 6:552–558.

95. Touquet VLR, Carruth JAS. Review of the treatment of port wine stains with the argon laser. Lasers Surg Med 1984; 4:191–199.

96. Brauner G, Schliftman A, Cosman B. Evaluation of argon laser surgery in children under 13 years of age. Plast Reconstr Surg 1991; 87:37–43.

97. Landthaler M, Haina D, Waidelich W, Braun-Falco O. A three-year experience with the argon laser in dermatotherapy. J Dermatol Surg Oncol 1984; 10:456–461.

98. Keller GS, Doiron D, Weingarten C. Advances in laser skin surgery for vascular lesions. Arch Otolaryngol 1985; 111:437–440.

99. Greenwald J, Rosen S, Anderson RR, et al. Comparative histological studies of the tunable dye (at 577 nm) laser and argon laser: The specific vascular effects of the dye laser. J Invest Dermatol 1981; 77:305–310.

100. Malm M, Rigler R, Jurell G. Continuous wave (CW) dye laser vs CW argon laser treatment of portwine stains (PWS). Scan Plast Reconstr Surg Hand Surg 1988; 22: 241–244.

101. Landthaler M, Haina D, Brunner R, et al. Effects of argon, dye, and Nd:YAG lasers on epidermis, dermis, and venous vessels. Lasers Surg Med 1986; 6:87–93.

102. Scheibner A, Wheeland RG. Argon-pumped tunable dye laser therapy for facial port-wine stain hemangiomas in adults—A new technique using small spot size and minimal power. J Dermatol Surg Oncol 1989; 15:277–282.

103. Scheibner A, Wheeland RG. Use of the argon-pumped tunable dye laser for port-wine stains in children. J Dermatol Surg Oncol 1991; 17:735–739.

104. Rotteleur G, Mordon S, Buys B, et al. Robotized scanning laser handpiece for the treatment of port wine stains and other angiodysplasias. Lasers Surg Med 1988; 8:283–287.

105. Mordon SR, Rotteleur G, Buys B, Brunetaud JM. Comparative study of the "point-by-point technique" and the "scanning technique" for laser treatment of port-wine stain. Lasers Surg Med 1989; 9:398–404.

106. McDaniel DH, Mordon S. Hexascan: A new robotized scanning laser handpiece. Cutis 1990; 45:300–305.

107. Chambers IR, Clark D, Bainbridge C. Automation of laser treatment of port-wine stains. Phys Med Biol 1990; 7:1025–1028.

108. Anderson RR, Parrish JA. Microvasculature can be selectively damaged using dye lasers: A basic theory and experimental evidence in human skin. Lasers Surg Med 1981; 1:263–276.

109. Anderson RR, Jaenicke KF, Parrish JA. Mechanism of selective vascular changes caused by dye lasers. Lasers Surg Med 1983; 3:211–215.

110. Garden J, Tan O, Parrish J. The pulsed dye laser: Its use at 577 nm wavelength. J Dermatol Surg Oncol 1987; 13:134–139.

111. Van Gemert MJC, Welch AJ, Amin AP. Is there an optimal laser treatment for port wine stains? Lasers Surg Med 1986; 6:76–83.

112. Garden JM, Tan OT, Kerschmann R, et al. Effect of dye laser pulse duration on selective cutaneous vascular injury. J Invest Dermatol 1986; 87:653–657.

113. Nelson J, Applebaum J. Clinical management of portwine stain in infants and young children using the flashlamp-pulsed dye laser. Clin Peds 1990; 29:503–508.

114. Ashinoff R, Geronemus RG. Flashlamp-pumped pulsed dye laser for port-wine stains in infancy: Earlier versus later treatment. J Am Acad Dermatol 1991; 24:467–472.

115. Tan OT, Gilchrest BA. Laser therapy for selected cutaneous vascular lesions in the pediatric population: A review. Pediatrics 1988; 82:652–662.

116. Tan OT, Sherwood K, Gilchrest BA. Treatment of children with port-wine stains using the flashlamp-pulsed tunable dye laser. N Engl J Med 1989; 320:416–421.

117. Reyes BA, Geronemus R. Treatment of port-wine stains during childhood with the flashlamp-pumped pulsed dye laser. J Am Acad Dermatol 1990; 23:1142–1148.

118. Goldman L, Taylor A, Putnam T. New developments with the heavy metal vapor lasers for the dermatologist. J Dermatol Surg Oncol 1987; 13:163–165.

119. Dinehart SM, Waner M, Flock S. The copper vapor laser for treatment of cutaneous vascular and pigmented lesions. J Dermatol Surg Oncol 1993; 19:370–375.

120. Pickering J, Walker E, Butler P, et al. Copper vapor laser treatment of portwine stains and other vascular malformations. Br J Plast Surg 1990; 43:272–282.

121. Walker E, Butler P, Pickering J, et al. Histology of portwine stains after copper vapor laser treatment. Br J Dermatol 1989; 121:217–223.

122. Lancer HA. Clinical summary of copper vapor laser treatment of dermatologic disease: A private practice viewpoint. Am J Cosmet Surg 1991; 8:1–4.

123. Neumann RA, Knobler RM, Leonshartsberger H, Gebhart W. Comparative histochemistry of port-wine stains after copper vapor laser (578 nm) and argon laser treatment. J Invest Dermatol 1992; 99:160–167.

124. Noe JM, Finley J, Rosen S, Arndt K. Post-rhinoplasty "red nose:" Differential diagnosis and treatment of laser. Plast Reconstr Surg 1981; 67:661–664.

125. Dicken CH. Treatment of the red nose with the argon laser. Mayo Clinic Proc 1986; 61:893–895.

126. Dicken CH. Argon laser treatment of the red nose. J Dermatol Surg Oncol 1990; 16:33–36.

127. Key JM, Waner M. Selective destruction of facial telangiectasia using a copper vapor laser. Arch Otolaryngol Head Neck Surg 1992; 118:509–513.

128. Wheeland RG, Applebaum J. Flashlamp-pumped pulsed dye laser therapy for poikiloderma of Civatte. J Dermatol Surg Oncol 1990; 16:12–16.

129. Lowe NJ, Behr KL, Fitzpatrick R, et al. Flash lamp pumped dye laser for roascea-associated telangiectasia and erythema. J Dermatol Surg Oncol 1991; 17:522–525.

130. Polla L, Tan O, Garden J, et al. Tunable pulsed dye laser for the treatment of benign cutaneous vascular ectasia. Dermatologica 1987; 174:11–17.

131. Goldman MP, Fitzpatrick RE. Pulsed-dey laser treatment of leg telangiectasia: With and without simultaneous scloerotherapy. J Dermatol Surg Oncol 1990; 16:338–344.

132. Koerber WA Jr, Price NM. Salabrasion of tattoos. A correlation of the clinical and histological results. Arch Dermatol 1978; 114:884–888.

133. Clabaugh W. Removal of tattoos by superficial dermabrasion. Arch Dermatol 1968; 98:515–521.

134. Wheeland RG, Norwood OT, Roundtree JM. Tattoo removal using serial tangential excision and polyurethane membrane dressing. J Dermatol Surg Oncol 1983; 9:822–826.

135. Scutt RWB. The chemical removal of tattoos. Br J Plast Surg 1972; 25:189–194.

136. Bailey BN. Treatment of tattoos. Plast Reconstr Surg 1967; 40:361–371.

137. Groot DW, Arlette JP, Johnston PA. Comparison of the infrared coagulator and the carbon dioxide laser in the removal of decorative tattoos. J Am Acad Dermatol 1986; 15:518–522.

138. Apfelberg DB, Maser MR, Lash H, et al. Comparison of argon and carbon dioxide laser treatment of decorative tattoos: A preliminary report. Ann Plast Surg 1985; 14:6–15.

139. Bailin PL, Ratz JL, Levine HL. Removal of tattoos by CO_2 laser. J Dermatol Surg Oncol 1980; 6:997–1001.

140. Reid R, Muller S. Tattoo removal by CO_2 laser dermabrasion. Plast Reconstr Surg 1980; 65:717–728.

141. Taylor C, Gange W, Dover J, et al. Treatment of tattoos by Q-switched ruby laser: A dose response study. Arch Dermatol 1990; 126:893–899.

142. Taylor C, Anderson R, Gange R, et al. Light and electron microscopic analysis of tattoos treated by Q-switched ruby laser. J Invest Dermatol 1991; 97:131–136.

143. Sigrist MW, Kneubuhl FK. Laser generated stress waves in liquids. J Acoust Soc Am 1978; 64:1652–1663.

144. Boulnois JL, Photophysical processes in recent medical laser developments: A review. Lasers Med Sci 1986; 1:47–66.

145. Watenebe S, Flotte TJ, McAuliffe DJ, et al. Putative photoacoustic damage in skin induced by pulsed ArF excimer laser. J Invest Dermatol 1988; 90:761–766.

146. Goldman L, Blaney DJ, Kindel DJ, et al. Effect of the laser beam on the skin: Preliminary report. J Invest Dermatol 1963; 40;121–122.

147. Goldman L, Wilson RG, Hornby P, et al. Radiation from a Q-switched ruby laser: Effect of repeated impacts of power output of 10 megawatts on a tattoo of man. J Invest Dermatol 1965; 44:69–71.

148. Reid WH, McLeod PJ, Ritchie A, et al. Q-switched ruby laser treatment of black tattoos. Br J Plast Surg 1983; 36:455–459.

149. Vance CA, McLeod PJ, Reid WH, et al. Q-switched ruby laser treatment of tattoos: A further study. Lasers Surg Med 1985; 5:179.

150. Taylor CR, Gange RW, Dover JS, et al. Treatment of tattoos by Q-switched ruby laser. Arch Dermatol 1990; 126:893–899.

151. Scheibner A, Kenny G, White W, Wheeland RG. A superior method of tattoo removal using the Q-switched ruby laser. J Dermatol Surg Oncol 1990; 16:1091–1098.

152. Reid W, Miller I, Murphy M, et al. Q-switched ruby laser treatment of tattoos: A 9 year experience. Br J Plast Surg 1990; 43:663–669.

153. Taylor CR, Anderson RR, Gange RW, et al. Light and electron microscopic analysis of tattoos treated by Q-switched ruby laser. J Invest Dermatol 1991; 97:131–136.

154. Anderson RR, Geronemus R, Kilmer SL, et al. Cosmetic tattoo ink darkening: A complication of Q-switched and pulsed-laser treatment. Arch Dermatol 1993; 129:1010–1014.

155. Goldstein N. Complications from tattoos. J Dermatol Surg Oncol 1979; 5:869–878.

156. Biro L, Klein WP. Unusual complications of mercurial (cinnabar) tattoo. Arch Dermatol 1967; 96:2.

157. Kyanko NE, Pontasch MJ, Brodell RT. Red tattoo reactions: Treatment with the carbon dioxide laser. J Dermatol Surg Oncol 1989; 15:652–656.

158. Brodell RT. Retattooing after the treatment of a red tattoo reaction with the CO_2 laser. J Dermatol Surg Oncol 1990; 16:771.

159. Ravits HG. Allergic tattoo granuloma. Arch Dermatol 1962; 86:287–289.

160. Schwartz RA, Mathias EG, Miller CH, et al. Granulomatous reaction to purple tattoo pigment. Contact Derm 1987; 16:199–202.

161. Koranda FC, Norris CW, Diestelmeier MF. Carbon dioxide laser treatment of granulomatous reactions in tattoos. Otolaryngol Head Neck Surg 1986; 94:384–387.

162. Anderson RR, Margolis RJ, Watenabe S, et al. Selective photothermolysis of cutaneous pigmentation by Q-switched Nd:YAG laser pulses at 1064, 532, and 355 nm. J Invest Dermatol 1989; 93:38–42.

163. Kilmer SL, Lee MS, Grevelink JM, et al. The Q-switched Nd:YAG laser effectively treats tattoos: A controlled, dose-response study. Arch Dermatol 1993; 129:971–978.

164. Kilmer SL, Anderson RR. Clinical use of the Q-switched ruby and the Q-switched Nd:YAG (1064 nm and 532 nm) lasers for treatment of tattoos. J Dermatol Surg Oncol 1993; 19:330–338.

165. Fitzpatrick RE, Ruiz-Esparza J, Goldman MP. The alexandrite laser for tattoos: A preliminary report. Lasers Surg Med 1992; 4S:72.

166. Tan OT, Lizek R. Alexandrite (760 nm) laser treatment of tattoos. Lasers Surg Med 1992; 4S:72–73.

167. Ohshiro T, Maruyama Y: The ruby and argon lasers in the treatment of naevi. Ann Acad Med Singapore 1983; 12:388–395.

168. Polla LL, Margolis RJ, Dover JS, et al. Melanosomes are the primary target of Q-switched ruby laser irradiation in guinea pig skin. J Invest Dermatol 1986; 89:281–286.

169. Dover JS, Margolis RJ, Polla LL, et al. Pigmented

guinea pig skin irradiated with Q-switched ruby laser pulses. Arch Dermatol 1989; 125:43–49.

170. Murphy GF, Shepard RS, Paul BS, et al. Organelle-specific injury to melanin-containing cells in human skin by pulsed laser irradiation. Lab Invest 1983; 49:680–685.

171. Hruza GJ, Dover JS, Flotte TJ, et al. Q-switched ruby laser irradiation of normal human skin. Arch Dermatol 1991; 127:1799–1805.

172. Ohshiro T, Maruyama Y, Makajima H, Mimi M. Treatment of pigmentation of the lips and oral mucosa in Peutz-Jeghers syndrome using ruby and argon lasers. Br J Plast Surg 1980; 33:346–349.

173. Ashinoff R, Geronemus RG. Q-switched ruby laser treatment of labial lentigos. J Am Acad Dermatol 1992; 27:809–811.

174. Goldberg DJ. Benign pigmented lesions of the skin: Treatment with the Q-switched ruby laser. J Dermatol Surg Oncol 1993; 19:376–379.

175. Goldberg DJ, Nychay SG. Q-switched ruby laser treatment of nevus of Ota. J Dermatol Surg Oncol 1992; 18:817–821.

176. Geronemus RG. Q-switched ruby laser therapy of nevus of Ota. Arch Dermatol 1992; 128:1618–1622.

177. Thibault P, Wlodarczyk J. Postclerotherapy hyperpigmentation: The role of serum ferritin levels and the effectiveness of treatment with the copper vapor laser. J Dermatol Surg Oncol 1992; 18:47–52.

178. Tan OT, Morelli JG, Kurban AK. Pulsed dye laser treatment of benign cutaneous pigmented lesions. Lasers Surg Med 1992; 12:538–542.

179. Goldman MP. Postsclerotherapy hyperpigmentation: Treatment with a flashlamp-excited pulsed dye laser. J Dermatol Surg Oncol 1992; 18:417–422.

180. Holmdahl K. Cutaneous hemangiomas in premature and mature infants. Acta Paediatr 1955; 44:370–379.

181. Morelli J, Tan O, Weston W. Treatment of ulcerated hemangiomas with the pulsed tunable dye laser. Am J Dis Child 1991; 145:1062–1064.

182. Ashinoff R, Geronemus RG. Capillary hemangiomas and treatment with the flash lamp-pulsed dye laser. Arch Dermatol 1991; 127:202–205.

183. Sherwood KA, Tan OT. The treatment of a capillary hemangioma with the flashlamp pumped-dye laser. J Am Acad Dermatology 1991; 22:136–137.

184. Garden JM, Bakus AD, Paller AS. Treatment of cutaneous hemangiomas by the flashlamp-pumped pulsed dye laser: Prospective analysis. J Pediatr 1992; 120:555–560.

185. Goldberg DJ, Sciales CW. Pyogenic granuloma in children. J Dermatol Surg Oncol 1991; 17:960–962.

186. Wheeland RG, Bailin PL, Norris MJ. Argon laser photocoagulative therapy of Kaposi's sarcoma: A clinical and histologic evaluation. J Dermatol Surg Oncol 1985; 11:1180–1185.

187. Tappero JW, Grekin RC, Zanelli GA, Berger TG. Pulsed-dye laser therapy for cutaneous Kaposi's sarcoma associated with acquired immunodeficiency syndrome. J Am Acad Dermatol 1992; 27:526–530.

188. Basford JR. Low-energy laser therapy: Controversies and new research findings. Lasers Surg Med 1989; 9:1–5.

189. Mester E, Korenyi-Both A, Spiry T, et al. Stimulation of wound healing by means of laser rays. Acta Chir Acad Scien Hung 1973; 14:347–356.

190. Kana JS, Hutschenreiter G, Haina D, Waidelich W. Effect of low-power density laser radiation on healing of open skin wounds in rats. Arch Surg 1981; 116:293–296.

191. Surinchak JS, Alago ML, Bellamy RF, et al. Effects of low-level energy lasers on the healing of full-thickness skin defects. Lasers Surg Med 1983; 2:267–274.

192. Hunter J, Leonard L, Wilson R, et al. Effects of low energy laser on wound healing in a porcine model. Lasers Surg Med 1984; 3:285–290.

193. Abergel RP, Meeker CA, Lam TS, et al. Control of connective tissue metabolism by lasers: Recent developments and future prospects. J Am Acad Dermatol 1984; 11:1142–1150.

194. Lyons RF, Abergel RP, White RA, et al. Biostimulation of wound healing in vivo by a helium-neon laser. Ann Plast Surg 1987; 18:47–50.

195. Longo L, Evangelista S, Tinacci G, Sesti AG. Effect of diodes-laser silver arsenide-aluminium (Ga-Al-As) 904 nm on healing of experimental wounds. Lasers Surg Med 1987; 7:444–447.

196. Abergel RP, Lyons RF, Catsel JC, et al. Biostimulation of wound healing by lasers: Experimental approaches in animal models and in fibroblast cultures. J Dermatol Surg Oncol 1987; 13:127–133.

197. Braverman B, McCarthy RJ, Ivankovich AD, et al. Effect of helium-neon and infrared laser irradiation on wound healing in rabbits. Lasers Surg Med 1989; 9:50–58.

198. Fava G, Marchesini R, Melloni E, et al. Effect of low energy irradiation by He-Ne laser on mitosis rate of HT-29 tumor cells in culture. Lasers Life Sci 1986; 1:135–141.

199. Karu TI, Kalendo GS, Letokhov VS, Lobko JJ. Biostimulation of HeLa cells by low-intensity visible light: Stimulation of DNA and RNA synthesis in a wide spectral range. Il Nuovo Cimento 1984; 3:309–318.

200. Boulton M, Marshall J. He-Ne laser stimulation of human fibroblast proliferation and attachment in vitro. Lasers Life Sci 1986; 1:125–134.

201. Lam TS, Abergel RP, Meeker CA, et al. Laser stimulation of collagen synthesis in human skin fibroblast cultures. Lasers Life Sci 1986; 1:61–77.

202. Pasarella S, Dechecchi MS, Quagliariello E, et al. Optical and biochemical properties of NADH irradiated by high peak power Q-switched ruby laser or by low power CW He-Ne laser. Bioelectrochem Bioenerg 1981; 8:315–319.

203. Castro JD, Abergel RP, Meeker CA, et al. Effects of the Nd:YAG laser on DNA synthesis and collagen production in human skin fibroblast cultures. Ann Plast Surg 1983; 11:214–222.

204. Abergel RP, Meeker CA, Dwyer RM, et al. Nonthermal effects of Nd:YAG laser on biological functions of human skin fibroblasts in culture. Lasers Surg Med 1984; 3:279–284.

205. Haas AF, Isseroff RR, Wheeland RG, et al. Low-energy helium-neon laser irradiation increases the motility of cultured human keratinocytes. J Invest Dermatol 1990; 94:822–826.

206. Robinson JK, Garden JM, Taute PM, et al. Wound healing in porcine skin following low-output carbon dioxide laser irradiation of the incision. Ann Plast Surg 1987; 18:499–505.

207. Garden JM, Robinson JK, Taute PM, et al. The low-

output carbon dioxide laser for cutaneous wound closure of scalpel incisions: comparative tensile strength studies of the laser to the suture and staple for wound closure. Lasers Surg Med 1986; 6:67–71.

208. Abergel RP, Lyons R, Dwyer R, et al. Use of lasers for closure of cutaneous wounds: experience with Nd:YAG, argon and CO_2 lasers. J Dermatol Surg Oncol 1986; 12: 1181–1185.

209. Abergel RP, Lyons RF, White RA, et al. Skin closure by Nd:YAG laser welding. J Am Acad Dermatol 1986; 14: 810–814.

210. Dougherty TJ, Kaufman JE, Goldfarb A, et al. Photoradiation therapy for the treatment of malignant tumors. Cancer Res 1978; 38:2628–2633.

211. McCaughan JS, Guy JT, Hawley P, et al. Hematoporphyrin-derivative and photoradiation therapy of malignant tumors. Lasers Surg Med 1983; 3:199–209.

212. Evensen J, Sommer S, Moan J, et al. Tumor localizing and photosensitizing properties of main components of hematoporphyrin derivative. Cancer Res 1984; 44:482–486.

213. Berns MW, McCullough JL, Porphyrin sensitized phototherapy. Arch Dermatol 1986; 122:871–874.

214. Carruth JAS. Photodynamic therapy: The state of the art. Lasers Surg Med 1986; 6:404–407.

215. Pennington DG, Waner M, Knox A. Photodynamic therapy for multiple skin cancers. Plast Reconstr Surg 1988; 82:1067–1071.

216. Bernstein EF, Friauf WS, Smith PD, et al. Transcutaneous determination of tissue dihematoporphyrin ether content—A device to optimize photodynamic therapy. Arch Dermatol 1991; 127:1794–1798.

217. Henderson BW, Dougherty TJ, Malone PB. Studies on the mechanism of tumor destruction by photoradiation therapy. Prog Clin Biol Res 1984; 170:601–612.

218. Gluckman JL, Waner M, Shumrick K, et al. Photodynamic therapy. Arch Otolaryngol Head Neck Surg 1986; 112:949–952.

219. White WE, Hunter JR, Van Woerkom L, et al. 120-fs terrawatt $Ti:Al_2O_3/Cr:LiSrAlF_6$ laser system. Opt Let 1992; 17:219–221.

220. Frederickson KS, White WE, Wheeland RG, Slaughter DR. Precise ablation of skin with reduced collateral damage using the femtosecond-pulsed, terawatt titanium-sapphire laser. Arch Dermatol 1993; 129:989–993.

221. Steinert RF, Puliafito CA, Trokel S. Plasma formation and shielding by three ophthalmic neodymium-YAG lasers. Am J Ophthalmol 1983; 96:427–434.

222. Yashima Y, McAuliffe JD, Jacques SL, Flotte TJ. Laser-induced photoacoustic injury of skin: Effect of inertial confinement. Lasers Surg Med 1991; 11:62–68.

223. Wyman A, Duffy S, Sweetland HM, et al. Preliminary evaluation of a new high power diode laser. Lasers Surg Med 1992; 12:506–509.

Chapter 4

Applications of Lasers in Gastroenterology

Norman S. Nishioka, MD

Medical Services, Gastrointestinal Unit, Massachusetts General Hospital and Department of Medicine, Harvard Medical School, Boston

INTRODUCTION

In many ways gastroenterology is ideally suited for the use of laser technology. Due to advances in gastrointestinal endoscopic technology and endoscopic techniques, both the upper and lower gastrointestinal tracts can be readily accessed in a safe and relatively noninvasive fashion. Furthermore, because light of many wavelengths and intensities can be transmitted through small diameter fibers and these fibers can be readily inserted through the instrument channels of endoscopes, light can be delivered to the mucosal surfaces of the gastrointestinal tract in a straightforward manner. For these reasons, gastroenterology was one of the earliest subspecialties to examine the use of lasers. Lasers were introduced into gastroenterology in the early 1970s for the arrest of gastrointestinal hemorrhage. Although initially used as therapeutic devices, recent investigations have begun to explore the use of light as a diagnostic tool. Despite the attractiveness of using lasers, they are not yet used by all gastroenterologists. There are many reasons for the continued specialized nature of using lasers in gastroenterology, but the most significant reasons are the large capital investment required to acquire current laser systems and the availability of less expensive devices to accomplish many of the same goals.

In this article the current uses of laser technology in gastroenterology are reviewed. Emphasis is placed on the current utilization and future directions of lasers in gastrointestinal endoscopy. Applications of laser technology that are no longer widely used are either omitted or given only cursory description. This article is not intended to be an exhaustive review of all aspects of the use of lasers in gastroenterology nor is it meant to provide instruction in the practice of laser endoscopy. The reader is referred to one of the many excellent treatises on these subjects. The article is divided into three major sections: therapeutic uses of lasers, diagnostic applications, and future directions.

THERAPEUTIC USES OF LASERS
Tumor Ablation

There are two general approaches to tumor ablation with lasers. The more common approach is the the use of a *thermal method* that converts laser light energy into heat that vaporizes tissue. In contrast, *photodynamic therapy* utilizes light to activate a previously administered drug and convert it into a cytotoxic compound that ultimately results in tumor necrosis. In both approaches, the overall goal is to remove sufficient tissue to reestablish a lumen of adequate diameter to relieve obstructive symptoms. Cure of the tumor is in general not a realistic objective. The greatest experience has been in the palliation of esophageal cancer, but obstructing lesions of the large intestine, stomach, and biliary tree also can be treated.

Thermal methods. The most frequent use of lasers in gastroenterology today is probably as a way to vaporize tumors. As noted above, the laser energy is absorbed by the tissue and converted to heat. If the heating rate is sufficient, the tissue is vaporized. However, tissue vaporization is not necessary to produce a successful clinical outcome. Coagulative thermal injury below the surface of the tumor can produce significant amounts of necrotic tissue that either spontaneously sloughs or can be mechanically debrided 48–72 hours later. Although many lasers could be used for this application, the most commonly used laser for tumor debridement remains the continuous wave Nd:YAG laser. It is available in high powers (up to 100 Watts), and the deep penetration of light at this wavelength (1.06 μm) produces deep thermal injury and hence excellent hemostasis.

Esophageal cancer. Relief of malignant dysphagia is the most common gastrointestinal use of the Nd:YAG laser in most centers. Although there are numerous other approaches to palliating esophageal cancer, endoscopic laser therapy has the advantage that it can be used after failure of a surgical procedure and in patients who have previously received chemotherapy or radiation therapy. The procedure was first described by Fleischer in 1982 (1). The laser energy is typically administered to the lesion through a 600-μm core diameter quartz fiber in either a contact or noncontact mode. Establishment of an adequate lumen to provide improvement in dysphagia typically requires one or two sessions and can be accomplished on an outpatient basis in many instances.

Numerous studies have demonstrated that endoscopic laser therapy is effective in the palliation of esophageal cancer [1,2]. Although technical success can be achieved in the majority of cases, not all patients obtain significant improvement in their dysphagia. In one prospective study of patients with advanced esophageal cancer, luminal patency was achieved in 97% of patients, although only 70% were able to ingest sufficient calories to maintain homeostasis [3]. As would be expected, the poorer the functional status prior to endoscopic laser therapy, the poorer the func-

tional result. Several factors have been identified as predictive of a poor technical result. In general, submucosal tumors, tumors in the proximal esophagus and at the gastroesophageal junction, especially those with sharp angulation, and those > 5 cm are the most difficult lesions to treat [4].

Endoscopic laser ablation of esophageal cancer has been compared to other methods in several trials. A prospective but nonrandomized study comparing the Nd:YAG laser to endoscopic intubation for palliation of esophageal cancer has been published by Loizou and co-workers [5]. Among patients with tumors of the thoracic esophagus, there was no significant difference in the improvement of dysphagia between the two groups. For tumors crossing the cardia, intubation appeared to provide better relief of dysphagia than laser ablation. However, among patients palliated over a long period (>3 months), the mean dysphagia grade was significantly better in the laser-treated group. Those patients required a greater number of procedures, but overall had a lower complication rate. In another non-randomized study, Jensen and co-workers [6] compared the Nd:YAG laser to the BICAP (electrocautery) tumor probe for palliation of esophageal cancer. They found no difference between the two groups in terms of dysphagia relief during a follow-up period of 16 weeks. However, there appeared to be a difference between the two techniques when the physical characteristics of the lesion being treated were considered. The authors concluded that the BICAP tumor probe and Nd:YAG laser were comparable for the treatment of circumferential tumors, but that the Nd:YAG laser was superior for treating noncircumferential lesions because of its ability to be directed endoscopically [6].

In general, the intent of the endoscopic laser therapy is to improve the quality of life rather than to alter mortality, and thus mortality has not been affected by Nd:YAG laser therapy in most studies. However, small studies have been reported in which patient survival appeared to be prolonged. For example, Karlin reported a retrospective case control study in which those patients with esophageal cancer who were treated with endoscopic laser therapy had a significantly longer median survival than case control subjects [7].

The major complication arising from endoscopic laser therapy is esophageal perforation. The reported rates vary between 0 and 10% [8]. Other complications that can result from endoscopic laser therapy include the formation of tra-cheo-esophageal fistulas, bleeding, low-grade fever, and odynophagia. The complication rates arising from laser therapy do not appear to be significantly different than those associated with other treatment methods.

Large intestine. Just as lasers can be used to palliate tumors of the esophagus, so too they can be used to ablate tumors of the large intestine. Although surgery remains the treatment of choice for most patients with colorectal cancer, a small fraction of patients are inoperable or very poor operative risks and may require nonsurgical palliative treatment. In particular, those patients with obstruction, bleeding, pain, or mucous discharge might benefit from endoscopic laser therapy. The technique and laser parameters used for palliating tumors of the large intestine are similar to those used for the treatment of esophageal cancer.

Numerous experiences with endoscopic laser therapy for palliation of colorectal tumors have been published. Unfortunately, the studies vary widely in the technique used, indications for the procedure, length of follow-up, criteria for success, and location and size of tumor. This wide variability in the published experience makes it difficult to assess the true utility of lasers in this clinical setting. These studies have been thoughtfully analyzed by Mathus-Vliegen [9] in 1991. In general, patients with bleeding as their predominant symptom respond the best to laser therapy and can expect a success rate of ~90%. Endoscopic laser therapy has only a 75% success rate for patients with predominantly obstructive symptoms. There have been several reports of successful treatment of early colorectal cancers in patients who either refused surgery or who were poor operative risks [10]. Complication rates have been reported to vary between 0 and 13% with mortality rates between 1 and 3% [9].

Photodynamic therapy. Photodynamic therapy (PDT) has been used to treat a variety of tumors within the gastrointestinal tract. By far the most common application has been for the palliation of advanced esophageal cancer, and this likely will be the first application of PDT to be approved by the FDA. Numerous photosensitizers have been used in humans, and an even greater number are in various stages of development, the greatest clinical experience being with porfimer sodium (Photofrin™). Two schemes are commonly employed in the illumination step of PDT. The most common approach is intraluminal illumina-tion in which a cylindrical diffusing tip is placed within the residual lumen of the tumor and the tumor is irradiated from the luminal aspect. In the interstitial approach, a fiber is placed in direct contact with the tumor or within the tumor parenchyma itself. Both systems are capable of delivering adequate doses of light to the tumor and in any given situation, one may be technically more convenient.

Esophagus. Although numerous patients with esophageal cancer have been treated by PDT, there are few well-controlled trials. In a small number of patients with advanced esophageal cancer, Heier and co-workers [11] randomized patients to receive either PDT with porfimer sodium or Nd:YAG laser therapy. There were no differences between the groups in terms of tumor length, diameter of the residual lumen, number of treatments, initial Karnofsky performance scale, or long-term survival. However, there was a statistically significant difference in the duration of the clinical response (67 days for the porfimer sodium group and 44 days for the Nd:YAG laser group). In addition, there was a greater improvement in the Karnofsky performance scale at 1 month among the patients who received PDT, suggesting that the rapidity of improvement was superior with PDT [11]. Treatment with PDT had the further advantages of no smoke produced during the procedure and the relative lack of chest discomfort experienced by patients. The authors also felt that PDT was technically much less demanding to deliver successfully. The complications were similar among both groups with the exception of an 18% incidence of skin photosensitivity in the PDT group.

Although the experience with PDT in treating esophageal cancer has largely been with a palliative intent, there have been efforts to cure esophageal cancer at early stages. In an interesting report by Overholt [12], two patients with early adenocarcinoma arising in Barrett's esophagus were treated with PDT with porfimer sodium. Although the follow-up period was brief, both patients were tumor-free following therapy and in one patient there was a significant distal migration of the squamocolumnar junction [12]. In a survey of Japanese medical centers, 11 patients with early esophageal cancer who had been treated with PDT were identified. Nine of the patients (82%) were disease-free one year following therapy [13].

Stomach. The treatment of gastric cancer with PDT has been largely ignored, although there have been limited attempts to treat patients with early gastric cancer. In a survey of Japanese medical centers, 30 patients with early gastric cancer who either refused surgery or who were deemed to be a poor operative risk received PDT with porfimer sodium. Twenty-eight (93%) of the patients were apparently disease-free at 1 year [13]. Although quite preliminary, these results suggest that PDT may have a limited role in the management of patients with early gastric cancer who are not eligible for surgical resection. Although there are few studies to provide guidance, many investigators feel that PDT also has the potential to treat dysplastic lesions of the gastric mucosa as well as small, focal recurrences following surgery.

Colorectal cancer. There have been isolated reports describing the palliation of colorectal cancer by means of PDT. Barr reported an experience with ten patients with advanced colorectal cancer who were considered inoperable [14]. All lesions were < 5 cm in length. Two patients with small lesions (anastomotic recurrence) were disease-free at 28 months. All three patients with obstructive symptoms had improvement in symptoms, and two of the four patients whose main complaint was bleeding improved. One of the two patients with diarrhea as a predominant symptom improved.

Biliary tree. McCaughan et al. reported a case of a 57-year-old woman with cholangiocarcinoma of the common bile duct [15]. PDT with Porfimer Sodium was delivered on numerous occasions over 4 years. Although the treatment did not cure the tumor, some extent of palliation was achieved. Because of the limited treatment options for patients with biliary cancer, PDT may prove to be a welcome addition to the treatment arsenal.

Future Directions. The use of PDT is clearly in its infancy. In the near future, at least one photodynamic agent will likely become widely available in the United States for clinical use. This will undoubtedly increase the clinical experience and expand the number of diseases for which it is used. However, one would also expect that further experience will lead to a refinement of the indications for its use to those patients most likely to benefit from it. Studies comparing PDT to other treatment modalities both in terms of outcome and cost are also needed. Newer photodynamic agents with the promise of greater selectivity and tumor cytotoxicity and a lower incidence of side effects will also improve the safety and efficacy of PDT as a whole. More compact and less expensive laser sources should also become available in the near future, making PDT available to more centers. Finally, delivery devices will have to be refined to ensure that the delivery of light an be made in a simple, reproducible, predictable, and reliable manner.

Bleeding

Ulcers. The use of lasers to halt gastrointestinal hemorrhage was first attempted in the early 1970s [16]. Although both the argon and Nd:YAG lasers have been used to treat gastrointestinal hemorrhage from peptic ulcers, the Nd:YAG laser has proven itself to be superior and is thus almost exclusively used for treating major hemorrhage in this setting [17,18]. Therapeutic endoscopy is typically performed in the emergent or semiemergent setting but is only performed after adequate fluid resuscitation has occurred. Typically, Nd:YAG laser energy is delivered to the ulcer through a quartz fiber in a noncontact mode. Laser powers of 70–90 Watts with exposure durations of 0.5–1 s are typical. Several applications are made around the base of the ulcer bed in the area of the bleeding point. Many investigators find that the prior injection of epinephrine into the ulcer decreases the likelihood of bleeding during the procedure and improves the overall outcome. Numerous controlled trials of Nd:YAG laser therapy for treating hemorrhage from peptic ulcers have been reported. However, each study varies in the technique used, the types of lesions treated (visible vessel, active bleeding, stigmata of recent hemorrhage, etc.), and the timing of the procedure. This has resulted in a wide variation of conclusions. In some studies, the recurrence of bleeding, the need for surgery, and overall mortality did not vary between control and treatment groups [19]. However, some of the studies with negative results have been criticized for including patients at low risk of rebleeding who are unlikely to benefit from a therapeutic intervention. In a prospective trial of the combination of epinephrine injection and laser in carefully selected patients with bleeding peptic ulcers, Rutgeerts demonstrated a reduction in emergency surgery and mortality in the treated group [20]. Similarly, Swain randomized 138 patients with bleeding from peptic ulcers and stigmata of recent hemorrhage at endoscopy to receive laser therapy or conservative management. Overall, the need for emergency surgery was reduced and the mortality rate of treated patients was 1% compared with 12% in the control group.

The major complications of laser photocoagulation are perforation and aggravation of bleeding. Perforation has been surprisingly rare with an incidence of <1%. Aggravation or precipitation of bleeding during the procedure has been reported to occur in as many as one-fourth of patients. However, most bleeding can be subsequently arrested by further laser therapy.

Despite the successful use of lasers to arrest hemorrhage from bleeding peptic ulcers in many studies, the use of lasers in this setting has fallen out of favor because of the widely held perception that alternate technologies such as the heater probe and bipolar electrocoagulation devices can produce similar results at much less expense. Matthewson [21] reported a study in which 143 patients with bleeding peptic ulcers and stigmata of recent hemorrhage were randomized to receive Nd:YAG laser photocoagulation, heater probe, or conservative treatment. The rebleeding rate among laser-treated patients was significantly less than control patients, whereas there was no statistical significance between the heater probe-treated and control groups. In a similar type of trial, Rutgeerts [22] compared the efficacy of Nd:YAG laser and bipolar electrocoagulator after injection of epinephrine and found no statistical significance between the two modalities. Thus the exact role of lasers for treating bleeding from peptic ulcers remains controversial.

Vascular malformations. There are numerous types of vascular malformations within the gastrointestinal tract, but the predominant lesions responsible for hemorrhage are angiodysplasia and the malformations associated with hereditary hemorrhage telangiectasia (HHT), also known as the Osler-Weber-Rendu syndrome. Surgical resection of vascular malformations has not proven an effective therapy for bleeding from these lesions because of the high morbidity and mortality rate and the high recurrence rate following surgery. Furthermore, in instances where the lesions are distributed throughout the gastrointestinal tract, particularly in HHT, surgical resection of all involved areas is often impossible. Because of these limitations, various forms of endoscopic therapy have been attempted. These include laser photocoagulation, heater probe, electrocautery, and injection therapy. The argon laser and Nd:YAG laser are the most commonly used lasers for treating vascular lesions. A pulsed dye laser operating at 577 nm [23] has also been used in a limited number of patients, although clinical results have not yet been reported.

The argon laser is an attractive alternative for the treatment of vascular lesions because the blue-green wavelength is strongly absorbed by hemoglobin within tissue. This results in relatively shallow (0.3 mm) penetration of the light into tissue. Thus the risk of perforation is usually low provided that relatively short laser exposures are used, although the superficial penetration does result in the creation of a shallow ulcer. However, portions of those vessels located within the submucosa may not be coagulated to any significant degree. Several uncontrolled studies examining the utility of argon laser photocoagulation for the treatment of vascular malformations have been reported. One large series of 50 patients was reported by Waitman [24]. During a follow-up period that ranged between 6 months and 4 years, two-thirds of patients had no recurrence of bleeding. In another series, Jensen and co-workers [25] observed a significant reduction in bleeding episodes and transfusion requirement without significant complications.

The Nd:YAG laser penetrates tissue to a greater degree than the argon laser. Thus the Nd:YAG laser has the theoretical advantage of reaching and coagulating vessels within the submucosa. For obvious reasons, the laser settings must be such that actual tissue vaporization/ablation is avoided. Typically, the working distance between fiber end and target and laser power and laser exposure are adjusted so that the laser induces a white area of coagulation. Numerous uncontrolled studies of the use of the Nd:YAG laser for treating vascular malformations have appeared in the literature. For example, Rutgeerts [26] reported the results of 57 patients with lesions in the upper and lower gastrointestinal tract treated with Nd:YAG laser. Both the frequency of bleeding episodes as well as the number of blood transfusions required were significantly decreased following therapy. The subset of patients with angiodysplasia has the most dramatic response with >80% of patients being free of further bleeding. Patients with HHT did the poorest, and all patients had further episodes of bleeding. As would be expected, the greater the number of lesions, the less likely laser photocoagulation was successful in preventing further bleeding. Perforation was seen in 4% of patients and delayed massive hemorrhage in 2%. Johnston reported that 19 of 22 (86%) patients treated by Nd:YAG laser had either complete control of bleeding or a significant reduction in bleeding, although they and a high complication rate with delayed hemorrhage in three patients and evidence of perforation in four patients [27].

As mentioned previously, multipolar electrocoagulation, heater probe, and injection sclerotherapy have also been used to treat vascular malformations of the gastrointestinal tract. Promising results have been reported with all modalities, and it may be that comparable results will ultimately be demonstrated for each method. A large, randomized, placebo-controlled trial of one or more treatment modalities is still lacking and would be of great utility in deciding the optimal modality for treating vascular lesions.

Other vascular lesions. Several reports have suggested that laser photocoagulation is an effective therapy for bleeding from antral vascular disease (watermelon stomach). For example, Gostout and co-workers [28] reported their experience with 13 patients who were treated with the Nd:YAG laser. Endoscopic as well as hematological improvement was seen in 12 of the patients (92%). No complications were noted [28]. The argon laser appears to be as effective as the Nd:YAG laser for treating these lesions that are predominantly in the mucosal layer [29].

Bleeding from radiation-induced vascular lesions also appears to respond to laser photocoagulation. Viggiano reported an experience with 47 patients with hematochezia from radiation-induced rectosigmoid vascular lesions [30]. All patients had failed medical therapy. Following laser photocoagulation with the Nd:YAG laser, the number of patients experiencing daily hematochezia fell from 85% to 5% and the mean hemoglobin level increased from 9.7 gm/dl to 11.7 gm/dl. No significant improvement was seen in six patients (13%). The authors concluded that endoscopic laser photocoagulation should be considered in patients with radiation-induced hematochezia prior to surgery.

Interstitial Laser Coagulation

Laser-induced thermal necrosis has been used successfully to coagulate metastatic lesions within solid organs, particularly the liver [31]. The laser energy is typically delivered by one or more laser fibers placed directly into the metastasis under ultrasound guidance. A low-power laser, frequently a Nd:YAG or diode laser, is used to heat the tissue. Ultrasound, magnetic resonance imaging (MRI) and dynamic computed tomography (CT) have been used to monitor the expanding zone of necrosis during irradiation. A large series was reported by Amin and colleagues [32].

They treated 55 liver metastases in 21 patients with a low power Nd:YAG laser inserted under ultrasound guidance. Complete necrosis of the metastasis was possible in 21 (38%) of the lesions. In 45 (82%) lesions, necrosis of >50% of the tumor volume was possible. Lesions greater than 4 cm in diameter were in general more difficult to treat. No significant complications occurred [32].

Although interstitial laser coagulation appears promising as a means of palliating metastatic lesions within solid organs, there are several other competing methods. Cryotherapy, high energy ultrasound, interstitial radio frequency or microwave energy, injection of alcohol, and interstitial radiotherapy are alternate methods that are capable of producing equivalent results. The precise role of the laser-based technique relative to the other modalities is the subject of ongoing investigations.

Lithotripsy

A wide variety of laser systems have been shown capable of fragmenting biliary calculi, and several of them have been used to fragment common duct stones in humans. The most commonly used lasers to fragment biliary stones are listed in Table 1. It should be noted that although a wide variety of laser parameters can be used for lithotripsy, the fragmentation efficiency is in fact dependent upon the laser parameters chosen [33]. For example, longer pulse durations are in general less efficient, and it has been demonstrated that very long pulse durations (seconds) result in the melting of stones rather than fragmentation per se [34]. However, clinically acceptable fragmentation rates have been achieved with pulse durations varying from 20 nanoseconds to 2 milliseconds (a factor of 100,000), and therefore there appears to be much latitude in the choice of laser parameters. Of practical importance is the observation that optimal fragmentation efficiency requires that the laser fiber be in direct contact with the stone. In addition, it has been demonstrated that immersion in water significantly increases fragmentation rates and therefore, performing the procedure in an aqueous environment can dramatically improve the efficiency of laser lithotripsy [35].

The majority of clinical experience with laser lithotripsy of biliary calculi has been confined to stones lodged within the common bile and intrahepatic ducts. Ell et al. [36] have reported their use of a pulsed Nd:YAG laser to treat patients with large common duct stones. The laser

TABLE 1. Most Commonly Used Lasers for Lithotripsy

Laser	Wavelength	Pulse duration
Tunable dye	504	1 μs
Q-switched Nd:YAG	1,060 nm	20 ns
Pulsed Nd:YAG	1,060 nm	2 msec

pulses were transmitted through a 200-μm diameter quartz fiber, and the procedure involved direct visualization of the stone through a choledochoscope inserted perorally. They were able to completely clear the common bile duct in two-thirds of patients.

A multicenter trial of the pulsed tunable dye laser operating at a wavelength of 504 nm with a pulse duration of 1 μs has been reported [37]. A total of 25 complex patients with stones that did not respond to standard nonoperative treatment underwent an attempt at laser lithotripsy. The laser energy was applied through a quartz fiber that was placed under direct vision with a choledochoscopes passed percutaneously or passed through a special "mother" duodenoscope or under fluoroscopic guidance. Some degree of fragmentation was seen in 23 cases (92%). Twenty (80%) of the patients subsequently had their ducts completed cleared of stones. There were no significant complications. The authors concluded that laser lithotripsy appeared to be a safe but technically challenging alternative to surgery in patients with large and difficult bile duct stones.

An interesting technical development has been reported by Ell and co-workers [38]. In this system, an optical detection system is used to determine whether the fiber is against a stone or tissue [38]. If the system determines that the fiber is against tissue, the laser pulse is terminated before a significant amount of laser energy can be delivered. These investigators were able successfully to treat nine patients under fluoroscopic control in the absence of direct visualization of the stone with a choledochoscope. The duct was completely cleared of stones in eight patients (89%). Although the clinical experience is limited, this system appears has the potential to simplify the delivery of laser energy and may help to broaden the number of patients approached by laser lithotripsy.

The clinical role of laser lithotripsy is uncertain at present. The devices are expensive and in most centers laser lithotripsy is reserved for those common bile duct stones that have not responded to more conventional therapy such as sphincter-

otomy, basket retrieval, and mechanical lithotripsy. Thus as presently implemented, laser lithotripsy is used in only a very small minority of patients with common bile duct stones. In addition, there are several technical challenges to be met before laser lithotripsy will become widely accepted. Reliable, small, portable, and inexpensive laser systems would make the technology much more practical. More importantly, the design and fabrication of delivery devices that reliably place laser fibers into direct contact with calculi without the need to directly visualize the process through an endoscope would greatly simplify the procedure.

DIAGNOSTIC USES OF LASERS

Most laser applications in gastroenterology rely upon the ability of light to alter tissue and thereby produce a therapeutic effect. However, in recent years there has been growing interest in using lasers as diagnostic devices, an area of investigation that has been termed "optical diagnostics." The overall goal of optical diagnostics is to provide diagnostic information about tissue by using light in a probing, yet nondestructive fashion. Because endoscopic diagnosis is predicated upon the ability of the endoscopist to identify abnormal tissue within a background of normal tissue, optical diagnostic methods might improve the diagnostic accuracy of endoscopy. Although a wide variety of optical techniques can be used to probe tissue, the methods explored to date have been based upon conventional laboratory spectroscopic methods such as diffuse reflectance spectroscopy and fluorescence spectroscopy. Numerous clinical applications of these spectroscopic modalities have been explored including distinguishing malignant from benign tissue, monitoring metabolic state, and measuring local drug concentration. Of the various techniques, fluorescence spectroscopy has generated the most interest and is discussed briefly here. Reflectance spectroscopy and laser Doppler velocimetry are two optical diagnostic techniques familiar to most readers and have been well described in the literature. They are beyond the scope of this article.

Laser-Induced Fluorescence

Fluorescence spectroscopy is a powerful laboratory tool that is widely used in chemistry, physics, biochemistry, and biophysics to characterize chemical and physical processes in materials. Although tissue is a complex, heterogeneous mixture of a large number of molecular species containing numerous potential fluorophores, in actual practice, the observed fluorescence signals are typically dominated by just a few fluorophores. This makes the fluorescence signals from tissue relatively featureless. The systems used to acquire fluorescence signals in vivo typically utilize a compact laser such as a pulsed nitrogen laser or helium cadmium laser as the source of the excitation light. The excitation light is transmitted through a small diameter quartz fiber that is passed through the instrument channel of an endoscope. The induced fluorescence is captured by the same fiber and transmitted back to an optical analyzer, frequently consisting of a grating polychromator and optical multi-channel analyzer. The end result is a measurement of the fluorescence intensity as a function of wavelength for a fixed excitation wavelength. Once the fluorescence signal is acquired, the information is transferred to a computer for further analysis [39].

Because fluorescence spectroscopy is used to probe the composition and physiological state of systems in the laboratory, it is reasonable to hypothesize that tissue autofluorescence would be useful as an nondestructive in vivo tissue probe of metabolic state. For example, Chance and co-workers [40] have used laser-induced fluorescence to monitor tissue redox state in vivo by utilizing the fact that NADH is a strongly fluorescent compound, whereas NAD is not. Although this technique has proved to be useful for many metabolic studies [41], its widespread implementation has been limited by its inability to provide quantitative information and its sensitivity to tissue components such as blood. The sensitivity of fluorescence to tissue composition makes it reasonable to hypothesize that laser-induced autofluorescence might be a valuable means of determining tissue type. This approach was first described by Alfano et al. [42]. They used blue (488 nm wavelength) light from an argon ion laser to excite urinary tract tissue in vitro. They showed that spectral features were present in subcutaneously implanted rodent bladder and prostate cancers that were not evident in normal tissues [42].

Although there are many gastrointestinal problems that could be approached by optical diagnostic methods, the problem that has received the greatest attention thus far has been that of distinguishing polyp type. The problem of correctly identifying polyp type is an interesting research area to test optical diagnostic techniques not only because it is an important clinical problem but because the studies may provide insight into how to identify neoplasia and dysplasia, problems of widespread interest. Using a helium cadmium laser to produce ultraviolet (wavelength 325 nm) fluorescence excitation, Kapadia and co-workers examined resected colon polyps and derived an algorithm for discriminating neoplastic from normal colonic tissue using a multivariate linear regression analysis [43]. They were able to identify adenomatous polyps with a sensitivity and specificity of 100% and 99%, respectively. However, using a similar system, Yashke et al. [44] could not identify a consistent laser-induced autofluorescence signature to distinguish between normal and abnormal tissue. In a study limited to small (<5 mm) adenomatous polyps, Richards-Kortum et al. [45] used a laboratory spectrofluorimeter to examine the excitation-emission spectra of surgically excised colons from patients with familial adenomatous polyposis. By analyzing excitation-emission matrices, they identified several promising excitation wavelength regions for differentiating normal from adenomatous tissue with an accuracy >95% [45]. Marchesini and co-workers [46] have examined laser-induced fluorescence in biopsy specimens of colonic mucosa using blue excitation light (410 nm wavelength) to excite fluorescence. Using a multivariate linear regression analysis, they achieved a sensitivity and specificity of 81% and 90%, respectively, for discriminating neoplastic from non-neoplastic mucosa.

These in vitro studies have subsequently led to in vivo studies of laser-induced fluorescence. Schomacker and co-workers [47] used a pulsed nitrogen laser (wavelength 337 nm) to excite fluorescence in patients found to have polyps at the time of routine diagnostic colonoscopy. After resection, the polyps were classified by pathological analysis. The fluorescence data from the 35 hyperplastic and 49 adenomatous polyps were subjected to a multivariate linear regression analysis. The resulting algorithm was able to correctly classify 80% of hyperplastic polyps and 86% of adenomatous polyps. This corresponded to a predicative value positive of 86% and a predictive value negative of 80%. These predictive values were comparable to the accuracy of clinical pathology using independent review by two senior pathologists as the gold standard [47]. Cothren et al. [48] reported their experience with laser-induced autofluorescence in 20 patients. Based upon their in vitro work, which suggested that an excitation wavelength of 370 nm would optimally distinguish between normal and adenomatous tissue [45], Cothren et al. used a nitrogen-pumped dye laser system to excite tissue autofluorescence at this wavelength [48]. Thirty-one adenomatous polyps, four hyperplastic polyps, and 32 normal areas were measured. Adenomatous polyps could be correctly distinguished from normal mucosa in 97% of instances. However, the number of hyperplastic polyps was too small to make firm conclusions about the ability of the technique to differentiate between adenomatous and hyperplastic polyps [48].

In summary, laser-induced autofluorescence appears to be capable of distinguishing between polyp types with an accuracy comparable to clinical pathology. If these studies can be confirmed by others, laser-induced autofluorescence would become a useful adjunct to diagnostic colonoscopy. However, at this point, the clinical experience is insufficient to recommend widespread clinical implementation. Although the technique appears to hold clinical promise, it is far from optimized. The fluorophores responsible for producing the signals remain unknown and only a limited number of excitation wavelengths have been examined in vivo. The optimal wavelength in any given situation is unknown and the optimal means of analyzing the data and producing an discriminating algorithm remain elusive. Optical diagnostic techniques might be greatly enhanced by exogenously administered fluorescence compounds that selectively localize within specific tissues [49]. For example, a number of compounds developed for use in photodynamic therapy appear to be selectively taken up and retained by neoplastic tissue. If these compounds can be used at doses that are nontoxic, they might become useful adjuncts to the diagnostic capabilities of laser-induced fluorescence. Other techniques such as Raman spectroscopy and near-infrared spectroscopy have been examined only in a cursory fashion but carry tremendous potential for identifying tissue type and tissue constituents. Optical diagnostics remains a fertile area of research and appears to possess vast potential for enhancing gastrointestinal endoscopy.

FUTURE APPLICATIONS OF LASERS IN GASTROENTEROLOGY

It is impossible to predict future applications of lasers in gastroenterology with any certainty but as noted throughout this review, many current applications continue to be the basis of ongoing investigations. These studies will likely lead to improved outcomes of laser-based methods as well as a better appreciation for the optimal role of laser technology in the endoscopic management of patients. The development of new applications will undoubtedly be spurred on by the introduction of new laser sources and new delivery devices as well as an improved understanding of the interactions of light with tissue, photosensitizing drugs, and biological systems.

REFERENCES

1. Fleischer D, Kessler F, Haye O. Endoscopic Nd:YAG laser therapy for carcinoma of the esophagus: A new palliative approach. Am J Surg 1982;143:280–283.
2. Pietraffita J, Dwyer R. Endoscopic laser therapy of malignant esophageal obstruction. Arch Surg 1986;121:395–400.
3. Mellow MH, Pinkas A. Endoscopic laser therapy for malignancies affecting the esophagus and gastroesophageal junction: Analysis of technical and functional efficacy. Arch Intern Med 1985;145:1443–1446.
4. Fleischer D, Sivak MV. Endoscopic Nd:YAG laser therapy as palliation for esophagogastric cancer: Parameters effecting initial outcome. Gastroenterology 1985;89:827–831.
5. Loizou LA, Grigg D, Atkinson M, Robertson C, Bown SG. A prospective comparison of laser therapy and intubation in endoscopic palliation for malignant dysphagia. Gastroenterology 1991;100:1303–1310.
6. Jensen DM, Machicado G, Randall G, Tung LA, English-Zych S. Comparison of low-power YAG laser and BICAP tumor probe for palliation of esophageal cancer strictures. Gastroenterology 1988;94:1263–1270.
7. Karlin DA, Fisher RS, Krevsky B. Prolonged survival and effective palliation in patients with squamous cell carcinoma of the esophagus following endoscopic laser therapy. Cancer 1987;59:1969–1972.
8. Fleischer D. The Washington symposium on endoscopic laser therapy. Gastrointest Endosc 1985;31:397–400.
9. Mathus-Vliegen EMH. Treatment modalities in colorectal cancer. In: Krasner N, ed. "Lasers in Gastroenterology." New York: Wiley-Liss, 1991:151–177.
10. Lambert R, Sabben G, Guyot P, Chavaillon A, Descos F. Cancer of the rectum: results of laser treatment. Laser Surg Med 1984;3:342.
11. Heier S, Rothman K, Heier L, et al. Final results of a randomized trial: photodynamic therapy vs. Nd:YAG laser therapy. Gastroenterology 1993;104:A408.
12. Overholt B, Panjehpour M, Tefftellar E, Rose M. Photodynamic therapy for treatment of early adenocarcinoma in Barrett's esophagus. Gastrointest Endosc 1993;39:73–76.
13. Suzuki H, Miho O, Watanabe Y, et al. Endoscopic laser therapy in the curative and palliative treatment of upper gastrointestinal cancer. World J Surg 1989;13:158–164.
14. Barr H, Krasner N, Boulos PB, Chatlani P, Brown SG. Photodynamic therapy for colorectal cancer: a quantitative pilot study. Br J Surg 1990;77:93–96.
15. McCaughan JS, Mertens BF. Cho C, Barabash RD, Payton HW. Photodynamic therapy to treat tumors of the

extrahepatic biliary ducts: A case report. Arch Surg 1991;126:111–113.

16. Fruhmorgen P, Bodem F, Reidenback HD, et al. The first endoscopic laser coagulation in the human gi tract. Endoscopy 1976;7:156–157.

17. Swain CP, Bown SG, Storey DW, et al. Controlled trial of argon laser photocoagulation in bleeding peptic ulcers. Lancet 1981:2:1313–1316.

18. Swain CP, Kirkham JS, Salmon PR, Bown SG, Northfield TC. Controlled trial of Nd:YAG laser photocoagulation in bleeding peptic ulcers. Lancet 1986;1:1113–1116.

19. Krejs GJ, Little KH, Westergaard H, Hamilton JK, Polter DE. Laser photocoagulation for the treatment of acute peptic ulcer bleeding: A randomized controlled clinical trial. N Engl J Med 1987;316:1618–1621.

20. Rutgeerts P, Vantrappen G, Broeckaert L, Coremans G, Janssens J, Geboes K. A new and effective technique of YAG laser photocoagulation for severe upper gastrointestinal bleeding. Endoscopy 1984;16:115–117.

21. Matthewson K, Swain CP, Bland M, Kirkham JS, Bown SG, Northfield TC. A randomized comparison of Nd:YAG laser, heater probe and no endoscopic therapy for bleeding peptic ulcer. Gut 1987;10:A1342.

22. Rutgeerts P, Vantrappen G, Van Hootgem P, et al. Nd:YAG laser photocoagulation versus multipolar electrocoagulation for the treatment of severely bleeding ulcers: A randomized comparison. Gastrointest Endosc 1987;33:199–202.

23. Nishioka NS, Tan OT, Bronstein BR, Farinelli WA, Richter JM, Parrish JA, Anderson RR. Selective vascular coagulation of the rabbit colon using a flashlamp-excited dye laser operating at 577 nanometers. Gastroenterology 1988;95:1258–1264.

24. Waitman AM, Graut DZ, Chateau F. Argon laser photocoagulation treatment of patients with acute and chronic bleeding secondary to telangiectasia. Gastrointest Endosc 1982;28:153.

25. Jensen DM, Machicado GM, Silpa ML. Treatment of GI angioma with argon laser, heater probe or bipolar electrocoagulation. Gastrointest Endosc 1984;30:134.

26. Rutgeerts P, VanGompel F, Geboes K, Vantrappen G, Broeckaert L, Coremans G. Long term results of treatment of vascular malformations of the gastrointestinal tract by Neodymium-YAG laser photocoagulation. Gut 1985;26:586–593.

27. Johnston JH. Complications follwoing endoscopic laser therapy. Gastrointest Endosc 1982;26:134–138.

28. Gostout CJ, Ahlquis DA, Radford CM, Viggiano TR, Bowyer BA, Balm RK. Endoscopic laser therapy for watermelon stomach. Gastroenterology 1989;96:1462–1465.

29. Bjorkman DJ, Buchi KN. Endoscopic laser therapy of the watermelon stomach. Lasers Surg Med 1992;12:478–481.

30. Viggiano TR, Zighelboim J, Ahlquist DA, Gostout CJ, Wang KK, Larson MV. Endoscopic Nd:YAG laser coagulation of bleeding from radiation proctopathy. Gastrointest Endosc 1993;39:513–517.

31. Masters A, Steger AC, Bown SG. Reviews: Role of interstitial therapy in the treatment of liver cancer. British J Surg 1991;78:518–523.

32. Amin Z, Donald JJ, Masters A, Kant R, Steger AC, Bown SG, Lees WR. Hepatic metastases: Interstitial laser photocoagulation with real-time US monitoring and dynamic CT evaluation of treatment. Radiology 1993;187:339–347.

33. Nishioka NS. Laser lithotripsy of biliary calculi. Seminars in Interventional Radiology 1988;5:202–206.

34. Watson GM, Wickham JEA, Mills ATN, Bown SG, Swain P, Salmon PR. Laser fragmentation of renal calculi. Brit J Urol 1983;55:613–616.

35. Nishioka NS, Levins PC, Murray SC, Parrish JA, Anderson RR. Fragmentation of biliary calculi with tunable dye lasers. Gastroenterology 1987;93:250–255.

36. Ell C, Lux G, Hochberger J, Muller D, Demling L. Laser-lithotripsy of common bile duct stones. Gut 1988;29:746–51.

37. Cotton PB, Kozarek RA, Schapiro RH, Nishioka NS, Kelsey PB, Ball TJ, Putnam WS, Weinerth J. Endoscopic laser lithotripsy of large bile duct stones. Gastroenterology 1990;99:1128–1133.

38. Ell C, Hochberger J, May A, Fleig WE, Bauer R, Mendez L, Hahn EG. Laser lithotripsy of difficult bile duct stones by means of a rhodamine-6G laser and an integrated automatic stone-tissue detection system. Gastrointest Endosc 1993;39:755–62.

39. Nishioka NS. Laser-induced fluorescence spectroscopy. Clinics in Gastrointestinal Endoscopy, 1994;4:313–326.

40. Chance B, Cohen P, Jobsis F, Schoener B. Intracellular oxidation-reduction states in vivo. Science 1962;137:499–508.

41. Salarma G, Lombardi R, Elson J. Maps of optical action potentials and NADH fluorescence in intact working hearts. Am J Physiol 1987;252:H384–H394.

42. Alfano RR, Tata DB, Cordero J, et al. Laser induced fluorescence spectroscopy from native cancerous and normal tissue. IEEE J Quantum Electronics 1984;QE-20:1507–1511.

43. Kapadia CR, Cutruzzola FW, O'Brian KM, Stetz ML, Enriquez R, Deckelbaum LI. Laser-induced fluorescence spectroscopy on human colonic mucosa. Gastroenterology 1990;99:150–157.

44. Yashke PN, Bonner RF, Cohen P, Leon MB, Fleischer DE. Laser-induced fluorescence spectroscopy may distinguish colon cancer from normal human colon. Gastrointest Endosc 1989;35:184.

45. Richards-Kortum R, Rava RP, Petras RE, et al. Spectroscopic diagnosis of colonic dysplasia. Photochem Photobiol 1991;53:777–786.

46. Marchesini R, Brambilla M, Pignoli E etal. Light-induced fluorescence spectroscopy of adenomas, adenocarcinomas and non-neoplastic mucoa in human colon. J Photochem Photobiol B: Biol 1992;14:219–230.

47. Schomacker KT, Frisoli JK, Compton CC, Flotte TJ, Richter JM, Deutsch TF, Nishioka NS. Ultraviolet laser-induced fluorescence of colonic polyps. Gastroenterology 1992;104:1155–1160.

48. Cothren RM, Richards-Kortum R, Sivak MV Jr, et al. Gastrointestinal tissue diagnosis by laser-induced fluorescence spectroscopy at endoscopy. Gastrointest Endosc 1990;36:105–111.

49. Bjorkman DJ, Brigham EJ, Peterson BJ, Straight RC. Photofrin II localization in rat cecum. Lasers Surg Med 1989;9:286–289.

Chapter 5

Lasers in Gynecology: Why Pragmatic Surgeons Have Not Abandoned This Valuable Technology

Richard Reid, MD, and Gregory T. Absten, MA

Gynecologic Laser Surgery, Sinai Hospital, Detroit, Michigan (R.R.); Gynecologic Endoscopy, Crittenton Hospital, Rochester, Michigan (R.R.); Department of Obstetrics & Gynecology, Wayne State University School of Medicine, Detroit, Michigan (R.R.); Advanced Laser Services Corp., Grove City, Ohio (G.T.A.); Ohio State University College of Medicine, Columbus, Ohio (G.T.A.)

INTRODUCTION

Understanding how radiant energy interacts with matter requires a brief look at atomic physics. Light is a traveling packet (photon) of electromagnetic energy, possessing both particle and wavelike properties. Light can be formed either by nuclear fusion (sunlight), nuclear fission (atomic bombs), or by changes in the electronic structures of atoms and molecules (gaslight, electric light, etc.). This latter mechanism is relevant to a discussion of lasers.

Atoms and molecules are quantum systems, wherein each electron orbit surrounding the nucleus represents a discrete energy level. When an atom or molecule is impinged upon by a suitable quantity of transmitted energy, one of these orbiting electrons will be pushed into a more distant orbit. This process is called "absorption" and corresponds to an increase in the kinetic energy carried by the displaced electron (Fig. 1) [1]. When the electron drops back to its original orbit—a process termed "spontaneous emission"—the excess kinetic energy is emitted as a photon of electromagnetic radiation (light). Spontaneous emission of light is a random process. Thus natural light contains multiple colors. Component waves travel in all directions and display different temporal phases.

Lasers are instruments in which a suitable medium is stimulated by an external energy source to emit an artificial energy known as *co-herent light*. "Coherent" means that the energy exists as a series of monochromatic, highly parallel energy waves, each sharing the same spatial and temporal phase (Fig. 2) [1,3]. Laser beams can therefore be focused to a spot much smaller than sunlight. Hence, energy densities can be concentrated sufficiently to coagulate or vaporize tissue.

Space does not permit a complete explanation of laser physics; however, a glossary of laser terminology is included at the end of this report.

INSTRUMENTATION: PRINCIPLES AND PRACTICALITIES
What Is a Laser?

Lasers have three basic elements—an active medium, a resonator cavity, and an excitation mechanism [4]. These three elements, together with safety and control adaptations, are secured within an outer console.

Lasers are characterized by their *active medium*. First, depending upon the physical state of this substance, lasers are described as solid, liquid, or gas. Second, because the spectrum of wavelengths emitted by each element is unique, lasers are also named by the active medium from which they were generated. It must be remembered that visible light is only one small portion of an electromagnetic spectrum that spans from the long wavelengths of radio to the very short waves of X-rays and beyond (Fig. 3). Theoretically, a laser

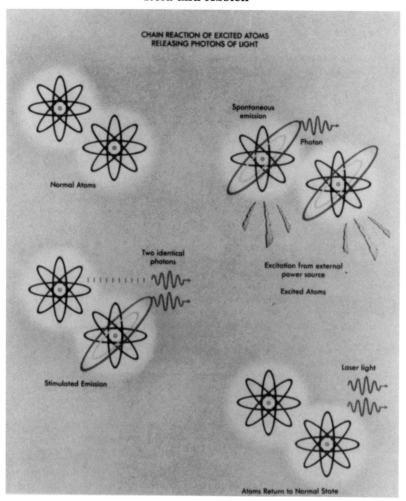

Fig. 1. Laser action relies on assembling a large population of atoms or molecules, excited by the absorption of energy from an external source. A small number of these excited atoms spontaneously release their energy into the laser medium, where they impact other excited atoms or molecules and stimulate the emission of identical photons, traveling in step with them. Release of additional photons increases the probability of stimulated emission, resulting in a chain reaction. This avalanche of light is the underlying process that creates a laser beam. (From Trost et al. [1], reprinted with permission.)

could be produced that would emit light at any point within the electromagnetic spectrum.

From the viewpoint of the physicist, all of these lasers share common properties, about which useful generalizations can be made. However, from the viewpoint of the physician, each laser in the medical armentarium was chosen because its emissions produce a unique tissue effect. Hence, the extent to which surgeons can generalize about different lasers is quite limited. That is to say, expertise garnered with one laser wavelength does not confer expertise with a different wavelength. Each instrument and each application must be learned specifically.

The second element of a laser is the *excitation mechanism*. For a quantum system to emit coherent radiation, the lasing medium must be "pumped" to "population inversion" by optical (e.g., a xenon or krypton lamp) or electrical energy (e.g., high voltage or radio frequency current). "Population inversion" refers to a situation in which there are more atoms or molecules in an upper level energy state than in one of the lower levels. Within a short time, some of these excited atoms or molecules will spontaneously return to the lower energy level, emitting the extra kinetic energy as a photon of electromagnetic energy. Some of these photons will strike atoms or molecules that are still at the higher level, thereby stimulating emission of a second photon that will be in the same temporal phase and propagated in the same direction.

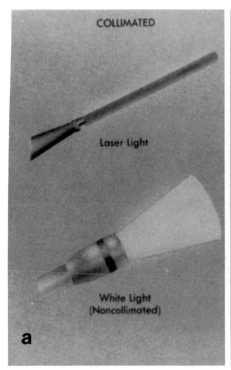
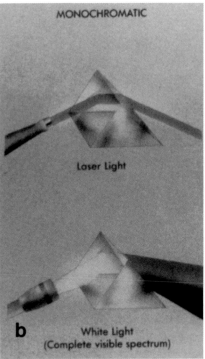
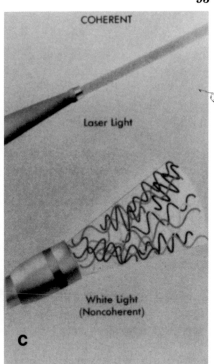

Fig. 2. **a:** Laser light may be highly collimated. This means that it can travel very long distances with minimal divergence. This property also allows laser light to be focused to very high intensity. **b:** Laser light may also be more monochromatic than any other light source. This means that it may consist of a very pure single color. **c:** Lasers also may be highly coherent. This means that the light waves travel in step with each other, crest to crest and valley to valley. (From Trost et al. [1], reprinted with permission.)

Laser efficiency ranges from fractions of a percent to as great as 30% [4]. Energy not converted to coherent light is generally transformed into heat, which must be dissipated by air cooling fans, water-to-air heat exchanger, or circulating tap water. Herein lies much of the cost and most of the noise that comes from operating the laser.

The third component is the *resonator,* an optical cavity that contains the active medium and a scheme to optimize stimulated emission. This is accomplished by placing co-axial mirrors at opposite ends of the optical cavity. Photons of light created by spontaneous or stimulated emission resonate back and forth by successive reflections from the end mirrors. With the release of each new photon, the rate of stimulated emission increases rapidly through an avalanche process. By making one of the mirrors partially transmissive, a portion of this energy will be given off as a laser beam (Fig. 4).

Laser Delivery Systems

The intense beam of monochromatic coherent light emitted from the partially transmissive end mirror must be delivered to the target. Several different delivery methods exist, depending upon wavelength, operating power, desired spot size, and accessibility of the target (Table 1). The two systems of importance to the gynecologist are reflection through articulating arms and transmission through fiberoptics or waveguides.

An *articulating arm* is a series of hollow tubes and mirrors. The laser beam is transmitted through each tube and is then reflected into the next tube by an appropriately angled mirror. This system provides excellent precision, particularly when adapted to an operating microscope. However, articulating arms are bulky, awkward, and expensive, and they require significant maintenance. Hence, articulating arms are really only used for the CO_2 laser, because this midinfrared radiation destroys the quartz or silica cores of optical fibers.

Waveguides are long, semiflexible steel tubes lined by ceramic tile. Laser energy is reflected down the tube by bouncing the beam off the lateral walls. This system delivers ~75% of input energy up to a maximum power of 40 W. The typical waveguides have 3 mm outer sheath

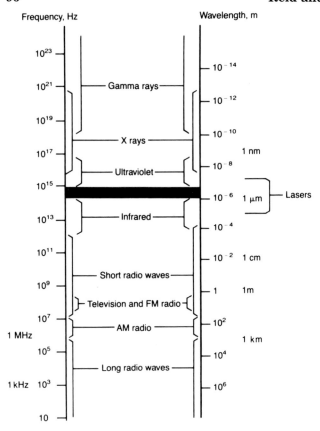

Frequency, Hz   Wavelength, m

Fig. 3. The electromagnetic spectrum. Lasers extend from the ultraviolet region through the entire visible region into the infrared region. (From Fuller [4], reprinted with permission.)

diameters, core diameters of 1 mm, and lengths of 40–50 cm. Hence, they fit through 5 mm trocar sleeves. Optically, the guide functions much as a true quartz laser fiber. It allows the operator to palpate a target and eliminates the need for aligning the beam down the operative channel. However, waveguides destroy the properties of coherence and collimation, making it hard to create a fine incision.

Fiberoptics are long, thin, flexible optical elements coated in opaque nylon or metal casings, which can capture and transmit visible and near infrared radiation down the length of the fiberoptic. Laser energy is transmitted along the fiberoptic by reflection off the opaque casing. Hence, the property of intense collimation is lost (Fig. 5). Rather, laser beams emerging from the tip of a flat cleaved fiberoptic diverge at an angle of about 12–15°. Thus, when the fiberoptic is held just above tissue, delivered energy will usually be of sufficient intensity to produce vaporization. Withdrawing the fiber a centimeter or two will

typically reduce delivered energy to the coagulation range.

In about the early 1980s, surgeons began replacing the flat, cleaved tip of a regular fiber with "hot tips" (variously termed adaptations such as sapphire "probes" or "crystals" and "sculptured tips") [5–8]. These adaptations produce a delivery device that expands the flexibility of laser performance, particularly that of the near infrared lasers. It should be stressed, however, that the predominant mechanism of action of these contact probes is quite different from that of a free beam [9]. Tissue effects derive not from direct beam absorption, but rather from the use of the laser energy to heat the crystal itself. The real point is that "hot tips" have added significantly to the versatility of the laparoscopist's armamentarium, by allowing visible and near infrared lasers to cut or coagulate, with much more favorable thermal effects than would be obtained from the same laser energy delivered through a bare fiber [6,9]. Tissue effects are not perfect; hence, hot tips should not be the first choice for surface applications. However, tissue effects are quite acceptable for endoscopic surgery (Table 2).

Rounding or sharpening the fiber tip completely disrupts the optical properties of the fiberoptic. Instead of being transmitted as a free beam (Fig. 6a), laser energy is reflected within the *sculptured fiber,* thus heating the tip to act like a "hot knife". Particularly when used in combination with the high frequency pulsed Nd:YAG laser, these sculptured tips can produce very fine and very rapid incisions, even within a pool of irrigating fluid.

Synthetic sapphire tips (actually, translucent ceramics) have evolved nicely for endoscopic use, incorporating such shapes as cone points, wedges, and rounded balls (Fig. 6b). Each geometric pattern dissects or coagulates tissue a little differently, and surgeons generally develop a personal preference for two or three shapes. One advantage of the sapphire probes over sculpted fibers is that they are bulkier—at the base, not the actual tip. Hence, sapphire tips act as thermal reservoirs to store heat for sustained vaporization. Both devices work well for fine dissection, but the bulkier tips are distinctly more efficient for dissecting thick or bloody tissues.

For efficient retention of the laser energy with the hot tip, all of these devices need some degree of surface discoloration. In a ritual known as "burning in," the fiber is held against blood or some noncritical tissue to heat and discolor the

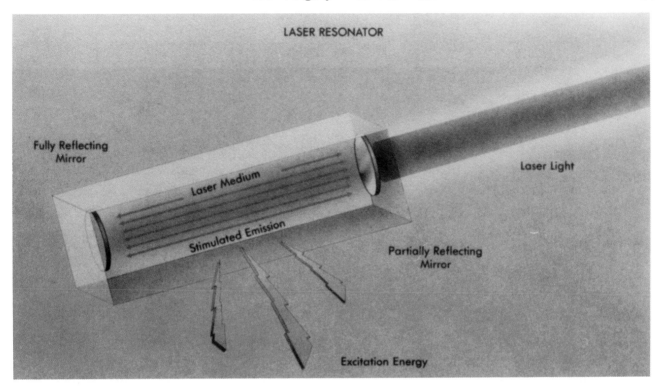

Fig. 4. A laser consists of an active medium that is raised to an excited state by an external energy source, such as a flash-lamp or an electric discharge. The resulting process of stimulated emission in the active medium produces an abundance of light photons, all at the same wavelength. A pair of mirrors at each end of the active laser medium reflects the light back and forth on itself, to increase the probability of stimulated emission. One of the mirrors allows a small fraction of the light to leak through, resulting in the output of a beam of laser light. (From Trost et al. [1], reprinted with permission.)

TABLE 1. Classifications of Laser Delivery Systems

Noncontact (free beam): Only the laser beam interacts with tissue → predominant optical effect.
- Articulated arm and lens system (CO_2 laser delivered through operating microscope or handpiece).
- Fiber-optic cable (argon laser delivered through endoscope).
- Waveguide (CO_2 laser through laparoscope).

Contact (hot tips): Energy concentrated at tip → cautery effect (+ partial transmission).
- Hot tips (sapphire, ceramic, metallic).
- Tapered fibers.

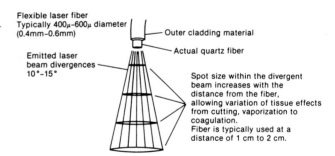

Fig. 5. Loss of collimation occurs as the laser beam diverges at a 10–15° angle from the quartz tip. Thus the spot size progressively enlarges the farther the laser travels from the quartz tip. (From Absten [9], reprinted with permission.)

"virgin tip." Once blackened, the hot tip will immediately cut with full efficiency. Alternatively, some manufacturers apply a special coating to the tip so as automatically to initiate this "burn-in" process.

Lasers Relevant to Gynecology

Thousands of wavelengths have been identified from hundreds of active materials. However, major gynecologic applications exist for only seven of these instruments.

Carbon dioxide. The CO_2 laser was developed in 1964 at Bell Laboratories by CKN Patel. It generates energy at a wavelength of 10.6 μm (10,600 nm), which is in the midinfrared region of the electromagnetic spectrum. The resonant cavity contains a mixture of CO_2, argon, and helium. The active medium, however, is CO_2 gas. The other two gases are included to improve laser efficiency.

TABLE 2. Physical Characteristics and Surgical Properties of Four Major Situations in Which Lasers Are Used

	High-power CO_2 laser	Visible and near-infrared	Hot tips sculptured fibers	Low-power CO_2 laser
Absorption length	Very short	Long	No direct laser-tissue interaction occurs	Very short
Scatter	Negligible	High	No direct laser-tissue interaction occurs	Negligible
Chromophore	Water molecules	Wavelength specific (e.g., Nd:YAG-protein; visible beam-hemoglobin or melanin)	No direct laser-tissue interaction occurs	Water molecules
Color selectivity	Nil	High	Nil	Nil
Method of beam delivery	Articulated arm and mirrors	Fiber-optic cable	Fiber-optic cable	Articulated arm arm and mirrors
Vaporization efficiency	Very high	Low	Moderate	Moderate
Wound characteristics	Clean crater with negligible subjacent thermal injury	Small crater with wide zone of adjacent photo-coagulation	Desiccated crater with extensive subjacent conduction burn	Carbonized crater with extensive subjacent con-duction burn
Width of tissue damage	Same as diameter of incident beam	Determined by scatter (many times wider than incident beam, but constant for a given wavelength)	Moderately wider than incident beam (typically, about 1 mm on each side)	Determined by exposure time and crater temperature (i.e., much wider than crater diam-eter)
Depth of tissue damage	Same as crater depth	Determined by extinction length and tissue color, but constant for that wavelength	Determined by tip temperature and speed of movement (typically, about 1 mm)	Determined by exposure time and crater temperature
Basis of depth control	Visual estimate of crater depth	Knowledge of extinction length for that wavelength	Crude visual estimate of crater depth	No reliable method (depth of coagu-lation necrosis $\neq$ crater depth)
Precision	Very high	High	Moderate	Low to dangerous
Comparability to good electrosurgery	Superior	Deep coagulation (superior)	Inferior	Markedly inferior
Hemostatic properties	Limited, but valuable	High/very high	High	High (but not worth the additional conduction burn)
Surgical applications	1. Precise but blood-less thermal incision of aqueous tissues 2. Precise shallow depth ablation of aqueous tissues	1. Selective destruction of pigmented lesions (e.g., FPDL for vulvodynia) 2. Deep but controlled coagulation of diseased epithelium (e.g., Nd:YAG endometrial ablation) 3. Incision/ablation in areas of difficult access (e.g., argon laser in endoscopy)	Crude thermal dissection in noncritical areas	Nil (obsolete)

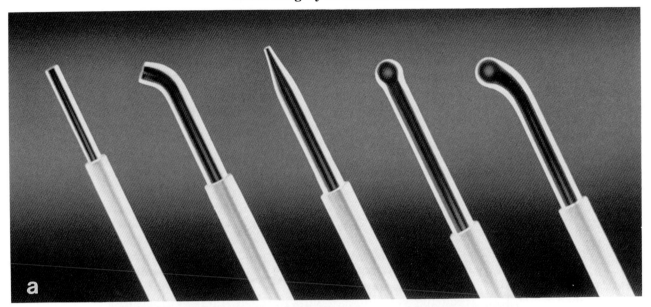

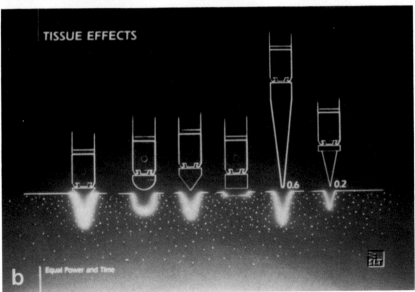

Fig. 6. **a:** Sculptured fibers (illustration courtesy Surgimedics/ESP, The Woodlands, TX). **b:** Sapphire tips: How they deliver heat (illustration courtesy Surgimedics).

In the conventional design of CO_2 lasers, a gas mixture flows through a hollow laser cavity where the CO_2 gas mixture is energized by high voltage electrical discharge. This stimulates emission of coherent light, but it results in disassociation of the active CO_2 molecule into carbon monoxide and a free oxygen radical. This fractured CO_2 molecule is no longer able to produce coherent light and must be either pumped away or recombined. Lasers that replenish used CO_2 with fresh CO_2 molecules are called "flowing gas systems." Historically, they carried the advan- tages of reliable, steady output and easy genera- tion of high powers. However, gas pumps make the laser bulky and noisy and add substantially to operating costs (because of the continuous need to purchase new cylinders of specially mixed gases). Sealed tube lasers are a newer technology that eliminates the need for replacement of the gas mixture. In the past, sealed tube lasers were ex- cited by direct current. This is an inefficient mechanism, which often sacrificed operating power. However, a newly developed excitation mechanism using radio frequency current (the

Ultrapulse™) has produced a laser capable of sustaining average powers in superpulsed mode that were hitherto unobtainable [9].

Nd:YAG. The neodymium:glass laser was discovered in 1961; however, the low thermal conductivity of glass posed operating problems. Hence, neodymium was doped into yttrium aluminum garnet and placed in a reflective optical cavity with krypoton arc flashlamps as the excitation source. Nd:YAG lasers emit near infrared radiation at 1.06 μm, with an operating power up to 120 watts. Early model Nd:YAG lasers required 230 volts, three phase electricity, and water cooling. However, there are now more efficient models, which utilize 115 volt power sources and air cooling. In addition to operating the Nd:YAG laser in continuous wave manner, this instrument can be configured to operate in superpulsed or Q-switched mode, thus producing very different types of tissue interactions.

Erbium:YAG. In the future, erbium:YAG lasers may allow even more precise surgery upon aqueous tissues [10]. The Er:YAG laser emits high energy pulses of midinfrared light with a wavelength of 2,940 nanometers (2.9 μm). The peak absorption of light in water occurs in the 2.9 μm range, making the Er:YAG laser energy even more highly absorbed in aqueous tissues than CO_2 laser energy (at 10.6 μm). The combination of high water affinity and high fluence pulses produces an exceptionally narrow zone of damage around the vaporization crater. Hence, the Er:YAG has been tried for corneal resculpting, a task generally reserved for the excimer laser. The Er:YAG laser is also very highly absorbed by osseous minerals, making it a highly precise drill and saw for bone surgery and dentistry.

Holmium:YAG. The most recent addition to the growing array of surgical lasers is the holmium:YAG laser, which emits 0.25 millisecond pulses of midinfrared energy (2.1 μm). The laser medium is holmium, a rare earth element, within an yttrium aluminum garnet crystal. The holmium:YAG laser is excited by a xenon arc flashlamp and currently produces up to 100 watts of laser power. Like the CO_2 laser, Ho:YAG energy is strongly absorbed by water, making it a useful tool for ablating most soft tissues. Unlike the CO_2 laser, Ho:YAG energy can be delivered through a flexible optical glass fiber, and can be operated effectively in an aqueous environment [1]. The Ho:YAG laser has proven very useful for arthroscopic treatment of torn menisci, articular degeneration, and synovial disease. The same proper-

ties also make this laser highly attractive to the advanced laparoscopic surgeon. Although Ho:YAG energy has a slightly longer absorption length than CO_2 energy, the strongly pulsed nature of the laser emission and the freedom from "thermal blooming" allow the Ho:YAG fiber to make a finer incision than an endoscopically delivered CO_2 beam.

Argon ion. The first laser emission from a gaseous ion was observed at Bell Laboratories in 1963. Within a year, >150 ionic emission lines were discovered, mainly coming from the noble gases (neon, argon, krypton, and xenon). Exposure of one of these gases to high electrical current densities ionized the gas molecule, resulting in two characteristic laser bands: a 488 nm (blue) and 514 nm (green). The high electrical current necessary for the ionization of the argon gas results in considerable dissipation of heat. Thus argon lasers tend to be inefficient. Large argon ion lasers can develop up to 15 watts; smaller ophthalmic models typically emit only 3–4 watts.

KTP. Passing Nd:YAG energy through a potassium titanyl phosphate (KTP) crystal doubles the frequency of transmitted laser light. However, since frequency is the inverse of wavelength, physicians generally think of the KTP laser emission as having half the wavelength (532 nm, 1,064 nm) of the parent Nd:YAG energy (532 nm). This method of beam generation is substantially more efficient than the argon ion laser; hence, air-cooled KTP lasers can easily generate powers of 20 watts. KTP laser energy is more highly absorbed by hemoglobin than is the argon laser. Moreover, KTP laser light is emitted as a high frequency train of pulses. The interval between pulses is so short that the KTP beam appears quasicontinuous to the naked eye. Nonetheless, the combined effect of greater color selectivity and some interpulse cooling does indeed reduce secondary heat conduction.

Dye lasers. A variety of liquid dyes are used in dye lasers as the laser medium and a very bright light (e.g., a xenon arc flashlamp or an argon laser) as the excitation source. Wavelength varies from 400–700 nm, depending upon the particular dye selected. Power output typically ranges to 5 watts. Three types of dye laser are important in genitourinary medicine.

1. A flashlamp excited dye laser utilizing Rhodamine 585nm dye (Candela SPTL 1A) emits 300–450 microsecond pulses of 585 nm energy. This wavelength (yellow light) has extreme af-

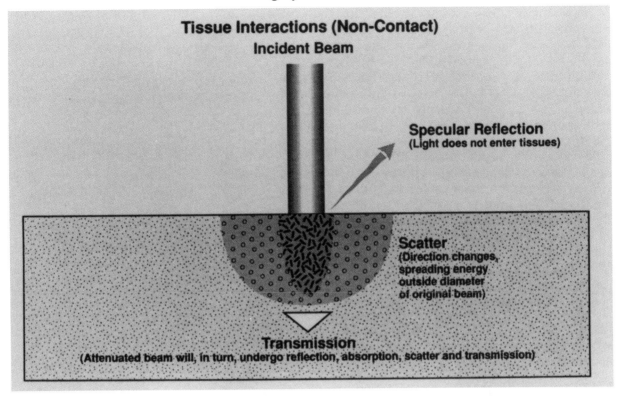

Fig. 7. Generic diagram of events at the site of laser impact. (From Reid [209], reproduced with permission.)

finity for hemoglobin and hence can be used as an instrument for selective destruction of abnormal blood vessels.

2. A flashlamp excited dye laser utilizing Coumarin dye (Candela MDL) emits ultrashort but extremely powerful (140 mJ) pulses of visible green energy. Pulsed dye lasers at 504 nm can literally fracture kidney stones, thus eliminating the need for an open surgical procedure. The laser vaporizes and ionizes segments of the stone to produce a plasma. The plasma is confined by the irrigant used during ureteroscopy and instantaneously reaches high pressures to generate a shock wave that fragments the stone. Because the 504 nm wavelength lies between the major two absorption bands of hemoglobin, less damage results to the ureteral wall if the laser energy is misguided. The combination of wavelength, pulse duration, and small-diameter fiber determines the size of the stone fragments produced by laser treatment.

3. A tunable dye laser emits 630 nm energy (red light) used to cause a photochemical reaction on a drug used in experimental cancer therapy.

FACTORS INFLUENCING LASER CHOICE

Choosing the best laser for a given surgical application depends on four things: (1) the absorptive characteristics of the tissue to be destroyed, (2) the wavelength of the emitted radiation, (3) the temporal parameters of the delivered energy, and (4) the mechanism of beam delivery.

Absorptive Characteristics

Electromagnetic radiation that impinges upon tissue can be reflected, scattered, absorbed, or transmitted (Fig. 7). Generically, any matter that impedes the passage of light causes nonspecific heating. Selective surgical advantage, however, depends on the presence of suitable chromophores (molecules capable of absorbing the incident radiation and converting it to heat). The potential for therapeutic advantage depends on the ratio of "target" vs. "competing" chromophores. A high ratio will facilitate selective destruction of diseased cells, whereas a low ratio will predispose to excessive damage of adjacent tissues.

The target chromophores for CO_2, Er:YAG, and Ho:YAG lasers are *water molecules*. Hence, this wavelength offers a useful method for the photovaporization of any tissue that has a high water content (epithelium, connective tissue, brain, or muscle). In contrast, CO_2 laser energy is poorly absorbed by nonaqueous tissue (fat, bone). On such tissue, CO_2 lasers produce diffuse conduction burns or actual flaming rather than a photovaporization crater. However, infiltration with an adequate volume of aqueous fluid (e.g., dilute vasopressin solution) will allow the CO_2 laser to cut subcutaneous fat or breast tissue.

The target chromophores for Nd:YAG radiation are *proteins* and *red or black pigment* molecules. Therefore, this instrument is an excellent tool for deep destruction of the diseased wall of a hollow viscus (e.g., endometrial ablation for menorrhagia, bladder wall coagulation for superficial cancers). Nd:YAG is also valuable for coagulation of heavily vascularized tissue (e.g., hepatic resection, transection of uterine septae). However, the very characteristics that make this wavelength useful for the above purposes also disqualify bare fiber Nd:YAG for use as an instrument of delicate surgery.

Absorption of argon, KTP, and flashlamp excited laser energy is color dependent, thus providing a potential for selective destruction of cells containing endogenous chromophores or light sensitive drugs. Lasers from the visible portion of the electromagnetic spectrum generally target *hemoglobin* as a means of selectively sclerosing blood vessels (Fig. 8). Their usefulness depends on the ratio of target (oxyhemoglobin) to competing chromophores (melanin or mitochondrial enzymes).

Relatively low levels of 630 nm red light from a tunable dye laser can be used to activate *human porphyrin derivative* (HPD), releasing toxic levels of single oxygen molecules [11]. Since HPD is selectively concentrated within malignant cells, this strategy could potentially destroy both nonresectable nodules and microscopic tumor deposits within any area that can be adequately illuminated. The promise of new, more selective HPD derivatives may increase the therapeutic advantage by making phototherapy a useful adjunct to any type of tumor debulking surgery.

Wavelength

The second consideration is wavelength, since this parameter defines the tissue interaction, color dependence, and irradiance volume.

Tissue interaction. Beam energy is in-

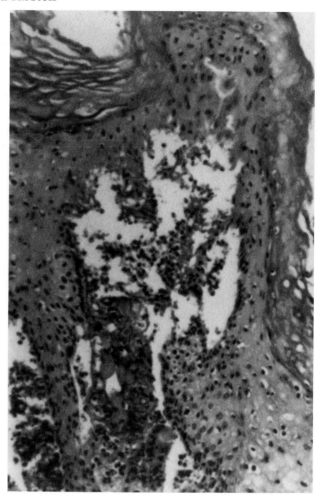

Fig. 8. Photomicrograph showing the extent to which absorption or transmission can be influenced by the presence of target chromophores. This condyloma has been irradiated with a beam from a flashlight-excited dye laser, resulting in transmission (without significant heating) through nonpigmented tissues but highly concentrated absorption (and thermal disruption) within blood vessels. (From Reid [209], reproduced with permission.)

versely proportional to wavelength. Absorption of high-energy photons (gamma rays, X-rays, and ultraviolet light) produces electron excitations that may result in ionization, dissolution of covalent bonds, and the formation of reactive molecular fragments. Excimer lasers, with a wavelength in the ultraviolet range, can photovaporize tissues by ionization rather than by thermal interaction. At the other end of the electromagnetic spectrum, the longer wavelengths of radio waves have too little energy for medical applications. Thus most surgical lasers come from the middle of the electromagnetic spectrum (the visible light and infrared regions). Such photons have insuffi-

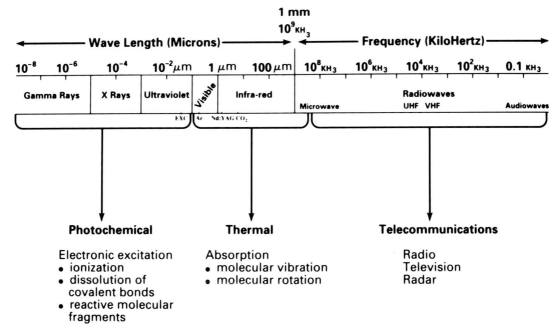

Fig. 9. Different types of tissue interaction that occur with laser energy from various points in the electromagnetic spectrum. (From Reid et al. [26], reproduced with permission.)

cient energy to induce ionization. Instead, absorption of visible light (dye, argon, KTP) and infrared (Nd: YAG, Er:YAG, Ho:YAG, and CO_2) photons increases molecular vibration or molecular rotation, leading to heat production at the impact site (Fig. 9).

Color dependence. Wavelength also determines whether absorption will be color-dependent (argon, KTP, dye, Nd: YAG) or color-independent (excimer, Er:YAG, Ho:YAG, CO_2) (Fig. 10). The physical basis of *color dependence* is easily understood by considering how light is reflected or absorbed by materials that the human eye can see. Sunlight contains all the colors in the rainbow, mixed together to appear as "white" light. Conversely, a red-colored object appears red because it absorbs the other colors in the rainbow but reflects away the red wavelengths. These red wavelengths travel to our retinas, where the reflected light is identified by our cone cells as red. In fact, "colored" objects absorb opposite colors best. "White" objects tend to reflect all visible light and "black" objects show heightened affinity for all visible wavelengths. Hence, when green or yellow laser light is used to irradiate blood vessels traversing a pale background, there is automatically a degree of preferential absorption by the red colored hemoglobin. However, this selectivity is too low for true surgical advantage.

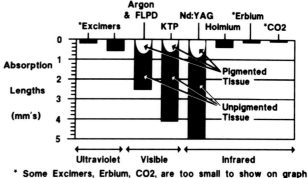

Fig. 10. Absorption lengths for the most important medical laser for those falling within the visible and near-infrared portions of the spectrum. Absorption lengths in pigmented vs. unpigmented tissues are compared. (From Laser Tissue Interaction: A Surgeon's Guide, Coherent, Palo Alto, CA, 1991, with permission.)

In addition to nonspecific color affinity, there are specific wavelengths which resonate with pigment molecules, producing a marked increased in energy absorption. Selectivity of laser–tissue interactions can therefore be amplified to the point of genuine surgical advantage. Two strategies are used. First, the surgeons must choose a wavelength that maximizes target (e.g. oxyhemoglobin) but minimizes background (e.g. dermis) absorption peaks (Fig. 11). Second, selectivity can be further refined by rapidly pulsing the laser energy. Incident light corresponding to a specific absorption peak is absorbed more quickly than light of a non-specific wavelength. Hence delivering an ideal wavelength over a shortened absorption interval can amplify selectivity of absorption within target molecules by many fold.

The opposite property—*color independence*—also needs some explanation. Midinfrared radiation is absorbed by water molecules, but not by such complex organic molecules as pigment, protein or nucleic acids. In short, CO_2, Er:YAG, or Ho:YAG energy is totally "color blind." Hence, the common practice of using blackened speculae for CO_2 laser surgery is naive. Any reduction in heat reflection off instruments comes from sandblasting the surface, so as to disrupt the mirror-like properties displayed by any polished metal.

Irradiance volume. Light striking tissue may be reflected, scattered, absorbed, or transmitted. Wavelength is the principal determinant of the qualitative differences in the tissue transfers functions of the various lasers [4]. Back scatter (reflection) and forward scatter occur with visible and near infrared beams, but not with midinfrared. Absorption length also varies markedly, according to wavelength (see Fig. 10). As described by Beer's law, the proportion of an incident beam that is transmitted through a tissue slab is determined from the equation:

$$I_x = (I_0 - I_r) \, e^{-\alpha}$$

where I_x = absorption intensity, I_0 = intensity, I_r = reflected intensity, and $e^{-\alpha}$ = the absorption coefficient of the incident energy as determined by wavelength. Simply stated, Beer's law says that the intensity of an incident light attenuates exponentially as it travels through tissue—hence, lasers are capable of unique surgical advantage.

By algebraic manipulation, Beer's law can be transformed into an equation that relates light absorption to the tissue thickness within which this interaction will occur. This equation becomes:

$$I_t = I_0 \cdot 10^{-\alpha x}$$

where I_t = transmitted intensity, I_0 = incident intensity, α = the absorption coefficient of the incident energy as determined by wavelength, and x = the thickness of tissue irradiate. If tissue thickness is set at $x = 1/\alpha$, Beer's law is reduced to the formula:

$$I_t = I_0 \cdot 10^{-1}.$$

Since 10^{-1} equates with one-tenth, this simplified formula describes the *extinction length;* namely, the distance from the tissue surface at which the incident beam has been reduced to 10% of its initial intensity. In other words, *the critical volume of tissue needed to absorb 90% of the incident radiation is defined by the reciprocal of the absorption coefficient.* This concept of critical volume is the fundamental concept that physicists use in predicting the patterns of tissue interaction characteristic of each laser [2].

From the surgeon's perspective, a closely related parameter—the *absorption length*—is perhaps more useful. Correlating histologic features of the laser wound to delivered energy has shown that the most dramatic tissue effects occur during the absorption of the first 63% (rather than 90%)

Fig. 11. Ratio of target (oxyhemoglobin) to background (melanin) absorption. Of the three oxyhemoglobin peaks, the second (532 nm) corresponds to KTP light (not shown) and the third (578 nm) corresponds to SPTL-1 dye laser light. By contrast, the two argon bands fall within one of the oxyhemoglobin absorption troughs. (Illustration courtesy Candela Lasers, Wayland, MA.) See insert for color representation.

Fig. 14. Hexascan. **a:** (See page 108.) The hexascan handpiece containing the computerized mechanism for "point by point" beam delivery. **b:** (See page 108.) Variously sized hexagonal fields that can be selected. When treating large areas, one normally uses the full 13 mm hexagon. The lower right figure shows how the treatment pattern allows tissue to cool between impacts. Thus by selecting a pulse width of two or three times the thermal relaxation time of the vessels (dependent upon vessel diameter), the erythrocytes within the vascular lumen can be heated just long enough for heat to diffuse to the vessel wall and perivascular collagenous cuff, but not long enough to burn adjacent structures. **c:** (See page 105.) A large port wine stain of the left forearm, prior to treatment. **d:** (See page 105.) The same patient, after initial hexascan photothermolysis. (Illustrations courtesy Lihtan Technologies, San Rafael, CA.) See insert for color representation.

Fig. 20. (See page 105.) Vascular rebound at the site of a vestibulectomy incision. See insert for color representation.

Fig. 21. (See page 105.) **a:** Incapacitating hypervascularity and failure to re-epithelialize of the right side of a vestibulectomy incision, 6 months postsurgery. **b:** Appearances 2 months later, showing re-epithelialization and early shrinkage of the rebound vessels. Subsequently, all redness faded, and the patient was able to return to work and resume coitus. See insert for color representation.

Fig. 22. (See page 105.) **a:** FEDL pulse captured on camera. **b:** Extreme vestibulitis, prior to FEDL photothermolysis. **c:** Intraoperative view showing immediate bruising at sites of impact. **d:** Successful outcome, 4 months after FEDL treatment. See insert for color representation.

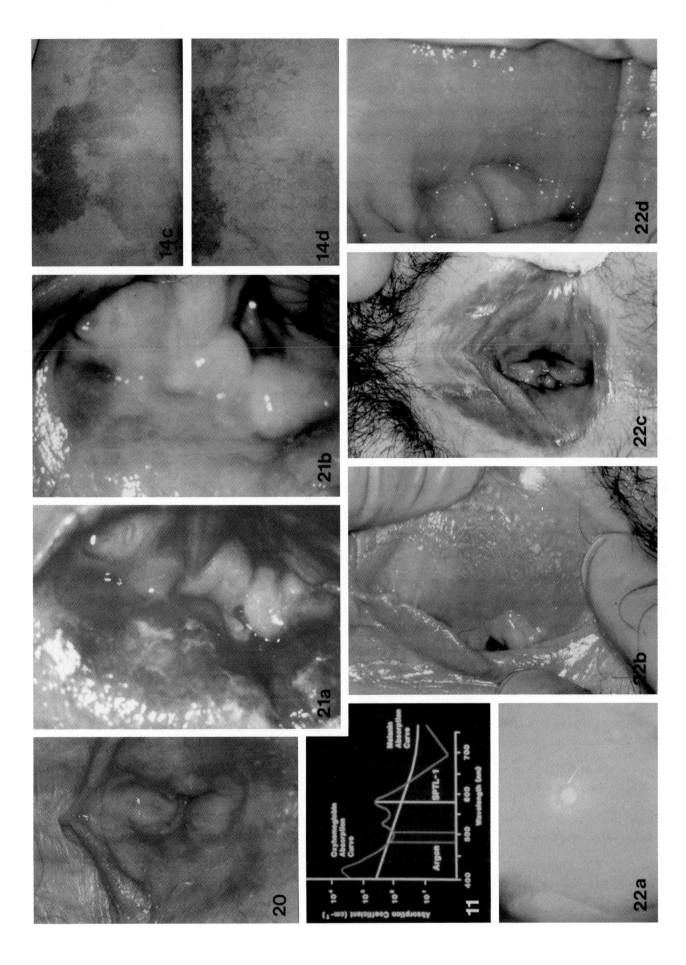

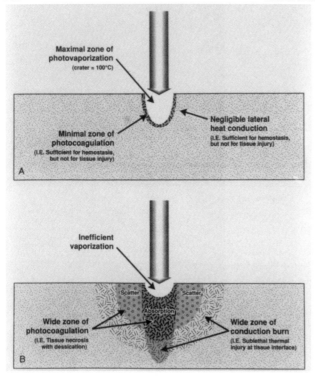

Fig. 12. Laser tissue interactions in four actual surgical situations. **A:** Short absorption length laser used at high fluence. **B:** Long absorption length laser used at adequate fluence. **C:** Contact tip laser. **D:** Short absorption length laser in which potential surgical advantage is lost because of low fluence. (From Reid [209], reproduced with permission.)

of the delivered energy. There are ~2.3 absorption lengths in each extinction length [1].

From the surgical perspective, laser–tissue interactions fall into two classes: short absorption length and long absorption length. Energy from *short absorption length* lasers is neither deeply transmitted nor extensively scattered. Rather, there is highly concentrated absorption, resulting in explosive disruption due to (1) flash boiling of intracellular and extracellular water and (2) heating to incandescence of any anhydrous tissue remnants (mainly proteins and nucleic acids). This zone of vaporization is surrounded by a narrow zone of thermal necrosis and by a second zone of sublethal thermal injury (Fig. 12a). Conversely, energy from *long absorption length* lasers is both deeply transmitted and widely scattered, resulting in a large but predictable zone of coagulation necrosis (Fig. 12b). Finally, the useful but imperfect tissue interaction of contact tips (Fig. 12c) and the potentially disastrous effects of unskilled CO_2 laser usage (Fig. 12d) are shown for comparison.

Temporal Parameters

Limiting secondary heat conduction. In molecular terms, lateral heat conduction within tissue is a relatively slow event. The time taken for absorption of radiant energy (i.e., for the conversion of electromagnetic energy into increased molecular vibration and oscillation) is almost too small to be imagined. In contrast, the transfer of increased kinetic energy from the *impact site* (i.e., the critical volume of tissue needed to absorb the incident radiation) to the *wound bed* (i.e., initially unaffected tissues adjacent to the absorption site) takes ~600 μsec in dermis. The slowness of this process—known as "thermal relaxation" to physicists—can be exploited to surgical advantage. Indeed, limiting the time during which laser energy strikes target tissue can be more important than the wavelength used. Rapid vaporization using ultrarapid pulsing techniques can dramatically reduce thermal relaxation, thereby increasing therapeutic efficacy. Alternatively, thermal diffusion can be controlled with robotized scanning de-

SwiftLase™ Operating Principles

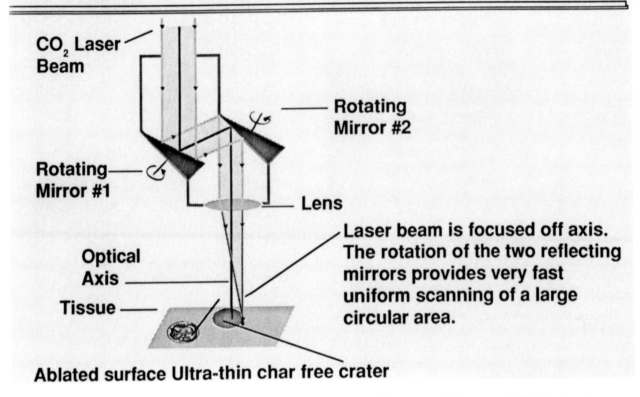

CO₂ Laser Beam

Rotating Mirror #2

Rotating Mirror #1

Lens

Optical Axis

Laser beam is focused off axis. The rotation of the two reflecting mirrors provides very fast uniform scanning of a large circular area.

Tissue

Ablated surface Ultra-thin char free crater

Fig. 13. Diagram of Swiftlaser system for robotized delivery of a rapidly moving, high-powered CW CO_2 laser beam.

vices that move very intense beams across tissue very rapidly.

The Xintec™ Nd:YAG laser is a good example of how *ultrarapid pulsing* can be exploited directly to overcome disadvantages that would have occurred if the same wavelength had been used as a low power continuous wave beam. As explained earlier, the conventional Nd:YAG produces deep tissue coagulation. Conversely, the Xintec™ laser pulses the Nd:YAG energy at very high frequency, just as is done with the rapid superpulse mode on a CO_2 laser. These rapid pulses of Nd:YAG energy create clean incisions with very narrow zones of lateral thermal damage. Unlike the CO_2 laser, this pulsed Nd:YAG energy can be delivered endoscopically to the operative site by quartz fibers, suitable for either contact or noncontact use.

Examples of *robotized scanning devices* that allow delivery of otherwise uncontrollable power densities of laser energy are provided by the Swiftlase™ and the Hexascan™. The Swiftlase™ uses a computer-controlled, motorized, oscillating mirror to move a high energy CO_2 beam very

quickly—too quickly for deep penetration to occur (Fig. 13). Because hand-eye coordination is quite finite, this operating speed could never be replicated with a manually controlled laser. Likewise, the Hexascan™ is a robotized scanning device that safely controls very high energy argon, KTP, or dye laser beams. This device links together a series of high intensity impacts within the scanned field, such that the edges of the spot of each laser pulse are not allowed to overlap (Fig. 14). Irradiated fields are configured as six-sided hexagons so that they can be fitted together without overlap, like building blocks. This is an improvement over manual application of the laser in that each field receives a uniform power density. In contrast, attempting to treat the same area manually with circular spots inevitably produces areas that are either double-dosed or left untreated.

When lasers are pulsed at very high energy densities, the linear relationship between energy and tissue temperature gives way to a nonlinear effect. That is to say, tissue interactions produced by extreme energy densities change from thermal

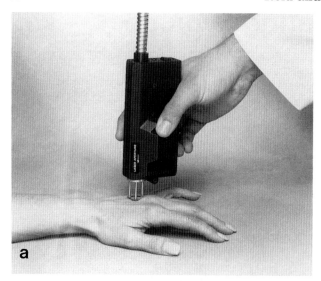

Fig. 14a. (Legend appears on page 104.)

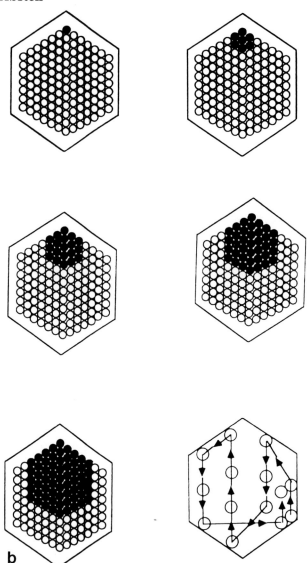

Fig. 14b. (Legend appears on page 104.)

(linear) to acoustic (nonlinear) (see Fig. 37). *Acoustic interactions* produce concussive shock waves that snap and tear rigid tissues. Lasers designed to exploit these concussive effects are sometimes called "cold-cutting" lasers, because there is no heat generation at the impact site. Examples are the laser lithotripsy, used to fragment renal stones, and the Q-switched Nd:YAG, used to fracture secondary cataracts that form behind prosthetic eye lenses.

Superpulsed CO_2 lasers. When using the CO_2 laser to excise or ablate delicate structures, optimal tissue effects depend upon two requirements: pulsed generation of the laser energy and sufficient power per unit pulse to produce single pulse vaporization.

Pulsed generation of the laser energy. Excellence with the laser assumes that almost all of the delivered energy will be harnessed to produce the desired *surgical objective* (vaporizing disease), rather than *unwanted morbidity* (heating adjacent tissue). Fulfilling this assumption requires that energy be delivered in pulse widths shorter than the thermal relaxation time and that the interpulse intervals be long enough to allow cooling of the impact site (by re-radiating most of the residual heat back to the atmosphere). A duty cycle (ratio of on:off time) of ~1:2 or 1:3 may be ideal. Conversely, as pulse width progressively exceeds 600 μsec, more and more of the delivered laser energy diffuses out of the intended target zone. Thus the benefit:morbidity ratio falls, as energy that should have produced localized photo-

vaporization contributes instead to an ever-widening zone of lateral photocoagulation.

Single pulse vaporization. Fourier's heat conduction relationship states that

$$PD = C_t \frac{\Delta T}{\Delta r}$$

where PD is the power density of the incident radiation, ΔT is the resultant change in tissue temperature, Δr is the distance (radius) from the laser impact center, and C_t is the thermal conductivity of that tissue. Thus until tissue mass is lost by explosive disruption, temperature rise will con-

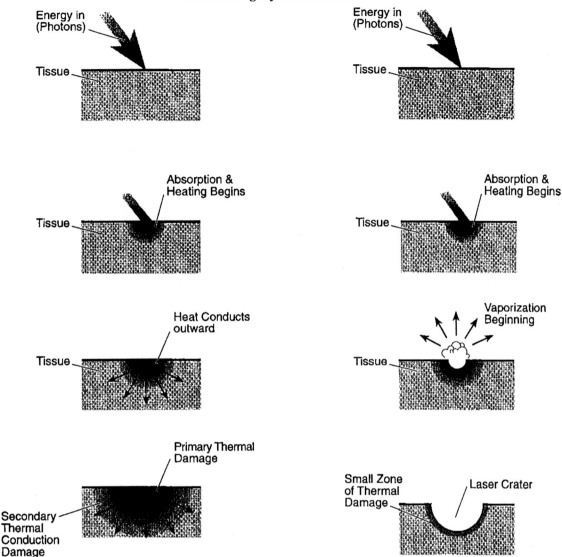

Fig. 15. Fourier's corollary. Until fluence exceeds the vaporization threshold, delivered energy can only leach into the wound bed, with potentially diastrous surgical complications.

Fig. 16. Beer's Law. Once fluence exceeds the vaporization threshold, heat no longer accumulates at the surgical site. Instead, heat from previous pulses exits the impact crater with the laser plume. Thus there is no major heat conduction into the wound bed, producing rapid healing and minimal cicatrization of the end result.

form to a linear ($\Delta T/\Delta r$) rather than an exponential, ($e^{-\alpha}$) model (Fig. 15) [4]. Simply stated, absorption of radiant energy at pulse energies below vaporization threshold results in widespread heat conduction into the wound bed. Conversely, if pulse energy is kept above the vaporization threshold ($\sim 4J/cm^2$ for dermis), laser:tissue interactions are dictated by Beer's law, rather than Fourier's corollary. Energy absorption for each pulse is now heavily localized within the critical volume, thus exceeding the sublimation point (Fig. 16). Most of the delivered heat then exits the impact site by convection (as steam and incandescent particles) and radiation (as emitted photons).

The combination of rapid pulsing and single pulse vaporization confines tissue damage to a sharply marginated crater, the volume of which is determined by the optical penetration depth of that wavelength (Fig. 17). Width of coagulation necrosis at the crater margin can be restricted to 70 μm or less. By comparison, the zone of coagulation necrosis increases to 170 μm for a 2 millisecond pulse and 750 μm for a 1/20 second pulse [12].

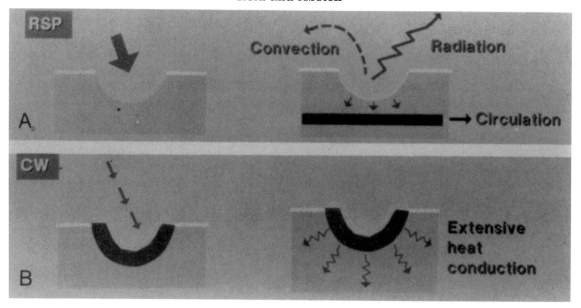

Fig. 17. **A:** A superpulsed laser of sufficient fluence to produce clean vaporization of the impact site plus effective cooling during the interpulse interval. **B:** With lower power continuous wave there is extensive desiccation of the crater (result-ing in a higher conduction gradient) plus prolonged heating (resulting in significant lateral thermal diffusion). (From Reid [208], reproduced with permission.)

Mechanism of Beam Delivery

An understanding of the strengths and limitations of each laser-tissue interaction is the key to rational surgery (see Table 2). For example, argon and KTP lasers have been promoted for a full range of gynecologic procedures, including cervical and vulvar ablations—such suggestions are at variance with the laws of physics. Likewise, although it is surgically feasible to excise or ablate genital neoplasia by delivery of laser-heated tips, such surgery essentially amounts only to an improved form of hot cautery. In either instance, tissue interaction is necessarily inferior to what could have been achieved with a high fluence CO_2 laser. A realistic knowledge of laser physics thus begets a fairly robust rule of thumb. Whenever ready surgical access permits easy beam delivery via an articulated arm, the CO_2 laser should be the automatic choice for any operation on aqueous tissue. Conversely, in endoscopic surgery, the advantages of flexible fiberoptic delivery may exceed the disadvantages that otherwise attend wavelengths with longer absorption lengths.

There is, however, an important biological difference between the healing mechanisms of mesothelial (mesodermal) and cutaneous (ectodermal) wounds. Vulvar wounds heal by epithelial ingrowth from the wound edge—taking 7–10 days for a sutured incision vs. weeks to months for an unrepaired defect. Conversely, reepithelialization of peritoneal wounds occurs by direct metaplasia within the exposed connective tissues [13]. The presence of a large raw area does not per se produce intraperitoneal complications; however, ischemia (e.g., from tight sutures) is a potent source of adhesion formation. Hence, despite theoretic differences between the various visible and infrared lasers, all of the fiberoptically delivered wavelengths produce satisfactory results within the abdominal cavity.

The choice between argon, KTP, contact Nd:YAG, Ho:YAG, and CO_2 lasers is generally determined by the experience and training of the user. Some surgeons like the speed and no-touch precision of the laparoscopically adapted CO_2 laser. Blind spots and difficulties in maintaining uniform mechanical pressure through the endoscope are thus avoided. Other surgeons are frustrated by the plume and by difficulties in keeping the CO_2 laser beam in alignment.

GYNECOLOGIC APPLICATIONS FOR ARGON, KTP, AND DYE LASERS
Endoscopic Use of Fiberoptic Visible Light Lasers

The argon laser (488 and 514 nm) was one of the first types of lasers used in medicine. It was introduced for selective photocoagulation of proliferating blood vessels arising on the ischemic retinae of aging diabetics. Ophthalmology remains the main application of the argon laser. However, such properties as excellent transmissibility within quartz fibers and a very small focal spot have made this instrument useful to the laparoscopist, as a hemostatic dissector and a photocoagulator. Fiberoptically delivered argon or KTP energy is probably the technically easiest modality to control, allowing the surgeon to accomplish several tasks without the distraction of having to change instruments. Hence, argon and KTP lasers have a shorter learning curve than the laparoscopically adapted CO_2 laser. To the laparoscopist, the argon and KTP lasers can be used interchangeably. The KTP laser (532 nm) emits a Kelly green beam with greater affinity for hemoglobin than blue-green argon light. This improved thermal precision is of major benefit in dermatologic applications (such as treating vulvodynia), but it is of no practical importance to the endoscopist.

Surgical techniques for fiberoptic lasers. Both lasers can be delivered efficiently through 400 or 600 μm fibers, and both can be used as noncontact (free beam) or contact (sculptured fibers) tools. The 600-μm fiber is the "general" use fiber because it is stiffer, easier to control, and has the largest spot size. However, the smaller spot size of the 400-μm fiber is useful for making fine incisions such as during laparoscopic treatment of ectopic pregnancy or for tubal infertility [14,15].

Noncontact technique depends upon the rapid predictable decline in power density, which occurs over distance as transmitted laser energy diverges from a flat-cleaved fiber tip. By moving the fiberoptic to a position of moderate defocus, 8–12 watts of power can photocoagulate moderate-size blood vessels within a vascular adhesion; then, by "tromboning" the fiber to a position just above the target surface, the same fiberoptic can cut right through the coagulated adhesion. Conversely, pulling the fiber even farther away would allow the surgeon to photocoagulate bleeding vessels safely without concomittant vaporization. This principle is generally implemented by passing the fiberoptic through a suction irrigator, so that an oozing vascular bed can be simultaneously rinsed and coagulated.

Contact technique offers more efficient cutting and reduced forward scatter. Hence, areas requiring coagulation are generally treated first, before contact cutting with a sculptured or carbonized fiber. Surgical techniques for all hot tips are the same. Contact cutting is initiated by first firing the laser and then immediately moving the fiber tip into tissue contact (Fig. 18a). Delay beyond 2 seconds or so will burn out the tip. It should be emphasized that the activated fiber is allowed to "float" through tissue at its own speed; attempts to mechanically force the cutting action are thermally inefficient and risk breaking the fiber. Finally, the fiber is withdrawn with the laser still activated, to prevent the hot tip from welding itself to the incised tissues. If the tip does stick, the laser must be activated before attempting to pull the fiber free.

Surgeons should understand that hot tips have a "sweet spot"—the last couple of millimeters—which does all of the work. Tips should never be inserted deeper than this "sweet spot." If the rate of incision is too slow, the power is turned up to the maximum tolerated by that tip (5–25 watts) and the desired depth reached by multiple passes. Once the surgeon develops a feel for this technique, the laser can be continuously fired while the tip is repeatedly lifted and reapplied to tissue—provided that the time off tissue is very brief.

Advantages and disadvantages of fiberoptic delivery. Significant *advantages* are: (1) Fiberoptic transmission, permitting energy delivery either down the central channel of an operating laparoscope or through the central aperture of the Nezhat-Dorsey suction irrigator [16]. (2) User friendly operating characteristics, including automatic beam alignment and rapid defocus beyond the immediate target. (3) Long absorption length, creating cogulation rather than vaporization; hence, green light lasers are strongly hemostatic and generate little smoke. (4) Color-dependent absorption, allowing energy delivery through a pool of irrigating fluid.

Significant *disadvantages* are: (1) Relative inefficiency of photovaporization, making tissue incision with these wavelentghs a relatively slow event. (2) Deep transmission and extensive forward scatter, such that tissue necrosis will occur ~2 mm beyond the visually apparent crater margin; hence, there is a reduced safety margin in the vicinity of vulnerable structures (e.g., ureter, great vessels).

Selective Photothermolysis for Vulvodynia

Idiopathic vulvodynia (vulvar vestibulitis syndrome and pruritic papillomatosis) is a chronic and distressing problem that has in-

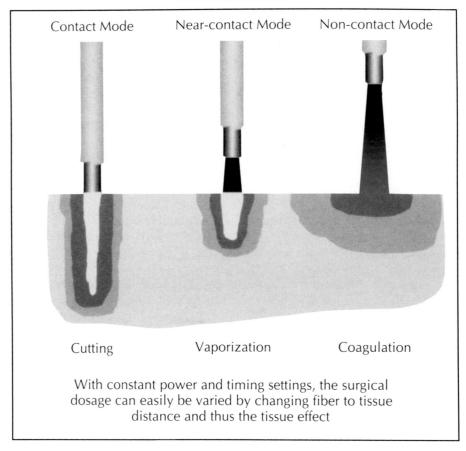

Contact Mode   Near-contact Mode   Non-contact Mode

Cutting   Vaporization   Coagulation

With constant power and timing settings, the surgical
dosage can easily be varied by changing fiber to tissue
distance and thus the tissue effect

Fig. 18. The more efficient, less thermally diffused nature of the contact cutting technique.

creased in prevalence over the last decade. Disability varies markedly from person to person. Milder cases suffer nuisance-level (but persistent) vulvar burning and loss of sexual pleasure. Severe cases report severe restriction or even total inability to have vaginal intercourse, often accompanied by constant vulvar pain that is severe enough to dominate daily activities. Treatment has been problematic. There are no specific therapies and no effective symptom-controlling, anti-inflammatory agents. Topical 5 fluorouracil (5FU) cream is often curative in pruritic papillomatosis but seldom helps established vestibulitis [17]. Success has been reported within an uncontrolled trial of alpha interferon, injected thrice weekly into the vulvar connective tissues over 4 weeks [18]. However, others have found that any clinical benefits are too transient to justify the pain and inconvenience of this regimen as monotherapy (Campion, pers. comm.; Reid, unreported data). Hence, the mainstay of conventional treatment for patients with macroscopically visible foci of painful erythema has remained cold knife

resection of the minor vestibular glands and the adjacent hymen, with closure by downward advancement of the vaginal mucosa [19]. Woodruff's localization of the main sites of pain to the minor vestibular glands and his recognition that excision could cure some patients were valuable advances. However, vestibulectomy has several unsatisfactory aspects: cosmetic appearances are disfiguring (Fig. 19), success rates approximate 50% and, symptoms can be dramatically worsened by the phenomenon of postoperative neo-angiogenesis (Fig. 20). In search of a more reliable, less mutilating surgical approach, we have explored a variety of laser therapies.

The first point to make about lasers is what not to do. Surgery with the CO_2 laser is a gamble. Some treatments secure a major reduction in symptoms, but others trigger neo-angiogenesis (Fig. 20) and incapacitating vulvar pain (Fig. 21a). In 1987, foci of proliferating telangiectatic surface blood vessels were eradicated by argon laser photocoagulation in five patients (Fig. 21b) [17]. However, continuous wave blue-green argon

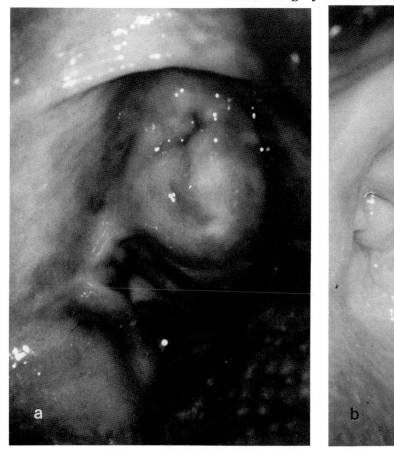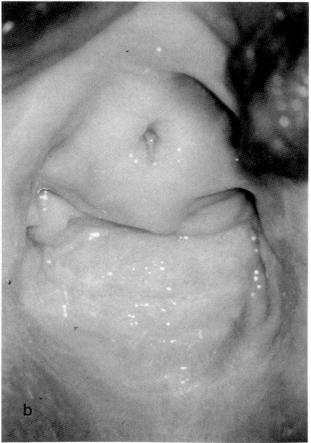

Fig. 19. **a:** Long-standing vestibulitis surrounding the skenes and minor vestibular glands. **b:** Successful control of symptoms by vestibulectomy. However, cosmetic appearance is disappointing.

beam has such poor selectivity for hemoglobin that damage to the adjacent stroma was almost as severe as that within the ectatic vessels, leading to considerable morbidity and protracted healing. Nonetheless, this observation had one important corollary. Long-term clinical remission in these five patients indicated that the blood vessels within these fields of reactive erythema were actual mediators of the chronic pain, rather than nonspecific sentinels of some other underlying process. The explanation for this phenomenon lies in the observation that vulvodynia represents a chronic, self-sustaining pain loop, mediated through the afferent and efferent sympathetic nerves supplying genital tissues of cloacal origin (vestibule, trigone and urethra, Bartholin's glands) [20]. That is, destruction of the chronically inflamed surface vessels (and the activated sympathetic nerves that surround them) offers a therapeutic window. Each time this pain loop is

broken, a proportion of individuals will remain in stable clinical remission [21].

Instrumentation. The flashlamp excited dye laser (FEDL) and the hexascan delivered argon or KTP lasers have been designed specifically for the destruction of small blood vessels within the superficial dermis. Both instruments have proven efficacious and nonmorbid tools for permanently blanching portwine stains of nongenital skin [22–24].

The safety and efficacy of the *flashlamp excited dye laser* are predicated upon several distinctive physical properties. First, yellow light with a wavelength of 585 nanometers (0.6 μm) has strong selectivity for the third oxyhemoglobin absorption peak. Second, peak powers are high enough to allow single pulse destruction of the target blood vessels. Third, since the ultrashort pulse widths are less than the thermal relaxation time, secondary thermal conduction from heated

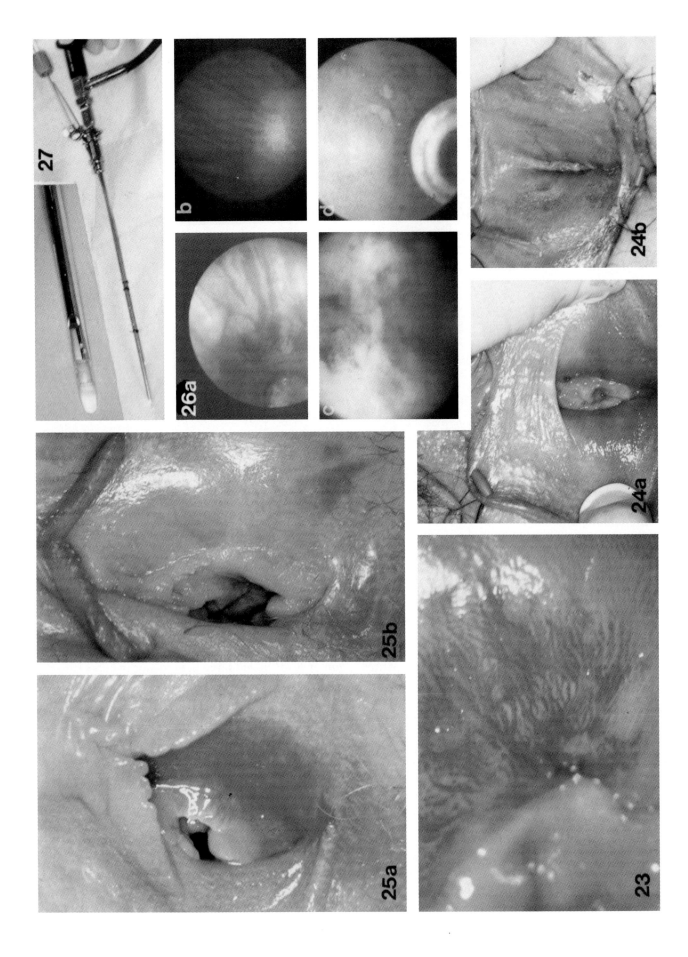

vessels within the impact site is reduced. Last, the high pulse energy permits the use of very large spot sizes, thus nullifying the problems caused by intense scattering of incident laser light within the dermis.

The hexascan is a robotized laser beam delivery device designed to reduce the secondary heat conduction that generally mars the dermatologic application of continuous wave yellow or green light to subcutaneous vascular lesions. The underlying principle is the inclusion of a computer-controlled scanner in the handpiece. Thus laser energy is systematically delivered as a series of small, nonoverlapping spots—distributed within a hexagon-shape area. Because each spot has time to cool before another impact is delivered in that part of the hexagon, there is no heat buildup at the operative site.

Surgical technique. Treatment of cutaneous portwine stains are generally performed without anesthesia. For a number of reasons, we found it necessary to treat vulvodynia patients in the operating room under general or regional anesthesia. First, obtaining sufficient exposure for effective energy delivery required extreme eversion of the vestibular epithelium (using a series of traction sutures). Second, targeting the deep dermal vessels required firm compression of the surface microcirculation, using specially constructed transmissive spatulae. Third, the impact of laser light upon areas of symptomatic hyperemia is acutely painful, perhaps indicative of the release of vasoactive peptides during thermal damage to the target vessels.

Through trial and error, FEDL energy levels were narrowed to a range of 8.0–10.0 joules per square centimeter (depending upon anatomic location and complexion type). Since 10% of the incident energy is reflected or scattered by the spatula, these settings deliver ~7.25–9 J/cm^2 at the tissue surface. Areas of erythema were then sequentially lased, using a hand probe with a 5 mm spot. Energy dosage was judged against two clinical endpoints. Within areas containing dilated stem vessels, power was adjusted to the point where a palpable vibration could be felt through the compressive spatula. For tissues without visible stem vessels, the clinical endpoint was a dark purpuric change, visible within 5 minutes of irradiation (Fig. 22).

Energy levels and clinical endpoint for the hexascan delivered lasers proved quite different. Equivalent power settings were 14–18 J/cm^2 for the KTP and 16–22 J/cm^2 for the argon laser. Again, energy is delivered through a compressive plastic footplate, thus reducing irradiance levels at tissue by ~10%. Unlike the FEDL laser, there are essentially no immediately visible tissue changes in epithelium treated with the hexascan. However, when seen at the 1 week follow-up visit, most patients show slight ecchymosis and a yellowish discoloration of the treated areas.

Results of therapy. Response to surface laser ablation of symptomatic hyperemia depends principally upon whether or not there is a second pain focus within the underlying Bartholin's glands. For women with surface-only disease, response rates (complete remission or significant partial improvement) exceed 90% after an average of 1.9 treatments. Conversely, among women in whom digital palpation of the Bartholin's fossae produced a sharp lancinating pain that was recognizably different from the burning hyperalgesia evoked by Q-tip palpation of the vestibular mucosa, complete response rates to FEDL or hexascan photothermolysis remained <4% (Fig. 23) [20].

Little difference has been found in response rates for FEDL versus hexascan photothermolysis. From the clinical perspective, however, the hexascan is best suited for initial treatment of patients with diffuse hyperemia (see Fig. 25), whereas the FEDL is most valuable for completing the destruction of the erythematous areas sur-

---

Fig. 23. Refractory pain loop, located deep within the right Bartholin's gland. See insert for color representation.

Fig. 24. **a:** Extreme vestibulitis, immediately prior to treatment with the hexascan adapted argon laser. **b:** Intraoperative view, showing some epithelial edema but no ecchymosis (contrast with Fig. 22c). See insert for color representation.

Fig. 25. **a:** Incapacitating surface vestibulitis, concentrated principally around the hymenal edge. **b:** Same patient after serial FEDL. photothermolysis disappearance of the hypervascularity is almost always associated with resolution of symptoms. See insert for color representation.

Fig. 26. **a:** Extreme hypervascularity of the urethral mucosa, showing dilated, hyperemic, branching vessels of variable caliber. **b:** Laser beam in position to fire. **c:** Effect of cytoscopically directed argon laser, producing ecchymosis and vascular occulation with minial epithelial damage. **d:** Long-term result, after healing, showing a pale, non-irritated mucosa. See insert for color representation.

Fig. 27. Standard cystoscope, modified by passing the angled delivery device *below* the lens, allowing the emitted KTP beam to diverge en route to its target on the opposite side of the urethral lumen. See insert for color representation.

rounding the Skene's and Bartholin's ducts (Fig. 24). Paradoxically, the FEDL is required for the treatment of rebound neo-angiogenesis that follows vestibulectomy or superficial CO_2 photovaporization. Indeed the hexascan must be avoided in these patients, since it carries a risk of further exacerbating these unstable surface vessels, thus further increasing vulvar pain.

Cystoscopic Photothermolysis for Urethrodynia

About 5% of patients with vulvar vestibulitis syndrome also have chronic urethral burning, a condition we have termed "urethrodynia." In normal women, the urethral mucosa projects a delicate pink hue, behind which lies a longitudinal palisade of uniform caliber submucosal arterioles and venules. However, in symptomatic women, urethroscopy shows an intensely red mucosal surface and a somewhat chaotic pattern of dilated submucosal stem vessels. Classic features of chlamydial or bacterial urethritis (such as purulent discharge or diverticulum formation) must be ruled out. Empiric preoperative treatment with doxycycline (100 mg b.i.d. for 10 days) is probably a wise precaution.

At *urethroscopy,* helpful diagnostic features are: (1) vasculature showing a haphazard branching pattern, as secondary channels dilate to shunt blood between the normally longitudinal network of submucosal vessels, (2) prominent variations in caliber, as areas of relative vasoconstriction give way to areas of extreme vascular engorgement, and (3) partial obscuring of these dilated submucosal vessels by areas of extreme mucosal hyperemia (Fig. 26). *Urodynamic testing* can also yield confirmatory evidence: (1) static urethral pressure profilometry may show painful spasm within the underlying urethral smooth musculature, and (2) the filling cystometrogram evaluation of the bladder musculature may show detrusor instability (urge incontinence), lowered sensation of maximum capacity (sensory urgency), or decreased bladder wall compliance (interstitial cystitis) [25].

Based upon the belief that the urethral pain look was probably emanating from hyperalgesic sympathetic nerve fibers surrounding these engorged submucosal vessels, we modified a cystoscope to allow precise photocoagulation of this vascular network under video control. In this instrument, the outer metal sheath was replaced by a 30 Fr. plastic tube with one closed end. By passing an irrigation tube through the righthand port

of a standard operative bridge, this closed plastic tube functioned as a water-cooling jacket. In addition, the relatively large diameter of this tube served to compress and blanche the hyperemic mucosa, making the network of symptomatic submucosal vessels more visible (and hence more accessible to incident laser energy). A KTP laser beam is then delivered via a side-firing quartz fiber (600 μm). This side-firing fiber is passed through the lefthand port of the cystoscopic bridge and brought forward to a point behind and just beyond the tip of a 30° lens (Fig. 27). Advantages of the side-firing fiber in this arrangement are: (1) the red HeNe aiming beam is clearly visible within the center of the video monitor, (2) the surgeon's view, however, is not obstructed by the outer metal casing of the quartz fiber, and (3) having the fiber *behind* the lens allows the KTP beam to continue to diverge as it travels from the exit point on the side-firing fiber to the mucosa on the opposite side of the urethral lumen. Spot diameter therefore broadens from 0.5 μm at the point of emergence, to 1.7 mm at the point of impact. Adjusting power output to 2.5 watts produces the desired power density of 135 w/cm^2 at the mucosal surface. At this power density, the target vessels are rapidly photocoagulated, with minimal explosive disruption. Thus the clinical endpoint is slight vascular shrinkage and a rapid color change (from bright red to dark purple). Aiming at a desired target is relatively easy, because the beam can be moved both horizontally (by rotating the side-firing laser from side to side around the long axis of the cystoscope lens) and vertically (by "tromboning" the cystoscope lens in and out within the plastic tube).

GYNECOLOGIC APPLICATIONS FOR THE CO_2 LASER

The use of CO_2 lasers has expanded enormously over the last decade, particularly as applied to the male and female genital tracts. Results have been generally good, and there is widespread belief that surgical success is essentially guaranteed by the technical sophistication of this instrument. Unfortunately, such beliefs are ill-founded.

Advantages and Disadvantages of CO_2 Lasers

Certainly, because of the affinity of water for midinfrared radiation, energy from the CO_2 laser displays several unique surgical properties: (1) diseased volumes can be vaporized under precise visual control, (2) there is little or no mechanical contact with the intended target, (3) heat propagation to adjacent tissue can be minimal, (4) microorganisms at the impact site will be automatically destroyed, and (5) vessels <0.5 mm (arterioles) will be thermally sealed. However, these surgical advantages occur only in the hands of experienced laser surgeons [26].

Low fluence CO_2 lasers conform to the thermal model described by Fourier's heat conduction relationship, rather than the optical model stipulated in Beer's law (see Fig. 12d). Hence, these outmoded devices produce wounds as bad (or even worse) than hot cautery or cryosurgery. Devastating thermal injuries can occur with improper use of the laser. The authors are aware of one ileal burn (during laser conization), one rectovaginal fistula, two vesicovaginal fistulae, several third-degree burns of vulvar or perianal skin (Fig. 28), and many serious cervical deformities (Fig. 29). Laser hazards result principally from the surgeon's lack of sophistication, rather than from the somewhat remote risk of accidental mishap [26]. Collagen damaged by secondary heat conduction can remain "mummified" in the dermis for many months, where it further delays healing and promotes fibrosis [27].

Before re-epithelialization can begin, heat-damaged tissue must be remodeled, either by sloughing of coagulation necrosis or by biochemical repair of sublethally injured cells. For as long as dermis is exposed to air, more and more fibroblasts are activated, resulting in increasing collagen deposition. Simply stated, the degree of wound cicatrization is directly proportional to healing time, which is in turn directly proportional to sophistication of energy delivery [28].

Based on the laws of physics and the realities of wound healing, certain firm generalizations can be offered. Superpulsed laser energy of adequate fluence has two unique benefits: the least attainable zone of coagulation necrosis (70 μm) and the sharpest (exponential) falloff in secondary heat conduction. The least depth of obligatory coagulation attainable with constant current electrosurgical loops is ~300 μm; moreover, heat conduction attenuates on a linear gradient. By comparison, low fluence CO_2 lasers can produce zones of eschar and sublethal injury that extend millimeters (or even centimeters) beyond the vaporization crater. It is not an overstatement to say that limiting lateral thermal injury is the essence of expertise and that failure to contain conducted heat is the source of most laser-associated morbidity.

Physical Principles Governing CO_2 Laser Surgery

Laser surgery is defined as "tissue destruction through direct thermal effects of intense electromagnetic radiation." Selective destruction of disease foci must be accomplished by radiant heat. Diffuse, poorly controlled burns, and a wide zone of sublethal injury are not acceptable.

The following six physical principles describe how to distribute incident energy and control the extent of tissue destruction (Table 3).

1. Use of an acceptable temporal mode. As noted above, meeting the optical ideal stipulated by Beer's law requires that laser energy be delivered in a train of rapid pulses, with each pulse having sufficient fluence to produce single pulse vaporization. CO_2 lasers from the 1980s, capable only of operation in continuous wave (CW), are now obsolete. No matter how skillful the surgeon, tissue effects from CW lasers reflect the laws of thermal diffusion, wherein heat damage declines along a linear (rather than exponential) gradient. Preferred temporal modes are as follows:

Rapid superpulse. In the 1980s, best tissue effects were provided by a form of rapid superpulse generated high voltage electrical excitation of a flowing gas laser tube. In this mode, the laser tube can generate a peak pulse of 500–700 watts, with a pulse duration of ~300 μs (Fig. 30). Unfortunately, such a high voltage electrical discharge ionizes the CO_2 gas, thus producing a longer than desired refractory period (~3 ms), while new gas is pumped into the tube. Herein lies the main disadvantage of conventional rapid superpulsing. The long refractory period reduces average operating power to about one-third of that attainable from the same laser tube used in the CW mode. This limitation made it impractical to treat large volumes of diseased epithelium with this temporal mode. Therefore, rapid superpulse was generally reserved for situations in which small tissue volumes needed to be treated with maximal precision.

Chopped wave. In the high voltage, flowing gas lasers of the late 1980s, the best compromise between the high precision of rapid superpulse and the high power of continuous wave was obtained from electrically pulsing the resonator to emit broad, flat pulses, with no refractory interval between pulses (Fig. 31). This compromise is commonly referred to as "chopped wave." Con-

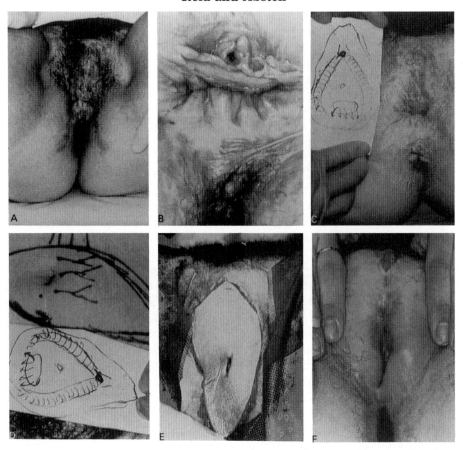

Fig. 28. Use of transverse abdominal muscle (TRAM) flap to reconstruct the vulva of a patient injured by poor laser technique (low power via a hand probe). **A:** Macroscopic view of the vulva, showing how the labia minora were sloughed off because of excessive thermal damage. The result is a markedly deformed appearance in which the vestibule has undergone keratinization because of the loss of the moistening labia minora. Moreover, dense scarring of the underlying tissue produced pain during any attempt at coitus or even vigorous walking. **B:** Exposed, keratinized, desensitized vaginal introitus. **C:** Planning the area of skin needed to reconstruct the vulva. **D:** Planning the TRAM flap, to be based on the left inferior epigastric artery. **E:** Transposition of this myocutaneous flap through a tunnel to the left side of the glans clitoris. The flap has been rotated 90% counterclockwise so that the periumbilical defect is positioned over the introitus and the left hypogastric skin is at the apex of the vulva. **F:** Appearance after a second operation 3 months later, during which the excess fat was removed from the center of the flap, giving better anatomic definition to the result. If so desired, similar improvements can be made at the right and left lateral margins to simulate the normal vulvar contour even more closely. (From Reid [208], reproduced with permission.)

sider the electrical pulsing of a 120-watt laser tube, manipulated so that the ratio of on:off time will never exceed 5:1. When used at the highest duty cycle, maximal output would be 100 watts (120 × 5/6). Conversely, selecting a 1:11 duty cycle would produce an output of only 10 watts (120 × 1/12). Because the peak power of each pulse is not amplified, an electrically pulsed laser tube does not have a refractory phase when used in chopped mode. Therefore, repetition rate can be increased to virtually any frequency. However, as pulse frequency approaches a duty cycle of 2:1, heat accumulation at the impact site becomes ex-

cessive and the clinical effects will resemble those of continuous wave laser. The best compromise is a duty cycle of ~1:1, producing both acceptable power (60 watts) and adequate cooling (preservation of about half of the interpulse interval).

Ultrapulse. The Ultrapulse™ is an enhanced version of the conventional superpulse CO_2 laser, generated by exciting a sealed tube laser excited with radio frequency (RF) electrical discharge. The difference between conventional rapid superpulse and Ultrapulse™ is that the latter maintains optimal power for the entire duration of the laser pulse. In contrast, electrically generated

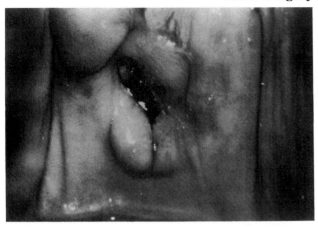

Fig. 29. Marked cervical deformity produced by unskilled laser surgery. A focus of CIN remains at the external os. (From Reid [209], reproduced with permission.)

rapid superpulse quickly hits peak power, but output fades rapidly for the remainder of the pulse (Fig. 32). Hence, a 100-watt Ultrapulse™ laser is able to generate higher energies in each pulse, typically 200 millijoules for an Ultrapulse™ vs. only 75 millijoules for conventional rapid superpulse. That is to say, it requires five RSP pulses to do the same work as one ultrapulse. Higher energies per pulse allow the laser to be operated at the same average power in the Ultrapulse™ and CW mode; hence single pulse vaporization can be achieved with both narrow and broad spot sizes. Char-free tissue effects can be extended to the widefield ablation of large disease volumes. The advantages of being able to maintain an optimal temporal mode throughout the power range (100 watts) make this RF excitation mechanism the model of choice for future CO_2 laser tube design.

2. With continuous wave lasers, use high powers to shorten exposure times. The formula for energy delivered to tissue is:

$$\begin{array}{ccc} \text{delivered energy} = \text{operating power} \times \text{exposure time.} \\ \text{(joules)} \qquad \text{(watts)} \qquad \text{(seconds)} \end{array}$$

A given amount of energy will destroy the same mass of tissue, regardless of energy delivery rate. In either case, irradiating with 100 watts for 1 second or 10 watts for 10 seconds will deliver 100 joules of infrared energy. However, different rates of energy delivery produce profoundly different surgical effects.

Using pulsed lasers of sufficient fluence, thermal damage is a function of the optical prop-

erties $(1/\infty)$ of the incident energy. A cold, clean, char-free tissue response will therefore occur at any operating power. In contrast, when pulse duration exceeds thermal relaxation time, a large proportion of the delivered energy will diffuse out of the vaporization crater [12]. Hence, heat accumulates at the surface of the impact crater—tissue damage now becomes primarily a function of exposure time. Low rates of energy delivery prolong exposure time and therefore increase lateral heat conduction (see Fig. 17). Surgeons tend not to realize the dangers of using lasers at low-power settings and are therefore reluctant to employ high powers as a way to shorten exposure times. This error was rampant in many of the gynecologic laser courses of the 1980s. However, if the experienced surgeon cannot obtain good results with 10–20 watts, the novice has no chance of obtaining an excellent result with such low wattage. The safety margin (between mediocre vs. calamitous results) is very narrow at low wattages. Because tissue killed by conducted heat appears normal at the time of injury, the unwary surgeon can produce a third-degree burn without realizing this (Fig. 33).

The potential magnitude of this error is reflected within our own material, as technique and instrumentation evolved. Up until 1984, there were no effective methods for reliably "flattening" energy distribution within the incident laser beam. Therefore, surgical control depended upon the choice of low powers (<30 watts of continuous wave energy), delivered at relatively low power densities (450 W/cm^2) [29]. However, when we began to control surgical effects by manipulating beam geometry (see below), we noticed that continuous wave laser at maximal power (80 watts) produced better results [28]. Healing times were reduced by an average of 3 days (Fig. 34) and complication rates fell from 10.3% to 6.5%. Subsequent availability of a laser that delivered rapid superpulse and chopped modes reduced surgical morbidity even further. Healing times for patients treated to a shallow plane decreased from 17 to 10 days, whereas healing from a deep plane decreased from 22 to 16 days (Fig. 35). Postoperative pain was greatly reduced and the incidence of heat-related complications decreased from 10.3% to 5.3%.

Ideally, CW lasers should never be used. However, if no other wave form is available, the surgeon may have no option. In this case, choice of realistic operating powers is absolutely critical. As a rule, effective photovaporization of a cervical

TABLE 3. Six Physical Principles Underlying Surgical Expertise With the CO$_2$ Laser

Parameters concerned with minimizing thermal diffusion

1. Use rapid superpulse or chopped wave, rather than continuous wave, thus preventing thermal relaxation between pulses.
2. Avoid carbonization of the impact crater by single pulse vaporization, and by keeping power density above 750 W/cm^2, wiping away debris, performing ablations with the operating microscope, and not caramelizing extravasated blood.
3. Minimize duration of thermal diffusion, by using high power settings (to deliver the necessary energy as rapidly as possible).

Parameters influencing control

4. Tailor pulse fluence or average power density to individual hand-eye speed.
5. Control beam geometry by incremental focus and defocus of the microslad, using tightly focused spots for incision and rounded beams for ablation.
6. Maintain high power in delicate situations, using shuttered pulses to maintain surgical control.

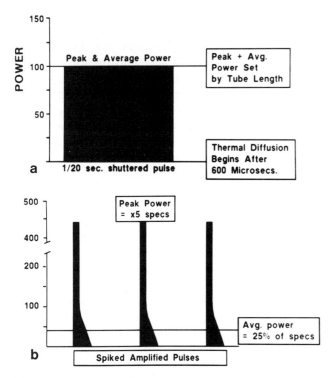

Fig. 30. Power-time characteristics of a 0.5-ms shuttered pulse of continuous wave laser energy (**a**), and a 0.5-ms burst of superpulsed laser energy (**b**), comprising (say) 15 pulses of 300 ms duration. (From Reid [208], reproduced with permission.)

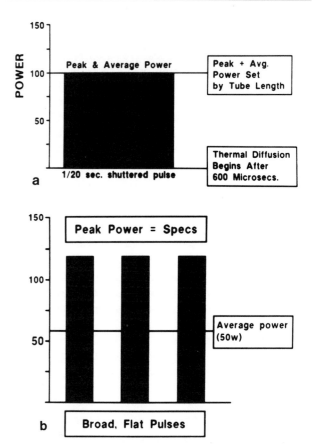

Fig. 31. Power-time characteristics of a 0.5-ms shuttered pulse of continuous wave laser energy (**a**) and a 0.5-msec burst of chopped wave (duty cycle 1:2) (**b**). (From Reid [208], reproduced with permission.)

lesion with a CW laser requires at least 25 watts of power. Paradoxically, because vulvar epithelium is more susceptible to injurious thermal effects, the safe photovaporization of vulvar and vaginal lesions with a CW laser requires at least 40 watts of power.

3. Avoiding carbonization within the laser crater. If surgical lasers emitted parallel beams of uniform intensity, power output would be the major factor in controlling tissue effects. However, CO$_2$ laser tubes used in medicine usu-

ally have diameters of 1–2 cm, producing beams that are too wide for direct surgical use. To limit incision width, the emergent beam must be focused to a small diameter, thereby increasing power density within the focal spot by as much as 10,000 times (see Fig. 3). Although intensity varies substantially from point to point within the

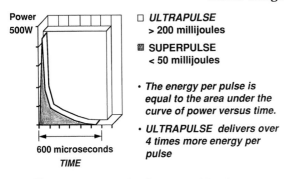

Fig. 32. The energy per pulse determined by the area under the curve (power × time). Ultrapulse delivers four times as much energy as convention rapid superpulses.

focal spot, the surgical effects of increasing effective beam power by focusing are best quantified by estimating average energy intensity within the central 86% of the incident beam.

Tissues irradiated at low-power densities have a low proportion of photovaporization. Hence, most of the delivered heat remains in the wound rather than rising with the laser plume. Moreover, slow heating of tissues will evaporate much of the water content. Thus even when the threshold for actual photovaporization is reached, steam formation is not sufficient to cleanly remove such anhydrous components as protein and nucleic acids. Continued irradiance of these desiccated tissues will lead to carbonization. Temperatures within the carbonized impact crater will rise well above 100°C, thereby increasing the conduction gradient (Fig. 36).

Irrespective of whether one uses pulsed or continuous mode, carbonizing the laser crater will inevitably produce a conduction burn, similar to or worse than burns seen with electrocautery or cryosurgery. This error generally arises in one of four ways: (1) excessive defocus of the laser beam allows average power density to fall below 750 W/cm^2 and beam geometry assumes a "watch glass" contour, (2) attempting ablative surgery with a hand probe, (3) failing to wipe accumulated debris from the laser crater, and (4) irradiating a bleeding point at low-power density, thus caramelizing hemoglobin at the surface but not coagulating the underlying vessel wall (see controlling intraoperative bleeding later in this section under Photovaporization of Vulvar and Anal Epithelium).

4. Tailoring power density to surgical requirements. Power output from the laser tube must be distinguished from power density within the focal spot. Power output—the speed of energy

delivery within the unfocused beam—is the major factor in determining how long the surgery will take. Hence, use of high powers was once of enormous importance in limiting the length of time over which thermal diffusion could occur. However, power output is not important in surgical control. In contrast, power density—average power within the focal spot—is the major factor in controlling the surgical effects of the delivered beam, irrespective of temporal mode or emitted power. That is to say, power density controls both the qualitative interaction and the speed of cut.

Type of tissue interaction. Different types of tissue interaction are produced by beams of different intensities (Fig. 37). Very low levels of energy delivery heat tissues just enough to destroy proteins, thus permitting their use for tissue welding. Beams with an energy intensity of 100 W/cm^2 cause tissue removal by photovaporization; however, carbonization limits the usefulness of this effect at the lower end of this range (<750 W/cm^2). Power densities >10,000 W/cm^2 cause ultrarapid photovaporization, suited to thermal incision rather than shallow ablation. Finally, extremely high power densities (>10^6 W/cm^2) result in plasma formation and acoustic shock waves, producing mechanical tearing of tissues, rather than thermal denaturation.

Speed of cut. This is critical because hand-eye coordination is limited. When using the laser to make deep thermal incision, power densities of >50,000 W/cm^2 are easy to control, requiring about the same speed of movement as cutting with a sharp knife. When the objective is to ablate a wide field of epithelium to a shallow depth, average power density must be kept below the 2,000 W/cm^2 range, since higher levels require excessively rapid hand movements. Nonetheless, if the laser is equipped with a proper defocusing device, these limitations should not prevent the expert from using any medical laser at full power (Table 4). Broadening spot diameter can make power outputs of 10–1,000 watts equally manageable. In contrast, focusing a 10-watt beam to a spot diameter of 0.2 mm would produce an average power density of 25,000 W/cm^2, making it impossible for even the most adroit surgeon to use such a beam for surface ablation.

Precise calculation of average power density is complex [1,4]. However, for clinical purposes, a sufficiently accurate approximation is given by the formula:

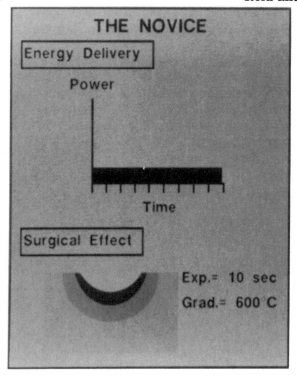
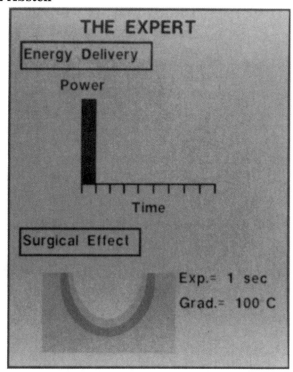

Fig. 33. Novice laser surgeons erode the potential advantages of the CO_2 laser through the use of low rates of energy delivery, resulting in both prolonged durations of lateral heat conduction and higher crater temperatures. Only the expert, using maximal rates of energy delivery, is successful in minimizing thermal energy to adjacent tissues. (From Reid [208], reproduced with permission.)

$$PD = \frac{110 \times W}{d^2} \ \ W/cm^2$$

where W = the power output shown by the in-line power meter on the laser console (in watts), d = the measured diameter (in mm) of the imprint left by a 10-watt, 0.1-second pulse on a moistened tongue depressor [30]. Since the area of a circle varies according to the square of its radius, any change in spot size will have a quadratic effect upon energy intensity within the focal spot. In contrast, increasing or decreasing the power output from the laser tube exerts only a linear effect upon power density. Despite the importance of average power density the influence of this parameter is often misstated. Minor variations have a negligible effect upon actual surgical control. Considerations of power density serve to set the incident beam with a broadly appropriate range. However, manipulating power density is not a useful method for fine control of the surgical beam.

5. Adjusting beam geometry to control

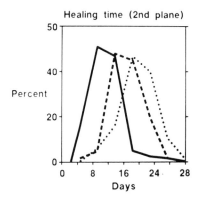

Fig. 34. Reduction in healing time attributable to improved heat control strategies. Healing from a superficial level (second plane). Superpulse and chopped wave are shown as the solid line, high-power continuous wave as the slashed line, and low-power continuous wave as the dotted line. (From Reid et al. [28], reproduced with permission.)

crater shape. Even within the unfocused beam emitted from the laser tube, there is substantial variation in energy intensity from point to point

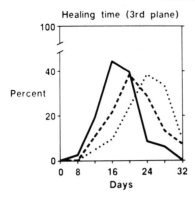

Fig. 35. Reduction in healing time attributable to improved heat control strategies. Healing from a deeper level (third plane). Superpulse and chopped wave are shown as the solid line, high-power continuous wave as the slashed line, and low-power continuous wave as the dotted line. (From Reid et al. [28], reproduced with permission.)

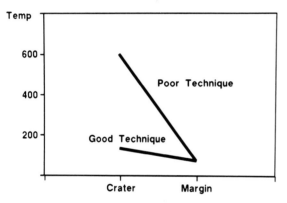

Fig. 36. Comparison of the thermal conduction gradients from a noncarbonized (top) and a carbonized (bottom) crater. With a lower irradiance level, here is a relatively thick zone of tissue heated above the coagulation threshold but below the vaporization threshold. Because such a coagulum is relatively anhydrous, this residue is no longer capable of vaporization. Rather, subsequent photons carbonize and heat this residue to crater temperatures of the order of 600°C. (From Reid [209], reproduced with permission.)

within the focal spot. Obviously, these differences in energy intensity will affect the shape of the resultant crater at the impact point. Points of higher intensity, usually the center of the beam, will vaporize more tissue per unit time than points of lower energy intensity (usually situated at the beam periphery). In other words, the actual shape of the impact crater will be a mirror image of the energy profile of the incident beam.

The degree of variation in energy intensity

within the raw beam is amplified many times by the focusing that occurs within the beam delivery system (Fig. 38). At points of extreme defocus, the energy profile will have an excessively flat geometry (Fig. 39). Therefore, *point z* produces a "watch-glass" defect crater characterized by excessive coagulation, minimal vaporization, and substantial heat accumulation at the operative site.

Sharp focusing will concentrate the vast majority of incident photons at the center of the focal spot. Energy absorption at *point x* greatly exceeds the thresholds for both coagulation and vaporization, producing a narrow, deep crater shaped like a golf tee.

Between these two extremes (points X and Z in Fig. 39), there is a region of defocus—*point Y*—that will create a "rounded" beam geometry. "Rounding" means that the energy profile has been flattened to the point where beam amplitude is about half the spot diameter. Therefore, the volume of tissue destruction conforms to one-half of an imaginary sphere, with crater depth approximating one radius and spot diameter approximating two radii. In defocusing to point Y, incident energy has to be balanced against the area of the focal spot. Using superpulse, the fluence of the beam must be kept above the vaporization threshold for the volume of target tissue needed to absorb this energy (i.e., the critical volume). Otherwise, even superpulsed beams will cause tissue charring. With continuous wave beams, it is even more important to maintain favorable balance between sublimation and thermal coagulation. Thus in either instance, beam geometry must be rounded so as to produce a shallow crater (like an ice cream scoop).

The ability progressively to defocus beam geometry until this hemispheric shape is reached is a crucial but neglected aspect of surgical control (Fig. 40). Incisions are always made with a tightly focused beam, and shallow photovaporization is always done with a beam defocused to the point of hemispheric geometry. These considerations hold true at all anatomic sites and for all surgical situations. Any XY hybrid will be too blunt for optimal cutting (resulting in a three-dimensional incision), yet too sharp for controlled photovaporization (resulting in bleeding from the vessels transected at the crater base). Similarly, any YX hybrid will produce an unfavorable ratio of coagulation:photovaporization—resulting in carbonization and excessive thermal injury.

In the past, beam geometry was controlled

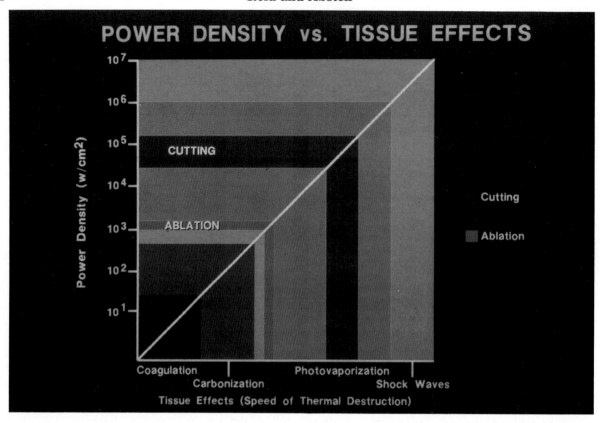

Fig. 37. Different qualitative effects (shown on the X axis), produced by different power densities (shown as a log scale on the Y axis). At low levels of irradiance ($<$750 W/cm^2), tissue heating is generally insufficient to reach the threshold of vaporization; hence, coagulation predominates over sublimation. However, at irradiance levels of 1,000 W/cm^2 to 500,000 W/cm^2, the rate of tissue healing is sufficient to ensure a predominance of vaporization. Beyond 500,000 W/cm^2, there is electron stripping (analagous to a lightning bolt), resulting in acoustic shock waves and tissue tearing. Although photovaporization occurs across a wide range of irradiance levels, the clinical realities of beam control dictate that both ablation and incision be done within quite narrow limits. (From Reid [209], reproduced with permission.)

TABLE 4. Factors Involved in Controlling Speed of Cut

Surgical objective	Factor crucial to optimal outcome	Factor essential to surgical control
Incision	Turn laser to narrowest available spot size.	Adjust speed of cut by turning power up or down.
Ablation	Turn power output to maximum.	Adjust speed of ablation by incremental defocus.

by mismatching the focal lengths of the optical and laser lenses (e.g., 300 mm visual and a 200 mm laser lens). However, modern lasers are equipped with microslad defocusing devices, which contain both converging and diverging lenses (Fig. 41). Incisions are done at the point of "zero defocus" where both lenses are in apposition and behave like a single convex lens (Fig. 42a). Epithelial ablation is done by incrementally winding the microslad to progressive points of de-

focus, until a 1/10-second impact leaves an approximately hemispherical crater on the tongue blade (Fig. 42b).

6. Gated pulses to improve delicate surgical control. Because quality of outcome with a CW laser depends directly upon the speed of energy delivery, surgeons must not decrease operating power as a control strategy in delicate situations, such as for the destruction of a lesion on the glans clitoris. Instead, the same temporal mode

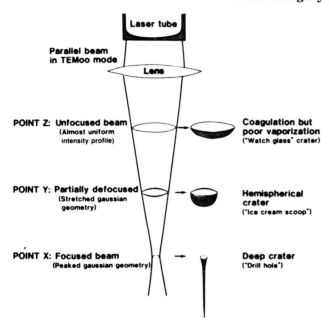

Fig. 38. Effect of defocusing on beam geometry. Whereas incisions are best made with a tightly focused beam (point X), surface ablation should always be done at a point of partial defocus (point Y). Fully defocused beams cause extensive char, with negligible penetration (point Z) and therefore have no surgical applications. (From Reid et al. [107], reproduced with permission.)

and operating power are maintained, but gated into 1/10–1/20-second bursts (Fig. 43). This strategy permits ample reaction time between pulses, thereby allowing the surgeon to continue using high rates energy delivery.

Some readers confused "gated pulse" with "superpulse." *Gated pulse* simply means placing a mechanical shutter or an electronic timer to interrupt the energy delivery to the target. In other words, gating is only an aid to hand-eye control. Unfortunately, gated pulses (e.g., 100–200 ms) are much longer than thermal relaxation times (e.g., 0.6 ms). Hence, gated pulsing does nothing to reduce lateral heat conduction. *Superpulsing* connotes the compression of energy within the laser tube, so as to produce higher peak powers than could be generated in CW steady-state emission. As such, superpulsing promotes char-free surgery. Superpulsed laser beams are no more difficult to use than CW beams and can be controlled just as easily by the strategy of gating.

Ablation or Excision of the Cervical Transformation Zone

Role of HPV infection. Although cancer can arise at any site within the lower genital tract, the metaplastic epithelium at the squamo-columnar junction has the greatest propensity for malignant transformation. Even in women who develop multifocal anogenital malignancies, disease generally arises first within the transformation zone [31,32]. Now that molecular biologists have resolved the early sources of testing artifact, it has become clear that the basic cellular transformation leading to *cervical intraepithelial neoplasia* (CIN) is initiated by infection of immature squamous metaplasia with an oncogenic human papillomavirus (HPV) [33–36]. The early genomic region of the oncogenic HPVs, but not the nononcogenic HPVs, provides all the means for inducing cellular immortality and for evoking an aneuploid chromosome complement in tissue culture (Fig. 44) [37,38]. Transfection with oncogenic HPV DNAs can immortalize human keratinocytes in cell culture, and further growth of these immortalized cells on collagen rafts or in nude mice can produce histologic patterns essentially identical to CIN 3 (Table 5) [39–43]. In clinical situations, the progressive potential of precursor lesions has been largely defined by HPV type [43–46].

Whether these HPVs also play a role in promoting progression from the precursor state to invasive disease is less certain. There have been reports of HPV-immortalized cells acquiring invasive properties simply by continued growth in vitro for 2–4 years, without exposure to additional carcinogens [40]. Within naturally occurring cervical neoplasia and cancer-derived cell lines, the HPV genome is consistently transcribed [47], albeit with striking differences at different points in the pathologic spectrum. Compared with the apparently "balanced" transcription seen in low-grade lesions (where both early and late regions are represented), invasive cancer cells show two marked differences—increased expression of the two viral transforming genes (E6 and E7) and no detectable late gene expression [36]. E6 and E7 proteins coded by oncogenic HPV types antagonize two important tumor suppressor proteins, p53 and pRB, thereby deregulating cell growth [37,38]. Finally, the integration of HPV genetic sequences into the host genome usually occurs just as the cell develops invasive properties [47]. For integration to occur, the HPV episomes are linearized in a way that typically preserves E6/E7 expression, but abolishes the negative regulatory effects of the E2 gene. The end result is a permanent mutation in the cellular genome, which is transmitted to all progeny cells during subse-

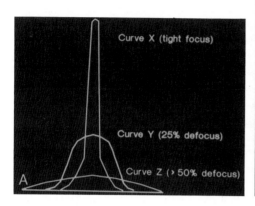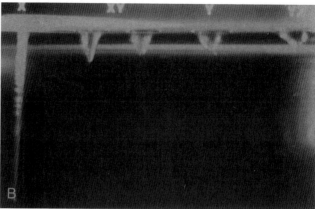

Fig. 39. **A:** Three schematic intensity profiles showing beam geometry at sharp focus (point X), partial focus (point Y), and complete defocus (point Z). **B:** Impact craters made by a laser beam at different points of focus and fired into the cross cut end of a plexiglass block. The craters are now viewed at right angles to the direction in which the laser beam traveled. Point X is the correct geometry for incision, and point Y is correct for shallow ablation. Hybrids XY and YZ are not suitable for surgical use. (From Reid [209], reproduced with permission.)

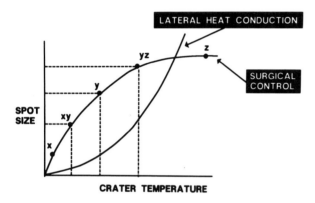

Fig. 40. How increasing ease of surgical control is paid for by increasing desiccation of the impact site (and hence, increasing heat conduction). Point Y (the point of initial "rounding") attains good control and acceptable heat conduction. Further increases in spot size (point YZ) substantially increase thermal injury, yet gain only modest improvement in surgical control. Conversely, insufficient defocus (point XY) produces too much bleeding for the slight additional reduction in crater temperature. (From Reid [209], reproduced with permission.)

quent mitotic divisions. Of course, malignant promotion from CIN 3 to invasive cancer probably involves multiple factors. Certainly the significant pool of chronic latent infection in otherwise healthy individuals and the low progression rate of untreated high-grade intraepithelial lesions indicate that this equation involves more than just the simple acquisition of an oncogenic HPV infection (Table 6) [43,47,48].

Basic treatment philosophy. The prevalence of morphological disorders of cervical epithelium greatly exceeds the eventual incidence of invasive cancer [49–51]. In the past, carcinoma in situ (CIS) was seen as a definite malignancy that was not yet invasive, for which a full measure of anticancer therapy (including radiation) was sanctioned [52]. In the 1950s and 1960s, cone biopsy was done with diagnostic rather than therapeutic intent. Unfortunately for women at that time, hysterectomy was considered mandatory in patients with CIS. In contrast, "dysplasia" was seen as a nonspecific epithelial alteration needing no special treatment or follow-up. In 1966, Kolstad et al. [53] showed that by attention to the margins of resection, the protection against eventual invasive cancer afforded by therapeutic conization was comparable to that afforded by hysterectomy.

Experience soon confirmed that colposcopically directed punch biopsies provided an accurate noninjurious method of obtaining a histologic diagnosis in patients with abnormal Papanicolaou smears. As an extension of the trend to treat CIS by excisional cone biopsy instead of hysterectomy, small localized lesions were managed by physical destruction of the abnormal transformation zone using cryosurgery, electrocoagulation diathermy, or the CO_2 laser. The use of these modalities has been found to be safe if a strict protocol is followed (Table 7) [54].

Efficient transformation zone destruction

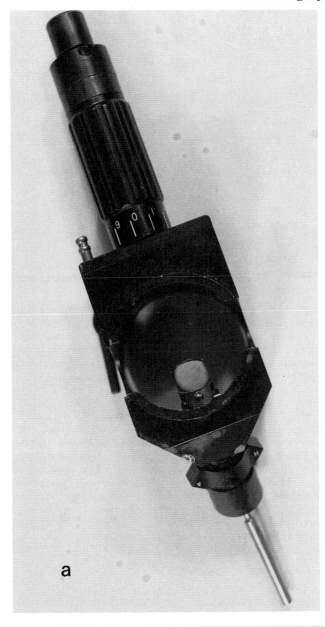

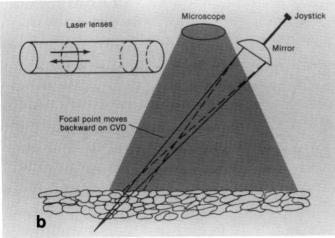

a

b

provides efficient and cost-effective prophylaxis against subsequent malignant progression. However, the spread of colposcopic methods of an ever-increasing number of gynecologists, and lately to family physicians or nurse practitioners, has had some negative aspects. In the 1980s, there were several articles reporting deaths from invasive cancer following outpatient therapy of premalignant lesions [55–57]. Analysis of the clinical details from these series has shown that the majority of mishaps are attributable to major breaches in compliance with the triage rules. Most glaringly, 45 of 99 cases reported by Townsend et al. [55] had cryosurgery or hot cautery for "chronic cervicitis" without prior colposcopic examination and biopsy. Of 66 women in two series who did undergo colposcopic examination, major triage errors included treatment without biopsy, failure to assess adequately the endocervical canal, ablative therapy for lesions extending deeply into the cervical canal, failure to evaluate further a positive endocervical curettage, and failure to act upon a colposcopic suspicion of possible invasion.

Patients with abnormal cervical cytology can be subdivided into two clear groups—high and low grade. High-grade (CIN 2–3) lesions represent a homogeneous population of permanently premalignant epithelium, generally as a result of genetic injuries induced by oncogenic HPV infection [33–43]. If left untreated, more than one-third will progress to invasive cancers within a decade [59]. Fortunately, such lesions can be recognized reliably by expert histologists and to a lesser extent, by expert cytopathologists. Treatment of CIN 2–3 is mandatory but can generally be accomplished by outpatient methods. Conversely, low-grade biopsies (CIN 1 and flat condyloma) comprise a heterogenous mixture of many different conditions, rather than a single pathologic entity. In essence, the histologic features represent a nonspecific tissue response to recent injury, be that infection by an oncogenic HPV virus, a nononcogenic HPV or repair of a nonspecific injury. Regression rates greatly exceed progression rates. Historically, low-grade cytologic abnormalities were therefore followed by repeating the Pap smear every 6 months, until three consecutive negatives were obtained. There is,

Fig. 41. **a:** Actual microslad defocusing device. The numbered ring can be rotated to create incremental defocus of the laser beam. **b:** How moving the joystick on a universal joint can rotate the laser mirror and thus move the laser beam within the optical field.

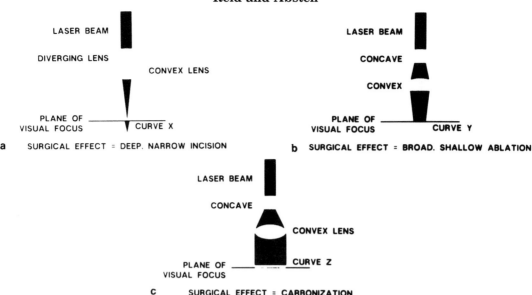

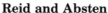

Fig. 42. Various settings attainable with the microslad. **a:** Cutting beam geometry. At the point of "zero defocus," the diverging and converging lenses are in opposition, thus behaving like a single convex lens. Hence, the laser energy reaches the plane of visual focus as a narrow beam that is also completely focused, producing a drill-like crater (corresponding to curve X in Fig. 40A). **b:** Partial defocus to a vaporizing power density. Used at this point of partial defocus ("position 4") the diverging lens is now separated from the converging lens such that the laser beam reaches the visual plane in partial defocus. Whether such defocus reflects a laser beam that is still converging toward focus or one the is diverging away from focus is of no surgical importance. What does matter is that for an incident power of 60 watts, point 4 on this Sharplan Industries microslad, produces an approximately hemispherical impact crater on a tongue blade. Higher powers require that the lenses be even farther separated (e.g., point 5 for 100 watts), whereas lower powers require less separation (e.g., point 3 at 30 watts). After using a tongue blade to find the beam geometry that approximately corresponds to curve "Y" (see Figs. 39a, 40) the surgeon can now make some trial impacts on the tissues. If the tissue crater shows a tendency to carbonization, the microslad must be turned back to a position of tighter focus, thus raising power density to a safer level. In contrast, if the impact crater has a prominent central depression (corresponding to an XY hybrid shown in Figs. 39b, 40), then the beam geometry needs to be further flattened by turning the microslad to a position of greater defocus. **c:** Partial defocus to an unacceptably low power density. (curve Z in Figs. 39a, 40). A surgeon committing his error nullifies the advantages of rapid superpulsing, chopped wave, or rapid energy delivery. There is excessive coagulation but inefficient vaporization. Because there is no significant vaporization, the accumulated heat remains in the wound rather than rising with the plume. Moreover, subsequent photons carbonize this coagulated anhydrous tissue, creating an excessive thermal gradient for heat diffusion. (From Reid [209], reproduced with permission.)

however, one major fallacy in this protocol. Approximately one in five women with low-grade Pap smears will be found to have high-grade dysplasias at the time of colposcopy [60]. Moreover, several longitudinal studies examining the natural history of untreated mild dysplasia were marred by instances of progression to invasive cancer [61–64]. Hence, authorities of the 1970s and 1980s generally recommended that women with low-grade smears be sent for colposcopic triage. As a natural progression of this policy, empiric destruction of the transformation zone was championed as a pragmatic and cost-effective alternative to serial follow-up. In reality, neither option is satisfactory. Long-term cytologic follow-up of LGSIL represents systematic undertreatment of the small fraction that might progress and empiric destruction of all LGSILs represents systemic overtreatment of the large fraction that would never progress. For the present, the latter protocol is the best choice, but since introduction of the Bethesda system, its value has been compromised by overreferral [65,66]. In the future, improved methods of virus testing probably will be used to triage low-grade lesions into one of two groups—early precursor or harmless mimic [33].

Recently, the winds of change also have begun to blow from another quarter. Now that cervical excision biopsies can be easily performed in an office setting, some have advocated a "see and treat" protocol [67,68]. The rationale for immediate loop electrosurgical excision of the transformation zone allows the first visit to be both diag-

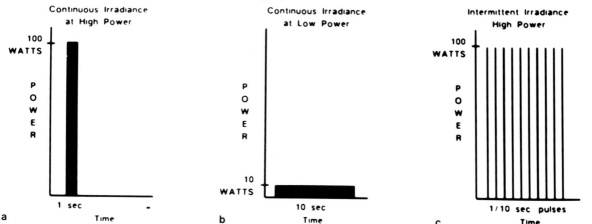

Fig. 43. Value of intermittent pulses as a means of maintaining surgical control in delicate situations. **a:** 100 joules delivered by irradiating with 100 watts for 1 second satisfies the requirement of rapid energy delivery, but may be hard to control. **b:** 100 joules delivered as 10 watts for 10 seconds causes too much lateral heat conduction. **c:** 100 joules delivered by 10 shuttered pulses of a 100-watt beam, each pulse lasting for one-tenth of a second. (From Reid [76], reproduced with permission.)

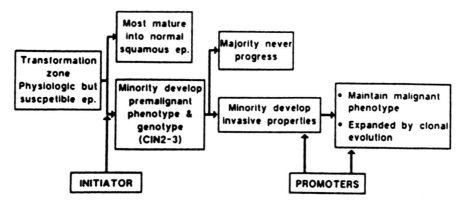

Fig. 44. Diagrammatic representation of the standard model for the pathogenesis of solid tumors. Initiators transform physiologic but susceptible squamous metaplasia into permanently altered precursor epithelium. In contrast, promotors act at various other points in this cascade, such as developing invasive properties, maintaining a malignant phenotype, or favoring clonal expansions. (From Reid, Lorincz [43], reproduced with permission.)

nostic and therapeutic. The weakness of this strategy is that the indication for surgery is now based on a screening test (the abnormal Papanicolaou smear), rather than on a diagnostic evaluation (a directed biopsy). In specific settings (e.g., in clinics for indigent women), benefits outweigh disadvantages. However, within a typical private practice, where less-experienced colposcopists are evaluating mainly low-grade abnormalities in young and compliant women, the "see and treat" philosophy will lead to substantial overtreatment, additional morbidity, and unnecessary cost.

Surgical geometry of the transformation zone. The human cervix is a cylinder of fibromuscular tissue, which averages ~3.5 cm in length and ~2.5 cm in diameter. The upper and middle thirds of the cervical canal are lined by Müllerian-derived columnar epithelium, continuous with the endometrium proximally. The peripheral part of the ectocervix is covered by squamous mucosa, continuous with the vulvar skin caudally. The glycogenated, stratified squamous epithelium derives embryologically as an upgrowth from the endodermal portion of the primitive cloaca. This endodermal-Müllerian boundary is generally located on the cervical portion, thus exposing a variable area of fragile columnar epithelium to the harsh acid environment of the vagina (Fig. 45) [69]. Repeated chemical burning results in activation of specialized cells called stromal reserve cells. Over time, this phenomenon produces the *transformation zone*—a donut

TABLE 5. HPV Infection Linked to Progression From CIN 2–3 to Invasive Cancer*

1. Cross-sectional data show strong, consistent relationship between specific HPV types and both precursor and invasive disease.
2. HPV-immortalized human cells can eventually develop tumorigenic (invasive) properties with long-term culture.
3. Animal papillomaviruses of analogous genetic organization produce invasive cancers in several species.
4. Viral genome (especially E6 and E7) is continuously transcribed within cancer cells and cervix-cancer-derived cell lines.
5. E6 and E7 viral proteins bind two cellular "antioncogenes" (p 53 and p RB) that control cell growth rates.
6. HPV DNA is episomal in benign lesions but integrated into the cellular genome of most cancer cells.
7. Integration destroys the viral negative control gene (E2) but preserves the transforming genes (E6 and E7).

*CIN = Cervical intraepithelial neoplasia. Reprinted with permission from Reid, et al. [208].

TABLE 6. Evidence of HPV Infection Linked to Pathogenesis of CIN 2–3*

1. Cancer-associated HPVs are found in 90% of CIN 2–3 vs. 10% of normal women, yielding a relative risk estimate of 80:1.
2. CIN 1 is indistinguishable from condyloma, but viral cytopathic effect decreases with increasing levels of premalignant transformation.
3. Noninfected cervical epithelium becomes senescent after ten passages in cell culture; however, cervical keratinocytes are immortalized by oncogenic HPV infection.
4. Histologic features of CIN 2–3 can be reproduced in vitro and in vivo by oncogenic HPV infection of previously normal human keratinocytes.
5. Progressive potential of minor cervical atypia is influenced by HPV type.

*CIN = cervical intraepithelial neoplasia. Reprinted with permission from Reid, et al. [208].

TABLE 7. Triage Rules

1. *Exclude invasive cancer*
   - Colposcopist able to recognize invasive cancer.
   - New squamocolumnar junction entirely visible.
   - Document canal status (colposcopy, cytobrush, ECC).
2. *Restricted indications for conization*
   - Suspected microinvasive squamous carcinoma.
   - Adenocarcinoma in situ.
   - CIN[a]-2 or -3* on portio, but new squamocolumnar junction not definable.
   - Unexplained significant cytology (>CIN 2).
3. *Most conservative therapy compatible with safety*
   - Cone biopsy = "therapeutic," not "diagnostic."
   - Hysterectomy reserved for rare indications
   - Remaining cases treated by transformation zone ablation.
   - Treatment planned by topography, not histologic grade.

*Cervical intraepithelial neoplasia.

shaped field of reserve cell proliferation, showing varying degrees of squamous maturation. If maturity (as judged histologically by the degree of differentiation in the epithelial layers) is reached under physiologic conditions, the risk of subsequent squamous cancer is remote. Conversely, cumulative genetic injury to activated reserve cells can deviate squamous metaplasia towards malignant change.

Defining the boundaries. Obviously, the original squamocolumnar junction (OSCJ) represents the distal transformation zone margin. In adults, the OSCJ is generally camouflaged by a proximally advancing field of squamous metaplasia. The new squamocolumnar junction (NSCJ) is readily recognized through the colposcope, but its significance is poorly understood (Fig. 46). Many colposcopists erroneously believe the NSCJ to be the upper limit of the transformation zone. In truth, the NSCJ is just above the middle of the transformation zone! It is generally known that distal to the NSCJ, one finds mature cornified metaplastic squamous epithelium. However, *it is a crucial, but poorly understood fact that squamous metaplasia is also found on the proximal side of the NSCJ,* although the cells within this less mature field of squamous metaplasia have not yet manifested layered differentiation. Hence, this boundary between highly reflective (differentiated) and nonreflective (undifferentiated) epithelium can be seen through the colposcope.

In younger women, the upper limit of squamous metaplasia (ULSM) is generally located ~1 cm into the canal (Fig. 47). During the peri- and postmenopausal years, the transformation zone tends to involute into the endocervical canal, thus moving the ULSM much closer to the histologic internal os. Because squamous neoplasia arises in the more mature half of the transformation zone, the NSCJ provides the clinical basis for designat-

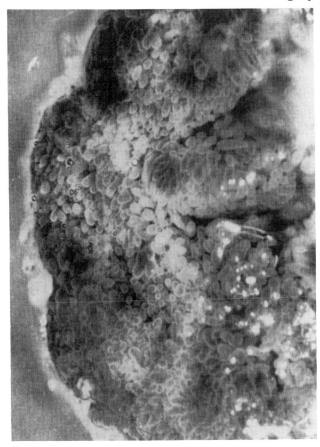

Fig. 45. Original squamocolumnar junction. The boundary between smooth original squamous epithelium and villous cervical columnar epithelium is very sharp, indicating the collision of two different tissues during embryogenesis.

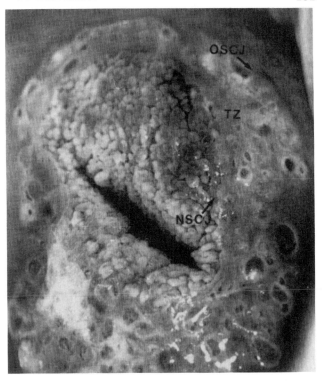

Fig. 46. New squamocolumnar junction. Progressive squamous metaplasia has transformed the OSCJ into a squamo-squamous (rather than squamo-columnar junction). The advancing edge of cornification withing this field is seen as a sharp line, called the new squamo-columnar junction by colposcopists. Squamous cancer arises between the NSCJ and the OSCJ, but adenocarcinoma arises between the NSCJ and the midcanal.

ing a colposcopic examination as "satisfactory" vs. "unsatisfactory" (Fig. 48). However, one of the most important elements in safe triage is the appreciation that cervical adenocarcinoma arises in the field of immature metaplasia located between the NSCJ and the ULSM (Fig. 49).

The most practical approach to setting treatment margins lies through a thorough understanding of the geometry of the transformation zone and the dynamic variations in this geometry over a woman's life. To this end, it is helpful to subdivide the various patterns into six discrete levels (Fig. 50).

Level 1. The colposcopic NSCJ is completely visible on the cervical portio, and the external os is completely surrounded by a concentric ring of villous columnar epithelium. Such patients will not have disease within the canal. The endocervical curettage (ECC) can be safely omitted for level 1 lesions.

Level 2. The colposcopic NSCJ is still visible on the cervical portion but adjoins immature squamous metaplasia rather than villous columnar epithelium. The risk of an unrecognized endocervical extension is negligible and again, ECC can be either omitted or replaced by a cytobrush sample from the lower canal. Level 1 and level 2 lesions are equally suited to either ablative or excisional therapies.

Level 3. The colposcopic NSCJ is at or just inside the external os, but is easily visualized within the distal 4 mm of the canal by using an endocervical speculum. Historically, untold thousands of such lesions have been treated by ablative methods. This practice is safe—provided that the triage rules (including canal sampling) are carefully followed. However, in modern office practice, the comfort of being able to send the distal 1 cm of the canal for histologic assessment has pushed the pendulum of surgical opinion away from laser or cryosurgical ablation and toward

The Anatomy of the Transformation Zone

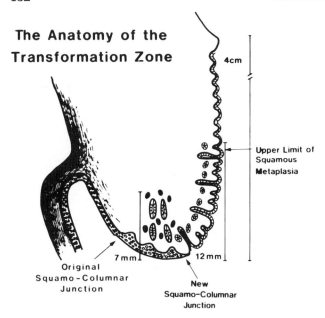

Fig. 47. The true anatomy of the transformation zone. The original squamocolumnar junction represents an embryologic boundary between an upgrowth of vaginal endoderm and a downgrowth of endocervical mesoderm. The original squamo-columnar junction denotes the distal margin of the transformation zone, but its location in adults is camouflaged by the proximal migration of squamous metaplasia. The advancing edge of this new squamous epithelium is readily recognized through the colposcope. Many colposcopists erroneously believe that this new junction is the upper limit of the transformation zone. In reality, the new junction represents only a boundary between mature and immature metaplasia. The proximal border of the transformation zone is the upper limit of squamous metaplasia (the point at which immature squamous metaplasia abuts a circumferential ring of unaltered columnar epithelium). (From Reid [76], reproduced with permission.)

loop excision. Certainly, less experienced colposcopists should definitely opt for office excision rather than simple destruction. Even for experienced gynecologists, occasional cases of unsuspected adenocarcinoma in situ (ACIS) will be detected by loop excision.

Level 4. The colposcopic NSCJ extends >5 mm above the external os. As such, the NSCJ can often be seen with an endocervical speculum. Nonetheless, with high-grade lesions extending to this level, the risk of occult invasive or ACIS within the canal is substantial. Hence, it is mandatory that a narrow cylinder of endocervical canal be removed for for histologic examination. The ideal depth of excision in level 4 lesions is ~1.5 cm. Such a specimen can be excised in the office by either laser minicone or electrosurgical

loop excision, (e.g., one full and one half pass with a 1 × 1 cm insulated electrode). However, the frequency of finding CIN at the apical margins is higher in level 4 lesions; hence, for more worrisome lesions, formal excisional cone under anesthesia should be considered.

Level 5. The NSCJ has receded deeply within the canal and cannot be visualized; this is typical of lesions in perimenopausal and postmenopausal women. In level 5 lesions, the greater portion of the transformation zone is completely out of colposcopic range. Hence, safe triage generally requires removal of a 2 cm cylinder of endocervix by formal diagnostic conization, even if hysterectomy is to be performed in the future. Such surgery is better done with a focused laser beam (or even a cold knife) rather than an electrosurgical loop.

Level 6. In patients treated by previous excisional conization, the visualization of an apparent NSCJ can no longer be relied upon. There is now a real possibility of an iatrogenic skip lesion. Hence, a high-grade smear warrants excision of a narrow cylindrical cone. Conversely, in patients in whom "satisfactory" lesions had been previously treated by cryosurgery or laser, a epeat transformation zone ablation can still be performed—provided that the entire NSCJ is visible.

Satisfactory colpscopies: The "cowboy hat" concept. Twenty years ago, pioneers of the various ablative methods had to make an empirical choice as to where to place their upper margins of destruction. In the United States, early advocates of cryosurgery decided that removal of the metaplastic epithelium in the lower canal would lead to cervical stenosis. Hence, they selected flat probes and advised against freezing the columnar epithelium adjacent to the external os. At the same time, the Australian pioneers of electrodiathermy observed that both initial failures and late recurrences were reduced by extending the therapeutic margins to include the entire field of metaplastic epithelium, rather than just the mature TZ distal to the NSCJ. Fears that the destruction of the lower centimeter of the canal might provoke cervical stenosis or infertility have proved groundless, largely because the cervix has an ability fully to regenerate the removed tissue. Hence, regardless of treatment modality, for lesions in which the NSCJ is satisfactorily seen, ablation or excision should conform to a "cowboy hat" pattern (rather than a flat cylinder) (Fig. 51). Within this cowboy hat, the peripheral disc

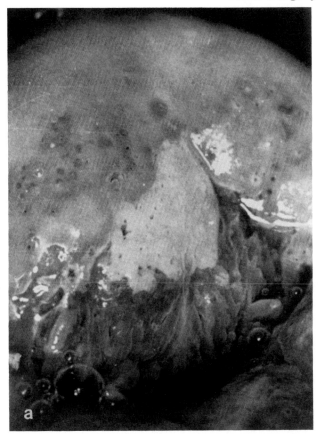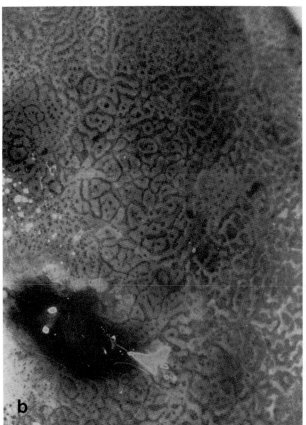

Fig. 48. **a:** Satisfactory colposcopy. This small CIN 3 is easily seen, bordering a field of physiologic squamous metaplasia in the lower canal. **b:** Unsatisfactory colposcopy. Extreme mosaic pattern on the ectocervix goes "out of range" into the cervical canal.

should have a vertical depth of 5–7 mm and a lateral diameter proportionate to the width of the lesion to be destroyed. The central cylinder requires an additional vertical depth of ~5 mm (high enough to reach the upper limit of squamous metaplasia), and a lateral diameter of ~1 cm (wide enough to encompass the endocervical crypts).

The defect regenerates by a downgrowth of columnar epithelium and loose connective tissue from the midcanal (Fig. 52). Once this downwardly growing tongue abuts the lateral margin of the treatment crater, the open surface is then covered by an ingrowth of squamous epithelium from the cervical portio (Fig. 53). This phenomenon is reflected in the pattern of subepithelial vessels that radiate from the peripheral treatment margin to the new external os. However, this regenerative capacity has limits—a vertical height of ~2 cm and a lateral diameter of about the same. Causes of cervical stenosis after cryo-

surgery, CO_2 laser or loop excision are: (1) treatment depth > 2 cm, (2) treatment diameter > 2 cm, (3) excess thermal damage to adjacent tissues, (4) repeated treatments (especially hot cautery), and (5) specific patients (DES exposed, perimenopausal, lactating women).

Unsatisfactory colposcopy: Role for laser excisional conization. If there were no reason to do otherwise, having the entire lower canal available for histology might make routine cone biopsy an ideal approach. However, such overuse of aggressive cone biopsy would be expensive and morbid. Historically, complications from cold knife cone ranged up to 12%, depending upon the volume of tissue excised. Hence, British and American gynecologists restrict conization to patients with lesions extending into the canal, cases in which there is a definite suspicion of occult invasion, unexplained high-grade cytologic atypia, and smears showing abnormal glandular cells (Table 8) [54].

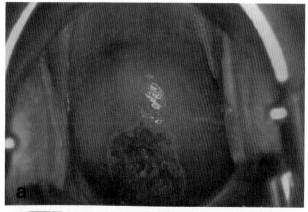

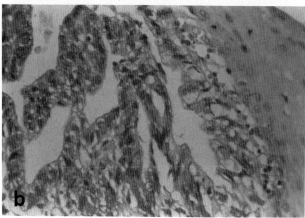

Fig. 49. **a:** Colpophotograph of a young woman with adeno-carcinoma in situ cells on Papanicolau smear. The pathology is located at the small white patch at 1 o'clock on the NSCJ. **b:** Biopsy of this area showing a small adenocarcinoma. (Illustration courtesy of EJ Wilkinson, MD.)

Unfortunately, excisional cone surgery performed with low-powered laser units, using incompletely focused beams and poorly refined surgical techniques, often yielded specimens with too much thermal damage for histologic examination. However, by using acceptable laser settings, such errors are completely avoidable. For the skilled laser surgeon with adequate equipment, it is always possible to do a better excisional cone by laser than by cold knife, as noted below.

1. The mechanics of beam delivery allow great flexibility in the geometry of the excised specimen. Choice of a cylindrical (rather than conical) shape avoids the need to sacrifice a significant proportion of the cervical fibromuscularis (Fig. 54). Thus the risks of cervical deformity, incompetence or stenosis are minimal, even with the need to resect a 20–25 mm cylinder of diseased canal.

2. Choice of a cylindrical geometry obviates the risk of cutting across diseased cervical crypts at the apex of the specimen.
3. Provided that lateral heat conduction is minimized by skillful technique, heat effect will be restricted to the stromal margin. Healing of the defect is both rapid and predictable; the excised cylinder of disease tissue is replaced by a downgrowth of submucosa and columnar epithelium from the midcanal. The end result is a pliable cervix with no net tissue loss.
4. Avoidance of a significant eschar and the prophylactic application of Monsel's solution to the conization bed reduces the risk of secondary hemorrhage to <1%.

Laser excisional conization: Choice of geometry. When conization is done, the width and length should be tailored to the indication and lesion topography. Thus the least injurious excision that will provide clear surgical margins can be planned (Table 9) [70].

Traditional broad, deep cone. Excision of a cone-shape specimen with a diameter and depth of 2–3 cm has the disadvantage of removing a large portion of the fibromuscularis (Fig. 55a). Large cones carry a relatively high complication rate and predispose to a deformed, incompetent cervix [71]. Therefore, this pattern (Fig. 56) [72] should be reserved for uncommon situations in which conization is being done to decide between whether a subsequent hysterectomy will be simple or radical.

Long cylindrical cone. For levels 5 and 6 lesions with no portio extension, excision of a long central cylinder (base = 1.5–2.0 cm; vertical depth = 2.0–2.5 cm) will provide adequate histology, at minimal morbidity (Fig. 55b). Long cylindrical cones are *much* easier to excise with the CO_2 laser than with the cold knife (Fig. 57) [72].

Combination excisional and ablative cone. The most common indication for conization is a broad-based level 4 lesion that extends out of range within the cervical canal. Occult invasion within the endocervical extension can be safely excluded by central laser excision. Morbidity is minimized by vaporizing rather than excising the peripheral extension (Figs. 55c, 58) [73,74].

"Minicone." The "minicone" was designed for patients in whom there is a little suspicion of a significant canal lesion but in whom the criteria for ablation of the transformation zone were not met. In the mid-1980s, surgeons began excising a cylinder with a vertical height of up to 1.5 cm,

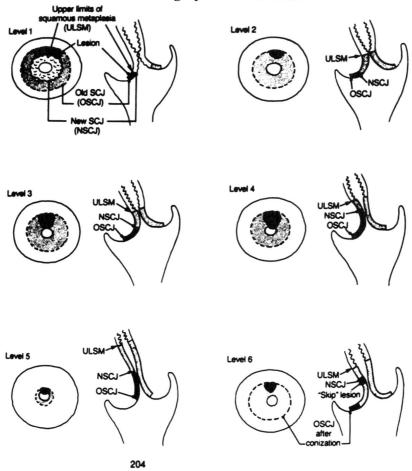

204

Fig. 50. System for categorizing the level of the transformation zone. The shaded area represents the transformation zone. (From Hacker [124], reproduced with permission.)

using the CO_2 laser through a bivalve speculum under local anesthesia (Fig. 55d) [75]. However, the wide availability of electrosurgical loops has sounded the death knell of the laser "minicone."

Surgical techniques. Although the cervix is resilient, *transformation zone ablation* should be done by the best technique available in that medical setting. The rapid superpulse and Ultra-pulse™ are major technologic advances and give better results than older, continuous-wave machines. However, if a CW laser is to be used, the surgeon should ensure adequate power outputs (>25 watts) and high-power densities (750–2,000 w/cm²). Beam geometry is partially defocused (point Y) to suit the specific surgical objectives of layered tissue removal [76]. Although laser destruction of ectocervical epithelium is relatively painless, vaporization within the cervical canal requires effective pain relief. Because paracervical block does not always provide complete anes-

Relation of "Cowboy Hat" to Cervical Anatomy

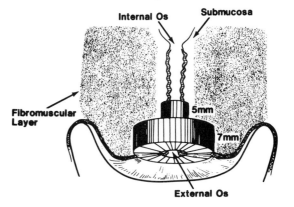

Fig. 51. Destruction of the transformation zone in a "cowboy hat" configuration. The diameter of the peripheral disc corresponds to the peripheral margin of the lesion being treated, whereas the diameter of the central cylinder reflects the depth of the endocervical crypts. (From Hacker [124], reproduced with permission.)

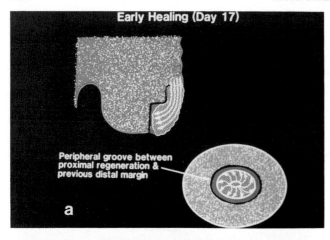

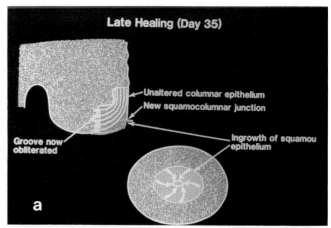

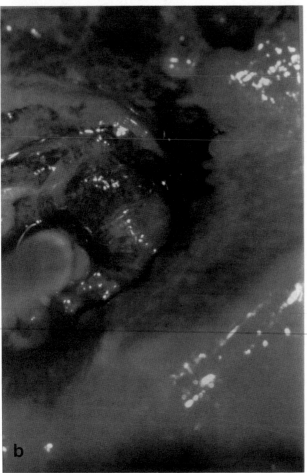

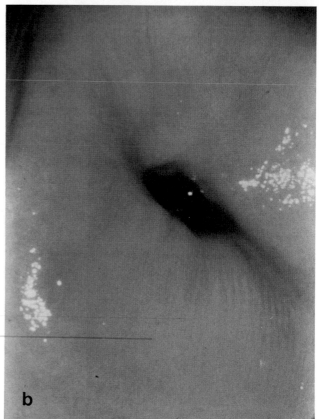

Fig. 52. Early healing. **a:** Healing begins by downgrowth of a "button" of glandular tissue from the endocervical margin. **b:** Groove between the "button" and the crater margin is visible in this colpophotograph taken at the 2-week visit. The canal is seen in the center of this glandular downgrowth, and is being moved with a Q-tip.

thesia, it is easier and more reliable to infiltrate just beneath the cervical mucosa with a dental syringe and a 27-gauge needle.

Fig. 53. Late healing. **a:** Once the crater is filled in, the activated squamous epithelium at the lateral margin grows across the healing "button." **b:** Colpophotograph 5 weeks after laser surgery. The linear pattern reflects the presence of vascular ingrowth during the process of epidermization.

The operation is performed as follows [77]: The cervix is stained with 25% Lugol's iodine (full-strength solution diluted 1:3 with tap water) and the peripheral margin is outlined with the laser before the iodine stain fades (Fig. 59a,b). Using a tight circular movement of the joystick

TABLE 8. Indications for Cervical Conization

1. Inability to visualize the new squamocolumnar junction.
2. CIN[a] 2–3 on ECC.
3. Colposcopic suspicion of occult invasion, even if target biopsies show only CIN[a] 3.
4. Significant discrepancy (2 grades) between the cytology and the histology.
5. Cytologic suspicion of adenocarcinoma in situ.
6. Microinvasion on the punch biopsy.

[a]Cervical intraepithelial neoplasia.

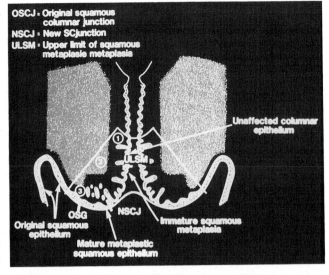

(circles have no beginning and no end), the peripheral portion of the transformation zone is ablated to a depth approximating 7 mm (Fig. 59c,d). The central button surrounding the external os is then destroyed for a distance of ~12 mm along the axis of the cervical canal (Fig. 61e,f). Finally, attention is given to making sure that the crater walls are evenly and vertically destroyed. To avoid inadvertent burns at the introitus, the Graves speculum blades should be opened as wide as is comfortable, and the axis of the vaginal canal should be kept parallel with that of the laser beam [26].

For *excisional conization,* the operation can be performed with either a handpiece or an operating microscope, depending on the laxity of the cervical ligaments. In patients who have a narrow vagina and cervix with minimal descent (e.g., nulliparous postmenopausal females), difficult exposure can be overcome by using the remote control afforded by the operating microscope. Lateral sutures are of no value and may cause additional morbidity. After repeat colposcopy, the cervix is infiltrated with a vasopressor (vasopressin 1:50 dilution) and the direction of the cervical canal carefully established. Provided the larger cervical arterioles are first vasoconstricted, excisional conization with the CO_2 laser should be bloodless.

The incision is made with a highly focused beam (point X) using a power density of at least 50,000 w/cm^2. After the initial cut, the central button is kept under continuous traction, using a Campion hook. Countertraction is provided by opening the Grave's speculum widely. Facility of dissection depends upon mobilizing the intended specimen for a full 360° around its circumference. If difficult exposure is being encountered, the reason is invariably because of failure to free the central cylinder over a 10–20° arc. For the right-handed surgeon, this residual bridge of stroma is usually at about the "7 o'clock" position.

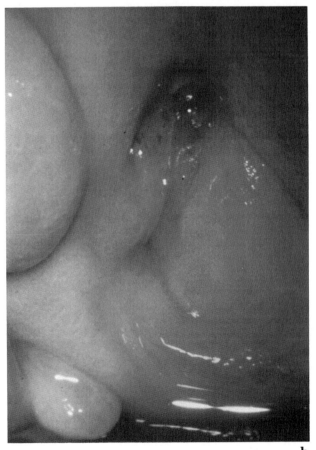

Fig. 54. **a:** Diagram showing the three disadvantages of a conical geometry: (1) the need to aim above the lesion apex, thus sacrificing some normal canal, (2) the inevitable cross-cut that removes some of the cervical fibromuscularis, (3) the need to start wide on the portio, so as to encompass crypt extensions beneath the lesion margin. **b:** Cryptophotograph showing the bad clinical outcome of a broad, deep cone.

TABLE 9. Attributes of Four Conization Geometries*

	Traditional broad, deep cone	Long cylindrical cone	Combination cone	Short minicone
Geometry and usual dimensions	Excision of a cone-shaped specimen with a basal diameter and vertical height of 2–3 cm.	Excision of a long central cylinder with a basal diameter of 1½–2 cm and a vertical height of 2–3 cm.	Excision of a long central cylinder (base = 1–2 cm, height = 1½–2 cm) and vaporization of peripheral areas to appropriate depth (7 mm proximal to OSCJ and 1 mm distal to OSCJ)	Excision of a shallow cylinder with a basal diameter of 1–1½ cm and a vertical height of 1–1½ cm.
Advantage	Entire lesion available for histology.	Provided there is minimal extension on to portio, all of the abnormal epithelium is available for histology.	Although most of ectocervical lesion is vaporized, lower half of canal is still available for histology.	Small cylinder of canal for histology. Done under local anesthesia in office setting.
Disadvantage	Removes large portion of fibromuscular layer predisposing to a deformed, incompetent cervix.	Removal of >20 mm of cervical canal can result in stenosis.	Removal of >20 mm of cervical canal can result in stenosis.	Only useful for shallow lesions (<15 mm).
Complication rate	Highest	Intermediate	Intermediate	Minimal
Objective	To obtain complete histology on a broad, deep lesion, when there is a strong suspicion of occult invasion.	To obtain full histologic assessment of the cervical canal, when colposcopy shows there is no lesion on the peripheral part of the ectocervix.	To obtain complete histology of the canal, where the possibility of invasion in the ectocervical extensions can be safely excluded by target biopsy.	To obtain histology on a small segment of the distal canal, where there is no suspicion of a significant canal lesion but the circumstances for transformation zone ablation are not fulfilled.
Indications	Cytologic suspicion of invasion or abnormal glandular cells, where abnormal colposcopic changes extend onto the peripheral ectocervix. Punch biopsy showing possible microinvasion. Colposcopic suspicion of abnormal vessels, in a patient with a positive smear or a target biopsy showing high-grade CIN. Colposcopic examination shows a large, coarse, complex lesion extending into the cervical canal.	Cytologic suspicion of invasion or abnormal glandular cells, where there is no colposcopic extension to the peripheral ectocervix. A definitely positive endocervical curettage and no lesion on peripheral ectocervix. Unexplained cytologic atypia predictive of CIN-2 or greater. Suspected microinvasion in pregnancy. Significant cytologic atypia following previous excisional cone for high-grade CIN.	Broad based, minor or moderate grade colposcopic atypia where the NSCJ extends >4mm into the canal. A positive endocervical curettage complicating a lesion that otherwise appeared suitable for treatment by transformation zone ablation. Broad-based minor or moderate grade ectocervical lesions in which target biopsy fails to explain the degree of abnormality predicted at cytology. Any broad-based lesion showing cytologic or histologic evidence of CIN-2 or -3 in a peri- or post-menopausal woman, even if the NSCJ appears to be within colposcopic range.	Minor but unexplained cytology, especially when the cervical os is narrowed. An unexpectedly positive endocervical curettage in a young patient with a minor lesion and a satisfactory colposcopic examination. An endocervical curettage with isolated fragments of dysplastic epithelium, suggestive of possible contamination from an ectocervical focus.

*OSCJ = original squamocolumnar junction; NSCJ = new squamocolumnar junction; CIN = cervical intraepithelial neoplasia.

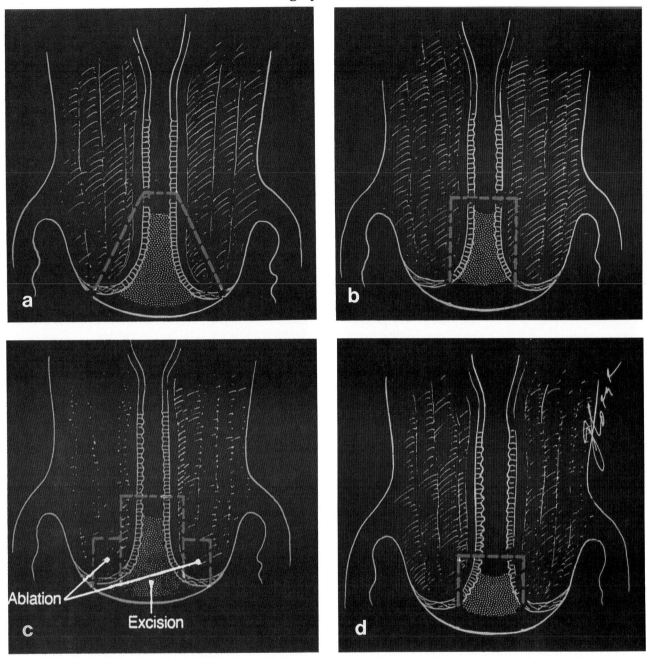

Fig. 55. Conization geometry. **a:** broad deep cone; **b:** long cylindrical cone; **c:** combination ablation and excisional cone; **d:** "minocone." (From Reid [54], reprinted with permission.)

Once the perimeter of the central cylinder has been deepened to the desired depth, the surgeon must decide how he or she is going to amputate the apex. Our general preference in cases with generous surgical access is to use a tonsillar snare. Otherwise, one can pull sharply downward on the Campion hook and use the laser to "chisel" across the apex of the intended specimen. A canal cytology sample is then collected, as additional information on the status of the apical margin. In women over age 35, a dilatation and curettage (D&C) should be performed to exclude squamous intraepithelial neoplasia in the upper endocervical canal (or, rarely, in the endometrium). Monsel's solution is then applied as prophylaxis against secondary hemorrhage during the ensuing 2 weeks.

Results of therapy. Complete removal of

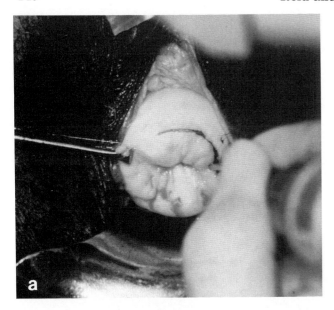 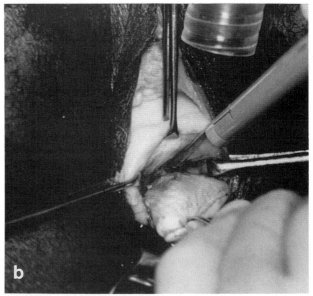

Fig. 56. **a:** Parous patient with genital prolapse, who had malignant glandular cells found at cytology. A broad deep conization is being done, to be followed by vaginal hysterectomy or Wertheim's hysterectomy, depending upon histology. **b:** Cutting with a focus laser beam is entirely bloodless.

the abnormal transformation zone by any method should be effective if used skillfully and with a good understanding of the natural history of cervical neoplasia. Physicians who make mistakes with one modality generally make the same mistakes with another. Tissue that is frozen to death should be just as dead as tissue that is electrocuted, irradiation, or cut to death. Hence, it seems fatuous to argue that one modality would be significantly more effective than another. Experience has long confirmed that for all methods that remove the lower 1 cm of the cervical canal, primary success rates approximate 95% (Table 10). Repeat therapy, when indicated, generally raises success rates to >99% [78,79].

Traditionally, treatment of cervical lesions hinged upon whether or not the triage rules were met. "Satisfactory" lesions were managed by ablative methods and "unsatisfactory" ones by conization. The availability of modern electrosurgical generators has blurred this distinction. However, attempts to overutilize the electrosurgical loop have had a deleterious effect upon cure rates. It is true that any residual disease will undergo spontaneous regression in about two-thirds of the time [80]. However, the converse must not be forgotten—namely, that women in whom CIN 3 extends to the apical margin are ~18 times more likely to have a positive Pap smear in the

future [81]. Thus, gynecologists should continue to respect the fact that some lesions still need formal conization, preferably by CO_2 laser excision.

Invasive cancer after outpatient therapy. No one should die of invasive cancer as a consequence of inappropriate conservatism in diagnosis or treatment. Of particular concern are the reports of invasive cancer occurring in women who have had ablative therapies [55–57]. Unlike cancers after previous conization or hysterectomy, two-thirds of these tumors appear within 12 months and >90% are diagnosed within 2 years, suggesting that an invasive cancer was missed during the initial triage.

Invasive cancer after previous therapy may occur in one of the three ways discussed below.

Failure to detect occult invasion at initial triage. The colposcopic appearance of an overt invasive cancer reveals an ulcerated or exophytic tumor covered with necrotic epithelium and punctuated by abnormal tumor vessels. Warning signs that safeguard against overlooking invasive cancer are listed in Table 11.

Invasion within persistent CIN. Any treatment that leaves a residual focus of CIN within the depths of a cervical crypt could predispose to the subsequent occurrence of an invasive cancer. In addition, failure to destroy the oncogen-exposed immature metaplasia immediately proxi-

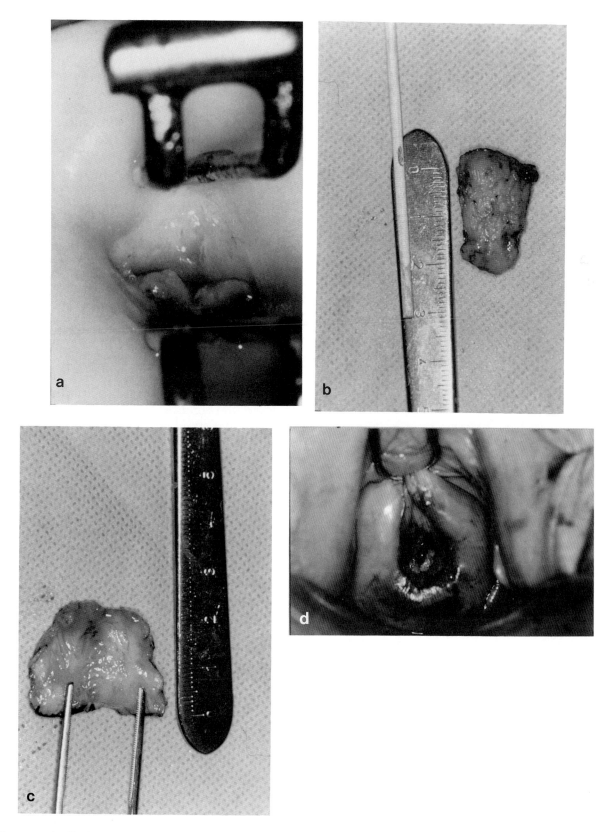

Fig. 57. **a:** Dull white epithelium without a vascular pattern, indicative of a high grade dysplasia. Only the distal portion of the transformation zone is visible, even when displaying the with an endocervical speculum (level 5). **b:** 2-cm cylindrical cone, showing negligible thermal effect on the stromal margin. **c:** Cone open at "3 o'clock," showing the arbor vitae of the endocervical canal, free of any thermal artifact. **d:** Conization crater; use of a cylindrical geometry allows each excision of the lower half (2 cm) of the endocervical epithelium and submucosa, with minimal sacrifice of cervical fibromuscularis. Thus, the cervix will heal without deformity and be at little risk of obstetric incompetence.

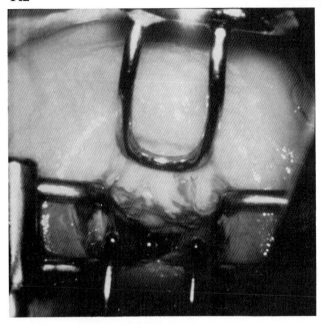

Fig. 58. High-grade endocervical lesion, merging with a low-grade portio lesion.

mal to the NSCJ might permit potentially neoplastic epithelium to remain viable within the cervical canal [78]. Hence, the importance of the "cowboy hat" model for transformation zone ablation [76].

Malignant progression in adjacent vaginal epithelium. About one-third of the invasive cancers that have developed after therapy for CIN have occurred in the original squamous epithelium of the vaginal vault [52]. Hysterectomy does not offer complete protection against subsequent cancer and may complicate matters by burying islands of HPV infected squamous epithelium beneath the vaginal scar (Fig. 60).

Photovaporization of Vulvar and Anal Epithelium

The lower anogenital tract encompasses large areas of squamous mucosa and specialized hair-bearing skin that share a common origin from the endodermal and ectodermal portions of the cloaca. Over the years, these elements are exposed to similar environmental carcinogens [82–84]. When squamous neoplasia does occur, disease is often *multicentric* (involving several distinct anatomic sites within the lower tract) and *multifocal* (originating at several discrete foci within each anatomic site). Hence, management is often very difficult. In particular, multifocal and multicentric disease is not easily resolved by resective surgery. However, since most lesions can be as-

sessed colposcopically, destructive techniques allow the removal of large tracts of surface epithelium without sacrificing the underlying connective tissues. For the gynecologist with sufficient training in laser biophysics and sufficient clinical training to exclude occult cancer, CO_2 laser will produce results that are not attainable with the cold knife.

Two patterns of vulvar neoplasia. Over the last decade, there has been a substantial increase in the prevalence of *vulvar intraepithelial neoplasia (VIN)*, particularly of the multifocal variety in young women. Invasive carcinoma of the vulva is often associated with preinvasive disease, and progression from VIN to invasive cancer has been observed, most frequently in immunosuppressed and elderly women [85]. Progression risk is estimated at ~10%.

Crum [86] suggested there are two patterns of vulvar cancer. Multifocal vulvar cancers appear to be HPV-associated; conversely, solitary nodular tumors generally arise in areas of chronic irritation and repair. In keeping with this hypothesis, Park [87] recently analyzed 36 women with VIN, including six in whom lesions progressed to invasive cancer. These authors described two dominant histological patterns: *Bowenoid* (warty) VIN, characterized by dyskaryotic acanthotic cells showing partial but disordered maturation (Fig. 61a), and a *basaloid* VIN, characterized by an epithelium composed completely of atypical immature parabasal cells (reminiscent of a classic carcinoma in situ of the cervix) (Fig. 61b). Within this retrospective cohort study, the bowenoid variety was associated with a higher frequency of HPV 16 detection (16/23 vs. 5/13) and a lower incidence of invasive carcinoma (3/23 vs. 3/13). The basaloid lesions were associated with chronic epithelial repair ("hyperplastic dystrophy"). It is emphasized that CO_2 laser ablation is only advocated for the management of the bowenoid VIN (Fig. 62). The basaloid (undifferentiated) variety has a different natural history and is not likely to respond to partial thickness destruction. Premalignant foci occurring in association with lichen sclerosus or lichen simplex chronicus always require excision (Fig. 63).

Anal and perianal neoplasias. Squamous carcinoma of the anus is an uncommon tumor that accounts for ~2% of cancers of the large bowel [88]. It typically occurs in the elderly and previously was seen more frequently in women. However, there has been a striking increase in ano-rectal cancer in young, never married Amer-

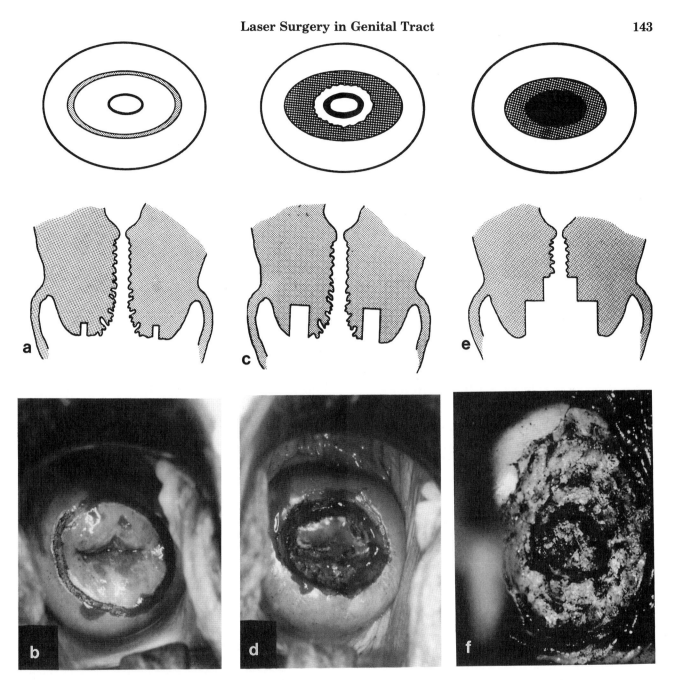

Fig. 59. Ablation of the peripheral transformation zone, forming a 7-mm gutter around the lower canal. (From Reid [77], reproduced with permission.)

ican men. The disease now occurs ~50 times more often in homosexuals than in heterosexual controls [89]. Both histologic and viral analyses confirm an association with papillomavirus infection, HPV 16 being the type most frequently isolated [89,90]. Local trauma, human immunodeficiency virus (HIV), and depressed immune function are all potential cofactors [91].

Precursor lesions for invasive carcinoma of the anus have been considered very uncommon, generally being detected as a chance finding during histologic examination of tissue excised for benign ano-rectal disease [88]. However, careful colposcopic examination of this region in women with multicentric squamous neoplasia will reveal *anal* or *perianal intraepithelial neoplasia ("AIN" or "PAIN")* in almost one-third of cases [92]. AIN and PAIN occur in two clinical forms. One form

TABLE 10. Success Rates for Cryosurgical Destruction of CIN* 3

Series	Patients	Successful initial treatment	Initial success rate
Ostergard [86]	250	210	84%
Kaufman [87]	126	103	82%
Popkin [88]	75	70	93%
Benedet [89]	365	316	87%
Hatch [90]	179	138	77%
Total	995	837	84%

	Failure rates after LEEP (recurrence within 1 year)		
Author	Patients	Failure after LEEP[a] (%)	Maximum Follow-up (months)
Murdoch et al. [84]	600	2.6	3
Prendiville et al. [123]	102	2.0	12
Bigrigg et al. [124]	1000	4.1	21
Luesley et al. [125]	616	4.4	6
Whiteley and Oláh [126]	80	5.1	6
Murdoch et al. [127]	1143	9.0	12
Wright et al. [129]	40	6.0	6

*Cervical intraepithelial neoplasia.
[a]Failure defined as either abnormal cytology and/or colposcopy or positive histology.

TABLE 11. Warning Signs to Safeguard Against Overlooking Invasive Cancer

1. Yellowish epithelium, especially areas that bleed when touched.
2. Colposcopically significant areas (index score ≥6 points) with an irregular surface.
3. Surface ulceration (particularly when bordered by acetowhite epithelium).
4. Atypical vessels (horizontal surface capillaries displaying a "tadpole" or "comma" shape; coarse subepithelial vessels showing an irregular caliber and a long, unbranched course).
5. Extremely coarse mosaicism or punctation, especially if there are wide, irregular intercapillary distances.
6. Large complex lesions (dull, "oyster-white" epithelium occupying 3 or 4 cervical quadrants and showing a mixture of high-grade colposcopic patterns).
7. High-grade colposcopic lesions extending >5 mm into the cervical canal.
8. CIN[a] 2 or 3 on a tangentially sectioned punch biopsy in which the basement membrane cannot be defined adequately.
9. Cytologic evidence of possible squamous carcinoma (CIS cells in large syncytial sheets, prominent nucleoli, bizarre cells, or a "dirty background").
10. Cytologic evidence of adenocarcinoma in situ.
11. Recurrent abnormal cytology in a patient previously treated for CIN[a] 3 (e.g., by cryosurgery, cone biopsy, or hysterectomy).
12. A Pap smear suggestive of HSIL in a postmenopausal woman or previously irradiated women.

[a]Cervical intraepithelial neoplasia.

occurs as plaques of thickened, keratotic, often discolored perianal skin. Although such lesions are generally visible to the unaided eye, they are much better appreciated through the colposcope, after soaking with 5% acetic acid (Fig. 64a). The other form occurs as premalignant change within macroscopic condylomata acuminata. Frequently the neoplastic transformation is unsuspected before histologic examination of representative lesions (Fig. 64b).

Proctoscopic examination of the anal canal and lower rectum will commonly reveal extensive acetowhite areas, some of which will also show significant histologic atypia. Men who have anal intercourse often develop large areas of squamous metaplasia between the dentate line and the proximal rectum. Somewhat analogous to the cervical transformation zone, this squamous metaplasia is very susceptible to infection by high-risk papillomaviruses [92].

Basic treatment philosophy. The clinical consequences of human papillomavirus (HPV) infection are highly individual. Perhaps 90% of exposed individuals never develop recognizable stigmata. When disease expression does occur, lesions may be unicentric or multicentric and disease extent can range from minute to massive. The clinical course varies from trivial and self-limiting to extensive and refractory.

To reconcile this "iceberg" concept with the realities of patient care, morphologic stigmata of HPV infection are best viewed as a cascade in which disease expression ranges from minimal to florid (Table 12) [53]. In a study of 160 women who had papillomavirus-associated diseases,

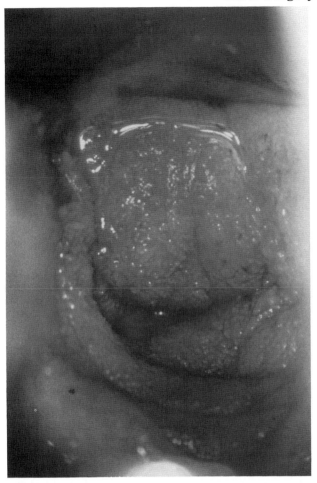

Fig. 60. A 48-year-old woman in remission from Hodgkin's disease, who was treated by abdominal hysterectomy for CIN 3. She presented 2 years later with an abnormal vault smear. Pressure from a cotton-tip applicator ruptured the vault scar, revealing a large, cavitating squamous cancer. The patient had total exenteration and survived.

HPV DNA was detected in 90% of actual lesions, in 69% of acetowhite epithelium surrounding these florid vulvar lesions, in 40% of the "normal" vaginal mucosa, and in 25% of unremarkable squamous metaplasia above that portion of the NSCJ demarcating the proximal margin of a high-grade CIN lesion [93]. This indicates that the presence of HPV genomic sequences is a necessary but insufficient cause for disease formation. Host factors are of equal or greater importance. Hence, HPV-induced diseases of the anogenital tract are best regarded as chronic, regional infections in which cell-virus interaction is regulated by local factors [94,95].

Aggressiveness of treatment must be coun-terbalanced with disease severity, e.g., benign, asymptomatic, subclinical vulvar or vaginal lesions do not require treatment. Therefore, the first objective is to differentiate important disease from the equivocal stigmata seen in at least one-quarter of patients (Fig. 65). Gynecologists must not be drawn into poorly considered therapy just because biopsy of an asymptomatic acetowhitening area is reported as "condyloma" or "HPV infection" by the pathologist. Treatment must be tied to realistic objectives such as the eradication of neoplastic foci, destruction of exophytic condylomas, control of infectivity, or relief of symptoms (Table 13). Treatment aimed at preventing "to and fro" reinfection in patients who are in monogamous relationships is probably misguided [96], and attempts to eradicate all HPV DNA from the genital tract are futile [97]. Rather, most patients can be easily managed by office methods [28]. However, for a small minority of problematic cases, the CO_2 laser is invaluable.

Management of specific disease patterns. Gynecologists will be concerned with focal condylomas of recent onset and with very extensive, refractory, and neoplastic disease.

Focal condylomas of recent onset. Gynecologists can choose from many therapies to manage the various HPV-associated diseases of the vagina, vulva, and anus (Table 14). Despite the CO_2 laser's precision, hemostatic properties, and afforded ease of access, using it as a simple "spot-welder" is not advantageous. Of 1,000 women with HPV-associated vulvar disease, 830 were managed by traditional office therapies that destroy exophytic condylomas [28]. Scissor excision is a useful way to obtain tissue for histology or HPV typing and for treating isolated condylomas. However, the technique is impractical within the vaginal or anal canal, as there is a risk of tissue denudation in patients with extensive disease. Although wide excision with primary closure can give acceptable results in difficult situations, the laser surgeon will always obtain better results.

The best general strategy for destroying external condylomas is the use of cytolytic chemicals. Because their use does not require local anesthesia, these chemicals are appropriate in all clinical settings, including birth control and sexually transmitted disease clinics. Because of an overly enthusiastic study conducted in 1944, which claimed control of penile warts in 96% of transient soldiers, 25% podophyllin resin is still commonly used [98]. However, subsequent

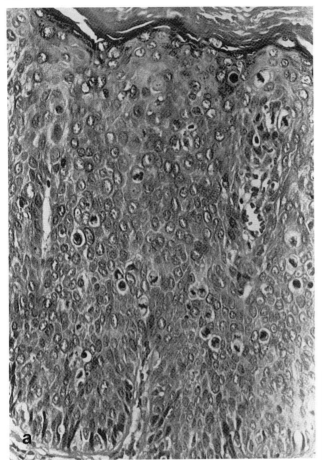

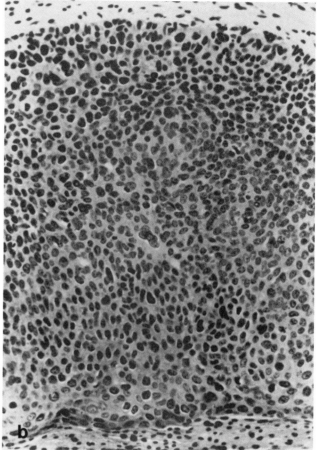

Fig. 61. **a:** VIN 2–3, Bowenoid pattern. Architectural disorganization is more prominent than cytologic abnormalities, and partial maturation presents. The lower two-thirds show crowded, vertically oriented, somewhat undifferentiated cells. Many mitotic figures are present, some of which are abnormal. The upper third shows partial differentiation, merging into a hyperkeratotic surface (not shown). (Illustration courtesy of EJ Wilkinson, MD) **b:** VIN 3, Basaloid pattern. Cytological atypia equal or exceed architectural disturbance. In this example, the lower two-thirds are completely replaced by undifferentiated basal cells, somewhat reminiscent of a CIN 3. Note the large multinucleated cell at center. The epithelial surface was parakeratotic. (Illustration courtesy EJ Wilkinson, MD).

trials of podophyllin have been disappointing; cumulative success rates have averaged from 20% to 40% after 3–6 months of therapy [99,100]. Trichloracetic acid is a effective as podophyllin, but it does not share the same risks of neurologic, myocardial, hepatic, renal, and embryologic toxicity. Moreover, since caustic agents are simple acid radicals that are not absorbed, trichloracetic acid may be used within the vagina and anus, even during pregnancy [101]. Podofilox (Condylox™), prepared by extracting the active lignan from crude podophyllin, represents another significant advance in topical therapy. The cytotoxic effects of podofilox are relatively specific to diseased tissue. Therefore, it has proven safe to allow self-treatment. Drug is applied for 3 days, followed by a 4-day rest period. Compared with crude podophyllin, self-application of the purified derivative has yielded improved success rates (80% vs. 40%) within shorter times [102].

Focal destruction of condylomas using electrocautery, cryosurgery, or localized laser ablation is another acceptable approach. In general, lesions on mucosal surfaces respond as well to cytolytic chemicals as to physical destruction. However, on the skin, surface keratin can impede the access of topical medications to the reservoir of HPV infection at the basal layers. Hence, actual physical destruction or removal is sometimes needed to remove stubborn cutaneous lesions. Al-

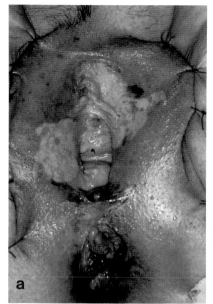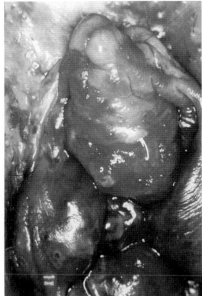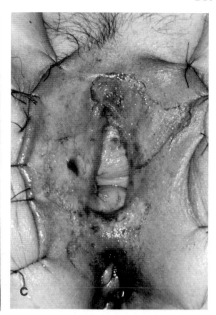

Fig. 62. **a:** Multicentric Bowenoid VIN 3, presenting as both white keratotic plagues and grayish-black maculopapular lesions. Although broadly suited for CO_2 laser ablation, the small ulcers on the right intralabial sulcus and the anterior hemorrhoid warrant excision for closer examination. **b:** Involvement of a prominent hemorrhoid, shown at hyper magnification. **c:** Combined laser ablation plus selective excision offers optimal cosmetic results without compromising patient safety.

though thermal methods require infiltration with local anesthetic, they are more effective than freezing [100]. If cryosurgery is to be used on the vulva, liquid nitrogen is preferable to nitrous oxide cooled cervical probes.

Very extensive, refractory, and neoplastic disease. The overwhelming majority of patients will be cured by destruction of the macroscopically apparent papillomas, without regard to the adjacent areas of acetowhite epithelium [28,96]. However, significant management problems arise with: (1) very extensive condylomas such as coalescent lesions occupying >30% of the vulvar surface (Fig. 66), (2) refractory disease that is unresponsive to >9 months of therapy (Fig. 67), (3) multifocal, multicentric intraepithelial neoplasias (Fig. 68), and (4) disease affecting such sensitive areas as the glans clitoris, urethra, or anus (Fig. 69).

The rationale for using the laser in difficult cases is to destroy the field of both clinically apparent and subclinical HPV-infected epithelium (Fig. 70). This strategy offers the best hope that the resurgent host-immune response will establish lasting dominance over the residual viral reservoir. If laser surgery is done skillfully, healing will occur from the unaffected keratinocytes in the underlying skin appendages, rather than by epithelial ingrowth from the wound edges (Fig. 71). Extended laser ablation is particularly helpful when "sanctuary sites" are extensively involved. Of course, this aggressive method must be reserved for the small subset of women who have special management problems.

Treatment of AIN and PAIN is essentially the same as for VIN, except that conservation of the normal tissues is even more vital. Although full-thickness excision with split-skin grafting can produce excellent cosmetic results, disruption of the nerve fibers within the lamina propria can lead to anal incontinence. Whenever possible, treatment should be by expert CO_2 laser photovaporization.

Helpful surgical strategies

Method of beam delivery. Simply observing optimal physical principles does not in itself guarantee success. Like other forms of surgery, a good outcome requires a combination of sound theoretic principles and practical strategies for implementing the surgical objectives [76]. In particular, success hinges upon whether the beam is

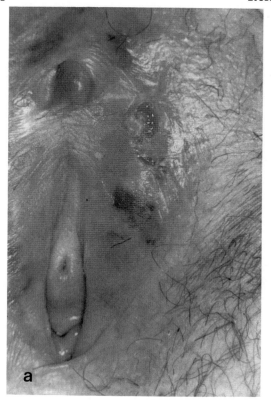

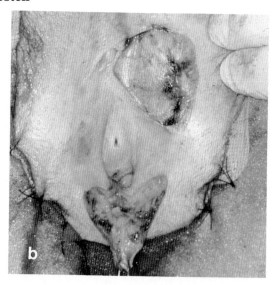

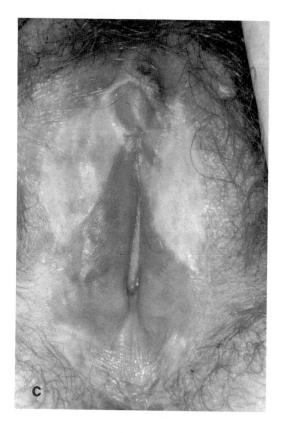

Fig. 63. **a:** Well-differentiated VIN 3 complicating longstanding lichen sclerosis in a 32-year-old woman. The shallow ulcer in the left interlabial sulcus showed superficially invasive squamous carcinoma, to a depth of <1 mm. Note the webbed contracture of the posterior fourchette. **b:** Wide deep excision, plus YV advancement flap. **c:** Healed result after split skin grafts. Note that a second, identical focus of invasion occurred in the right interlabial sulcus, after 6 months after treatment of the left side.

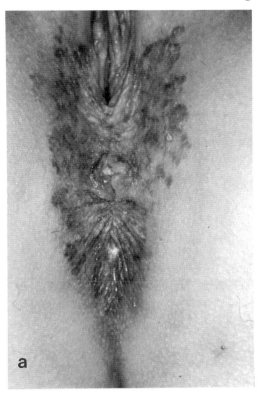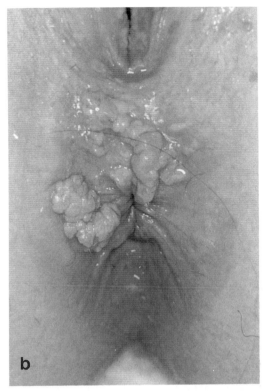

Fig. 64. **a:** Keratotic plague of PAIN 3. **b:** Papillary PAIN 3, potentially mistakable for benign condyloma.

TABLE 12. Varying Levels of Disease Expression

Well-developed Papillomavirus infections:
   Vegetative viral replication (benign condyloma and SPI[a])
   Nonproductive viral infection (Intraepithelial neoplasia
     and invasive cancer)
Low-grade Papillomavirus infections:
   Normal cell phenotype ("true latency")
   Minimal viral cytopathic effect (MEPI)

[a]Subclinical papillomavirus infection.

delivered by a hand-held probe or an operating microscope. Provided that the tip of the probe is kept in contact with the target, hand-held delivery systems can create ideal thermal incisions. However, attempting to perform surface ablation with a conventional hand probe is a mistake, for several reasons. (1) The focal plane is so narrow that even slight variations in lens-to-target distance will dramatically alter spot diameter, causing an exponential rise or fall in power density. (2) If the probe is held at an angle, the energy profile at the point of impact will have an oval, rather than circular distribution. Creating an "egg-shape" crater adds a further dimension to the difficulty of trying to ensure uniformity of power density. (3) Failure to use the operating microscope robs the surgeon of the benefit of anatomic landmarks, making depth control haphazard. (4) The unaided eye has insufficient visual resolution to permit surgical control over beams of >750 W/cm^2. In short, attempting to perform superficial ablation with a conventional hand-held probe may cause the surgeon to make nonuniform, poorly localized cuts at a power density close to the carbonization range. However, if the hand probe has a microslad defocusing device, some of these errors can be avoided.

Minimizing thermal damage by tissue cooling. Despite the application of optimal physical principles, there is always some heat conduction to adjacent tissues during laser surgery. However, thermal damage during vulvar laser ablation can be devastating. Thermal spread can be reduced by ~25% by simply chilling the tissues with iced saline [12]. Such measures reduce postoperative pain and swelling and allow for more rapid healing.

For cooling, use laparotomy packs soaked in a bowl of semifrozen saline slush, to which cephalosporin may be added. Chill the tissues before initial laser impact and at frequent intervals during surgery. Precooling acts as a buffer against

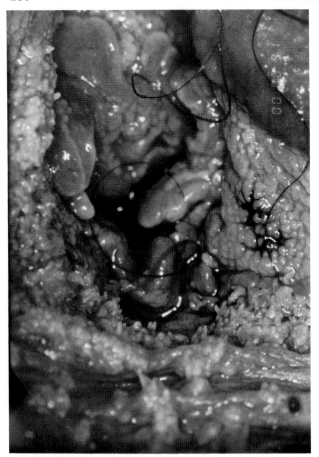

Fig. 65. Micropapillae seen in 25% of the normal population. (Reid [133], reproduced with permission.)

TABLE 13. Management Decisions for HPV-Associated Female Genital Disease

Differentiate definite disease from nonspecific micropapillary change.

Outline specific benefits from treatment.

Cervical disease requires transformation zone excision or ablation, rather than focal destruction of isolated lesions.

Vulvar and vaginal disease generally respond to focal lesion destruction, repeated until new lesions no longer develop.

Very extensive or refractory condylomas and multicentric intraepithelial neoplasia warrant destruction of both the visible lesions plus the adjacent subclinical reservoir.

Adjuvant interferon administration will markedly increase success rates for extended laser ablation.

burning, because diffused heat must first restore temperatures to a normal range before tissue injury can occur. Reapplying iced saline immediately after laser irradiation is also beneficial, because cooling breaks the cascade of continued tissue damage caused by vasoactive peptides released at the time of initial thermal injury.

Controlling intraoperative bleeding. With CO₂ lasers, it is far easier to prevent bleeding than to secure hemostasis once it occurs. During shallow depth ablation, the main preventive strategy is to accurately flatten the laser beam to the "point Y" (see Fig. 39). If tissue is to be excised with a focused beam, the principal strategy for preventing intraoperative bleeding is to inject a vasoconstrictor solution (e.g., 10 units of Vasopressin™ in 50 ml of 0.25% bupivacaine). If hemorrhage is encountered, the surgeon must distinguish partial transection of a small vessel from laceration of a much larger artery or vein. Most intraoperative bleeding arises from laser impact punching a hole in the side of a small vessel. Hence, tamponading the vessel with a dry cotton swab and relasing through the cotton bundle is an effective way to seal the vessel walls at the point of mechanical compression. However, if this maneuver is not successful, insert a hemostatic suture or apply Monsel's solution (ferric subsulphate) [26,77].

Good exposure and perpendicular beam impact. Expert control over the CO₂ laser requires good exposure and perpendicular beam delivery. Exposure on external surfaces is generally simple. Although it can be tedious continuously to reposition either the laser or the target, do not trade the accuracy of the microscopically adapted laser for the easy maneuverability of the hand-held delivery system.

Exposure within body cavities requires the correct instruments: pediatric nasal speculum for the urethra, right- and left-sided open speculae for the vagina, and suitable anoscope for the anus (Fig. 72). The angle of laser impact may be further improved by pressure with a cotton swab, traction with a Campion hook, or manipulation with a tenaculum (perhaps applied lateral to the central aperture).

The use of mirrors to help expose difficult areas of vaginal surface has not been useful. Visualization in a mirror is less detailed than with direct colposcopic viewing. Moreover, the mirror is rapidly fogged by steam and particulate debris from laser plume and requires constant wiping. The hand that would be used to hold the mirror is better employed flattening the vulvar folds or maneuvering the vaginal speculum.

Accurate delineation of treatment margins. The ability to set accurate margins for the excision or destruction of diseased tissue is essential for success. Obviously, failure to recognize the true extent of disease will adversely affect success rates.

Soaking the vulva with 5% acetic acid will

TABLE 14. Treatment Modalities for Mucosal and Cutaneous Condylomas*

Method	Advantages	Disadvantages	Clinical role
Traditional office methods for lesion eradication			
Scissor excision of isolated lesions	Obtains tissue for histology or viral typing. Removal of large papillomas may allow chemical destruction of remaining smaller lesions.	Cumbersome (local anesthesia, suture, instruments). Epithelial denudation and bleeding, if done to excess.	Baseline biopsy. Removal of large lesions.
Desiccant acids (85% trichloracetic acid in 70% alcohol)	Quickest and easiest method. Sterile instruments not required. Can be used on mucosal surfaces (vagina, rectum, mouth).	Requires weekly or second weekly office visits. Less effective for cutaneous (rather than mucosal) warts. Safe during pregnancy.	Highly effective for localized mucosal papillomas. Moderately effective for localized cutaneous lesions.
Crude podophyllin extracts (e.g., 25% podophyllin in benzoin)	None	Crude, nonstandardized mixture of toxins and active lignans. Rare but calamitous toxicity. No more effective than desiccant acids.	Obsolete
Podophyllotoxin ('Condylox')	Selective destruction of condylomatous areas, with sparing of normal epithelium. Self-application regimens are more effective than single-dose office therapies.	Cannot be used on highly absorptive surfaces (vagina, rectum). Contraindicated during pregnancy.	Highly effective for cutaneous condylomas. Effective for vulvar mucosal lesions of limited extent.
Localized physical destruction (hot cautery, liquid nitrogen, laser "spot welding")	Immediate eradication of papillomas.	Cumbersome (local anesthesia, special equipment). Time-consuming for physician. Local infection or scarring more common than with chemical methods.	Destruction of isolated refractory papillomas.
Cytolytic 5-fluorouracil regimens	Nonsurgical method of lesion eradication. Can forestall diffuse postoperative recurrence if therapy begins before extensive papilloma formation.	Painful alternative to skilled CO_2 laser photovaporization. Potentially teratogenic in pregnant women.	Effective for extensive, exophytic vaginal condylomas. Valuable postoperative "rescue" strategy.
Alpha interferon (as primary therapy)	Biological substances with documented antiviral and immunomodulatory actions. Nonsurgical method of lesion eradication.	Primary success rates have been disappointing and unpredictable. Intralesional regimens are slow, expensive, and painful. Systemic regimens require high dosages, with corresponding frequency of side effects.	Value as primary therapy not established. Valuable adjuvant.
Destructive methods requiring operating room therapy			
Segmental excision and primary closure	Tissue available for histology, if doubt exists.	Tissue removal is fundamentally undesirable.	Essentially outmoded by CO_2 laser surgery.
Extensive electrodiathermy ("Bovie" destruction)	Equipment readily available.	Morbid recovery and unacceptable scarring.	Outmoded in Western society.
Extended laser ablation	Can eradicate any volume of diseased epithelium, with negligible risk of scarring. Removes entire field of active HPV expression, irrespective of size, shape, or location. Anatomic methods of depth control allow destruction of VIN 3 within pilosebaceous ducts.	Requires sophisticated laser instrumentation and highly developed physician skills. Not appropriate for simpler cases. Cannot prevent subsequent reactivation of latent viral reservoir. Not an appropriate alternative to simpler methods.	Very extensive condylomas (coalescent papillomas occupying >30% of vulva and perineum). Refractory condylomas (disease not controlled by >9 months of office therapy). High-grade intraepithelial neoplasia (VIN 2–3 and PAIN 2–3).[a]
Method for controlling the residual viral reservoir			
Noncytolytic 5-fluorouracil regimens	Relatively inexpensive. Minimal systemic absorption. Effective in immunosuppressed patients.	Limited efficacy (especially in simpler cases). Poorly tolerated in patients of fair complexion. Distressing side effects (vaginal scarring, vestibular ulceration, possible vulvodynia).	An essential ingredient for the control of HPV disease in immunosuppressed patients.
Low-dose adjuvant interferon regimens	Biological substance with documented antiviral and immunomodulatory actions. Adjuvant effect documented in controlled trial.	Must monitor potential leukopenic and hepatotoxic effects. May not be effective in immunosuppressed patients. Theoretical risk or organ rejection in allograft recipients.	Probably indicated in immunocompetent patients with disease severe enough to warrant extended laser ablation.

*Source: Reid [132], reprinted with permission.
[a]VIN = vulvar intraepithelial neoplasia; PAIN = perianal intraepithelial neoplasia.

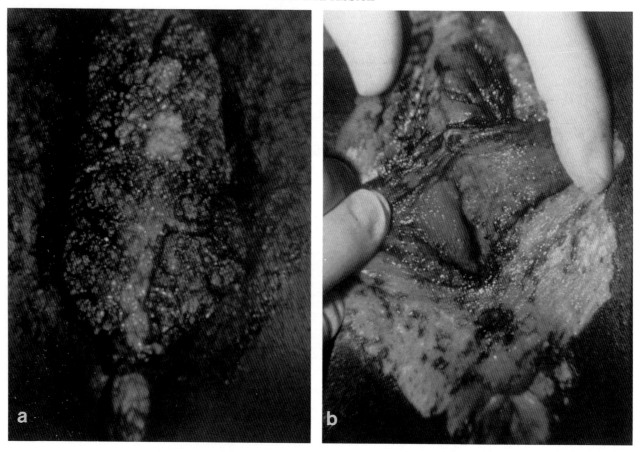

Fig. 66. **a:** Coalescent benign condylomas affecting the entire vulva. **b:** Extended laser ablation, to the first surgical plane.

usually produce prominent acetowhitening of skin that had appeared normal to the naked eye (Fig. 73). The clinical significance of acetowhite changes and vestibular micropapillae in women without obvious condylomas is confusing [103]. Although biopsy will usually show low-grade koilocytotic atypia, papillomavirus genomes are not generally detectable within these tissues [28]. In contrast, Southern blot hybridization of samples taken from acetowhite epithelium at the margins of exophytic condylomas or vulvar intraepithelial neoplasia (VIN) generally identified the same type of HPV DNA as found within the principal biopsies (Fig. 73d) [93]. One investigator correlated the risk of treatment failure with detectable HPV DNA at the lesion margin [104]. Moreover, the Koebner phenomenon (new warts at the treatment margins) is a well-recognized manifestation of the proclivity for the conversion from latent HPV infection to active expression during tissue regeneration (Fig. 74) [101,105]. Hence, there is little doubt that these adjacent

areas of acetowhite epithelium represent an important viral reservoir, at least among patients who have classical disease stigmata [105]. Destroying the surrounding subclinical HPV infection in difficult situations will produce higher surgical success rates.

Accurate depth control. Perhaps the major difficulty confronting the surgeon is how to control the depth of photovaporization. Depth control while ablating the cervical transformation zone is straightforward. The cylindrical nature of the resulting defect and the relatively large dimensions of the intended crater make it easy to control the depth of cervical ablation by actual measurements. However, in vaginal and vulvar surgery, depth of destruction is too shallow to control by measurement, particularly since the laser crater has no well-defined sides to act as reference points. Also, satisfactory healing of vulvar wounds depends on the preservation of the skin appendages, a task that is too delicate for reliance on crude measurements. Therefore, the surgeon

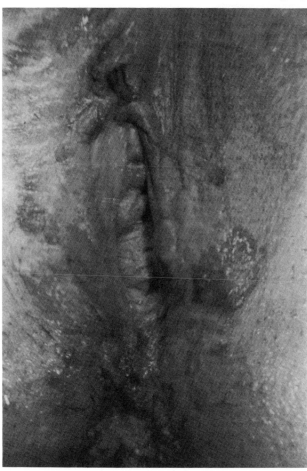

Fig. 67. Chronic condylomas in an immunosuppressed patient.

must learn to control depth according to the visual characteristics at the impact site [106].

From the surgical viewpoint, tissue destruction occurs through two distinct mechanisms: immediate photovaporization and delayed coagulation necrosis [30]. The depth of the photovaporization crater is controlled by hand-eye coordination. In contrast, the thickness of the zone of coagulation necrosis is variable, depending on laser settings. With a superpulsed laser used at adequate fluence, "what you see is what you get." In contrast, with CW lasers, much of the normal tissue on the wound surface will have suffered thermal destruction and will separate as an eschar, after activation of the host inflammatory response. Hence, if an expert has to photovaporize vulvar epithelium with a CW laser, crater depth must be judged so that the zone of thermal necrosis (rather than the zone of photovaporization) lies at the intended depth of penetration. This

level of precision requires the use of anatomic landmarks in the crater base to indicate the surgical plane of destruction (Table 15) [29,106].

Surgical planes

The first surgical plane. Destruction to the first plane removes only the surface epithelium down to the level of the basement membrane. This plane is reached by limiting penetration of the laser crater to the prickle cell layer. Destruction to this depth is accomplished by rapid oscillation of the micromanipulator, so that the helium-neon spot shows a roughly parallel series of lines. When done correctly, each pass of the laser beam will reveal bubbles of silver opalescence beneath the charred surface squames (Fig. 75a) and the maneuver will be accompanied by a distinct crackling sound.

Lasing to the prickle cell layer shears the basal cells from the basement membrane, thereby producing a plane of cleavage. These detached basal cells are easily removed with moistened gauze, thus exposing the smooth, intact surface of the papillary dermis (Fig. 75b). These wounds heal completely within 5–14 days, depending on the sophistication of energy delivery [28]. The cosmetic appearance and functional qualities of the healed wound are entirely indistinguishable from normal vulvar skin.

The second surgical plane. Destruction to the second surgical plane removes both the epidermis and the loose network of fine collagen and elastin fibers that make up the papillary dermis. This plane is reached by a similar set of rapid oscillations, moving the beam so quickly that the laser scorches (rather than craters) the exposed corium. When done correctly, the scorched surface should be rough and yellow in color, similar to the color of a chamois cloth (Fig. 76a). This clinical appearance indicates that the zone of coagulation necrosis will lie within the papillary dermis, with only minimal thermal injury to the underlying reticular dermis (Fig. 76b). The second plane is the preferred level of ablation for extensive condylomas. These wounds heal rapidly and also produce an end result indistinguishable from normal skin.

The third surgical plane. Destruction to the third surgical plane removes the epidermis, the upper portions of the pilosebaceous ducts, and the upper third of the reticular dermis. Correct depth control is associated with the recognition of three characteristic landmarks: (1) lasing to the midreticular layer uncovers coarse collagen bundles that can be seen through the operating micro-

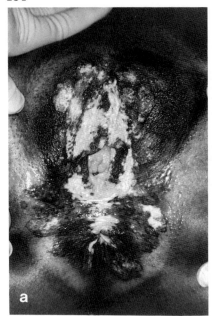 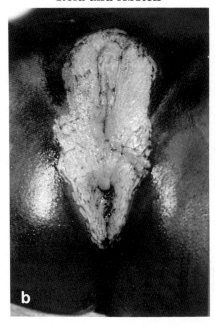 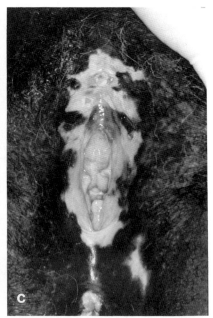

Fig. 68. **a:** Extreme Bowenoid VIN 3 in a 29-year-old woman. Occult invasion was ruled out by multiple colposcopically directed biopsies. **b:** Intraoperative view, showing extended laser ablation to the third surgical plane. **c:** Healed result—disease free, normal anatomy, and coital function, but some depigmentation.

scope as gray-white fibers, resembling waterlogged cotton threads, (2) wiping with iced saline reveals the bright, alabaster white color of these basal collagen plates (Fig. 77a), and (3) this maneuver also exposes a network of prominent arterioles and venules running horizontal to the epithelial surface (Fig. 77b).

The technique of micromanipulator control for lasing to the third plane is slightly different. The rapid, oscillating action gives way to a slower, more deliberate movement. Hand speed is coordinated to the visual recognition of a "fibrous grain" within the crater base. Moving the beam too rapidly will not expose these collagen bundles and moving the beam too slowly will uncover skin appendages within the deep reticular dermis. If uncovered, hair follicles and sweat glands will be seen through the operating microscope as tiny refractile granules that resemble grains of sand. The rationale for limiting destruction to the third surgical plane is to allow re-epithelialization by regeneration from the keratinocytes within these skin appendages. Exposing these structures within the crater base signals a third-degree burn in that area. Therefore, the third surgical plane is the deepest level from which optimal healing will occur.

The fourth surgical plane. Under rare circumstances, it may be necessary to produce a deliberate third-degree burn to destroy abnormal keratinocytes within the hair follicles or sweat glands. Because of its precision, the CO_2 laser can destroy the adnexal epithelium while preserving a layer of collagen fibers within the deep reticular dermis. Dermal regeneration produces a much better bed for skin grafting than either subcutaneous fat or granulation tissue. Hence, cosmetic and functional results are superior to those attained by skinning vulvectomy (Fig. 78).

Extended laser ablation of vulvar and perianal epithelium. After inducing anesthesia, carefully shave the perineum to facilitate colposcopy and to simplify postoperative care. Antiseptic solutions are not recommended because they impair the response of tissue to acetic acid. They are also unnecessary, because of the high temperatures attained at the laser site. Instead, soak the vulva and anus in 4–5% acetic acid for 1–2 minutes. Next, carefully examine the perineum with the colposcope. Outline the lesion borders before the acetic acid reaction fades. The viral reservoir lying between this outer margin and the hymenal ring is then destroyed en bloc, using the microscopically controlled technique for depth control. Except for long-standing condylomas, which can become pedunculated, most lesions have a flat base. Attempts to undercut condylomas that are not required for histologic examina-

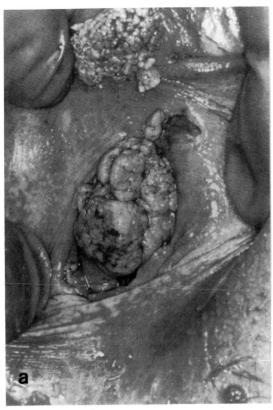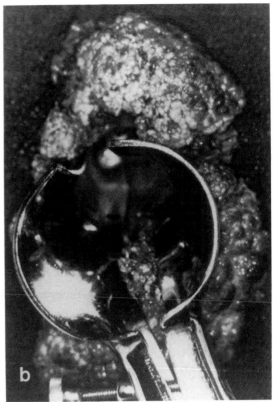

Fig. 69. **a:** Urethra: A large mass of condylomas distends and fills the external urethral meatus. A second papilloma occupies the entire surface of the glans clitoris. **b:** Anus: A large mass of perianal condylomas has occluded the anal canal. (From Reid [132], reproduced with permission.)

tion will produce unnecessary dermal defects. The best strategy is to umbilicate each condyloma by lasing the condyloma center and allowing tissue shrinkage at the laser impact site to pull the edge of the lesion into the operative field [29]. Initially, the vaporization crater should extend only to the level of surrounding skin. Then the adjacent areas of subclinical HPV infection are brushed and the operative field gently debrided with a moist gauze swab. Any residual epithelial fronds or capillary spikes are readily seen and can then be accurately destroyed by spot lasing. Healing will be rapid, and final appearance should be cosmetically indistinguishable from adjacent skin.

The frequency with which the epithelium of the skin appendages are colonized by HPV genomes is unknown. However, in the absence of neoplastic transformation, morphologic evidence of viral expression is never found below the basement membrane [107]. Hence, for benign condylomas, only the surface epithelium need be destroyed. In contrast, VIN 2-3 usually extends part way down the pilosebaceous ducts. Nonetheless,

depth of destruction should be evaluated preoperatively by examining representative histologic sections. Fortunately, foci of deep pilar extension are rare. Lasing to the midreticular level is adequate in most instances. Any focal areas of deep pilar extension must be surgically excised.

Postoperative care. Treatments are performed on an outpatient basis, except in extreme cases. Before being released from the recovery room, patients receive written postoperative instructions, a prescription for a narcotic analgesic, and an office appointment for the following week. Early postoperative pain can be reduced by icing the area and then infiltrating the treated areas with 0.25% bupivacaine. Late onset postoperative pain is greatly diminished by a suprapubic catheter with leg bag, worn until vestibular healing is virtually complete (generally 1–2 weeks). Care of the catheter is simple. The collection system is washed daily in household detergent, and one ounce of vinegar is added to the bag (to eliminate urine odor). The most important part of the postoperative regimen is to apply either silver sul-

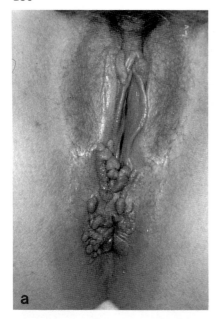
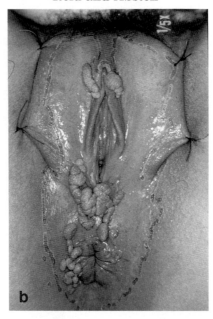
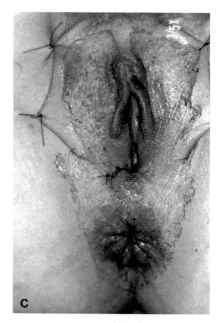

Fig. 70. **a:** Refractory, pruritic condylomas in a 22-year-old, insulin-dependent diabetic. **b:** Appearances after acetic acid soaks. The acetowhite skin was confirmed to represent subclinical papillomavirus infection rather than nonspecific change, by Southern blot hybridization showing HPV 6 in biopsies from both papilloma and subclinical areas. The intended margin of ablation has been marked with the CO_2 laser, before the acetowhite reaction could fade. **c:** With this volume of disease, extended laser ablation improves efficacy, but adds nothing to morbidity.

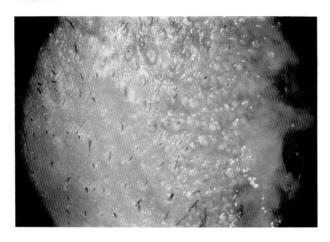

Fig. 71. The postero-inferior margins of an ELA wound at the 10-day postoperative visit. Healing is occurring by epithelial outgrowth from the skin appendages.

phadiazine cream or nitrofurazone soluble dressing, as prophylaxis against conglutination of denuded surfaces. Used cream should be washed off by taking a Sitz baths at least three times a day. Postoperative antibiotic therapy is not helpful, except as prophylaxis against urinary infection. However, preoperative reduction of vaginal flora with topical clindamycin, or metronidazole is prudent.

Patients must be seen weekly for 3 weeks to correct any early coaptation of adjacent raw surfaces (Fig. 79). Healing should be virtually complete within 14–21 days. Thereafter, have patients with refractory condylomas return every 2–4 weeks for the next 3 months, so that any focal recurrences can be controlled with caustic agents. Provided that the diagnosis is made before the formation of large condylomatous aggregations, diffuse recurrence can also be forestalled by applying 5-fluorouracil cream twice a week [28]. Because women with vulvar neoplasia or papillomavirus infections are at high risk for developing squamous neoplasia at other sites within the genital tract, annual Pap smears are mandatory.

Efficacy in benign condylomas. Of 1,000 women seen between 1982–1988, 117 had condylomas sufficiently extensive or refractory to justify extended laser ablation [28]. Seventy-nine (67%) of these women were controlled by a single laser ablation, and another 30 (26%) were controlled by either repeat surgery or the use of topical 5-fluorouracil as soon as recurrence appeared inevitable (Fig. 80). Treatment of the remaining 8 (7%) required deep laser destruction with skin grafting (prior to 1986). However, three patients (2%) never achieved lasting clinical remission.

Kaplan Maier cumululative survival analy-

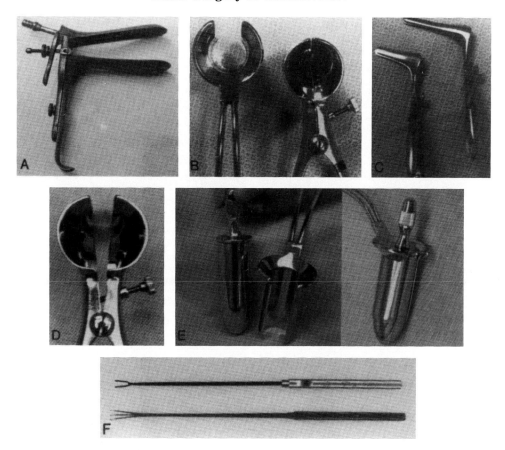

Fig. 72. Speculae used to secure exposure within the lower genital tract. **A:** Graves' speculum with suction port. **B** and **D:** Pair of anal speculae as seen from the surgeon's eye (top) and from above (bottom). **C:** Two pediatric nasal speculae for exposing the distal and proximal female urethra. **E:** Fixed anoscope, shown with the obturator in place and removed. **F:** Two-pronged and three-pronged Campion hooks. (From Reid [209], reproduced with permission.)

sis showed that 50% of recurrences occurred within the first 6 months. However, beyond 1.5 years, the tail of the survival curve becomes quite flat, indicating that these patients are in stable clinical remission (Fig. 81) It is emphasized that our measure of success referred to long-term freedom from clinical recurrence. In our opinion, the question of whether latent HPV DNA remains at the treatment site is irrelevant.

Our primary control rate of 67% indicates the strength and weakness of the CO_2 laser. If used skillfully, the laser can remove any volume of diseased tissue under fine control, with the added assurance of rapid healing without scarring. However, its weakness is that the laser cannot prevent reactivation of the latent viral reservoir within surrounding areas of surface skin, and perhaps within the skin appendages themselves. Therefore, the availability of an effective adjuvant antiviral therapy would be a natural complement.

Historically, *topical 5-fluorouracil* (5FU) was used in high dose regimens (e.g., daily for 5–10 days) to slough cutaneous condylomas [108]. Such cytotoxic doses have been abandoned because they are inefficient, poorly controllable, and extremely painful. Except for the treatment of intravaginal condylomas, destruction of exophytic papillomas is best done with the CO_2 laser.

In patients with renal allografts or other immune deficiencies, the lifelong use of low dose 5 FU (e.g., once weekly) is a prerequisite to disease control [109]. In 1986, Krebs [110] reported improved success rates (87% vs. 62%) in the group randomized to use biweekly topical 5-FU for 6 months. Thus the concept of forestalling viral re-expression with noncytotoxic doses of 5FU was extended to the treatment of immunologically competent women. Kreb's [110] conclusions were selectively confirmed by our group. Among 160 women treated by extended laser ablation for condylomas or VIN 2–3, low-dose 5 FU helped

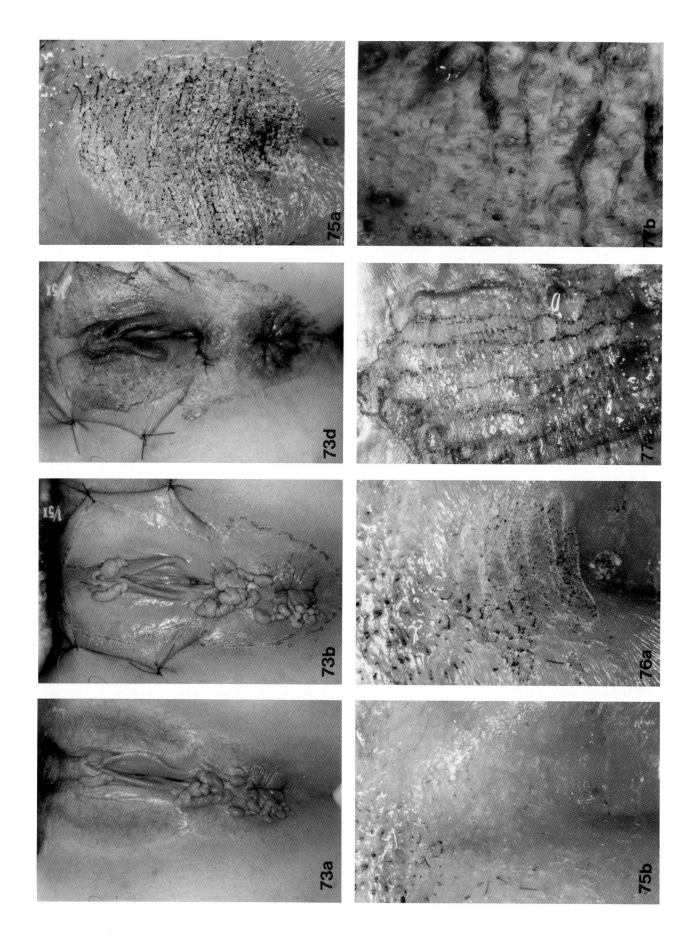

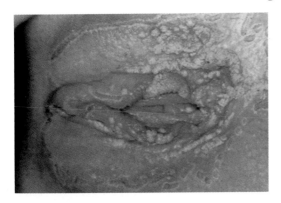
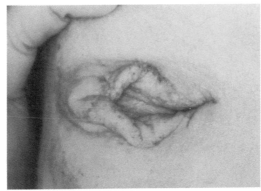

B

D

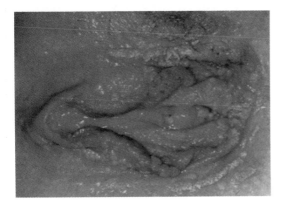
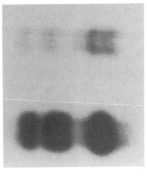

Lane 4
Lane 3
Lane 2
Lane 1

c

Fig. 73c.

Fig. 73. **a:** (see pg. 158) Extensive vulvar condyloma before vinegar soaking. **b:** (see pg. 158) View of the same patient after a 3-minute soak with 4.5% acetic acid, showing extensive subclinical HPV infection of the intervening skin. Biopsy samples from this area showed prominent histologic features of active albeit subclinical viral expression. **c:** (see above) Southern blot hybridization done under conditions of high stringency. (Courtesy A. Lorincz, PhD.) Samples from an exophytic condyloma (lane 1) and an area of adjacent acetowhitening (lane 4) contain the typical banded pattern of HPV DNA, whereas biopsies of nonacetowhite skin and normal vaginal mucosa (lanes 2 and 3) had no detectable signal. **d:** (see pg. 158) Extent of surgical destruction. Because healing occurs by epithelial regeneration from underlying skin appendages, healing time and postoperative discomfort are the same as that after local destruction of the exophytic condylomata alone. (From Reid et al. [28], reproduced with permission.) See insert for color representation.

Fig. 75. First surgical plane. (see pg. 158) **a:** View through the operating microscope after initial brushing with the laser. Beneath the charred remains of the surface squames can be seen the refractile remnants of plump keratinocytes within the proliferating zone of the epidermis. **b:** After wiping, the anatomically intact dermal surface is exposed. A small area

of third plane penetration is shown at top. (From Reid [132], reprinted with permission.) See insert for color representation.

Fig. 76. Second surgical plane. **a:** (see pg. 158) The exposed papillary dermis has been gently released, sufficient to scorch (but not cut) the dermal surface. At top, there is an area of third plane (white) and at bottom an area of first plane (pink). **b:** (see pg. 160) The papillary dermis shows coagulation necrosis (top), but the reticular dermis is unaffected (bottom). (From Reid [132], reprinted with permission.) See insert for color representation.

Fig. 77. Third surgical plane. **a:** (see pg. 158) Slower, more deliberate movement of the laser beam has vaporized the upper half of the dermis, revealing barely visible fibrous grain, representing the coarse reticular dermis collagen obscured by a thin layer of surface eschar. **b:** (see pg. 158) Different patient, after rinsing the surface eschar. The stark white color of the reticular collagen and the arcuate vascular arcades are characteristic of this depth. **c:** (see pg. 160) Biopsy from the base of such a wound, showing the presence of viable hair follicles that act as a source of epithelial regeneration. (From Reid et al. [107], reproduced with permission.) See insert for color representation.

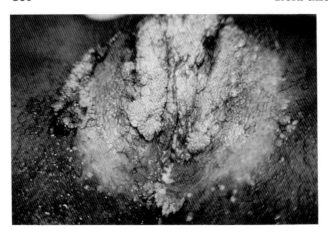

Fig. 74. Koebner response showing active viral expression within a field of pre-existing latent HPV infection as a result of healing. (From Reid [209], reproduced with permission.)

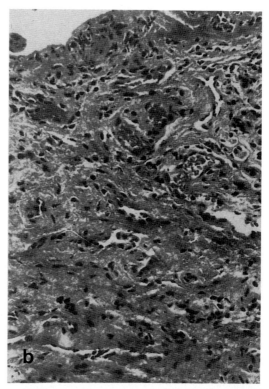

prevent postoperative recurrence in 76 high-risk women with two or more adverse factors (88% vs. 56%) (Table 16), but provided no protection against whatever in the 84 low-risk women (93% vs. 87%) (Fig. 82) [28].

Interferons are a group of immunomodulatory proteins, produced by all mammals, that have antiviral and antiproliferative properties [111]. Efficacy of alpha- and gamma-interferons against HPV infection has been documented [112,113]. However, even when used in high doses by intramuscular injection, primary treatment using systemic interferon as monotherapy has proven ineffective [114]. Dermatologic groups have shown that intralesional interferon can clear up to five warts. However, such regimens are impractical; they require two or three office visits per week over several weeks, produce substantial pain at the injection sites, and will clear only the lesions that are actually infiltrated [115,116].

In contrast, a subsequent open-labeled, randomized trial of systemic alpha-interferon used at 1 mU three times a week (one-sixth of the usual therapeutic dose) provided substantial protection against postoperative recurrence (Reid, unpub. data). Success rates in the interferon arm was 28 of 34 (83%), vs. 19 of 35 (54%) in the control arms (Fisher's exact test = 0.02) (Fig. 83). Moreover, 14 (78%) of 18 failures in the control arms and 2 of 6 failures in the study group were rescued from second laser surgery by crossover to either 1 mU or 3 mU of interferon, respectively.

Efficacy in VIN 2-3. Treatment of VIN is controversial, with recommendations ranging

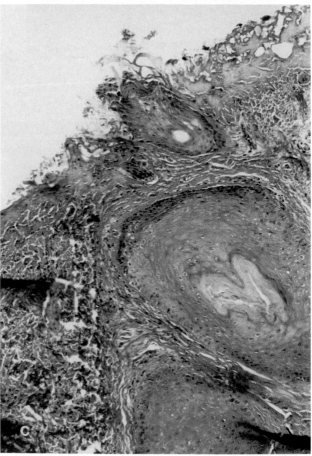

Figs. 76b and 77c. (Legends appear on page 159.)

TABLE 15. Summary of the Salient Features of the Four Surgical Planes in Vulvar Laser Surgery*

| Parameter | Surgical plane | | | |
	First	Second	Third	Fourth
Target tissue	Surface epithelium	Dermal papillae	Pilosebaceous ducts	Pilosebaceous glands
Zone of vaporization	Proliferating layer of epidermis	Superficial papillary dermis	Upper reticular dermis	Midreticular dermis
Zone of necrosis	Basement membrane	Deep papillary	Midreticular	Deep reticular
Type of healing	Rapid and cosmetic	Rapid and cosmetic	Slower but usually cosmetic	Needs grafting
Visual landmark	Opalescent epidermis debris (shiny pink after wiping)	Yellowish and nonreflectant (chamois cloth)	Stark white with arcuate vessels and fibrous "grain"	Skin appendages visible as "sand grains"

*From Reid [29], reprinted with permission.)

from wide excision to superficial "skinning" vulvectomy. The treatment originally proposed for "carcinoma in situ" of the vulva was wide local excision, but fear that the disease was preinvasive lead to widespread use of simple vulvectomy. However, most documented instances of invasion have occurred in immunosuppressed or elderly women [85,91]. In young patients, the risk of malignant progression is real (Fig. 84) [117]. Nevertheless, risks are not sufficient to justify such mutilating surgery. Moreover, recurrences after simple vulvectomy are common (Fig. 85).

Wide excision of small foci produces excellent results. However, multifocal or extensive lesions obviously cannot be managed by wide excision. In the past, the only reasonable alternative was skinning vulvectomy with grafting. Although a definite improvement over conventional vulvectomy, cosmetic and functional results of skinning vulvectomy are unpredictable. Fortunately, for bowenoid VIN 3, treatment with the CO_2 laser is an effective, nonmutilating alternative [28,96,118,120–122]. Success rates from reported series approximate 85% (Table 17).

Because occult invasion >1 mm carries a 10% risk of lymph node metastasis, there is little room for error [123]. The rate of invasive vulvar cancer associated with VIN has been reported to be as high as 8%; however, four-fifths of these were superficially invasive (<1 mm) [120]. When triage is restricted to physicians experienced in vulvar disease, the consensus view is that occult invasion can be excluded by careful colposcopy and liberal use of excisional biopsy [53].

Complications. Complication rates directly reflect surgical skill. In a series of 160 patients treated by extended laser ablation, major complications were related to thermal damage in the adjacent tissues [28]. The cumulative incidence of cellulitis, scarring, or secondary hemorrhage was 10.3% among those treated in low-power CW mode, but fell with pulsed temporal modes. Recovery and postoperative pain were also dependent on laser settings. Over a 6-year period, improvements in laser technique produced a 7-day reduction in mean healing times.

Although there were no instances of nonhealing or major scarring in this study, we have seen such problems in women treated elsewhere. The vulvar vestibule is like the palm of the hand: the surface epithelium is firmly fixed to the underlying fascia. Consequently, any loss of vestibular area (e.g., by lesion excision) or any reduction in fascial elasticity (e.g., by heat contracture) produce major impairment of coital function. Since the split skin grafting cannot correct for loss of fascial elasticity, restoration of cosmetic anatomy and good coital function generally require either a full thickness skin graft (Fig. 86) [124] or local skin flaps [125]. For posterior contracture, YV advancement flap [126] is easy, symmetric, and very effective (Fig. 87). Repair of central vestibular defects is probably best undertaken using local transposition skin flaps. Perhaps the most useful such method is the Martius flap, which allows the surgeon to mobilize and transpose interlabial sulcus skin, with or without the bulbocavernosus fascia (Fig. 88) [127–129]. In the event of extreme deformity affecting a large area, a considerable volume of hairless skin can be harvested by means of either bilateral arterialized medial thigh flaps (based on the terminal branches of the pudendal arteries) (Fig. 89) [130] or a central transverse rectus abdominus muscle (TRAM) flap (mobilizing abdominal skin based on the inferior epigastric artery) (see Fig. 29) [131,132].

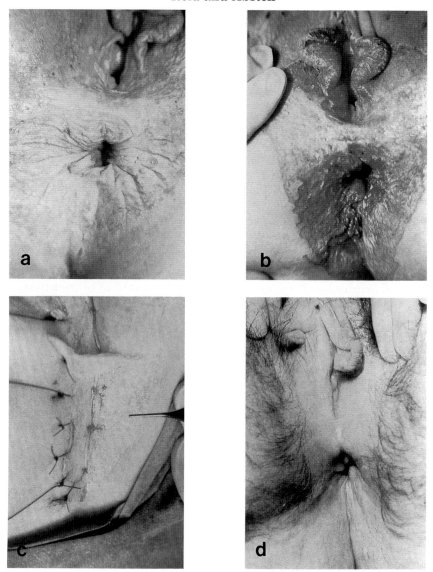

Fig. 78. Fourth surgical plane. **a:** Area of refractory perianal dysplasia that has failed three prior superficial laser vaporizations. **b:** Vaporization of the perianal skin to the fourth plane. Each of the craters represents a site at which a skin appendage was destroyed, whereas the intervening areas represent viable collagen bundles within the deep part of the reticular dermis. **c:** Same area 10 days later, showing the extent of dermal regeneration at the time of skin grafting. **d:** Final result. (From Reid [76], reproduced with permission.)

Photovaporization of Vaginal Mucosa

Although invasive carcinoma of the vagina is rare, there has been a definite increase in the prevalence of *vaginal intraepithelial neoplasia* (VAIN) over the last decade. VAIN has a well-defined potential for malignant progression. Indeed, about one-third of the invasive cancers detected after therapy for cervical neoplasia have occurred in the original squamous epithelium the vaginal vault [103,133]. Various treatment techniques have been advocated; however, no single method has been universally endorsed. Despite conflicting reports about the efficacy of ablative therapy for VAIN, this modality has one major advantage. The CO_2 laser is the only surgical method for destroying large areas of intricately contoured epithelium, without causing vaginal scarring or shortening [134,135].

Ablation of vaginal condylomas or VAIN 3.

Control of secondary heat conduction. The vaginal mucosa consists of a simple stratified squamous epithelium that is separated from the underlying muscularis by the lamina propria—a loose layer of connective tissue. Although the mucosa is folded into a myriad of rugae, there are no deep epithelial clefts as seen in the cervical transformation zone. Hence, the desired depth of destruction for both vaginal condyloma and VAIN is relatively shallow.

Good laser technique is crucial within the vagina. The authors are aware of two vesicovaginal fistulas that followed ablation "just to the level of the submucosa," because of excessive heat conduction from a carbonized crater. Adequate power densities are especially important for vaginal laser surgery. An oblique impact can inadvertently reduce a seemingly effective power density down to the carbonization range. Hence, extra care must be taken to manipulate the vaginal walls so that the beam impinges at no less than 60°. Whereas electrosurgery can adequately replace the laser for the ablation of the cervical transformation zone, the prudent surgeon should not even consider attempting loop excision or extensive fulguration of extensive VAIN 3.

Depth of destruction. Within the vagina, depth of destruction cannot be controlled by actual measurement. Therefore, vaginal laser surgery is always performed through the operating microscope, controlling depth by a system of anatomic landmarks. Ablation is performed in a stepwise fashion, removing a thin layer of tissue with each pass of the beam. Devitalization and shearing of the vaginal epithelium—*the first surgical plane*—is indicated by a pearly opalescent color, mixed with a small amount of brownish char (Fig. 90). Since the underlying lamina propria will now be obscured by this debris, maintaining visual orientation requires wiping with a saline soaked swab. Moreover, wiping away the debris from the base of the laser crater will expose any foci of still adherent basement membrane. Within the treated field, islands of intact vaginal epithelium may also persist because of the obscuring effect of the rugose folds. Hence, a sequence of repeated lasing and wiping must be maintained.

Because of the convoluted nature of the vaginal walls, the *second surgical plane* is hard to establish. However, a shallow *third surgical plane* is reached by re-lasing the exposed lamina propria, such that the beam leaves a definite furrow. Fibrous bundles, similar to those visible in the vulvar dermis, can now be seen in the base of each furrow. Since the vaginal mucosa has neither crypts nor appendages, further destruction is of absolutely no benefit. Healing occurs by ingrowth from the wound edge; because this is a mucosal surface, re-epithelialization is almost as rapid as on the vulva.

Techniques for better exposure. A number of anatomic and pathologic factors combine to complicate the management of VAIN. First, the vagina has a large surface area that tends to be obscured by the cervix, speculum blades, and various rugose folds. Displaying lesions within the fornices can be especially difficult, because of the distensible nature of the upper vagina. Second, the colposcopic features of VAIN 3 are highly variable and serious lesions are readily overlooked by the inexperienced observer. Therefore, to permit adequate manipulation of the vaginal speculum, extensive multifocal VAIN is best treated under general anesthesia. Staining with Lugol's iodine will help expose lesions that are difficult to detect.

The lateral vaginal walls are exposed between the open blades of a bivalve speculum. The anterior and posterior walls are treated by successive rotations and gradual withdrawal of the speculum. In the lower part of the vagina, a better angle of impact is obtained by aiming through the sides, rather than the central aperture, of the speculum (Fig. 91a). Once the entire circumference has been treated, withdraw the speculum and use moist gauze to wipe away epithelial debris. When the speculum is reinserted, the untreated areas are easily identified and can be ablated under direct vision.

Visualizing the vaginal vault always requires manipulation. If the uterus is intact, the epithelial folds within each of the vaginal fornices can often be flattened by pulling the cervix in the opposite direction. In easier cases, this is accomplished by using your left thumb on a rectal swab to apply pressure in an opposite fornix (Fig. 91b). Alternatively, a righthanded surgeon should apply a tenaculum through the left side of the speculum. By pushing or pulling the cervix, each of the vaginal cornices can be exposed. (Fig. 91c).

In a patient who has had a prior hysterectomy, the vaginal scar can be exposed by use of single or multiple pronged hooks (Fig. 91d). This maneuver is satisfactory for ablating benign condylomas (preferably after confirmation by virus testing). However, as discussed below, surgeons should *never* attempt to vaporize VAIN 3 involving a hysterectomy scar. To do so would be

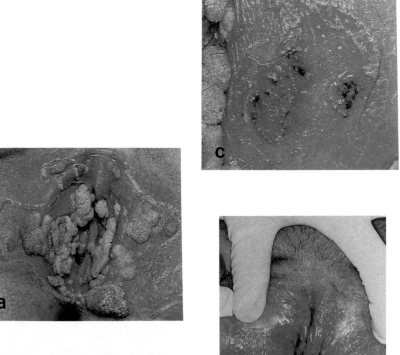

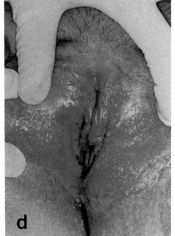

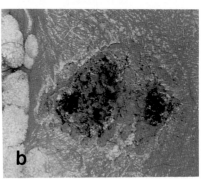

Fig. 79. Coaptation of the labia minora.

analogous to treating a level 5 CIN 3 with cryo-surgery.

Postoperative care. Because there are no skin appendages, the vagina is the slowest healing area within the lower genital tract. However, if the lamina propria is not excessively damaged by unskilled laser technique, complete re-epithelialization usually occurs within 4 weeks. Postoperative care is aimed primarily at preventing adhesions, vaginal shortening, or postoperative scarring. It may be helpful to have the patient insert an applicator of estrogen or antibacterial cream every other day. Occasionally, squamous re-growth can be inhibited by either granulation tissue or areas of columnar metaplasia. Cauterizing with 85% trichloroacetic acid or silver nitrate will reactivate the healing process.

Excision of vaginal intraepithelial neoplasia.

Role for excision. There are few risks associated with the CO_2 laser when the uterus is intact. However, this is not the case for the treatment of VAIN occurring after hysterectomy [136]. In a British series of 23 women with recurrent VAIN who were managed by laser vaporization, only six patients were disease-free 30 months after treatment [137,138]. Three women in whom VAIN 2-3 involved the vault scar developed invasive cancer in islands of buried vaginal epithelium. The most important single factor in preventing subsequent invasive cancer is to rule out occult malignancy before attempting laser ablation. We have used excisional techniques in the following circum-

Final result

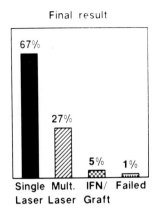
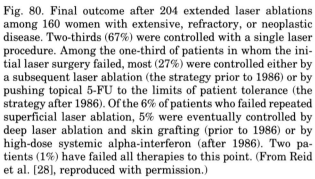
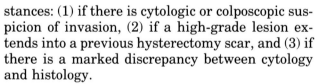

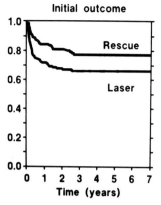

Fig. 80. Final outcome after 204 extended laser ablations among 160 women with extensive, refractory, or neoplastic disease. Two-thirds (67%) were controlled with a single laser procedure. Among the one-third of patients in whom the initial laser surgery failed, most (27%) were controlled either by a subsequent laser ablation (the strategy prior to 1986) or by pushing topical 5-FU to the limits of patient tolerance (the strategy after 1986). Of the 6% of patients who failed repeated superficial laser ablation, 5% were eventually controlled by deep laser ablation and skin grafting (prior to 1986) or by high-dose systemic alpha-interferon (after 1986). Two patients (1%) have failed all therapies to this point. (From Reid et al. [28], reproduced with permission.)

Fig. 81. Kaplan-Meier survival curve showing the curability of clinical control obtained by the initial laser ablation in 160 women. Of the failures, 50% occurred within 3 months and 95% within 18 months. The lower curve represents the patients who had no significant recurrences after their first surgery (immediate successes), whereas the higher curve (eventual successes) represents both immediate successes plus those rescued from a repeat laser ablation by various office therapies. These initial failures were recycled for repeat laser ablation, resulting in the eventual control of all but three women. (From Reid et al. [28], reproduced with permission.)

stances: (1) if there is cytologic or colposcopic suspicion of invasion, (2) if a high-grade lesion extends into a previous hysterectomy scar, and (3) if there is a marked discrepancy between cytology and histology.

Since lower genital tract neoplasia is often a multifocal problem, some areas may require excision for proper diagnosis, whereas other areas may be safely ablated. For example, we often combine excisional conization or excision of an obscured vaginal fornix with ablation of previously biopsied, multifocal areas of VAIN 3 on the vaginal walls. Before the advent of laser surgery, treating these lesions required extensive resection of vaginal mucosa. However, laser combination procedures obviate the need for wide excision and concomittant skin grafting [139].

Surgical technique. Irrespective of whether excision is performed with the CO_2 laser of the cold knife, this surgery is best done using the colposcope for magnification (Fig. 92a) [118]. For laser excision, we recommend a tightly focused beam of rapid superpulse energy at an average power of 40 watts. Infiltration with dilute vasopressin, at 1:50 dilution materially aids both hemostasis and the recognition of tissue planes. Dissection is done using the Campion hook for

traction and the pressure of a widely opened Grave's speculum for countertraction (Fig. 92b). The potentially vascular remnants of the cardinal-uterosacral ligaments are clamped and suture ligated (using Vicryl™ 0 on a 5/8 circle urology needle) (Fig. 94c). The peritoneal cavity is entered sharply and the vault resupported by taking deep bites of the retroperitoneal fascia with a prolene #1 pursestring suture. The transected edges of the vaginal scar are then sutured with everting vertical mattress sutures (Fig. 94d).

Results of treatment. The primary success rates for vaginal laser surgery have been lower than those for cervix or vulva. In a series of 98 cases of VAIN treated by photovaporization [140], an initial failure rate of only 11% was reported in women with unicentric disease, compared with 28% in patients with multicentric disease. Therefore patients with more difficult disease patterns need individualized management:

1. Unicentric VAIN with uterus in situ. Good results are readily attainable by laser photovaporization to the level of the lamina propria.
2. Multicentric VAIN with uterus in situ. Multicentric genital neoplasia is more difficult to cure, perhaps because such patients are more permissive hosts. Reassuringly, most recurrences were diagnosed within the first 6

TABLE 16. Results of Once-Weekly 5-Fluorouracil Treatment Used as Prophylaxis Against Disease Recurrence in the 76 Patients Who Had Two or More Adverse Factors*

Adjuvant usage	Controlled by a single laser surgery	Not controlled by initial laser ablation	Total
Laser plus 5 Fu	21 (87.5%)	3	24
Laser alone	29 (55.8%)	23	52
Total	50 (100%)	26	76

*Note: X^2 = 7.325: P < .01. (From Reid et al. [28], reprinted with permission.)

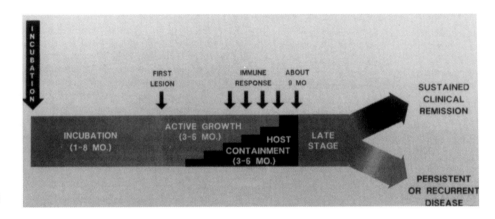

a

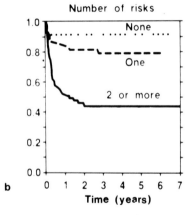

b

Fig. 82. Kaplan-Meier survival curve showing the cumulative effect of these various adverse factors upon treatment outcome. Two adverse factors shown as a solid line, one as a dashed line, and no factors as a dotted line. (From Reid [209], reproduced with permission.)

months following surgery. Eventual success rates of about 90% can be obtained by repeatedly re-treating initial failures [118]. After initial photovaporization, low-dose maintenance 5FU therapy can be used [141]. The usual regimen is to instill ~2 grams of 5 FU weekly for ~6 months. Two grams of 5 FU is delivered by filling one-quarter of a 10 ml Ortho applicator with the 5% cream and inserting it deeply into

the vagina at bedtime. Any residual cream must be carefully washed from the vulva upon waking to prevent chemical vulvitis. The patient should not have coitus while the 5 FU cream is in place and must not become pregnant while using the cream.

3. VAIN of the vault posthysteretomy. Whereas the CO_2 laser is ideal for treating vaginal lesions when the uterus remains in situ, VAIN

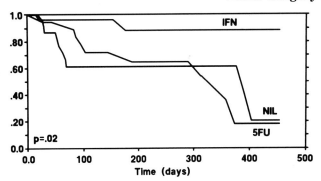

Fig. 83. Kaplan-Meier survival curve showing the significantly improved rates for clinical control attending the use of adjuvant interferon compared to laser plus 5-FU or laser alone (*P* < 0.01). (Reid [133], reproduced with permission.)

after hysterectomy often requires excision of the vault scar [142].

4. Recurrent VAIN after pelvic irradiation. Ruling out occult cancer in women with recurrent VAIN after prior radiation therapy mandates expert consultation. Therapy is also difficult, requiring both skilled local destruction and possibly 5 FU cream.

Microsurgical Resection of Bartholin's Glands

The most important step in the assessment of vulvodynia patients is to distinguish surface from deep pain loops. For those people who have *only surface pain,* the symptomatic vessels are selectively photocoagulated using either the hexascan or the flashlamp excited dye laser (FEDL) (see the third section under Selective Photothermolysis for Vulvodynia). Success rates of >90% can be anticipated within 3–5 treatment repetitions. Conversely, for patients with *surface plus deep pain loops,* it is impossible to control the surface component until the deep pain is also suppressed. Sometimes this can be done with regional interferon injection. However, for those people who do not respond to medical management, microsurgical removal of the Bartholin's glands appears unavoidable.

The surgical technique involves exposure with traction sutures, localization of the Bartholin's duct with the Sialogram catheter, and staining of this duct by instillation of toluidine blue (Fig. 93a). The dissection is done with the CO_2 laser. There are two essential planes that must be established. First, the plane between the Bartholin's duct and the vaginal adventitia on the me-

dial side (Fig. 95b), and second, the plane between the Bartholin's duct and the capsule of the vestibular body on the lateral side (Fig. 95c). Once these planes are established, it is possible to elevate the gland itself, allowing suture ligation of the vessels that emanate from the underlying urogenital diaphragm (Fig. 95d). Finally, the wound must be closed in layers inserting a couple of 3-0 vicryls into the dense vestibular fascia to safeguard against wound breakdown.

Gland resection can either lead directly to a clinical remission or can at least remove the troublesome deep pain loop so that additional surface treatment will then be successful (Fig. 94). Combining the initial and eventual successes, we have found that the combination of surface therapy plus gland resection will lead to success in ~90% of patients. These figures stand in sharp contradistinction to the 10% or less success that would come from persistent surface therapy in this subset.

For patients with *Bartholin's gland pain plus a tissue deficit* (e.g., prior vestibulectomy, or scarring from previous surface laser treatments), we find that the incisions made for gland removal will not heal well if closed by primary suture. Hence, in these patients, we must often resort to various reconstructive techniques to close the incision sites. Such techniques include: (1) skin grafting, usually full thickness graft, since split thickness neither prevents contracture nor replaces the lost dermis, (2) the transposition of random skin flaps from the interlabial sulci, or (3) creation of a specific axial flap (e.g., a pudendal-thigh fasciocutaneous flap).

Endoscopically Adapted CO_2 Lasers

The CO_2 laser can be connected to an operative laparoscope by a coupling device that transmits the beam down the operative channel of the instrument. The CO_2 laser offers the endoscopist several advantages: (1) the rapid photovaporization capacity of this wavelength provides an efficient thermal scalpel with reasonable hemostatic properties, (2) no-touch incision/ablation and operation by remote control can greatly facilitate endoscopic surgery upon an inaccessible target, (3) high water affinity allows the use of pooled irrigation fluid as a backstop, and (4) the short absorption length guarantees localization of thermal damage to a narrow, visually recognizable band. However, these advantages are counterbalanced by several troublesome disadvantages—

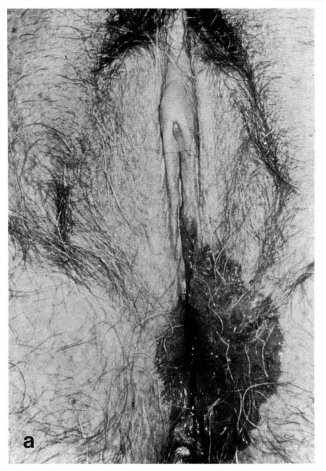 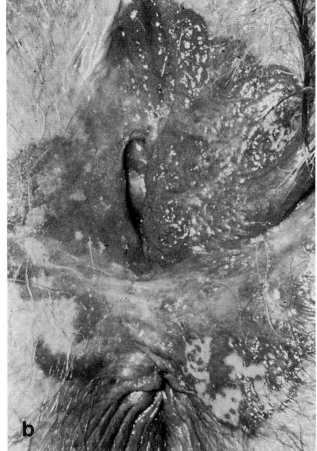

Fig. 84. **a:** Extensive VIN 3 lesion centered upon the left interlabial sulcus and extending both distal to the pilosebaceous line and proximal to the mucocutaneous line. **b:** Same lesion after 3 years without treatment. A large area of invasive squamous carcinoma has now arisen in the left interlabial sulcus. (Courtesy RW Jones, MD, Auckland, NZ.)

smoke formation, awkward beam delivery, and thermal blooming. Strategies for overcoming such impediments are summarized below.

Maintaining visibility. Good operative visibiity requires an extrabright helium:neon (HeNe) aiming beam (at least 5 mW), so as to remain visible upon a brightly illuminated video monitor. The large amount of smoke and steam produced during CO_2 photovaporization must be counteracted by always depressing the trumpet valve on the suction-irrigator, each time the laser foot pedal is activated [143]. In order to maintain the pneumoperitoneum with such frequent use of intra-abdominal suction, the surgeon must have a high-flow insufflation system (e.g., pressure regulated flow rates of at least 6 L/mm) [144].

Facile beam delivery. Our inability to transmit 10.6 μm energy fiberoptically is a major obstacle. Five years ago, the CO_2 laser was delivered to the endoscope by an articulating arm and then directed down the center of the operating channel by an inefficient joystick located on an awkward and bulky coupling device. Keeping the beam in alignment was an exercise in frustration. Any small change in the relationship of the coupling device and the endoscope produced a misaligned beam that bounced off the sides of the operating channel [145].

In search of a solution to this problem, some manufacturers fitted the CO_2 laser to a waveguide. This adaptation was certainly more facile; however, loss of the gaussian beam profile was too large a tradeoff. Cutting with a waveguide-delivered CO_2 laser requires that the operating laparoscope to be moved almost into contact with the intended target, thus robbing the surgeon of perspective at a most crucial time.

The best solution lay in redesigning the old

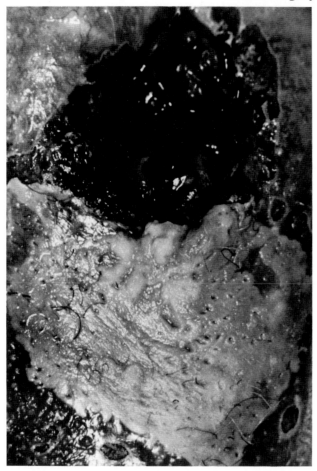

Fig. 85. Recurrence of VIN 3 at the lateral margin of a simple vulvectomy. (From Reid [133], reproduced with permission).

TABLE 17. Success Rates for Laser Ablation of VIN 3

Series	Success with one Treatment
Baggish & Dorsey [119]	31/35
Townsend [206]	31/33
Leutcher [207]	35/42
Campion & Singer [120]	44/50
Reid [28]	31/41
Total	172/201 (86%)

fashioned coupling device. The movable mirrors and joystick were replaced; instead, the articulating arm was fitted directly into the operating channel of the endoscope (Coherent, Palo Alto, CA; Herdeus Lasersonics, Milpitas, CA; Sharplan, Tel Aviv, Israel). Thus the laser and scope function as a long thermal scalpel, which cuts directly along the line of vision.

Limiting thermal blooming. Since the laser beam was itself generated from the carbon

TABLE 18. Concomitant Laparoscopy With Hysteroscopy

Absolute indications
  1. Resection with intrauterine septum
  2. Resection of significant fundal adhesions (Asherman's disease)
Relative indications
  1. Resection submucous myoma
  2. Endometrial ablation
  3. Performation or other complication

dioxide molecules, this 10.6 μm energy will resonate at the same frequency as the molecular bonds in the CO_2 insufflation gas. Hence, the laser beam is attenuated and distorted as it traverses the pneumoperitoneum, en route to the target. Power to tissue is reduced 30–50% with a 7.2 mm operating channel (12 mm scope) and 60% with a 6 mm channel (10 mm scope) [146]. These problems can be secondarily worsened by two procedural errors: not connecting the insufflation gas to the laser delivery channel and using low gas flow while lasing. Such errors allow the laser beam to heat the stagnant gas within the operative channel, producing a phenomenon known as "thermal blooming." Several operative problems result. First, the diameter of the focal spot enlarges dramatically—thus attenuating power density. Reich et al. [146] showed that unchecked thermal blooming kept power density below 800 w/cm^2, even with use of a 100-watt laser. CO_2 laser used through the operating channel of laser laparoscopes; in vitro study of power and power density losses. Second, divergence of the CO_2 beam also widens the He:Ne spot, reducing intensity to the point where the aiming beam can barely be seen on tissue. Third, the focal spot becomes unstable, leading the He:Ne light to "jump around." Fourth, using an alternative insufflation port also allows humid, smoky gas to flow back into the operative channel, coating the lenses and thus further exacerbating problems of beam transmission and image recognition. The solution is threefold: CO_2 must always be insufflated down the operative channel, high rates of gas flow must be maintained by some degree of downstream venting (e.g., by activating the suction-irrigator each time the laser is fired), and the superpulsed temporal mode should be used.

Recently, a CO_2 laser has been modified specifically for intra-abdominal use. The Ultrapulse 5000L™ (Coherent) uses the $^{13}CO_2$ isotope as the laser medium, thus creating a small shift in the emitted wavelength—from 10.6 to 11.1 μm. Since

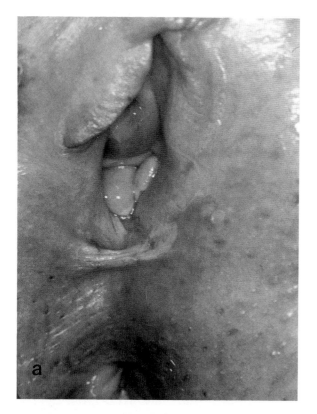

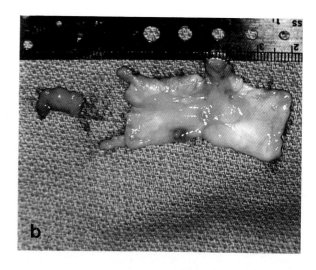

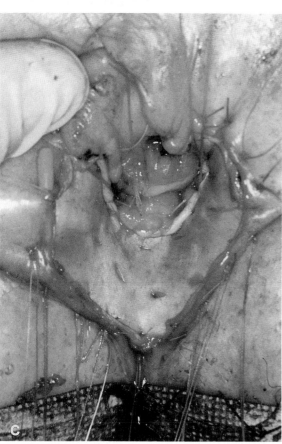

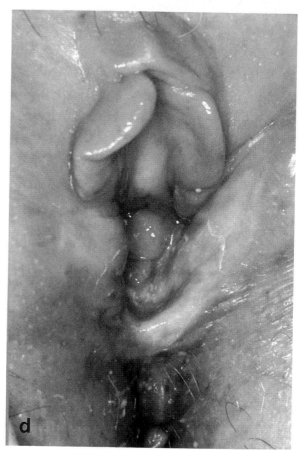

Fig. 86. **a:** Large field of carcinoma in situ of the posterior fourchette of an 80-year-old woman. Directed biopsy of an area of focal ulceration showed superficial invasion. **b:** Hemivulvectomy specimen. **c:** Reconstruction by full thickness skin graft, harvested from the anterior abdominal wall. The skin is then carefully de-fatted, cut to shape, and sewn on a dry recipient site. **d:** Final outcome.

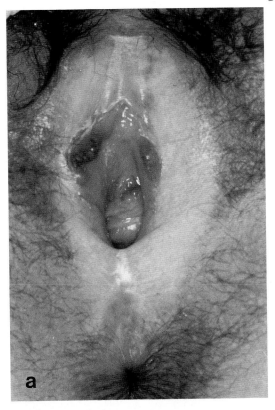

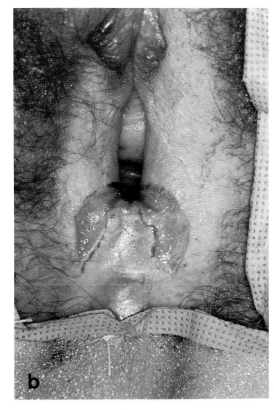

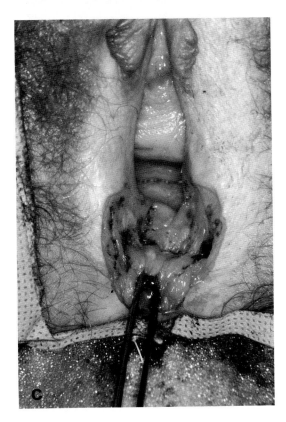

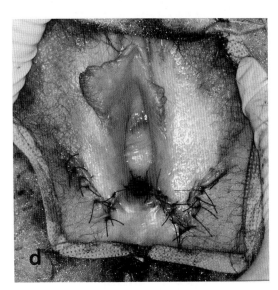

Fig. 87. **a:** Results of low-powered CO_2 laser, producing wide-spread epithelial atrophy and a "burnlike" contracture of the posterior fourchette. **b:** Fashioning an advancement flap, in the shape of an inverted "Y". **c:** Extending the mobilizing incision into the scarred perineal body. **d:** Closure by forwardly advancing the central tongue of the "inverted Y", and backwardly advancing the lateral angles of the "inverted Y".

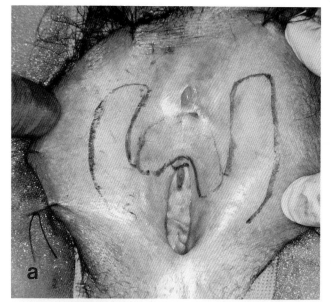

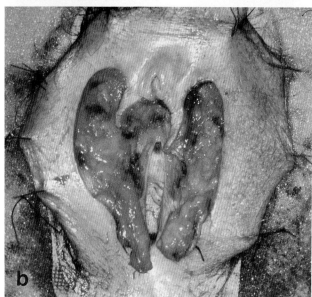

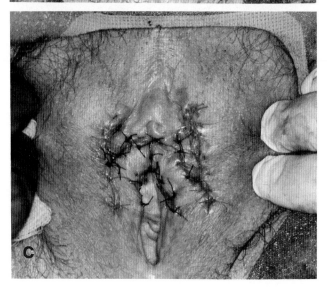

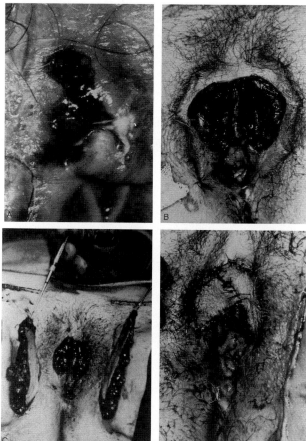

Fig. 89. Use of an arteriolized flap of medial thigh skin (based on the terminal branches of the pudenal artery) to allow clitoral conservation and restoration of normal anatomic appearance, after wide resection of the 0.5 mm, well-differentiated invasive squamous carcinoma arising in the skin overlying the shaft of the clitoris. **A:** Colpophotograph of the lesion, showing incipient ulceration and a bizarre mosaic vascular pattern. **B:** Resection of the anterior vulva to the pilosebaceous lines exposing the crura and shaft of clitoris as they arise from the pubic bone. **C:** Raising the flap of medial thigh and inguinal skin, by dissecting down to the fascia of adductor magnus. **D:** Transposition of the flaps, to restore anatomic integrity. (From Reid [132], reproduced with permission.)

Fig. 88. **a:** Elderly woman with focal invasive squamous cancer in the "boomerang-shaped" area between the clitoris and the urethra. This cancer arose within a field of long-standing lichen sclerosus, as shown by the webbed deformity of the posterior fourchette. Most of the benign epithelial changes have regressed with potent steroid therapy. **b:** Developing flaps that mobilize skin, fat, and bulbocaverosis fascia, to be transposed from the donor sites (lateral) to the recipient site (central). **c:** End result.

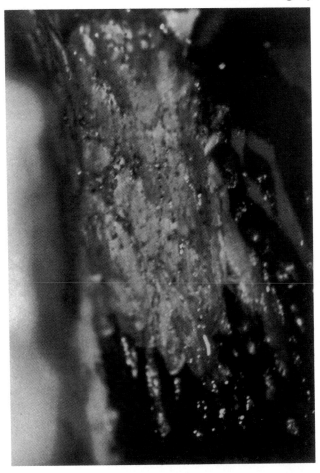

Fig. 90. First vaginal plane. After the epithelial debris is wiped away, the surface of the lamina propria appears as a shiny, white layer. (From Reid [132], reproduced with permission.)

the pneumoperitoneum does not contain significant quantities of this isotope, the 11.1 μm beam no longer resonates with the insufflation gas. Thus the laser beam will reach the target at full power and in tight focus [147].

GYNECOLOGIC APPLICATIONS FOR NEODYMIUM:YAG LASERS

Historically, hysteroscopy was a frustrating exercise. Difficulties arose from the thickness of the uterine walls, the small size of the cavity, and the tendency of the endometrium to bleed on contact [148]. Uterine distension was a major obstacle. Even then, early lens systems and restricted illumination yielded poor images. Finally, light bulbs were on the distal end of the telescope, where they produced a risk of thermal injury and were also prone to failure.

These problems were solved by a series of technical inventions: improvement of image quality by construction of a rod lens, development of a fiberoptic hysteroscope, improvements in distention techniques, and the introduction of lightweight high resolution cameras. Gynecologists of the 1980s quickly embraced the hysteroscope as a new diagnostic instrument, especially as a means of improving the accuracy and limiting the fiscal waste of the hospital D&C [149]. This search for more conservative diagnostic approaches to intrauterine disease inevitably led to the development of hysteroscopic biopsy forceps and hysteroscopic scissors and to the adaptation of rectoscopic electrosurgery instruments—all of which could be passed alongside the telescope and thus used within the uterus under direct visual control. However, the use of mechanical instruments within the uterine cavity is difficult; hence, operative hysteroscopists turned to thermal energy sources. Neuwirth [150] began adapting the urological resectoscopes in the early 1970s. The availability of optical fibers capable of transmitting intense energy levels also made it possible to couple the Nd:YAG laser to the operative hysteroscope, as a tool for both photovaporization and photocoagulation [151]. Electrosurgery was soon adapted for the same purpose [152] and has replaced the Nd:YAG at most centers [153,154].

Advantages and Disadvantages of Nd:YAG Lasers

Earlier discussion extolled the virtue of nonscattering short extinction length over extensively scattering extinction length lasers. However, when the surgical objective is to produce deep coagulation of highly vascular tissues, the opposite holds true. Consider the theoretic example of a small packet of CO_2 or Nd:YAG energy, each having a beam area of 1 mm^2. The very short extinction length (0.03 mm) of CO_2 laser light leads to intense heating of a small critical volume (only 3×10^{-2} mm^3)[76] (Fig. 95a) (4A). In the endometrial cavity, such a confined energy uptake would not reach the stratum basalis, and the hemostatic effects seen in cervical ablation would be overwhelmed by the size of the endometrial blood vessels. Conversely, even the unrealistically small packet of Nd:YAG photons described in this theoretic example would elicit a very different tissue effect. The extensive lateral and forward scatter would enlarge the effective surface area of the circular impact site to ~9 mm^2, and the longer extinction length of the shorter wavelength would extend the depth of coagulation to ~2 mm. Hence,

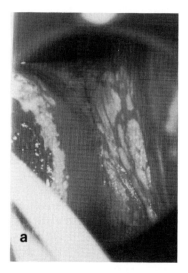
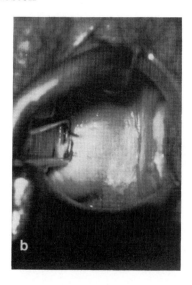
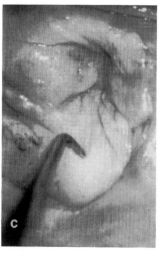
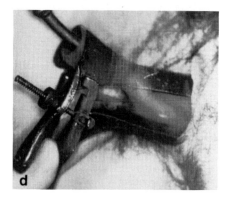

Fig. 91. Maneuvers for vaginal exposure. **a:** Distending the vaginal fornix by pressure on the opposite fornix with a rectal swab, held in position by the thumb of the hand that controls the speculum. **b:** Deviating the cervix by pushing or pulling with a tenaculum, applied lateral to the lateral blades of a Graves speculum. **c:** Exposing the vaginal vault scar with a skin hook. **d:** Improved exposure, by firing between lateral edges of the speculum blades. (From Reid [132], reproduced with permission.)

tissue damage from even these few photons of Nd: YAG energy would correspond to a cylinder with a critical volume ~18 mm^3 (see Fig. 97b). Compared to the small packet of CO_2 photons the dispersed energy absorption pattern of Nd:YAG energy would heat a 600 times larger tissue volume to much lower temperatures.

Endoscopically Adapted Nd:YAG Lasers

Like the argon and KTP lasers, Nd:YAG energy has dramatically different surgical effects,

depending upon whether or not the fiber is held in contact with the target tissue.

Noncontact use. In real life, noncontact delivered Nd:YAG energy penetrates to a depth of 4–6 mm. At usual operating power densities, the tissue effect is to create a deep but sharply defined zone of coagulation necrosis. This is reflected visually as a delayed blanching and/or "bubbling" of tissue (Fig. 96). At much higher powers, the Nd:YAG energy densities can reach the vaporization threshold. However, such vaporization cra-

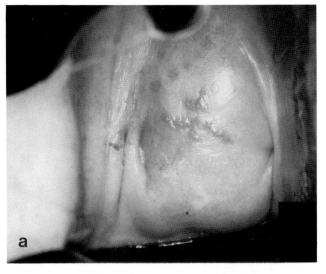

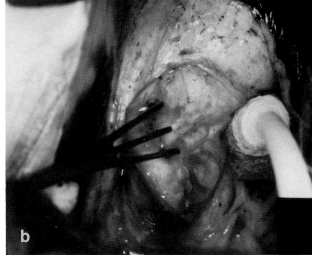

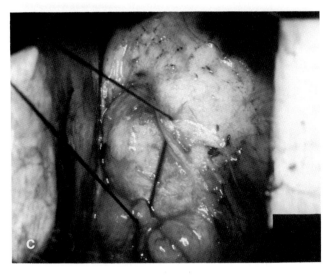

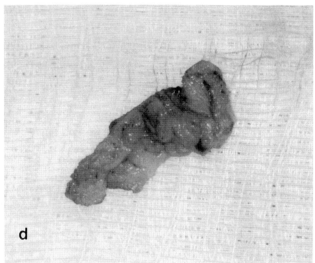

Fig. 92. **a:** Postmenopausal patient, status post-TAH for CIN 3, with a suspicious red patch involving the right vaginal angle. **b:** Wide field of surrounding VAIN 1–2 has been lased to the third plane. Centrally, the suspicious area is being laser-excised, using traction from a Campion hook and countertraction from a large cotton swab. The cul de sac peritoneum is seen beneath the excised specimen. **c:** Suturing the vaginal muscularis over the exposed peritoneum. **d:** Excised specimen.

ters are bounded by a several millimeter margin of coagulation necrosis. Cutting densities of Nd:YAG energy would be rational for hepatic transection but disastrous for fine surgical dissection of most soft tissues.

Contact use. Some laparoscopists feel that tissue contact provides a sense of touch, thus giving better surgical control. Contact tips create less smoke than a CO_2 laser, do not require a backstop, and may be used under fluid. Although tissue effects from the Nd:YAG are less precise, the differences are measured in microns. On the skin, such differences would be clinically important. However, within the abdomen, they are of no significance.

As a generalization, the diffuse patterns of tissue of the free beam Nd:YAG energy are ideal for operative hysteroscopy, whereas the confined tissue effects of the hot tips are much safer for the laparoscopist. There is one absolute rule: gas-cooled contact tips must never be inserted into the uterine cavity (see later under Complications of Operative Hysteroscopy).

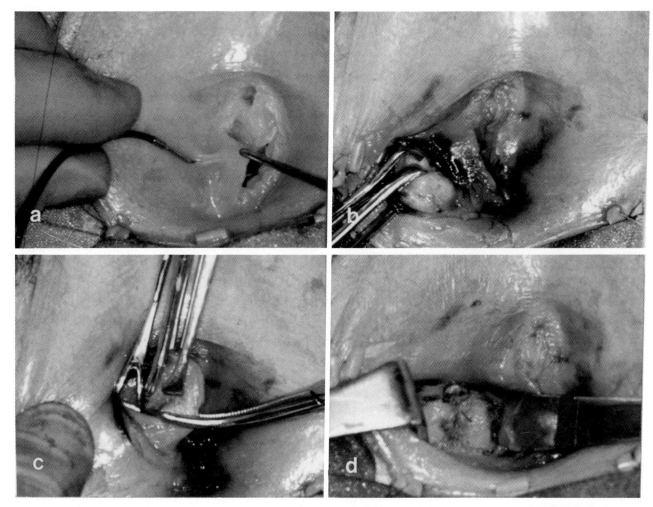

Fig. 93. **a:** Canullating the Bartholin's duct with a Sialogram canulla. **b:** Medial and lateral planes have been developed, and the Bartholin's gland is being elevated by a pair of baby Allis forceps. **c:** Clamping the deep (vascular) pedicule that attaches the Bartholin's gland to the underlying urogenital diaphragm. **d:** The cleaned-out Bartholin's fossa, showing pubococcygeus on the deep medial margin. See insert for color representation.

Endometrial Ablation with the Free-Beam Nd:YAG Laser

Hysterectomy is one of the most commonly performed major surgeries in the United States. Every year, >600,000 women undergo hysterectomy, costing ~ three billion dollars in direct health care expenses [149]. In Australia, 40% of women will have lost their uterus prior to menopause [155]; hysterectomy rates in the United States are at least as high. About one-third of hysterectomies are performed for such clear indications as endometrial hyperplasia, large leiomyomata, uterine prolapse, and pelvic cancer. However, the most common single indication for hysterectomy, accounting for perhaps 200,000 operations per year, is menorrhagia unrelated to myomas or malignancy [156]. Most such women have no other gynecologic complaint, and most such uteri show no pathologic change upon extirpation [157,158]. Hysterectomies for dysfunctional uterine bleeding are often done by open laparotomy, thus necessitating several days of hospitalization and at least 1 month of disability. Complication rates of 30% and greater have been reported; even worse, there is also a mortality rate of ~0.1% [159,160]. Thus advances in operative hysteroscopy spurred a renewed search for an alternative approach to disruptive menstrual bleeding, not associated with recognizable pelvic pathology.

In 1948, Asherman [161] described a syndrome of amenorrhea following traumatic curettage of the endometrium. Since that time, several investigators have sought to create an artificial

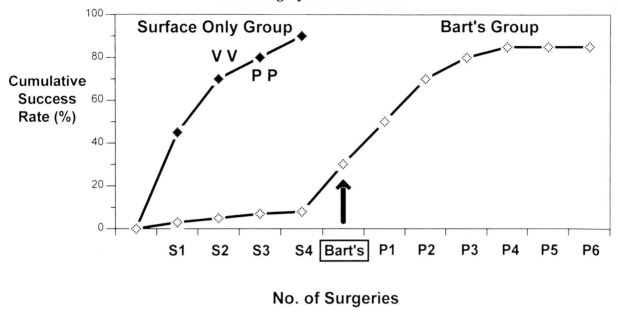

Fig. 94. Cumulative response rates for "surface only" (VV and PP) vs. "surface plus deep" (Bartholin's group). On the X axis, "S 1-4" refers to initial FEDL photothermolysis; "Bart's" refers to gland resection; "P 1-6" refers to post-resection repetition of FEDL photothermolysis. (From Reid et al. [20], with permission)

Asherman's syndrome, experimenting with both chemical and physical methods. The greatest obstacles facing past investigators were the regenerative capacity of the endometrium and the susceptibility of the upper cervical canal to cicatrization. The combination of incomplete endometrial destruction plus cervical stenosis generally leads to painful hematometra or uterine abscess formation. Goldrath [151] overcame the first of these obstacles by suppressing the ovarian cycle with danazol 800 mg per day for 3 weeks prior to surgery. Then, by expert and painstaking hysteroscopic technique, Goldrath used a hysteroscopically adapted Nd:YAG laser to ablate the stratum basalis of the corpus and fundus. The isthmus and upper canal were spared under direct visual control. The long absorption length of the Nd:YAG laser ensured relatively uniform endometrial photocoagulation, whereas the underlying myometrium acted as a backstop for any energy transmitted more deeply.

Indications for endometrial ablation. Endometrial ablation was introduced as an alternative to hysterectomy. Suitable candidates are women with problematic menstrual bleeding, who have failed conservative therapy and in whom malignant disease has been excluded. Endometrial ablation has been *especially useful* in: (1) dysfunctional uterine bleeding, as an isolated gynecolog-

ical problem, (2) menorrhagia complicated by other pelvic complaints, when the primary objective is to control bleeding yet avoid the disruption of resective surgery, (3) control of major uterine hemorrhage in women with significant medical (e.g., hemorrhagic diathesis) or surgical problems (e.g., morbid obesity, extensive incisional hernia, dense intra-abdominal adhesions), and (4) persistent postmenopausal bleeding that might otherwise prevent estrogen replacement therapy.

Potentially premalignant endometrial hyperplasia must be ruled out by hysteroscopy and vigorous endometrial biopsy, within 6 months of the planned procedure. Diagnostic workup should also include CBC, sex hormone, thyroid and clotting studies, and pelvic ultrasound. Preferably, the curettings should be viewed by an expert gynecologic pathologist. Atypical adenomatous hyperplasia and occult endometrial cancer are *absolute contraindications* to endometrial ablation. Although there is no good data implicating benign cystic hyperplasia as a bona fide precursor to endometrial carcinoma, the prudent surgeon should probably view any such finding as a sign for caution.

Relative contraindications to endometrial ablation are: (1) associated gynecologic problems, such as pelvic pain or significant utero-vaginal prolapse, (2) a large uterus (12 wks), (3) a dis-

Absorption characteristic CO_2 laser

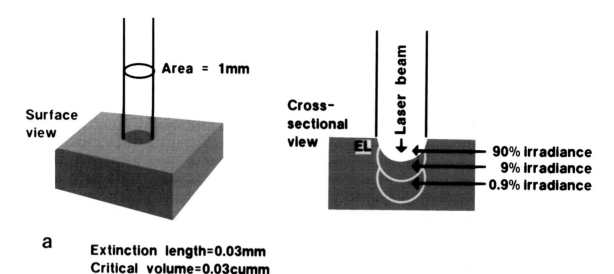

Absorption characteristics-Nd:YAG laser

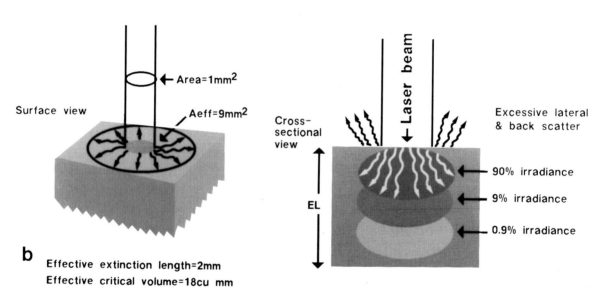

Fig. 95. Comparison of (a) CO_2 and (b) Nd:YAG absorption patterns.

torted uterine cavity, especially if endoscopic visualization is impeded, (4) actively growing intramural and subserosal fibroids, (5) pelvic inflammatory disease, (6) unresolved adnexal pathology, (7) a history of chronic anovulation in a young patient, because of concern about any endometrium that may remain, and (8) a significant family history of ovarian, breast, colon, and uterine cancer.

Severity of menstrual bleeding is highly subjective. Some women are incapacitated by a blood flow that would be perceived as normal by others [157]. Endometrial ablation is a quick, outpatient procedure with few complications, generally followed by prompt personal recovery and early return to work. Hence, there has been a tendency for endometrial ablation to be performed "on demand," as if it were an elective surgical procedure like tubal ligation, mammoplasty, or liposuction. This trend is undesirable. Endometrial ablation can cause serious complications, including death [162–165]. Moreover, statistics on the long-term

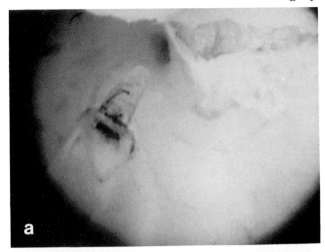

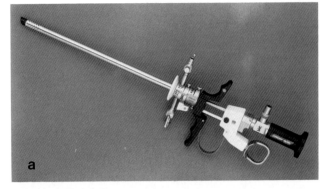

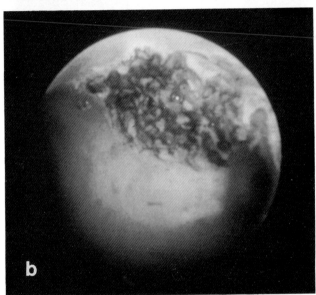

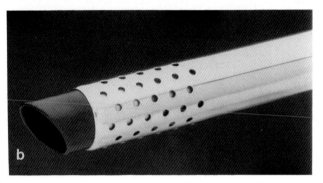

Fig. 97. USA Elite System Gynecologic 27 Fr Continuous Flow Resectoscope (U.S. Trademark of Circon Corp.). **a:** Assembled instrument. **b:** Distal end, showing outflow holes on both top and bottom of the outer sheath. (Photos courtesy of Circon Corp.).

safety of endometrial ablation are still being compiled. In particular, the cohort of women treated by endometrial ablation in the 1980s has not yet reached the mean age for endometrial adenocarcinoma (67 years). From the theoretical viewpoint, one would expect this surgery to lower subsequent cancer incidence, because the ablated endometrium is replaced by a single layer, cuboidal epithelium with sparse glands. Admittedly, isolated islands of endometrium may persist within the myometrium. However, such foci of adenomyosis are at negligible risk of neoplastic

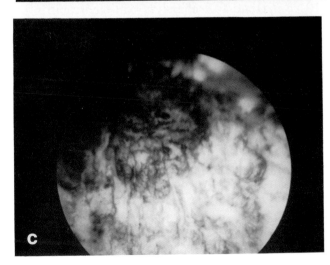

Fig. 96. **a:** Beginning Nd:YAG ablation of the endometrium. The laser fiber is pointing directly as the right tubal ostium. A light brown photovaporized furrow is surrounded by an extensive white area of white photocoagulated endometrium. **b:** The upper field shows extensive contact photovaporization effect, and the lower area shows non-contact photocoagulation. **c:** Final result. (Illustrations courtesy of MJ Campion, MD.)

WATER OVERLOAD (3.6L)

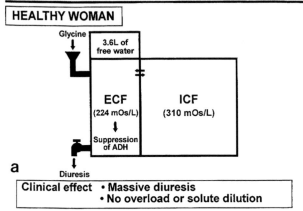

a

| Clinical effect | • Massive diuresis |
| | • No overload or solute dilution |

WATER OVERLOAD (3.6L)

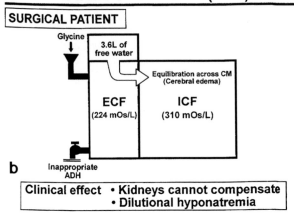

b

| Clinical effect | • Kidneys cannot compensate |
| | • Dilutional hyponatremia |

Fig. 98. **a:** Water overload in a healthy 60 Kg woman. The excess water is rapidly excreted by the kidney, before a chronic hypo-osmolar state can develop. (ECF = extracellular fluid; ICF = intracellular fluid). **b:** Water overload in a surgical patient. Inappropriate ADH secretion causes dilutional hyponatremia. Equilibration into the ICF causes swelling of the brain cells, with consequent risk of medullary coning or respiratory arrest.

transformation. The major areas of unresolved concern are that, if a uterine malignancy were to arise, impeded egress of any symptomatic bleeding and restricted diagnostic access to the endometrial cavity could significantly delay diagnosis. In such event, measurement of the thickness of the "endometrial stripe" by transvaginal ultrasound would probably be the most helpful strategy [166]. Until these issues are settled, it is prudent that endometrial ablation be done only as an alternative to indicated hysterectomy.

Preoperative preparation. Ablation is facilitated by preoperative induction of an hypoestrogenic state. Reducing the thickness of the *stratum functionalis* improves the likelihood that the delivered laser or electrical energy will en-

compass all viable endometrial rests within the *stratum basalis*. This is an important concept. During the healing phase, even small islands of viable endometrium can "swarm" across the denuded area, producing complete or near-complete endometrial regeneration. The most commonly used preoperative protocols are: (1) Danazol (Danocrine™), 400 mg twice daily for 4–6 weeks, (2) Medroxyprogesterone acetate (Provera™), 20–30 mg daily for 4–6 weeks, (3) Megestrol acetate (Megace™), 20–40 mg daily for 4 weeks, and (4) Leuprolide acetate (Lupron™), given as an initial 7.5 mg (1 vial) depot intramuscular injection during the second half of the menstrual cycle and followed by a second depot intramuscular injection of Lupron™ 3.75 mg 4 weeks later. Surgery is scheduled 2 weeks after this second injection. The Lupron™ regimen is preferred because it offers the most complete endometrial suppression, the lowest incidence of side effects, and is the only method that ensures patient compliance.

In the patient of child-bearing age, concomitant sterilization is recommended. Endometrial ablation reduces fertility; however, transcervical coagulation of the tubal ostia has been shown to have a high failure rate, irrespective of whether Nd:YAG laser energy or electricity is used [167, 168]. Pregnancies have been reported after endometrial ablation [169,170] and carry a risk of placenta accreta and intrauterine growth retardation.

Approximately 24 hours prior to surgery, 1–3 mm laminaria tents are placed through the cervix and checked to be above the internal os. A 10 cc syringe full of polymyxin-bacitracin ointment is inserted into the upper vagina and the laminaria packed in place by gauze swabs. Doxycycline 100 mg b.i.d. may be started at this time.

Choice of distending medium. Carbon dioxide gas is not useful for operative laparoscopy. First, admixture of gas and blood produces an opaque red froth that totally obscures vision. Second, despite the low flow rates built into hysteroscopic insufflators (100 ml/min), gas embolism might still occur because of the presence of open venous sinuses within the operative field. Third, the CO_2 gas has no cooling properties, thereby dictating that laser power would have to be kept below 25 watts. Hence, for operative hysteroscopy, the surgeon must choose between high and low viscosity fluids.

The *high viscosity* fluid used in hysteroscopy is Hyskon™ (Kabia Pharmacia, Piscataway, NJ). Hyskon™ is a solution of 32% dextran-70 in 10%

glucose. Dextrans are products of bacterial polymerization of glucose and are classified clinically according to the molecular weight (MW). Low MW (<50,000 daltons) are filtered through the kidney but not reabsorbed; hence, dextran 40 has sometimes been used as an osmotic diuretic. High MW dextrans were introduced into medicine as plasma volume expanders. As a distention medium, Hyskon™ has excellent optical properties, does not admix with blood, and requires only a simple delivery system. Hence, Hyskon™ is used extensively in diagnostic hysteroscopy—either in full strength or in a 1:1 dilution with saline. Dextran 70 can be used to perform either electrical or laser surgery. However, from the viewpoint of the operative hysteroscopist, Hyskon™ has three major disadvantages: (1) full-strength Hyskon™ is very sticky and will form a permanent bond that can glue instruments together and ruin video cameras, (2) heating high viscosity fluids produces large bubbles that significantly impede the surgeon's efforts to treat the anterior uterine wall, and (3) intravasation of as little as 100 ml of Hyskon™ may produce a dangerous combination of pulmonary edema plus acute renal failure.

For operative hysteroscopy, most surgeons use low viscosity fluids for distention of the uterine cavity, cooling of the fiberoptic or electric energy source, and removal of bloody debris. For Nd:YAG ablation, normal saline or Ringer's lactate is the only reasonable choice. However, electrosurgical current is dispersed by electrolyte solutions. Hence, for rollerball and resectoscopic surgery, the surgeon must choose an electrically inert solution, such as glycine 1.5% (a nonessential amino acid), sorbitol 3% (an inert 6 carbon carbohydrate) or Cytal™ (Abbott Laboratories, North Chicago, IL), a commercially available mixture of 2.7% sorbitol and 0.54% of mannitol. Fluid is delivered either by mechanical pump (e.g., the Zimmer™ pump), by constant pressure from an orthopedic tourniquet or by gravity pressure. Whichever method is chosen, risk of fluid overload is minimized by setting infusion pressure at the level that just maintains adequate distention and a clear operative field (usually 40–60 mmHg).

Instrumentation for operative hysteroscopy. Most panoramic telescopic lenses are 4 mm in diameter, with a viewing angle that is either "straight on" (0°) or "forward oblique" (30°). The telescopic lens fits through an operative sheath, which provides a means of delivering the distending/cooling medium, a channel for additional instruments, and a channel for the deflecting (Albaran) bridge. Original investigators used *intermittent-flow* urologic sheaths in which the valve is set either for inflow or for outflow. During inflow, egress of fluid, blood, and debris depends upon dilating the cervix to 1–2 mm wider than the outer diameter of the operative hysteroscope (i.e., to 27–31 Fr). Fluid balance was estimated by secondarily collecting outflow fluid into a waterproof drape placed beneath the patient's hips. Because accurate fluid records are so important, gynecologists should use a *continuous-flow* resectoscope, with an "inner sheath" to separate inflow from outflow. This modification increases the diameter of the outer sheath from about 6.3 mm (19 Fr) to ~8 mm (24 Fr). However, the advantage of a dedicated outflow valve to allow collection of used distending fluid, directly into a nest of suction canisters, more than outweighs the problems posed by a larger sheath diameter.

Light sources, light cables, and video monitoring systems are the same as used in laparoscopy, except that the lighting source for hysteroscopy does not have to be as intense. Video monitoring is also less important in hysteroscopy because the surgery is done in one plane, with the operator sitting down and looking straight ahead. If video is used, the camera operator must rotate the camera 180° when working on the anterior uterine wall in order to maintain proper orientation.

Operative procedure. Because prostaglandin release during endometrial destruction produces painful uterine contractions, endometrial ablation must be performed in the operating room under general or regional conduction anesthesia. The patient is positioned in lithotomy position, laminaria from the night before are removed and sterile washing is performed. Preparations are made to collect outflow fluid directly (by drainage to a suction canister) and indirectly (by placing a drape with a large plastic pouch to catch any additional runoff fluid).

The direction and length of the uterine cavity are carefully assessed by bi-manual examination. The cervix is grasped with a tenaculum and cervical dilation checked. Difficulty in insertion and removal of the hysteroscope is the prime reason for intraoperative perforation. Under continuous flow, the operative hysteroscope is advanced under vision, through the cervical canal, and into the endometrial cavity. The function of the continuous inflow and outflow systems is checked, the video camera is focused, and clarity of view established. The 600-μm fiberoptic is inserted through the operating channel of the hysteroscope and the Nd:YAG laser set at 50–60 watts of continuous wave laser power. The endometrial cavity is then carefully inspected for polyps, myomas, or suspect hyperplasia. If thick endometrium remains despite hormone suppression, it can be removed by suction curettage immediately prior to ablation.

The internal cervical os and the tubal ostia are specifically identified (Fig. 96a). Ablation is performed in a systematic manner. The internal os is first circumscribed to define the caudad limit of ablation. Inadvertently carrying the field of ablation into the upper cervical canal risks secondary hemorrhage and potential stenosis. Next, the fundus is ablated, from one tubal ostium to the other. Finally, the anterior and posterior walls are separately and systematically ablated. Restricted access and bubble formation make treatment of the anterior wall more challenging. Therefore, many surgeons prefer to treat the anterior wall first while anatomic orientation is still easy. Bubbles and debris can be removed by retroverting the uterus and flushing the cavity rapidly with distending media. The interference posed by bubbling and debris collection is reduced by the use of modern inflow/outflow pumps and by selecting a resectoscope adapted for gynecologic use, especially one with outflow holes at both top and bottom of the outer sheath (Fig. 97). Treated areas change in color from whitish pink to brownish black. Any areas that show extreme blackening represent carbon deposition, which may prevent adequate penetration of the Nd:YAG laser. In this event, the laser power should be checked and consideration given to re-stripping the end of the fiber.

Nd:YAG laser energy can be delivered using either a blanching (no touch) or dragging (touch) technique (Fig. 96b,c). There has been debate as to which technique is better [149,171]. In reality, the topography of the uterine cavity dictates that most surgeons will use a combination of both. The uterine fundus and cornua are most readily and safely approached using the blanching technique, with the fiber held ~1–3 mm above the surface as the laser is activated. The clinical endpoint is marked blanching and shrinkage of the endometrium as it is coagulated. Conversely, the anterior and posterior walls are less suitable for the blanching technique, because it is difficult to deliver the energy at right angles to the tissue. Instead, a dragging technique is used, such that the bare fiber indents the endometrium as it is drawn outward in a roughly parallel series of cephalad-caudad furrows

("mowing the lawn"). Obviously, to limit the risks of uterine perforation with an active energy source, the Nd:YAG must never be fired as the fiber is being advanced toward the fundus.

Intraoperative bleeding is occasionally encountered at the completion of the procedure. By slowing the inflow rate, bleeding sites can be identified and individually coagulated. Bleeding may also occur in the recovery room. This problem is managed by placing a Foley catheter and inflating with a small volume of fluid (typically ~6 ml), to tamponade the bleeding points. Care must be taken not to overinflate this balloon for fear of rupturing the uterus. The catheter is left in place for 4 hours and then deflated in the recovery room. Four hours is generally all that is needed to establish dependable hemostasis.

Concomitant laparoscopy. The indications for concomitant laparoscopy with hysteroscopy are outlined in Table 18. Laparoscopy is absolutely indicated in resection of intrauterine septae and for attempted lysis of intrauterine synechia in the fundal region. Relative indications include resection of sessile submucous myomas, during endometrial ablation, and in the investigation of perforation or other complication. Perhaps the best generalization is that laparoscopy should be done whenever it makes the surgeon feel more comfortable.

Laparoscopy is a procedure with a small but definite morbidity and even occasional mortality. Hence, one must question any decision to add laparoscopy to the planned endometrial ablation. Concomitant laparoscopy does, however, offer several important advantages. First, having a second surgeon watch the integrity of the uterus offers a degree of safety to those surgeons who are beginning endometrial ablation. Perforation is most reliably anticipated by turning laparoscopic illumination down to "twilight" levels and watching the uterine walls for any intense local transillumination from the hysteroscopic light source. Second, placing 500 ml of Ringer's lactate in the cul de sac surrounds the uterus with a buffer zone of coolant, which would protect intraperitoneal structures in the event of perforation with an active energy source. Third, concomitant laparoscopy is often indicated to occlude the fallopian tubes of women of child-bearing age undergoing endometrial ablation.

Results of Nd:YAG laser ablation of the endometrium. Assessing success of Nd:YAG laser ablation is subjective. Nonetheless, ~90% of people achieve the desired level of menstrual con-

TABLE 19. Complications of Operative Hysteoscopy Are Self-explanatory

A. *Trauma*
   1. Perforation during dilation
   2. Perforation with hysteroscope
   3. Perforation with energy delivery system
   4. Perforation due to distending medium
B. *Bleeding*
   1. Secondary to perforation
   2. Secondary to resectoscopic procedure
   3. Secondary to dilation
C. *Infection*
D. *Intra-abdominal Injury*
   1. Perforation with scope
   2. Perforation or trauma from instrumentation
   3. Trauma of energy delivery system
E. *Distending media mishaps*
   Distending media mishaps are much more common then have been reported and for this reason are presented in some detail.
F. *Anesthetic mishaps*
G. *Miscellaneous*
   1. Electrical burns
   2. Laser burns
   3. Fire
   4. Light cord burns

trol, ~70% report subsequent amenorrhea, 10% exhibit 1 or 2 days of hypomenorrhea, and ~10% have menstrual flow in keeping with a normal period [151,154]. Thus the procedure does fail in ~10% of cases, particularly in patients with associated fibroids or a large complex endometrial cavity. Endometrial ablation can be repeated. However, because of the distortion, scarring, thinning, and possible loculation of the endometrial cavity, second attempts are technically more difficult and more hazardous. As a generalization, laparoscopically assisted vaginal hysterectomy is probably preferable.

Some patients may consider very light bleeding for 1 or 2 days as treatment failure, whereas others will be greatly relieved by return to such a relatively normal menstrual flow. Ultimately, the patient's opinion as to the success or failure of the procedure is probably influenced by her expectations. During preoperative counseling, it should be stressed that hysterectomy offers the only guaranteed method of ensuring amenorrhea and that endometrial ablation is a conservative alternative that seeks to reduce menorrhagia rather than necessarily to induce amenorrhea.

Complications of operative hysteroscopy. Endometrial ablation through the operative hysteroscope is a major advance in gynecologic surgery. Complications associated with operative laparoscopy are essentially self-explanatory and are listed in Table 19. Sadly, during the developmental years, there have been a number of deaths, mostly from errors in the choice or control of the distending/cooling medium. In 1989, Baggish and Daniell [162] described two fatalities and two near fatalities from *gas embolism,* following inappropriate attempts at endometrial ablation using Nd: YAG powered artificial sapphire tips. *Because these probes are cooled by high volume, high pressure CO_2 gas flow, they must never be inserted into the uterine cavity!* In the event of cracking (e.g., from heat damage), large volumes of gas spill into the venous circulation, with catastrophic results.

Hyskon™ should not be used for operative laparoscopy—for technical as well as safety reasons. Intravasation of high MW dextrans into the transected uterine veins produces *increased oncotic pressure.* The plasma expanding effect of high MW dextrans is surprisingly powerful; each ml of intravasated Hyskon™ will increase blood volume by ten times its own volume. Thus absorption of 100 ml of Hyskon™ will increase plasma volume by 1 liter; absorption of 350 ml would double the blood volume of a 60 kg female [172].

High oncotic pressure states cause a dangerous combination of pathophysiologic disturbances—pulmonary edema and oliguria. Treatment begins with ventilatory support and an attempt at diuresis. However, neither loop diuretics nor simple dialysis resolves the underlying problems of increased oncotic pressure. Because dextran has a long half-life, pulmonary edema or renal failure can last for weeks. In refractory cases, plasmapheresis may be needed. In addition to the results of a hyperoncotic state, direct dextran toxicity can produce rare anaphylactic reactions [173,174] or disseminated intravascular coagulation [175,176].

Intravasation of low viscosity fluids produces a different set of disturbances—volume overload, water intoxication, and electrolyte imbalance. No matter how carefully input-output is monitored, intravasation of 500–1,000 ml is common. With a competent surgical team, however, fluid deficit will never be allowed to exceed 1,500 ml. *Volume overload* with 1.5 liters of lactated Ringer's solution is unlikely to produce serious sequelae in a healthy female; moreover, any high output left ventricular failure that might result will respond quickly to a loop diuretic (furosemide 40 mg). However, intravasation of 1.5 liters of salt-free fluid can produce *dilutional hyponatremia.* This little understood complication is by far the greatest danger facing the operative hysteroscopist. Indeed, perhaps the major advantage of the Nd:YAG laser over electrosurgical alternatives is that the laser surgeon can use electrolyte containing distending media.

Dangers of Dilutional Hyponatremia

Mechanism of water overload. At the moment of infusion, glycine 1.5% and sorbitol 3% are almost iso-osmolar with plasma. However, these organic molecules are soon metabolized—glycine to oxalate and ammonia; sorbitol to fructose and glucose—leading to water intoxication [164,172]. Because water molecules are highly diffusible, excess free water within the intravascular compartment equilibrates rapidly with interstitial and intracellular fluids. Water also moves relatively freely across the blood-brain barrier, leading to congestion and reduced blood flow within the cerebral capillary beds, and eventually to herniation of the brainstem through the foramen magnum [177].

Dangers facing the operative hysteroscopist. A hemolytic reaction following absorption of sterile water during a transurethral resection of the prostate (TURP) was first reported by Creevy [178] in 1947. Soon after, the resectoscope came into widespread use in the 1950s. The syndrome of dilutional hyponatremia became widely known among urologists. Nonetheless, a recent multicenter epidemiologic study showed that TURP still carries a higher mortality than open prostatectomy, principally because of hypotonic fluid absorption during the endoscopic resection [179]. When technologic advances in one specialty are transferred to another, there is always a danger that the lessons of morbidity will have to be re-learned by the new group. That is, the operative protocol is quickly assimilated, but knowledge as to recognition and response to unfamiliar complications often lags behind. From the very beginning of their training, urology residents are taught that water intoxication may lead to cardiovascular overload, respiratory collapse, and permanent brain injury. Experience acquired over decades by urologists must not be re-learned by gynecologic hysteroscopists, especially since the female brain has a diminished ability to adapt to hyponatremia.

Prevalence of hyponatremia. The reported prevalence of sodium:water imbalance is astounding. Dilutional hyponatremia is seen in ~1% of all hospital admissions [180], 4.4% of postoperative patients [181], and up to 41% of TURPs [182]. Healthy adults can remain in fluid electrolyte balance despite a challenge of up to 15 liters of water within a 24-hour period. Why, then, do certain subsets of hospitalized patients become hyponatremic after absorbing just a few liters of water? The answer lies in the fact that essentially all postoperative patients have raised plasma antidiuretic hormone (ADH) concentrations (Fig. 98). Inappropriately elevated ADH levels (fear, pain, restriction of oral fluids, vomiting, hypotonic infusions) impair the excretion of free water, thereby setting the stage for dilutional hyponatremia [181,183]. This unwelcome trend is dangerously accentuated by the scientifically unfounded habit of injecting vasopressin into the cervix at the time of endometrial ablation [165].

Arieff et al. [177] reported a series of 15 previously healthy women who underwent elective surgery and subsequently developed hyponatremia. In 8 of the 15 patients, the onset of seizure and respiratory arrest occurred without warning. These patients had been "lying in bed awake with only minor symptoms. Within a period of less than 10 minutes, these eight patients went from a state in which they were alert and talking to a grand mal seizure, which was soon followed by respiratory arrest." A subsequent case control study compared 65 cases of postoperative hyponatremic encephalopathy with 674 controls that had asymptomatic postoperative hyponatremia. Ayus et al. [184] concluded that men and women were equally likely to develop hyponatremia or hyponatremic encephalopathy (HNE) surgery. However, estrogen reduces the ability of the sodium-potassium pump within the cell membrane to extrude sodium from the intracellular compartment, as a means of forestalling brain swelling secondary to the water intoxication [184]. Of the 34 patients who developed permanent brain damage or died, 33 (97%) were women ($P < 0.001$). Of the women suffering brain damage, 25 (76%) were of child-bearing age ($P < 0.001$). Relative risk for death or permanent brain damage from HNE was thus 28 times higher in women compared with men (CI = 5 − 141), and 26 times higher in menstruant compared with postmenopausal women (CI = 11–62). In other words, if HNE does develop, menstruant women are ~25 times more likely to die or have permanent brain damage than either men or postmenopausal women [184].

Early recognition. Morbidity is not directly tied to actual serum sodium levels. Urologists have traditionally set a serum Na^+ of 120 mEq/liter as the threshold for active correction with hypertonic saline; however, it must be emphasized that women who dilute their sodium

TABLE 20. Signs and Symptoms of Hyponatraemia

Early hyponatraemic encephalopathy
- Headache
- Nausea
- Vomiting
- Weakness

Advanced hyponatraemic encephalopathy
- Impaired response to verbal stimuli
- Impaired response to painful stimuli
- Bizarre (inappropriate) behavior
- Visual hallucinations
- Auditory hallucinations
- Obtundation
- Urinary incontinence
- Faecal incontinence
- Hypoventilation

Very advanced hyponatraemic encephalopathy
(manifestations secondary to increased intracranial pressure)
- Decorticate or decerebrate posturing, or both
- Unresponsiveness
- Bradycardia
- Hypertension
- Altered temperature regulation (hypothermia or hyperthermia)
- Dilated pupils
- Seizure activity (focal or grand mal or both)
- Respiratory insufficiency
- Respiratory arrest
- Coma
- Polyuria (secondary to central diabetes insipidus)

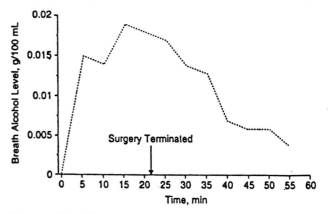

Fig. 99. Use of breath alcohol level to monitor a patient who showed rapid glycine absorption during endometrial ablation. (From Hultén et al. [187], reprinted with permission)

stores to this degree are at risk of sudden death. HNE has been reported in females with a serum Na^+ as high as 128 mEq/liter in females.

Since risks relate to the occurrence of hypoxic events in uncontrolled clinical situations [177], the key to preventing morbidity is early recognition. Ideally, dilutional hyponatremia should be detected in the recovery room, by comparing pre- and postoperative Na^+ levels [165]. In reality, most patients with asymptomatic hyponatremia are discharged undetected. Even in women who develop HNE, diagnosis is usually made on the second or third postoperative day, by which time treatment is more difficult and more hazardous. Arieff et al. [177] also observed that hyponatremia was not generally considered in the initial resuscitation of the 25 women reported in his initial series. Average delay was 16 ± 7 hours, mainly attributable to time spent in doing diagnostic studies—lumbar puncture, CAT scan, EEG, carotid and vertebral angiography, and even open brain biopsy [177].

The onus of recognition begins with the anesthesiologist. Hypothermia, tremulousness, dilated pupils, falling oxygen saturation, or slow emergence should immediately raise suspicions of

hypo-osmolarity [165]. Ideally, endometrial ablation should be done under spinal anesthesia (without too much sedation), so that the patient can articulate potential cardiac, pulmonary, or central nervous system symptoms during surgery. Signs and symptoms of developing HNE in the nonanesthetized patient are detailed in Table 20. Nausea, vomiting, headache, weakness, or inappropriate behavior are knife-edge warning signs in patients who received salt-free distending solutions at pressures above that of the venous circulation. Progression to the point of confusion, hallucination, hypoventilation, or obtundation is inherently hazardous.

Prevention of dilutional hyponatremia. For endometrial ablation with the Nd:YAG laser, distention with isotonic saline or lactated Ringer's solution obviates the problem. However, if electric current is to be used, a sorbitol-mannitol mixture (Cytal™, Abbot Laboratories, North Chicago, IL) or even isotonic mannitol (which will not be metabolized) are to be preferred over the traditional 1.5% glycine. Vasopressin must *not* be used—alleged benefits are unsubstantiated and the potential for deleterious events is extreme.

In post-TURP syndrome, absorption of hypotonic fluid has been related to: (1) area of tissue resected, (2) procedure duration, (3) irrigation pressure [185], and (4) the vascularity of the organ being treated. Surgeons should try to restrict infusion pressure to the 40–60 mmHg range [185]. For those using a gravity system, this corresponds to ~60–80 cm H_2O of fluid elevation. Resistance to fluid egress must be assiduously prevented, by ensuring that the outflow valve is open and by slightly overdilating the cervix. Difficulty in maintaining intrauterine pressure at these pump settings is an almost certain sign of occult perforation. Such an injury carries three dangers: (1) the risk of thermal injury to abdominal viscera, (2) the risk of concealed hemorrhage, and (3) the risk of delayed absorption of hypotonic fluid from an intra-abdominal pool.

Although meticulous intake-output totals must be kept, urologists have learned that undue reliance cannot be placed upon these measurements. Hence serum Na^+ should be checked preoperatively, intraoperatively at each 500 ml of irrigant deficit and 4 hours postoperatively. A recent report from Scandinavia showed that glycine irrigation deficits of up to 500 ml led to a mean decrease in serum Na^+ of 2.5 mEq/liter, compared to an average decrease of 8 mEq/liter in patients whose deficit was >500 ml [86]. A fluid deficit of 500 ml requires a loop diuretic and careful maintenance of normovolemia, by exact replacement of urine output with intravenous saline (to counteract any tendency to inappropriate ADH secretion). Surgeons should think about finishing at a deficit of 1,000 ml and must definitely terminate at deficits of 1,500 ml. Even in the absence of a measured deficit, there may be wisdom in adopting the urologic dictum of limiting resection time in TURP to 1 hour.

Recovery and measurement of irrigant are both difficult tasks. An ingenious Swedish team added 1% ethanol to the irrigant fluid, and monitored absorption by end title breath alcohol analysis [186]. Hulton et al. [187] showed that as little as 100 ml of absorbed irrigant could be detected (Fig. 99). This is an inexpensive, easily performed and nontoxic method for real-time monitoring of fluid absorption, using an AlcoSensor III™ (Intoximeters, St. Louis, MO). This protocol deserves serious consideration by other institutions.

Treatment of hyponatremia. Optimal management hinges upon diagnosing hypo-osmolality before increased intracranial pressure can occur. Asymptomatic hyponatremia is a benign disorder that requires only water restriction, diuretic, and careful replacement of renal output with isotonic saline. Serum Na^+ must be monitored; any downward trend *mandates* hospital admission. Traditionally, urologists have also managed symptomatic HNE by water restriction, unless serum Na^+ fell below 120 mEq/liter. Although not the wisest of choices, this protocol persisted because men often show no ill effect from even severe hyponatremia (<110 mEq/liter). However, in symptomatic women of child-bearing age, delayed correction of even modest hypona-

tremia (120–132 mEq/liter) carries a risk of sudden, irreversible collapse. Hence, HNE in women mandates immediate ventilatory support and urgent transfer to an ICU.

Another fallacy of traditional management has been a misplaced concern that excessively rapid correction of chronic hyponatremia might lead to central pontine myelinolysis [188]. In reality, the real dangers of allowing a woman to remain in acute hyponatremia vastly exceed the mainly theoretical risk of inducing this hyper-osmotic demyelination syndrome. Among patients with symptomatic hyponatremia complicating endometrial ablation, many deaths have been reported among patients treated expectantly with water restriction and loop diuretics. Conversely, hypertonic sodium chloride has been safely used to dehydrate the edematous brain in >170 consecutive patients worldwide [189]. All patients treated with hypertonic (514 mM) sodium chloride survived. When hypertonic saline administration is needed, 250–500 ml (514 mM) of this solution is delivered through a constant infusion pump over 24–48 hours. Furosemide is generally given concomitantly to promote net free water diuresis, without depletion of urinary $Na+$ levels [190]. The endpoint is either a plasma sodium level of 130 mEq/liter or the disappearance of symptoms—whichever comes first. Under no circumstances should serum Na^+ concentration be corrected back to physiologically normal values.

ADVANCED OPERATIVE LAPAROSCOPY
Revolution in Gynecologic Surgery

Experimental laparoscopy began in 1901 [191,192] and became popular among internists of the 1930s and 1940s as a diagnostic technique for liver disease and tuberculosis [148]. Laparoscopy was first used to diagnose an ectopic pregnancy in 1937 [193] and was popularized as an effective method of female sterilization in 1967 [194]. Laparoscopic adaptation of the CO_2 laser was introduced by Bruhat [195] in 1979; fiberoptic delivery of argon energy was described 4 years later [196]. In the succeeding decade, intra-abdominal gynecologic surgery has undergone a veritable revolution. Modern-day experts routinely treat ectopic pregnancies, endometriosis, adnexal masses, and intraperitoneal adhesions. Laparoscopic transection of the infundibulopelvic vessels has initiated a new era of vaginal hysterectomy. Techniques for retroperitoneal dissection now permit laparoscopic Burch urethropexy for stress incontinence

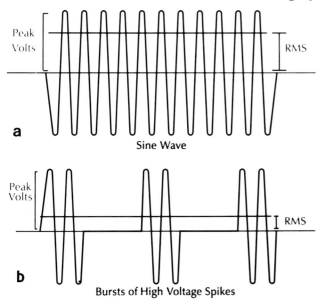

Fig. 100. Comparison of "cut" vs. "coag" wave forms. **a:** "Cut" represents a continuous wave of high current/low voltage electricity. **b:** "Coag" represents damped, high voltage/low current electricity.

and laparoscopic lymphadenectomy for gynecologic malignancy.

The advantages of treating significant intra-abdominal disease through the laparoscope, instead of by laparotomy, are dramatic. Postoperative recovery can be shortened from weeks to days, with correspondingly rapid return to work. The key requirement for minimally invasive surgery is the ability to perform facile, hemostatic dissection endoscopically. Of the multiple options that exist, thermal instruments have been used most extensively.

The laparoscopic use of monopolar electrosurgery dates to Raoul Palmer in the 1940s [197]. Monopolar (unipolar) electrosurgery requires modest capital outlay, is convenient to set up and use, and has the apparent advantage of familiarity. Even when the laparoscope is used as a means of tubal occlusion, rare but catastrophic intestinal burns occur. In 4,000 laparoscopies using unipolar electricity for tubal sterilization at the Johns Hopkins Hospital between 1969 and 1974, there were 12 intestinal burns [198]. None of these problems was attributable to a misapplication of the forceps to the surface of the intestine. Rather, the problem is now recognized to represent electrical capacitance.

In "electrically simple" environments, such as an open wound or within the uterine cavity, electrosurgery is very safe. However, within the "electrically complex" environment of the perito-

neal cavity, there is more to learn about electrosurgery than the laser. Unfortunately, errors are often lethal. Surgeons using monopolar current must be exquisitely sensitive to the possibility of inducing an electromagnetic field by passing a high voltage current through long, partly insulated trocars [199]. Operative laparoscopists must also have a clear understanding of the voltage and resistance relationship of the "cut" and "coagulate" settings (Fig. 100). The least risk of sparking or capacitance burns is about ×10 higher in the "coagulate" setting. Hence, most intraperiotenal monopolar electrosurgery is done with cutting current. By varying electrode size and shape, the surgeon can change tissue effects from incision to hemostasis. Specifically, by using the edge, a monopolar spoon electrode will incise cleanly and quickly; flipping it over onto its broad surface provides good electrodessication even though the instrument is left on full "cut" setting. If it is necessary to superficially fulgurate an oozing vascular bed, unipolar coagulation current can also be used. The broad side of the spoon electrode is held close to (but not in contact with) the intended target.

Comparison of Lasers and Electrosurgery

In response to deaths from monopolar electrical burns, several alternative energy sources were introduced. Semm [200] invented the endocoagulator, an electrical device in which current does not flow to tissue, but is distributed solely to the heating element of an endoscopic instrument (knife, probe, or forceps). Rioux and Cloutier [201] developed the bipolar forcep as a safer means for electrodessication of fallopian tubes, large vessels, or bleeding points. Even with bipolar coagulation, lateral thermal damage may spread for a surprising distance beyond the application site. The reason for this is that impedance between the two active electrodes increases as the target tissue is desiccated. Thus, in finding the path of least resistance, the current balloons laterally between the instrument jaws. Hence, when performing bipolar coagulation of the large vessels in the infundibular pelvic ligament, the Kleppinger forceps must be applied close to the mesovarium and the pedicle stretched medially in order to prevent thermal spread to the pelvic sidewall [202].

Partly to fill this void, lasers were adapted for endoscopic use. Comparing lasers and electrosurgery has two caveats. First, it is assumed that both are being used knowledgeably by informed users—after all, any surgical instrument can inflict serious injury in untrained hands. However, the likelihood of the laser getting out of control and perforating an adjacent structures is no greater than the risk associated with laparoscopic scissors or electrosurgery. Second, it must be emphasized that similarities exceed differences. Both are simply thermal instruments intended to extend the surgeon's "reach," thereby making it possible to replicate most laparotomy maneuvers through the endoscope. Success with either hinges principally upon laparoscopic skill, rather than upon the physical properties of thermal energy. Experts will secure comparable results with each method; beginners often fail with either one. In fact, accomplished surgeons often use several modalities during the same operation.

Because of their "high-tech" image, lasers have received much more attention than electrosurgery in terms of training and credentialing requirements for physicians. This distorted perspective has left many with the impression that lasers are more complex, more difficult to use, and more "dangerous"—especially because hospitals require no training or credentialing for the use of electrosurgery. In truth, there is more to learn about the correct and safe application of electrosurgery to laparoscopy. In contrast to the sharp margination of laser coagulation, thermal damage at electrosurgery follows the path of least resistance to current flow—a path is not always predicted by the laparoscopist. Considering the visual uncertainty of predicting immediate electrosurgical damage, the potential for stray current effect, the risk of unseen capacitance burns to the bowel, and the risk of "downstream" burns at sites of unintended high current density (faulty dispersive electrode, alternative pathway sites) the relative safety of the laser over monopolar electrosurgery is obvious.

Other arguments against the laser are equally specious. Proponents of electrosurgery have tended to emphasize the capital costs of the laser. However, most hospitals have already made this capital outlay. Operating costs for electricity and laser surgery are equivalent. In short, differences are largely artificial—the choice of instrument generally revolves upon individual preference of the surgeon.

In reality, neither electrosurgery nor the laser is absolutely required for skilled laparoscopy. However, both add a margin of safety, often under different circumstances. Lasers cannot rival the ability of electrosurgery to desiccate large vessels. The quintessential advantage of the laser over electrosurgery is the well-delineated, visually recognizable zone of damage surrounding the sites of incision or excavation. In contrast, it is very difficult to assess the extent of tissue damage produced by electricity. For example, an inadvertent intestinal perforation produced by stray laser energy can be safely managed by oversewing the defect. In contrast, anything more than a trivial burn to the intestinal wall requires segmental resection [203]. This property is an important consideration in delicate situations, such as uterosacral ligament transection. Contrary to prevailing misconception, the laser offers the greatest protection against thermal damage to the ureter or the adjacent vessels [204]. More patients have been injured with electrosurgical generators than by lasers. Thus it is likely that the pendulum of surgical opinion will one day swing back to the laser, not as the sole instrument for peritoneal dissection, but as a valuable tool within a varied armamentarium.

CONCLUSION

For certain selected purposes, lasers provide one of the safest and most versatile tools that a surgeon could ask for. Whether excising, ablating, or promoting hemostasis, the laser is of advantage only if the desired surgical objective can be achieved without concomitant secondary heat conduction. Over the last 15 years, misadventure arising from errors in energy configuration or surgical prudence has the largely theoretical risk of optical hazard, or injury to intended targets. Like all technological innovations, fulfilling the promise requires an understanding of the relevant physics, acquisition of new surgical skills to deliver this thermal energy, awareness of new sources of potential morbidity, and honing of medical judgment, particularly on the issue of when to revert to a more conventional approach.

REFERENCES

1. Trost D, Zacherl A, Smith MFW. Surgical laser properties and their tissue interaction. In: Smith MFW, McElveen JT, eds. "Neurological Surgery of the Ear." St. Louis, MO: Mosby-Yearbook, 1992, pp 131–162.
2. Lipow M. Laser physics made simple. Curr Prob Obstet Gyneco Infert 1986;9:441–493.
3. Polanyi TG. Laser physics: Medical applications. Ototlaryngol Clin North Am 1983;16:753.
4. Fuller TA. Physical considerations of surgical lasers. Obstet Gynecol Clin North Am 1991;18:391–405.
5. Daikuzono N, Joffe SN. Artificial sapphire probe for contact photocoagulation and tissue vaporization with the Nd:YAG laser. Med Instrum 1985;19:173–178.

6. Driscoll WG, Vaughan W. "Handbook of Optics." Optical Society of America. New York: McGraw Hill, 1978.

7. Joffe SN. The Neodynmium:YAG laser in general surgery. Contem Surg 1985;27:17.

8. Shirk GJ, Brumsted JR, Gimpelson RJ. Operative laparoscopy with the Nd:YAG laser in the treatment of endometriosis and pelvic adhesions. Lasers Surg Med 1991;11:297–300.

9. Absten GT. Physics of light and lasers. Obstet Gynecol Clin North Am 1991;18:407–427.

10. Wolbarsht ML, Esterowitz L, Tran D, et al. A mid-infrared (2.94 m) surgical laser with an optical fiber delivery system. Lasers Surg Med 1986;6:257.

11. Lele SB, Piver MS, Mang TS, et al. Photodynamic therapy in gynecologic malignancies. Gynecol Oncol 1989;34:350.

12. Walsh JT Jr., Flotte TJ, Anderson RR, Deutsch T. Pulsed CO_2 laser tissue ablation: Effect of tissue type and pulse duration on thermal damage. Lasers Surg Med 1988;8:108.

13. Perry CP, Daniell JF, Gimpelson RJ. Bowel injury from Nd:YAG endometrial ablation. J Gynecol Surg 1990;6:199–203.

14. Keye Wr Jr, Dixon J. Photocoagulation of endometriosis by the argon laser through the laparoscope. Obstet Gynecol 1983;62:383.

15. Keye WR Jr. KTP and argon laser laparoscopy. Obstet Gynecol Clinic North Am 1991;18:605–611.

16. Dorsey JH. Laser surgery for cervical intraepithelial neoplasia. Obstet Gynecol Clin North Am 1991;18:475–489.

17. Reid R, Greenberg MD, Daoud Y, et al. Colposcopic findings in women with vulvar pain syndromes: A preliminary report. J Reprod Med 1988;33:523–532.

18. Horowicz BJ. Interferon therapy for condylomatous vulvitis. Obstet Gynecol 1989;73:446.

19. Woodruff JD, Parmley TH. Infection of the minor vestibular gland. Obstet Gynecol 1983;62:609.

20. Reid R, Omoto KH, Precop SL, et al. Flashlamp excited dye laser of idiopathic vulvodynia is safe and efficacious. Am J Obstet Gynecol (in press).

21. McKay M. Vulvodynia: A multi-factorial clinical problem. Arch Dermatol 1989;125:256–262.

22. Tan OT, Carney M, Margolis R, et al. Histologic response of portwine stains treated by argon, carbon dioxide and tunable dye lasers: A preliminary report. Arch Dermatol 1986;122:1016–1022.

23. Garden J, Tan OT, Kerschmann R, et al. Effect of pulsewidth on vessel specific changes induced by a pulsed laser radiation. J Invest Dermatol 1986;87:653–657.

24. McDaniel DH, Mordon S. Hexascan: A new robotized scanning laser handpiece. Cutis 1990;45:300–305.

25. Karram MM. Urodynamics: Urethral Pressure Profilometry. In: Walters MD, Karram MM, eds. "Clinical Urogynecology." St. Louis, MO: Mosby, 1993, pp 89–101.

26. Reid R, Elson L, Absten GT. A practical guide to laser safety. Colposc Gynecol Laser Surg 1987;2:121–132.

27. Kamat BR, Carney JM, Ardnt KA, et al. Cutaneous tissue repair following CO_2 laser irradiation. J Invest Dermatol 1986;87:268.

28. Reid R, Greenberg MD, Daoud Y, et al. Superficial laser vulvectomy. IV. Extended laser vaporization and adjuvant 5-fluorouracil therapy of human papillomavirus associated vulvar disease. Obstet Gynecol 1990;76:439.

29. Reid R. Superficial laser vulvectomy. III. A new surgical technique for appendage-conserving ablation of refractory and very extensive condylomas. Am J Obstet Gynecol 1985;152:504–509.

30. Fuller TA. Laser tissue interaction: The influence of power density. In: Baggish M, ed. "Basic and Advanced Laser Surgery and Gynecology." New York: Appleton-Century, 1985.

31. Richart RM, Barron BA. A follow-up study of patients with cervical neoplasia. Obstet Gynecol 1969;105:386–393.

32. Coppleson M, Pixley E, Reid BL. Colposcopy—A Scientific Approach to the Cervix Uteri in Health and Disease, 3rd ed. Springfield, IL: Charles C. Thomas, 1986.

33. Munoz N, Bosch FX, Shah KV, Meheus A. "The Epidemiology of HPV and Cervical Cancer." International Agency for Research on Cancer. New York: Oxford University Press, 1992.

34. Schiffman MH, Bauer HM, Hoover RN, et al. Epidemiologic evidence showing that Human Papillomavirus infection causes most cervical intraepithelial neoplasia. JNCI 1993;85.

35. Koutsky LA, Galloway DA, Holmes KK. Epidemiology of genital human papillomavirus infection. Epidemiol Rev 1988;10:122–163.

36. Stoler MH, Rhodes CR, Whitbeck A, et al. Gene expression of HPV types 16 and 18 in cervical neoplasia. UCLA Symp Mol Cell Biol New Ser 1990;124:1–11.

37. Werness BA, Levine AJ, Howley PM. Association of human papillomavirus types 16 and 18 E6 proteins with p53. Science 1990;248:76.

38. Barbosa MS, Shlegel R. The E6 and E7 genes of HPV 18 are sufficient for inducing two stage in-vitro transformation of human keratinocytes. Onocogene 1990;43:1529–1532.

39. Woodworth CD, Doniger J, DiPaolo JA. Immortalization of human foreskin keratinocytes by various human papillomavirus DNAs corresponds to their association with cervical carcinoma. J Virol 1989;63:159–164.

40. McCance DJ, Kopan RI, Fuchs E, Laimans LA. Human papillomavirus type 16 alters human epithelial cell differentiation in vitro. Proc Natl Acad Aci USA 1988;85:7169–7173.

41. Hurlin PJ, Kauer R, Snit PP, et al. Progression of human papillomavirus type 18 immortalized human keratinocytes to malignant phenotype. J Proc Natl Acad Sci USA 1991;88:570–574.

42. Fuchs PG, Girardi F, Pfister H. Human Papillomavirus DNA in normal, metaplastic, preneoplastic and neoplastic epithelium of the cervix uteri. Int J Cancer 1988;41:41.

43. Reid R, Lorincz AT. Should Family Physicians test for human papillomavirus infection? An affirmative view. Am J Fam Pract 1991;32:183–188.

44. Campion MJ, McCance DJ, Cuszick J, Singer A. Progressive potential of mild cervical atypia: Prospective cytologic and virologic study. Lancet 1986;ii:237–240.

45. Koutsky LA, Holmes KK, Critchlow CW, et al. A cohort study of the risk of cervical intraepithelial neoplasia grade 2 or 3 in relation to papillomavirus infection. N Engl J Med 1992;327:1272–1278.

46. Weaver MG, Abdul-Karim FW, Dale G, et al. Outcome in mild and moderate cervical dysplasias related to the

presence of specific human papillomavirus types. Modern Pathol 1993;50:3709–3715.

47. Schelgel R. Papillomavirus in human cancer. Semin Virol 1990;1:297–306.

48. Cullen AP, Reid R, Campion MJ, Lorincz AT. An analysis of the physical state of different human papillomavirus DNAs in preinvasive and invasive cervical neoplasia. J Virol 1991;65:606–612.

49. Hensen D, Tarone R. An epidemiologic study of the cervix, vagina and vulva based on the Third National Cancer Survey in the United States. Am J Obstet Gynecol 1977;129:525.

50. Becker TM, Stone KM, Alexander ER. Genital human papillomavirus infection: A growing concern. Obstet Gynecol Clin North Am 1987;14:389–396.

51. Miller AB. Control of carcinoma of the cervix by exfoliative cytology screening. In: Coppleson M, ed. "Gynecologic Oncology," 2nd ed. London: Churchill Livingstone, 1992 pp. 543–555.

52. Coppleson M. Management of preclinical carcinoma of the cervix. In: Jordan JA and Singer A (eds) The Cervix Uteri. London, WB Saunders, 1976 pp. 453–474.

53. Kolstad P. Carcinoma of the cervix. Stage Ia. Diagnosis and treatment. Am J Obstet Gynecol 1969;104:1015.

54. Reid R. Preinvasive disease. In: Berek JS and Hatcher NF, eds. "Practical Gynecologic Oncology." Baltimore: Williams & Wilkins, 1994, pp 201–244.

55. Townsend DE, Richart RM. Diagnostic errors in colposcopy. Gynecol Oncol 1981;12:s259.

56. Webb MJ. Invasive cancer following conservative therapy for previous cervical intraepithelial neoplasia. Colpo Gynecol Laser Surg 1984;1:245.

57. McIndoe GAJ, Robson MS, Tidy JA, Mason WP, Anderson MC. Laser excision rather than vaporization: The treatment of choice for cervical intraepithelial neoplasia. Obstet Gynecol 1989;74:165–168.

58. Personal communication to Attila Lorincz from Keerti Shah, from an unpublished in situ study conducted in 1989 of CIN 3 lesions from New Zealand.

59. McIndoe WA, McLean MA, Jones RW, et al. The invasive potential of carcinoma in situ of the cervix. Obstet Gynecol 1984;64:451.

60. Montz F. Natural history of the minimally abnormal Pap smear. Obstet Gynecol 1992;80:385–388.

61. Fox CH. Biological behavior of cervical dysplasia and carcinoma-in-situ. Am J Obstet Gynecol 1967;99:960–974.

62. Richart RM, Barron BA. A follow up study of patients with cervical neoplasia. Obstet Gynecol 1969;386–393.

63. Evans AS, Monaghan JM. Spontaneous resolution of cervical warty dysplasia. The relevance of clinical and nuclear DNA features: A prospective study. Br J Obstet Gynecol 1985;92:165–169.

64. Koss LG, Stewart FW, Foote FW, et al. Some histological aspects of behavior of epidermoid carcinoma-in-situ and related lesions of the uterine cervix. Cancer 1963;16:1160–1211.

65. 1988 Bethesda system for reporting cervical/vaginal cytologic diagnoses. JAMA 1989;262:931–934.

66. Bethesda System for Reporting Cervical/Vaginal Cytologic Diagnoses. ACTA Cytol 1993;37:115–124.

67. Phipps JM, Gunasekera AC, Lewis BV. Occult cervical carcinoma revealed by large loop diathermy. Lancet 1989;ii:453.

68. Howe DT, Vincenti AC. Is large loop excision of the transformation zone (LLETZ) more accurate than colposcopically directed punch biopsy in the diagnosis of cervical intraepithelial neoplasia? Br J Obstet Gynecol 1991;98:588.

69. Pixley E. Morphology of the fetal and prepubertal cervicovaginal epithelium. In: Jordan JA and Singer A, eds. "The Cervix." Philadelphia: W.B. Saunders, 1976.

70. Reid R. The Treatment of HPV infection and intraepithelial neoplasia in females. Curr Probl Obstet Gynecol Fertil 1989;12:145–56.

71. Luesley D, McCrum A, Terry PB, Wade-Evans T. Complications of cone biopsy related to the dimensions of the cone and the influence of prior colposcopic assessment. Br J Obstet Gynecol 1985;92:158.

72. Jordan JA. Symposium on cervical neoplasia. I. Excisional methods. Colpo Gynecol Laser Surg 1984;1:271.

73. Dorsey JH, Diggs ES. Microsurgical conization of the cervix by carbon dioxide laser. Obstet Gynecol 1979;54:565.

74. Wright C, Davies E, Riopelle MA. Laser surgery for cervical intraepithelial neoplasia: Principles and results. Am J Obstet Gynecol 1983;145:181.

75. Indman PD. Conization of the cervix with CO_2 laser as an office procedure. J Repro Med 1985;30:388.

76. Reid R. Physical and surgical principles governing expertise with the carbon dioxide laser. Obstet Gynecol Clin North Am 1987;14:513.

77. Reid R. Symposium on cervical neoplasia. V. Carbon dioxide laser ablation. Colpo Gynecol Laser Surg 1984;1:291.

78. Reid R, Atkinson K, Chanen W, et al. Symposium on cervical neoplasia. VI. Differing views. Colpo Gynecol Laser Surg 1984;1:299.

79. Stanhope CR, Phibbs GD, Stewart GC, Reid R. Carbon dioxide laser surgery. Obstet Gynecol 1983;61:624.

80. Koss L. Carcinoma of Cervix Uteri. In: Koss L, ed. "Diagnostic Cytology." Pennsylvania: Lippencott, 1968, pp 170–236.

81. Jones DED, Creaseman WT, Dombroski RA, et al. Evaluation of the atypical pap smear. Am J Obstet Gynecol 1987;157:544–549.

82. Graham JB, Meigs JV. Recurrence of tumor after total hysterectomy for carcinoma in situ. Am J Obstet Gynecol 1952;64:1159.

83. Lee RA, Symmonds RE. Recurrent carcinoma in situ in the vagina in patients previously treated for in situ carcinoma of the cervix. Obstet Gynecol 1975;48:61.

84. Reid R, Campion MJ. The biology and significance of human papillomavirus infections in the genital tract. Yale J Biol Med 1988;61:307.

85. Buscema J, Woodruff JD, Parmley T, Genardry R. Carcinoma in situ of the vulva. Obstet Gynecol 1980;55:225.

86. Crum CP, Burkett BJ. Papillomavirus and Vulvovaginal Neoplasia. J Repro Med 1989;34s:566–571.

87. Wilkinson EJ, Friedrich EG jr. Diseases of the Vulva. In: Kurman RJ, ed. "Blaustein's Pathology of the Female Genital Tract." New York: Springer-Verlag, 1987.

88. McConell EM. Squamous carcinoma of the anus: A review of 96 cases. Br J Surg 1973;57:89.

89. McCance DJ, Clarkson PK, Dyson JL, et al. Human papillomavirus types 6 and 16 in multifocal intraepithelial neoplasia of the female lower genital tract. Br J Obstet Gynecol 1987;82:1101.

90. Daling JR, Weiss NS, Klopfenstein LL, et al. Correlates of homosexual behavior and the incidence of anal cancer. JAMA 1982;247:1988.

91. Frazer IH, Medley G, Crapper RM, et al. Association between anorectal dysplasia, human papillomavirus and human immunodeficiency virus in homosexual men. Lancet 1986;ii:657.

92. Campion MJ. Natural history and clinical manifestations of HPV infection. Obstet Gynecol 1988;14:363–388.

93. Reid R, Greenberg M, Jenson AB, et al. Sexually transmitted papillomaviral infections: I. the anatomic distribution and pathologic grade of neoplastic lesions associated with different viral types. Am J Obstet Gynecol 1987;156:212–222.

94. Lorincz AT, Reid R, Jensen AB, et al. Human Papillomavirus Infection of the Cervix: Relative Risk Association of 15 Common Anogenital Types. Obstet Gynecol 1992;79:328–337.

95. Jochmus I, Durst M, Reid R. Major histocompatibility complex (MHC) and HPV 16 E7 expression in high grade vulvar lesions. Hum Pathol 1993;24:519–524.

96. Reid R, Pizzuti DR, Daoud Y, et al. Superficial laser vulvectomy: VI. Host and viral factors influencing therapeutic outcome for human papillomavirus-associated disease (in prep.).

97. Riva JM, Sedlacek TV, Cunnane MF, Mangan CE. Extended carbon dioxide laser vaporization in the treatment of subclinical papillomavirus infection of the lower genital tract. Obstet Gynecol 1989;73:25.

98. Culp OS and Kaplan IW. Condyloma acuminata: 200 cases treated with podophyllin. An Surg 1944;120:251.

99. Hellberg D. The female patient—clinical diagnosis and treatment. Proc Int Sym 17th World Congress Dermatol. Berlin, May 1987.

100. Simmons PD. Podophyllin 10% and 25% in the treatment of anogenital warts. Br J Vener Dis 1981;57:208.

101. Schwartz DB, Greenberg MD, Daoud Y, Reid R. The management of genital condylomas in pregnant women. Obstet Gynecol Clin North Am 1987;14:589–599.

102. von Krogh G. Condyloma acuminata: An updated review. Semin Dermatol 1982;2:109.

103. Reid R. Laser therapy of human papillomavirus infections. In: Keye WR Jr, ed. "Laser Surgery in Gynecology and Obstetrics." Chicago: Yearbook, 1989.

104. Ferenczy A, Mitao M, Nagai N, Silverstein SJ, Crum CP. Latent papillomavirus and recurring genital warts. NEJM 1985;313:784–788.

105. Jensen AB, Kurman RJ, Lancaster WD. Tissue effects of and host response to human papillomavirus infection. Obstet Gynecol Clin North Am 1987;14:397–406.

106. Reid R, Elfont EA, Zirkin RM, Fuller TA. Superficial laser vulvectomy. II. The anatomic and biophysical principles permitting accurate control of the depth of dermal destruction with the carbon dioxide laser. Am J Obstet Gynecol 1985;151:261–271.

107. Reid R. Superficial laser vulvectomy. I. The efficacy of extended superficial laser ablation for refractory and very extensive condylomas. Am J Obstet Gynecol 1985;151:1047–1052.

108. Sillman FH, Sedlis A, Boyce JG. A review of lower genital intraepithelial neoplasia and the use of topical 5-fluorouracil. Obstet Gynecol Survey 1985;40:190.

109. Sillman FH and Sedlis A. Anogenital papillomavirus infection and neoplasia in immunodeficient women. Obstet Gynecol Clin North Am 1987;14:537–558.

110. Krebs HB. Prophylactic topical 5 fluorouracil following treatment of human papillomavirus associated lesions of the vulva and vagina. Obstet Gynecol 1986;68:837.

111. Trofatter KF. Interferon. Obstet Gynecol Clin North Am 1988;14:569–579.

112. Gall SA, Hughes CE, Mounts P, et al. Efficacy of human lymphoblastoid interferon in the therapy of resistant condyloma acuminata. Obstet Gynecol 1986;67:643.

113. Kirby P, Kiviat N, Beckman A, et al. Tolerance and efficacy of recombinant human interferon gamma in the treatment of refractory genital warts. Am J Med 1988;85:183.

114. Reichman RG, Micha J, Bonnez W, et al. A multicenter study of interferon alfa-nl (Wellferon) treatment for refractory condyloma acuminatum. [Abstract 96]. Proc 25th Interscience Conference on Antimicrobial Agents and Chemotherapy, September 29–October 2, 1985, p 106.

115. Eron LJ, Judson D, Tucker J, et al. Interferon therapy for condyloma acuminata. NEJM 1986;315:1059.

116. Friedman-Kien AE, Eron LJ, Conant M, et al. Natural interferon alpha for transmission of condyloma acuminata. JAMA 1988;259:533.

117. Jones RW, McLean MR. Carcinoma in situ of the vulva: A review of 31 treated and five untreated cases. Obstet Gynecol 1986;68:499–503.

118. Dorsey JH, Baggish MS. Multifocal vaginal intraepithelial neoplasia with uterus in situ. In: Sharp F, Jordan JA, eds. "Gynaecological Laser Surgery." Proceedings of the 15th Study Group of the Royal College of Obstetricians and Gynaecologists. Ithaca, NY: Perinatology Press, 1985.

119. Campion MJ, Singer A. Vulvar intraepithelial neoplasia: A clinical review. Genitourin Med 1987;63:147–152.

120. Chafee W, Ferguson K, Wilkinson EJ. Vulvar intraepithelial neoplasia (VIN): Principles of surgical therapy. Colpo Gynecol Laser Surg 1988;4:125.

121. Friedrich EG, Wilkinson EF, Fu YS. Carcinoma in situ of the vulva: a continuing challenge. Am J Obstet Gynecol 1980;136:880.

122. DiSaia PJ. Management of superficially invasive vulvar carcinoma. Clin Obstet Gynecol 1985;28:196.

123. Hacker NF. Vulvar cancer. In: Berek JS, Hacker NF, eds. "Practical Gynecologic Oncology," 2nd ed. Baltimore: Williams & Wilkins, 1994, pp 403–440.

124. Knapstein PG. Principles of reconstructive surgery. In: Knapstein PG, Friedberg V, Sevin B-U, eds. "Reconstructive Surgery in Gynecology." Stuttgart. Thieme, 1990, pp 1–10.

125. Hoskins WJ, Park RC, Long R, Artman LE, McMahon EB. Repair of urinary tract fistulas with bulbocavernous myocutaneous flaps. Obstet Gynecol 1984;63:588.

126. Daniel RK, Kerrigan CL. Principles and physiology of skin flap surgery. In: McCarthy JG, ed. "Plastic Surgery." Philadelphia: W.B. Saunders, 1990.

127. Barnhill DR, Hoskins WJ, Metz P. Use of the rhomboid flap after partial vulvectomy. Obstet Gynecol 1983;62:444.

128. Jervis W, Salyer KE, Vargas-Busquests MA, Atkins RW. Further applications of the Limberg and Dufourmentel flaps. Plast Reconstr Surg 1974;54:335.

129. Lister GD, Gibson T. Closure of rhomboid skin defects:

The flaps of Limberg and Dufourmentel. Br J Plast Surg 1972;25:300.

130. Wee JT, Joseph VT. A new technique of vaginal reconstruction using neurovascular pudenal-thigh flaps: A preliminary report. Plastic Reconstruct Surg 1989;83: 701–709.

131. Reid R, Dorsey JH. Physical and surgical principles of carbon dioxide laser surgery in the lower genital tract. In: Coppleson M, Monaghan JM, Morrow CP, Tattersall MHN, eds. Gynecologic Oncology, 2nd ed. London: Churchill Livingstone, 1992, pp 1087–1132.

132. Reid R. Laser surgery of the vulvar. In: Dorsey JH, ed. "Physical and Surgical Principles of Laser Surgery in the Lower Genital Tract." Obstet Gynecol Clin North Am 1991;18:491–510.

133. Graham JB, Meigs JV. Recurrence of tumor after total hysterectomy. 1952;64:1159.

134. Dorsey JH. Skin appendage involvement and vulval intraepithelial neoplasia. In: Sharp F, Jordan JA, eds. "Gynaelogic Laser Surgery." Ithaca, NY: Perinatology Press, 1986, p 193.

135. Stuart GC, Flagler EA, Nation JG, et al. Laser vaporization of vaginal intraepithelial neoplasia. Am J Obstet Gynecol 1988;15:240.

136. Soutter WP. The treatment of vaginal intraepithelial neoplasia after hysterectomy. Br J Obstet Gynecol 1988;95:961.

137. Woodman C, Jordan JA, Wade-Evans T. The management of vaginal intrepithelial neoplasia after hysterectomy. Br J Obstet Gynecol 1984;91:707.

138. Woodman C, Mould JJ, Jordan JA. Radiotherapy in the management of vaginal intraepithelial neoplasia after hysterectomy. J Obstet Gynaecol 1988;95(10):976.

139. Evans TN, Poland ML. Vaginal malformations. Am J Obstet Gynecol 1982;59(4):435–444.

140. Dorsey JH, Baker CH. Credentialing of the gynecologic laser surgeon. Colpos Gynecol Laser Surg 1984;1:179.

141. Krebs HB. The use of topical 5-Flourouracil in the treatment of genital condylomas. Obstet Gynecol Clinic North Am 1987;14:559–568.

142. Jordan JA, Sharp F. CO_2 laser treatment of vaginal intrepithelial neoplasia. In: Sharp F, Jordan JA, eds. "Gynaecological Laser Surgery." New York: Appleton, 1985, pp 181–188.

143. Nezhat CR, Nezhat FR, Silfen SL. Videolaseroscopy. The CO_2 laser for advanced operative laparoscopy. Obstet Gynecol Clin North Am 1991;18:585.

144. Semm K. Course of endoscopic abdominal surgery. In: Semm K, Friedrich ER, eds. Operative Manual of Endoscopic Abdominal Surgery. Chicago: Year Book, 1987, p 130.

145. Dorsey JH. Indications and general techniques for lasers in advanced operative laparoscopy. Obstet Gynecol Clin North Am 1991;18:555.

146. Reich H. Laparoscopic treatment of extensive pelvic adhesions, including hydrosalpinx. J Repro Med 1987;32: 754.

147. Adamson GD, Lu J, Suback LL. Laparoscopic CO_2 laser vaporization of endometriosis compared with traditional treatments. Fertil Steril 1988;50:704.

148. Gordon A. The history and development of endoscopic surgery. In: Sutton C, Diamond M, eds. "Endoscopic surgery for Gynaecologists." London: Saunders, 1993, pp 3–7.

149. Goldrath MH, Sherman AI. Office hysteroscopy and suction curretage: Can we eliminate the hospital diagnostic dilatation and curettage? Am J Obstet Gynecol 1985; 152:220.

150. Neuwirth RS, Amin JH. Excision of submucous fibroids with hysteroscopic control. Am J Obstet Gynecol 1976; 126:95–99.

151. Goldrath MH, Fuller TA, Segal S. Laser photovaporization of endometrium for the treatment of menorrhagia. Am J Obstet Gynecol 1981;140:14–19.

152. DeCherney AH, Polan ML. Hysteroscopic management of intrauterine lesions and intractable uterine bleeding. Obstet Gynecol 1983;70:668–670.

153. DeCherney AH, Diamond MP, Lavy G, Polan ML. Endometrial ablation for intractable uterine bleeding: Hysteroscopic resection. Obstet Gynecol 1987;77:591–594.

154. Townsend DE, Richart RM, Paskowitz RA, Woolfork RE. "Rollerball" coagulation of the endometrium. Obstet Gynecol 1987;679:679–682.

155. Selwood TS, Wood EC. Incidence of hysterectomy in Australia. Med J Aust 1978;2:201–204.

156. Easterday CL, Grimes DA, Riggs JA. Hysterectomy in the United States. Obstet Gynecol 1983;62:203.

157. Chimbira TH, Anderson ABM, Turnbull AC. Relation between measured menstural blood loss and patient's subjective assessment of loss, duration of bleeding, number of sanitary towels used, uterine weight and endometrial surface area. Br J Obstet Gynaecol 1980;87:603–609.

158. Grant JM, Hussein IY. An audit of abdominal hysterectomy over a decade in a district hospital. Br J Obstet Gynecol 1984;91:73–77.

159. Dicker RC, Greenspan JR, Strauss JT, et al. Complications of abdominal and vaginal hysterectomy among women of reproductive age in the United States. Am J Obstet Gynecol 1982;144:841–848.

160. Wingo PA, Huezo CM, Rubin GL, et al. The mortality risk associated with hysterectomy. Am J Obstet Gynecol 1985;152:803–808.

161. Asherman JG. Amenorrhea traumatica. J Obstet Gynecol Br Emp 1948;55:23.

162. Baggish MS, Daniell JF. Catastrophic injury secondary to the use to coaxial gas-cooled fibres and artificial sapphire tips for intrauterine surgery. Lasers Surg Med 1989;9:581–584.

163. Wood SM, Roberts FL. Air embolism during transcervical resection of endometrium. Br Med J 1990;300:945.

164. Baggish MS, Brill AI, Rosenweig B, Barbot JE, Indman PD. Fatal acute glycine and sorbitol toxicity during operative hysteroscopy. J Gynecol Surg 1993;9:137–143.

165. Arieff AI, Ayus JC. Endometrial ablation complicated by fatal hypoantremic encephalopathy. JAMA 1993; 270:1230–1232.

166. Fleischer AC, Dudley BS, Entman SS, et al. Myometrial invasion by endometrial carcinoma: sonographic assessment. Radiology 1987;162:307–310.

167. Brumstead JR, Shirk G, Soderline MJ, Reed T. Attempted transcervical occlusion of the fallopian tube with the Nd:YAG laser. Obstet Gynecol 1991;77:327–328.

168. Darabi KF, Richart RM. Collaborative study on hysteroscopic sterilization procedures. A preliminary report. In: Sciarra JJ, Zatacuni GI, Spiedel JJ, eds. "Risks, Ben-

efits and Controversies in Fertility Control." Hagerstown, N.J.: Harper & Row, 1978, 1149–53.

169. Maher PJ, Hill DJ. Transcervical endometrial resection for abnormal uterine bleeding—report of 100 cases and review of the literature. Aust New Zealand J Obstet Gynecol 1990;30:357–360.

170. Whitelaw N, Sutton C. Nine years experience of endoscopic surgery in a District General Hosptial. In: Sutton CJG, ed. "New Surgical Techniques in Gynaecology." Carnforth, Lancs: Parthenon, 1993.

171. Loffer FD. Hysteroscopic endometrial ablation with the Nd:YAG laser using a non-touch technique. Obstet Gynecol 1987;69:679.

172. Witz CA, Silverberg KM, Burns WN, et al. Complications associated with the absorption of hysteroscopic fluid media. Fert Steril 1993;60:745.

173. Ahmed N, Falcone T, Tulandi T, Houle G. Anaphylactic reaction because of intrauterine 32% dextran-70 instillation. Fertil Steril 1991;55-1014–1016.

174. Trimbos-Kemper TCM, Veering BT. Anaphylactic shock for intracavity 32% dextran-70 during hysteroscopy. Fertil Steril 1989;1053–1054.

175. Jedeikin R, Olsfanger D, Kessler I. Disseminated intravascular coagulopathy and adult respiratory distress syndrome: Life threatening complications. Am J Obstet Gynecol 1990;162:44–45.

176. Mangar D, Gerson JI, Constantine RM, Lenzi V. Pulmonary edema and coagulopathy due to Hyskon (32% dextran-70) administration. Anesth Analg 1989;68:686–687.

177. Arieff AI. Hypoantremia, convulsions, respiratory arrest and permanent brain damage after elective surgery in healthy women. NEJM 1986;314:1529–1535.

178. Creevy CD. Hemolytic reactions during transurethral prostatic resection. J Urol 1947;58:125–131.

179. Roos NP, Wennberg JE, Malenka DJ, et al. Mortality and reoperation after open and transurethral resection of the prostate for benign prostatic hyperplasia. NEJM 1989;320:1120–1124.

180. Anderson RJ, Chung HM, Kluge R, Schrier RW. Hypoatremia: A prospective analysis of its epidemiology and the pathogenic role of vasopressin. Ann Intern Med 1985;102:164–168.

181. Chung HM, Kluge R, Schrier RW, Anderson RJ. Postoperative hyponatremia: A prospective study. Arch Intern Med 1986;146:333–336.

182. Logie JRC, Keenan RA, Whiting PH, Steyn JH. Fluid absorption during transurethral prostatectomy. Br J Urol 1980;52:526–528.

183. Witz CA, Silverberg KM, Burns WN, et al. Complications associated with the absorption of hysteroscopic fluid media. Fertil Steril 1993;60:745.

184. Ayus JC, Wheeler JM, Arieff AI. Postoperative hyponatremic encephalopathy in menstruant women. An Int Med 1992;117:891–897.

185. McLucas B. Intrauterine applications of the resectoscope. Surg Gynecol Obstet 1991;172:425.

186. Istre O, Skajaa K, Schjoensby AP, Forman A. Changes in serum electroctyes after transcervical resection of endometrium and submucous fibroids with use of glycine 1.5% for uterine irrigation. Obstet Gynecol 1992; :218–222.

187. Hultén J, Sarma VJ, Hjertberg H, Palmquist B. Monitoring of irrigating fluid absorption during transurethral prostatectomy. Anesthesia 1991;46:349–353.

188. Norenberg MD, Leslie KO, Robertson AS. Association between rise in serum sodium and central pontine myelinolysis. Ann Neurol 1982;11:128–135.

189. Lyon RP, Mangar D, O'Connor TM, Corson SL, Morgenthaler A, Arieff AI, Ayus JC, Seidman DS. Letters to the editor: Hyponatremic encephalopathy after endometrial ablation. JAMA 1994;271:343–345.

190. Arieff AI. Management of hyponatremia. BMJ 1993; 307:305–308.

191. Kelling G. Uber Oesophagokopie, Gastrokopie and Koelioskopie. Munchner Medizinische Wochenschrift 1902; 49:22–24.

192. von Ott DO. Ventroscopic illumination of the abdominal cavity in pregnancy. Zhurnal Akrestierstova I Zhenskikh Boloznei 1901;15:7–8.

193. Hope R. The differential diagnosis of ectopic pregnancy by peritoneoscopy. Surg Gynecol Obstet 1937;64:229–234.

194. Steptoe PC. "Laparoscopy in Gynaecology." London: Livingstone, 1967.

195. Bruhat MA, Mage G, Manhes H. Use of CO^2 laser by laparoscopy. In: Kaplan I., ed. "Laser Surgery III." Proceedings of the Third International Congress on Laser Surgery. Tel Aviv: Jerusalem Press, 1979, p 225.

196. Keye WR, Dixon J. Photocoagulation of endometriosis by the argon laser through the laparoscope. Obstet Gynecol 1983;62:383–386.

197. Palmer R. La coelioscopie. Bruxelles-medical 1948;28: 305–312.

198. Wheeless CR Jr, Thompson BH. Laparoscopic sterilization: Review of 3,600 cases. Obstet Gynecol 1973;42:751.

199. Soderstrom RM. Basic Operative Technique. In: Soderstrom RM, ed. "Operative Laparoscopy: The Masters Techniques." New York: Raven Press, 1993, p 25.

200. Semm K. Instruments and equipment for endoscopic abdominal surgery. In: "Operative Manual for Endoscopic Surgery." Chicago: Year Book, 1987, p 46.

201. Rioux JE, Cloutier D. Basic principles of electrosurgery. Laparoscopy 1977;4:24.

202. Dorsey JH. The role of lasers in advanced operative laparoscopy. Obstet Gynecol Clinic North Am 1991;18: 545–553.

203. Thompson BH, Wheeless CR Jr. Gastrointestinal complications of laparoscopy sterlization. Obstet Gynecol 1975;41:669.

204. Osher SS. The argon laser in gynecologic operative laparoscopy. In: Soderstrom RM, ed. "Operative Laparoscopy: The Masters Techniques." New York: Raven Press, 1993, p 73.

205. Leutcher RS, Townsend DE, Hacker NF, et al. Treatment of vulvar carcinoma in situ with CO_2 laser. Gynecol Oncol 1984;19:314–322.

206. Townsend DE, Levine RV, Richart RM, et al. Management of vulvar intrapethial neoplasma by carbondioxide laser. Obstet Gynecol 1982;60:49–52.

207. Reid R. Physical and surgical principles governing carbon dioxide laser surgery on the skin. Dermatol Clin 1991;9:2.

208. Reid R. Lasers in gynecology. In: Dorsey JH, ed. "Physical and Surgical Principles of Laser Surgery in the Lower Genital Tract." Obstet Gynecol Clinic North Am 1991;18:429–474.

Chapter 6

Low Intensity Laser Therapy: Still Not an Established Clinical Tool

Jeffrey R. Basford, MD, PhD

Department of Physical Medicine and Rehabilitation, Mayo Clinic and Foundation, Rochester, Minnesota

INTRODUCTION

The basic tenet of laser therapy is that laser radiation (and perhaps monochromatic light) has a wavelength-dependent capability to alter cellular behavior in the absence of significant heating. Accelerated wound healing and hair growth were among the first effects reported, and early investigators believed that laser radiation "stimulated" biological processes. As a result, the phenomenon was initially termed "biostimulation." However, as it was found that low intensity radiation could inhibit as well as stimulate cellular activity, terminology changed. Today, the term "biostimulation" has been replaced with an array of nearly interchangeable descriptive phrases such as low intensity, low level, and low power, which emphasize the nonthermal, low energy characteristics of the approach. In practice, laser therapy typically involves the delivery of ≤ 1–4 J/cm^2 to treatment sites with lasers having output powers between 10 mW and 90 mW.

Whatever the terminology, clinical use and research in low energy lasers today owe much of their popularity to work begun in Hungary and the Eastern Bloc countries in the mid-1960s [1, 2]. Today, laser therapy is used worldwide to treat musculoskeletal injury, pain, and inflammation. Despite surveys showing routine use in >40% of physical therapy clinics in Great Britain and perhaps 30% of dental clinics in Scandinavia [3], acceptance in the United States is minimal and Food and Drug Administration (FDA) approval has not been granted for any indication.

The earliest laser therapy reports were enthusiastic and anecdotal, but contained no clear mechanism of action. In addition, their appearance, typically, in obscure (at least to the American reader) foreign language journals contributed to a general skepticism and lack of knowledge in the United States. Nevertheless, although laser therapy remains on the fringes of U.S. medicine, interest has increased here as well as abroad. Over the years, the early reports have been vastly expanded with new clinical and laboratory work.

There are two major areas of laser therapy research: the laboratory and the clinic. The laboratory presents the least ambiguous results.

TABLE 1. Cellular Function Altered by Low Energy Laser Irradiation

Cell Process	Effect	
Protein synthesis[4–7]	⇑	⇓
Cell growth and differenation[8–13]	⇑	⇓
Cell motility[14–16]	⇑	
Membrane potential and binding affinities[17–19]	⇑	
Neurotransmitter release[20]	⇑	
Phagocytosis[21,22]	⇑	
ATP syntheses[17]	⇑	
Prostaglandin synthesis[6]	⇑	

Here, although unsupported results do appear, the vast majority of published work finds clear evidence that laser irradiation alters animal and bacterial cellular processes in a nonthermal, wavelength-dependent manner (Table 1). The mechanism of this interaction is not established. However, mitochondrial respiratory chain components exhibit frequency-dependent action spectra, and many feel that the respiratory chain is at the base of any effects that laser therapy might have [8, 23]. Extension of this subcellular mechanism to the clinic is tenuous at best and is not pursued in this review.

The value of low intensity laser irradiation in the clinic is more arguable and is the focus of this review. Although most of the focus here is on reviewing clinical work, the laboratory findings outlined in Table 1 should not be ignored. They provide the scientific rationale of laser therapy and give an impression of the breadth of influences that laser irradiation can have on cellular processes.

Early laser therapy clinical work was usually anecdotal, unblinded, poorly controlled, and incompletely reported. Standards have improved markedly over the last decade. Current work remains more variable than might be desired, but it is almost uniformly better designed, better controlled, and more carefully blinded. As a result, this more recent work can be more effectively evaluated and this review restricts itself to the controlled and blinded studies of this last period. Studies indexed in the major medical indices may be overrepresented, but there have been attempts to review controlled and blinded work in nonindexed journals.

BACKGROUND

It is important to remember that medical treatment involving light and electromagnetic energy has roots extending back into antiquity. Thus, whereas it seems counterintuitive that laser irradiation, or for that matter light from any source, can have biological effects, the concept is not new. The Greeks, for example, believed that sunlight strengthened and healed. Later in the Middle Ages, sunlight was used to combat the plague, and by the late nineteenth century UV radiation was utilized to treat cutaneous tuberculosis (scrofula) [24]. Today, light, and electromagnetic energy in general, continue to have both new and established uses [25]. Light is used for the treatment of psoriasis, hyperbilirubinemia, and seasonal affective disorder (SAD). Electromagnetic energy is used for shortwave diathermy and stimulation of fracture healing [25]. With this in mind, the belief that electromagnetic fields, and laser radiation in particular, can alter biological processes seems neither farfetched nor surprising.

Laser therapy thus may be thought of as reestablishing light to a place of prominence in the physical therapy clinic with existing electromagnetic agents such as radio-frequency diathermy and infrared (IR) heat sources. This idea is correct, but it should be remembered that their uses are different. The radiofrequency and IR agents deliver as much as hundreds of watts to the patient and gain their effects by grossly heating tissue by as much as 5°C. The lasers used in laser therapy, however, have output powers, orders of magnitude smaller and associated temperature elevations ≤0.5–.75°C [5, 20, 26, 27]. These latter temperature changes are usually imperceptible and are far too low and localized to produce significant physiological effects.

Laser therapy has utilized large portions of the visible and infrared spectrums. Initial research emphasized (perhaps due to availability) the visible light of inert gas lasers such as the helium neon (HeNe), ruby, argon, and krypton (Table 2). More recently, gallium arsenide (GaAs) and gallium aluminum arsenide (GaAlAs) IR semiconductor laser diodes have become more available. There is a growing belief that these latter devices are particularly effective. Today, HeNe devices are still widely used, but the majority of work is done with GaAs and GaAlAs diodes with wavelengths between 820 nm and 904 nm (Table 2).

Laser therapy initially involved lasers with output powers ≤1 mW. Over the years, technology has improved and powers have increased. Today, treatments are performed with devices hav-

TABLE 2. Low Energy Lasers in Clinical Use

Laser	Wavelength(s) (nm)
Helium neon (HeNe)[a]	632.8 nm
Gallium aluminum arsenide (GaAlAs)[a]	820, 830 nm
Gallium arsenide (GaAs)[a]	904 nm
Neodymium-yttrim-aluminum garnet (Nd:YAG)[b]	1064 nm
Carbon dioxide (CO_2)[b]	10600 nm
Argon (Ar)[c]	488, 514
Krypton (Kr)[c]	521, 530, 568, 647
Ruby[c]	694

[a]Commonly used.
[b]Less commonly used, but still frequently reported.
[c]Frequently used in the past, now much less commonly.

TABLE 3. Low Energy Laser Treatment Parameters

Wavelength	Typically 632.8, 820, 830, or 904 nm
Powers	Average powers 10–90 mW (rarely a few hundred)
Waveform	Continuous wave, pulsed (1–4,000 Hz) Q-switched
Dosage/site	1–4 J/cm²
Regimen	Treatments of a few to 30s on a daily or alternate day schedule
Spot size	Variable: <1 mm² to defocussed and scanned beams covering the treatment area

TABLE 4. Treatment Approaches

Delivery techniques[a]:
  Single point
  Grid pattern
  Scanning (manual or automatic)
  Defocussed
  Point contact
Irradiation sites[a]:
  Over the lesion or painful area
  Peripheral nerves innervating the area of interest
  "Trigger points"
  Acupuncture or auricular therapy points
  Superficial sympathetic ganglia (e.g., stellate ganglion)
  Intravascular
  Ex-corporal with subsequent reinfusion
  Intraoperative
  Endoscopic
  In conjunction with photosensitizers

[a]Listed in approximate order of their frequency of use.

ing output powers between 10 and 90 (and occasionally even up to a few hundred) mW. Treatment times, however, have shortened as powers have increased and the radiant exposures delivered to treatment sites have usually remained near the 1–4 J/cm² levels established by the earliest investigators [1, 2].

Despite similarities of dose and a convergence in laser choice, significant differences persist between treatment approaches. Among these differences are pulse rate (continuous wave to 5,000 Hz), applicator placement (contact, non-contact), and the use of a single or a combination of wavelengths. Also of potential importance are the irradiance (power/unit area), beam divergence (3–8° or more for IR diodes), spot size, delivery (fiber optic, direct), polarity, and for pulsed devices, pulse duration and duty cycle. Table 3 summarizes some of the most common variations.

Discussion of laser therapy should ideally include all these parameters as well as information about site preparation, technique (Table 4), and number of treatments. Unfortunately, these details rapidly become unwieldy and will be sacrificed at times to improve intelligibility. The reader in need of more detailed information about specific clinical applications is referred to the appropriate references in the bibliography. Those with more interest in laboratory results may look at specific reviews [23, 28].

BIOPHYSICS OF LASER THERAPY

Two questions are obviously pertinent to laser therapy. First, which, if any, laser characteristics are essential in therapy? Second, can radiation penetrate deeply enough into tissue to produce the reported effects? Fortunately, laser radiation and tissue optics have been studied extensively and a great deal is known about each of these issues.

The characteristics of laser irradiation—coherency, collimation, and monochromaticity—have been examined in detail. In particular, coherency and collimation do not seem to be crucial since they are rapidly degraded by scattering as a beam passes through tissue. Supporting their relative lack of importance is the fact that both laser diodes (whose output is divergent and highly coherent in neither space nor time) and noncoherent light (from monochromatic sources) can alter biological processes. Monochromaticity, however, appears vital as investigators such as Karu et al. [8, 23] have shown that effects present with narrow bandwidth stimulation are absent with broad spectrum light.

There is a surprisingly large amount of information concerning the effects of radiation. For example, there is an optical "window" of sorts in the visible and IR portion of the spectrum, which extends from ~600 nm to 1,300 nm [29] and in-

TABLE 5. Conditions Reported as Treated With Laser Therapy

Inflammatory arthritis	Patellofemoral pain
Rheumatoid arthritis	Soft tissue wounds
Ankylosing spondylitis	Diabetic ulcers
Sjögren syndrome	Pressure sores
Osteoarthritis (degenerative joint disease)	Venous stasis ulcers
Knees	Surgical wounds
Thumb	Radiation dermatitis
Cervical spine	Stomatitis
Lumbar spine	Keloids
Periarthritis ("frozen shoulder")	Sports injuries
Tendinitis	Ankle sprain
Lateral epicondylitis (tennis elbow)	"Muscle pulls"
Medial epicondylitis	Buerger's disease (thromboangiitis obliterans)
Supraspinatus tendinitis	Headaches (vascular and muscular)
Bicipital tendinitis	Pruritus
Achilles tendinitis	Nerve repair
Neuropathic pain	Peripheral nerve repair
Carpal tunnel syndrome	Following neurosurgery
Diabetic neuropathy	Cranial nerve VII (facial nerve) repair
Radiculopathy	Trigger point (elevation of pain threshholds)
Postherpetic neuralgia	Sympathetic nervous system dysfunction
Occipital Neuralgia	Hemangiomas
Oro-facial pain	Tinnitus
Dental surgery	Immune modulation
Oral dysesthesia	Allergeric rhinitis
Trigeminal neuralgia	Leukemia
Temporomandibular pain	Bactericidal effects
Dental hypersensitivity	Pyronie's disease
Acute and chronic musculoskeletal pain	
Low back pain	
Tension myalgia	
Myofascial pain	

cludes most of the lasers currently used in laser therapy. As a result, although specific absorption characteristics may be important for particular lasers (e.g., hemoglobin, 488, 515 nm, for the argon laser; water, 10,600 nm, for the CO_2 laser), the commonly used (Table 2) HeNe, GaAIAs, and GaAs devices fall in a region of the spectrum without strongly absorbing chromophores and have better penetration capabilities than might be expected.

It is also important to remember that the attenuation of a laser beam is not an all-or-none phenomena. Rather, it is best described as an exponential decrease produced by the scattering and absorption that occur as light passes through tissue. Longer wavelengths are more resistant to scattering than shorter ones. For example, the red light (632.8 nm) of a HeNe laser penetrates 0.5–1 mm before losing 1/e (37%) of its intensity, whereas longer wavelength IR radiation will pen-

etrate ≥ 2 mm before losing the same fraction of its energy [29, 30].

Laboratory research suggests that radiant exposures of ≤ 0.01 J/cm^2 can alter cellular processes [8, 23]. Laser therapy typically involves exposures of 4 J/cm^2 per treatment, and six penetration depths are possible before an incident beam of 4 J/cm^2 is attenuated to the 0.01 J/cm^2 level. As this depth is equivalent to 0.5–2.5 cm, therapeutic amounts of energy can reasonably be expected to reach the superficial nerves, joints, and tissues typically treated with laser therapy. Treatment effectiveness at deeper sites seems more problematical; however, it should be recognized that a 1 mW HeNe beam easily transilluminates a finger.

CLINICAL TREATMENT

Laser therapy is used to treat an impressive assortment of conditions (Table 5). Regrettably, differing lasers, discordant techniques, variable research quality, and the dilution of effort produced by the sheer number of conditions investigated preclude objective evaluation of the discipline as an entity. In addition, evaluation of most trials is complicated by the waxing and waning of the conditions studied, frequent reliance on clinical diagnosis, and the semiquantitative nature of many treatment outcomes (e.g., lessening of pain or stiffness). The following sections review controlled clinical trials for some of the most intensively investigated laser therapy applications. Even with this focused approach, results often differ. Some studies will show benefits, but others that are equally well designed may show little or none.

Rotator Cuff Tendinitis

Rotator cuff tendinitis is a common, painful, and limiting soft tissue disorder of the shoulders, which often results from the wear and tear of repetitive trauma. The middle aged, the elderly, and the athlete are all affected, and conventional treatment involves a wide range of options, including heat, ice, rest, exercise, massage, nonsteroidal anti-inflammatories, and corticosteroid injections. Unfortunately, none of the approaches produces rapid or consistent benefits. In view of this lack of success and the superficial location of the rotator cuff, it is not surprising that laser therapy is viewed as an option.

Early investigators often listed shoulder tendinitis as one of many soft tissue conditions successfully treated with laser therapy. Unfortunately, the trials were generally open, and it was difficult to isolate patients with shoulder problems from those with other conditions. Recent studies, however, allow more rigorous evaluation. For example, England et al. [31] investigated 30 patients with supraspinatus or bicipital tendinitis of the shoulder. The subjects were divided into groups that received either treatment with a repetitively pulsed 3 mW 904 nm laser for 5 minutes, dummy laser treatment for the same duration, or nonsteroidal anti-inflammatory drugs. After six treatments, the laser subjects had improved significantly more than the other groups in terms of range of motion and lessened pain. It should be noted, however, that although the patients and investigators were blinded, the treating therapists were not. Thus a therapist bias for or against laser therapy could have influenced the findings.

Another recent study by Vecchio et al. [32] also considered shoulder tendinitis. This study randomized 30 patients to 3 J treatments at a maximum of five points with a 30 mW 830 nm CW laser or with an identically appearing inactive device for 16 sessions. Improvement in movement, strength, and lessened pain occurred in both groups, with no statistically significant advantage to either. Differences between this study and that of England et al. [31] include use of a different wavelength, longer term pain, more complete blinding, and a diagnosis of rotator cuff tendinitis rather than the more specific bicipital and supraspinatus tendinitis.

Animal studies, offer some support for tendinitis treatment. For example, in addition to the processes outlined in Table 1, tendons of tenotomized rabbits irradiated in vivo with 1 or 5 mJ/cm^2 of repetively pulsed HeNe laser radiation for 20 days show 0 collagen fibril production altered in ways that would seem to speed healing [4].

These discrepant results mirror a basic problem in evaluating laser therapy: similar but not identical diagnoses, treated with similar but not identical devices and similar but not identical methodologies produce different results. Although it would be desirable to establish the validity of laser therapy in general, all that can be legitimately inferred is that differing dosages, wavelengths, and study designs produce differing outcomes.

Rheumatoid Arthritis

Rheumatoid arthritis is frequently treated with low intensity lasers, perhaps because of the frequent involvement of superficial joints and a belief that laser therapy can modulate immune function and inflammation. In contrast to many other areas, a number of controlled and blinded studies are available. A variety of IR and visible lasers have been used with a large number of investigations finding a decrease in pain, swelling, medication use, and morning stiffness following treatment [33–38]. Benefits, nonetheless, are often quite modest, and even in investigations showing clinical benefits, effects on humoral quantities such as immune complexes, C-reactive protein (CRP), and sedimentation rates are variable. Other rheumatic diseases such as ankylosing spondylitis have been treated with HeNe and IR radiation with similar reports in terms of less pain, medication use, and stiffness [39].

Although most of the rheumatic disease studies present positive findings, almost all leave some questions in terms of rigor, data analysis, and sample size. Negative results also occur. In fact, one large, well-designed, multicenter study of 820 nm laser and superluminous diode irradiation on rheumatoid arthritis of the hands was terminated following midstudy data evaluation due to what the sponsor felt was an insufficient trend toward effectiveness. Another, somewhat earlier, multicenter study using a 0.95 mW HeNe laser was reviewed by a FDA panel in the mid-1980s. There was some evidence of benefit, but the panel did not recommend approval.

Neurological Conditions

The interaction of laser irradiation with nerve tissue is another area of intense research. Nerve growth and repair are important aspects of these studies, but Table 5 illustrates the important role of pain relief and analgesia. It is significant that, whereas analgesia may be produced by treating the injury itself, successful treatment of neuropathic and radicular pain (Table 5) may indicate that direct neurological effects are also important.

Clinical and animal studies provide significant information about this interaction. Physiological studies often [40–44], but not always [45, 46] show that laser irradiation can alter nerve conduction, repair, and evoked potentials. Rochkind et al. [47, 48], in particular, have intensively examined the effects of laser irradiation on neurological function and recovery after injury. These investigators have shown that ≤17 mW HeNe irradiation improves neurological viability and healing in rats and rabbits with both peripheral nerve and CNS injuries [47, 48]. This same group also finds that recovery in humans following surgical release of tethered spinal cords is improved if the operative site is exposed to radiation at the time of surgery [49].

Other experimental work gives inconsistent information about the consequences of irradiation on neurological behavior. Walker and associates [43, 44], e.g., reported that 1 mW HeNe laser irradiation lessens pain, suppresses clonus, and triggers action potentials. Similarly, Bork and Snyder-Mackler [42] find that radiation from the same laser can prolong superficial radial nerve distal latencies. Work by Basford et al. [45] and Wu et al. [46], with similar 1 mW HeNe lasers, nevertheless reproduced neither the prolonged superficial radial nerve latencies nor the action potential findings.

Work with somewhat higher power (30–60 mW) laser diodes at IR wavelengths between 820 and 830 nm shows alterations of several percent in superficial radial and median nerve distal latencies following 10–12 Joules of irradiation over the course of the nerves [40, 41, 50]. As alterations of these magnitudes can be easily produced with conventional ice and heat agents, their clinical significance remains uncertain [40–44, 47–49].

Carpal tunnel syndrome (CTS) is an extremely common and disabling repetitive stress injury that involves pain, inflammation, and altered neurological function in the relatively superficial distal median nerve. Conventional treatment involves rest, splinting, work modification, anti-inflammatory medications, corticosteroid injection, and, at times, surgery. As might be expected from this wide variety of approaches, response is often inadequate.

Laser therapy is advocated for this condition, and a large, well-designed, double-blinded, randomized-controlled multicenter study of 160 automobile workers with electrodiagnostically confirmed and clinically symptomatic carpal tunnel syndrome has recently completed its treatment phase [Good, ms. in prep.]. The workers were divided into two groups, each of which took part in an exercise and ergonomic modification program. One group, however, was treated with 90 mW array of three 830 nm CW laser diodes; the other received sham irradiation with an identically appearing device. Final results are not yet available, but it appears that both groups improved in such measures as grip strength. In addition, the laser group reportedly had a better return to work rate and demonstrated a statistically significant lessening symptoms relative to the control group. Other quantities such as nerve conduction velocities, distal latencies, and blood flow are being evaluated. If the final results are strongly positive, this study, due to its size and careful design, may serve as the basis of a FDA review.

Dental Surgery

Dentists and oral surgeons have applied laser irradiation to an assortment of painful and superficial conditions ranging from gingivitis and aphthous ulcers to craniomandibular pain and surgical wounds. As is true elsewhere, many reports have been anecdotal and the effects reported often difficult to compare [51–56]. Some studies show that irradiation improves wound healing following tooth extraction [51], craniomandibular pain [52], and dentinal hypersensitivity [55]. Other studies involving conditions such as pain and swelling following tooth extraction as well as chronic oro-facial pain have found no benefit [53, 54, 56]. A double-blinded study of chronic oro-facial pain by Hansen and Thoroe [3] found placebo more effective than repetitively pulsed 904 nm IR radiation combined with a visible red guidelight. 5-HIAA is often used as a marker for serotonin production, and it is interesting that the placebo group in this study had an increase in 5-HIAA urinary excretion similar to that in laser therapy responders in an earlier HeNe chronic pain study [57]. Other recent double-blinded investigations by Ferando et al. [58] and Masse et al. [59] find that 4 J 30 mW 830 nm laser and 2.5 minutes mixed HeNe (0.27 mW) and IR (80 mW) radiation neither lessens pain, reduces swelling, nor improves healing following tooth extraction. A recent study by In de Breakt [50] found that 1 J/cm^2 830 nm IR irradiation for 10 treatments did not alter wound healing or maxillary arch dimensions in beagles following surgery.

Many laser therapy proponents believe that irradiation is most effective in poorly vascularized, nutrient-deficient tissue and that multiple treatments at roughly daily intervals are necessary for maximal effectiveness. In addition, others suspect that treatment (perhaps by a humoral mechanism) produces "systemic" effects at sites distal to, as well as at, the point irradiated. Dental studies typically involve well-vascularized tissue, single treatments, and often have control and treatment sites in the same mouth. As a result, whereas the majority of the studies summarized here do not support the clinical utility of laser therapy, their generalization to other areas of treatment may be limited.

Wound Healing

The reports by Mester et al. in the late 1960s and early 1970s [1, 2] that 1–4 J/cm^2 of laser irradiation induced healing of chronic nonhealing soft tissue ulcers formed the genesis of clinical laser therapy. With time, these studies grew to include >1,000 patients but remained poorly controlled. As a result, despite their large size, impressive photographs, and reported cure rates of >70%, they did little to convince skeptics that laser therapy had any validity.

Laboratory work provides some support for the use of low intensity laser radiation in wound healing. Many investigations, although not uncontested [61], find that visible and IR radiation stimulates capillary growth and granulation tissue formation and alters cytokin production. Other studies show altered keratinocyte motility and fibroblast movement following irradiation [62]. Additional studies find that laser irradiation may either enhance, inhibit, or have no effect on the function of a variety of microorganisms and cells [10].

Animal studies also offer some basis for treatment. Improvements, particularly in the earliest phases of wound healing, have been reported following laser irradiation in many rabbit and rodent experiments [63–66]. The applicability of these findings to humans is unclear, since similar experiments with pigs, which have skin more similar to that of humans [67, 68], may show no benefit [69, 70].

Well-controlled and blinded human wound healing studies are extremely difficult to carry out due to the vagaries of wound size, patient characteristics, and the coincidental activities. Nevertheless, some are available. One, by Lundeberg and Malm [71], involved 46 individuals with venous ulcers. All patients were treated with a program of paste-impregnated bandages and compressive wraps. In addition, one-half received 4 J/cm^2 of 6 mW HeNe laser irradiation twice a week for 12 weeks, and one-half were treated with an inactive but otherwise identical device. No significant differences in healing were found between the groups at the end of the study. Another study involving venous ulcers found that the addition of 1 or 4 J/cm^2 of HeNe radiation to a program of twice-a-day compresses offered no advantage over compresses alone [72].

A recent survey of >500 Dutch health professionals [73]—dermatologists, as well as physicians and nurses working in nursing homes—is pertinent here. The participants were asked to rank a list of pressure sore treatments on a scale from "0" (harmful) to "10" (excellent). Pressure relief and patient education were ranked highly at 6.2–8.3. High protein diets, hydrocolloid dressings, and zinc oxide were ranked intermediately (5.0–5.6). Laser therapy was less well known and scored far lower at 1.5–3.1 [73].

Low Back Pain

Low back pain is another widespread and disabling condition whose many treatments are slow and not always more effective than rest and a gradual return to normal activity. Although its diffuse nature hinders objective evaluation, it is not surprising that laser therapy is used for its treatment.

Early work was anecdotal and poorly controlled. More recent investigations are more rigorous and systematic. One analysis by Klein and Eek [74], e.g., involved two groups of 20 subjects. All subjects received a standard exercise program. In addition, one-half were irradiated three times a week for 4 weeks with 1.3 J/cm^2 from an array of pulsed 904 nm diodes; the other half was identically treated with an inactive array. Both groups improved over the course of the study, but no statistical differences were found between them in any of the pain, disability, or range of motion parameters measured.

Patellofemoral Pain

Patellofemoral pain is routinely treated with activity restriction, ice, vastus medialis strengthening, knee sleeves, and nonsteroidal anti-inflammatories. Improvement is slow, often incomplete, and frequently at the cost of the patient being forced to alter his or her activities.

Laser therapy has advocates here also. Early trials were open and reported success with this as well as many other forms of musculoskeletal pain. Controlled studies are now more available. Rogvi-Hansen et al. [75], e.g., recently described the results of a double-blinded study of 40 individuals with arthroscopically documented chondromalacia patellae. Subjects received eight 10-minute treatments with either an active or a sham 1,000 Hz pulsed 17 mW GaAs laser. No statistically significant differences were found between the groups at the end of the 5-week study. There was, however, a trend toward laser effectiveness with about half the treated group and only 30% of the sham group "improving." How a larger study or one with less severe disease, would have fared is unclear.

Lateral Epicondylitis (Tennis Elbow)

Lateral epicondylitis is another common painful soft tissue condition thought to be associated with repetitive trauma. The patient complains of lateral elbow pain that is exacerbated by grasping. Physical findings are characterized by localized tenderness and pain when the elbow is extended and wrist or index finger extension resisted. The condition is chronic, relapsing, and responds slowly to a program of splints, heat, ice, epicondylar straps, massage, injection, and activity modification.

Laser therapy, perhaps due to the superficial location of the aponeurosis and the relatively slow response to conventional agents, is widely used to treat this disorder. Local as well as laser acupuncture treatment protocols have been examined in double-blinded studies. For example, two acupuncture studies by Haker and Lundeberg in 1990 [76, 77] showed no benefit following a single treatment with a HeNe, or with either single or 10 treatments from 0.07 and 12 mW pulsed GaAs IR devices. A double-blinded controlled study in 1992 of 30 subjects by Vasseljen et al. [78] found that eight 3.5 J/cm^2 local treatments with an 18 mW repetitively array of pulsed 904 nm IR diodes produced improvements in visual analog scale (VAS) scores and wrist extension strengths statistically significantly better in the treated patients than in the control group. However, even with these results, the investigators felt that the benefits were limited if irradiation was performed in isolation from other therapy.

Trigger Points

"Trigger points" (defined as points that produce a well-described pattern of referred pain when pressed upon) are a significant, albeit controversial, factor in musculoskeletal research. Laser therapy has been examined here also. One 1989 double-blinded controlled study by Snyder-Mackler et al. [79] involved 24 patients. The investigators found both a statistically significant reduction of pain and increased skin resistance (a proxy for altered sympathetic function) at the trigger points in the group that was irradiated with a 0.95 mW HeNe CW laser. Another study of 18 subjects by Olavi et al. [80] was performed with a higher power 904 nm IR laser. This investigation also found irradiation significantly increasing pain thresholds.

Acupuncture

Laser therapy is frequently used as an acupuncture or auriculotherapy technique with uncontrolled reports typically finding 80% + of the subjects improved or cured after treatment. Unfortunately, as the lateral epicondylitis studies of Haker and Lundeberg discussed above [76, 77] showed, controlled studies may produce less sanguine results. Other controlled studies of laser therapy as an acupuncture technique are also available. For example, a double-blinded study by Brockhaus and Elger [81] found needle acupuncture altered thermal pain thresholds, whereas similar treatment with a 10 mW repetitively pulsed HeNe laser did not. In contrast, King et al.

[82] used a 1 mW HeNe laser to treat 80 subjects in a controlled auriculotherapy evaluation. Although it is not clear how well the evaluators were blinded, these investigators found pain threshold increased a statistically significant 18% in the treated group.

Bactericidal Effects

Although early laser investigators reported alterations of bacterial growth following irradiation [2], the bactericidal effects of these devices has not received much clinical emphasis. Nevertheless, information is available. Thus, whereas McGuff and Bell [83] found that a .05 mW HeNe laser had no effect on bacteria such as *S. Aureus* and *P. Aeruginosa,* other groups using the same laser at 6–40 mW powers found that some bacteria were radiation sensitive [84, 85], but that a larger number were killed with similar exposures when exposed in the presence of dyes such as toluene blue and the phenylmethane classes [84, 85].

Safety

The dangers of high power lasers are well known and center on tissue destruction. The powers used in laser therapy are by definition too low to cause tissue damage by either heating or acoustic effects. Nonetheless, it seems possible that the same effects that are claimed to promote beneficial processes could also be detrimental. However, neither experience nor literature searches reveal substantive risk. Patients do comment at times about transient warmth or "tingling" during or shortly after treatment. However, in our experience this has occurred in both active and placebo subjects. It also seems pertinent that even though high power laser beams are surrounded by a low power penumbra, no unusual effects are reported from these beams either.

In practice, direct observation of a 1 mW HeNe (visible red light) beam can produce a headache even though beams of 5 mW neither stimulate nociocepters nor produce >0.1°C temperature changes in the cornea [86]. In any event, retinal hazard is a concern and the use of protective glasses and avoidance of looking directly at a beam, or its reflection, seem prudent. Although there is no proven risk, as far as I know, many investigators avoid treating pregnant women, cancer patients, acute hemorrhages, growth plates, and photosensitive skin as a general precaution.

Meta-Analysis

Although meta-analysis requires the grouping of dissimilar laser therapy regimens and conditions, it can be argued that this approach would provide a more objective overview of laser therapy than a review. This is arguable, but attempts have been made. Beckerman et al. [88] published an overview in 1992 that evaluated 36 randomized laser therapy studies of musculoskeletal pain and skin disorders (such as chronic ulcers). Despite the fact that >1,700 subjects were included, variability of study design and quality limited analysis. In fact, pooling was not possible. No decision about skin conditions was possible, and all that could be said about the musculoskeletal studies was that the "better" investigations showed a tendency for treatment to be more effective than placebo.

Gam et al. [88] presented another, even more recent, 1993 meta-analysis, which was more strenuously restricted than that of Beckerman et al. [87] and was limited to 23 musculoskeletal pain trials. No differences were found between active and placebo treatment in the studies that were deemed "adequately blinded"; only a 9.5% difference occurred in the "insufficiently blinded" subset. As the confidence intervals of both groups included "no effect," it is not unexpected that these authors concluded that low power laser therapy has no proven musculoskeletal effectiveness.

CONCLUSIONS

In 1986, an editorial about laser therapy by this author [61] had the grandiose and alliterative title "Laser Therapy: Hype, Hope or Hokum? At that time I concluded that clinical effectiveness was still unknown, but I hoped that within 5 years we would have definitive information. The definitive answer has not yet appeared, but some progress has been made. Much of the "hype" has dissipated and methodical, dispassionate, reproducible, controlled studies have become more common. Another significant change has been the relative standardization of the field with a commonality of lasers (IR diodes or HeNe) and radiant exposures of 1–4 J/cm^2.

What does all this tell us? A few conclusions seem possible. One conclusion is that laboratory studies support the concept that laser irradiation can modify cellular processes in a wavelength-dependent, nonthermal manner. Another is that intensities sufficient to produce these effects on cells can be delivered to the superficial joints and tissues typically treated with laser therapy. Nevertheless, whether on a category-by-category approach as was done in this review, or at best by meta-analysis, high quality trials still show marginal clinical effectiveness. Laser therapy may be particularly effective for neurological applications, and it may be here that it has the best potential to move from the laboratory to the clinic.

REFERENCES

1. Mester E, Spiry T, Szende B, Tota JG. Effect of laser rays on wound healing. Am J Surg 1971; 122:532.
2. Mester E, Mester AF, Mester A. The biomedical effects of laser application. Lasers Surg Med 1985; 5:31.
3. Hansen HJ, Thoroe U. Low power laser biostimulation of chronic oro-facial pain: A double-blind placebo controlled cross-over study in 40 patients. Pain 1990; 43:169–179.
4. Enwemeka CS. Ultrastructural morphometry of membrane-bound intracytoplasmic collagen fibrils in tendon fibroblasts exposed to He:Ne laser beam. Tissue Cell 1992; 24:511–523.
5. Lam TS, Abergel RP, Meeker CA, Castael JC, Dwyer RM, Uitto J. Laser stimulation of collagen synthesis in human skin fibroblast cultures. Lasers Life Sci 1986; 1:61–77.
6. Mester E, Toth N, Mester A. The biostimulative effect of laser beam. Laser Basic Biomed Res 1982; 22:4.
7. Lyons RF, Abergel RP, White RA, Dwyer RM, Castel JC, Uitto J. Biostimulation of wound healing in vivo by a helium-neon laser. Ann Plast Surg 1987; 18:47.
8. Karu TI. Photobiological fundamentals of low-power laser therapy. IEEE Journal of Quantum Electronics 1987; QE-23:1703.
9. Rood PA, Haas AF, Graves PJ, Wheeland RG, Isseroff RR. Low-energy helium neon laser irradiation does not alter human keratinocyte differentiation. J Invest Dermatol 1992; 99:445–448.
10. Quickenden TI, Daniels LL. Attempted biostimulation of division in *saccharomyces cerevisiae* using red coherent light. Photochem Photobiol 1993; 57:272–278.
11. Karu TI. Molecular mechanism of the therapeutic effect of low-intensity laser radiation. Lasers Life Sci 1988; 2:53–74.
12. Van Breugel HHFI, Bar PR. He-Ne laser irradiatin affects proliferation of cultural rat Schwann cells in a dose dependent manner. J Neurocytol 1993; 22:185–190.
13. Abergel RP, Dwyer RM, Meeker CA, Lask G, Kelly AP, Uitto J. Laser treatment of keloids: A clinical trial and an in vitro study with Nd:YAG laser. Lasers Surg Med 1984; 4:291.
14. Sato H. Landthaler M, Haina D, Schill WB. The effects of laser light on sperm motility and velocity in vitro. Andrologia 1984; 16:23.
15. Deckelbaum LI. Scott JJ, Stetz ML, O'Brien KM, Sumpio BE, Madri JA. Bell L. Photoinhibition of smooth muscle cell migration: Potential therapy for restenosis. Lasers Surg Med 1993; 13:4–11.
16. Wollman Y, Rochkind S. Muscle fiber formation in vitro is delayed by low power laser irradiation. J Photochem Photobiol B Biol 1993; 17:287–290.
17. Passarella S, Casamassima E, Molinari S, et al. Increase of proton electrochemical potential and ATP synthesis in rat liver mitochondria irradiated in vitro by helium-neon laser. FEBS Lett 1984; 175:95.
18. Kubasova T, Kovacs L, Somosy Z, Unk P, Kokai A. Biological effect of He-Ne laser investigations on functional and micromorphological alterations of cell membranes, in vitro. Lasers Surg Med 1984; 4:381.
19. Passarella S, Casamassima E, Quagliariello E, Caretto G, Jirillo E. Quantitative analysis of lymphocyte—Salmonella interaction and effect of lymphocyte irradiation by helium-neon laser. Biochem Biophys Res Comm 1985; 130:546.
20. Fork RL. Laser stimulation of nerve cells in aplysia. Science 1971; 171:907–908.
21. Young S, Bolton P, Dyson M, Harvey W, Diamantopoulos C. Macrophage responsiveness to light therapy. Lasers Surg Med 1989; 9:497–505.
22. Karu TI, Ryabykh TP, Fedoseyeva GE, Puchkova NI. Helium-Neon laser-induced respiratory burst of phagocytic cells. Lasers Surg Med 1989; 9:585–588.
23. Karu TI. Photobiological fundamentals of low-power laser therapy. IEEE J Quant Elect 1987; 23:1703.
24. Licht S. "History of Ultraviolet Therapy in Therapeutic Electricity and Ultraviolet Radiation," 2nd ed. New Haven, CT: Elizabeth Licht 1967, pp 191–212.
25. Basford JR. Physical Agents and Biofeedback in Rehabilitation Medicine: Principles and Practice. In: DeLisa JA, ed. Philadelphia: J.B. Lippincott, 1988, pp 257–275.
26. Vizi ES, Mester E, Tizza S, Mester A. Acetylcholine releasing effect of laser irradiation on Auerbach's plexus in guinea pig ileum. J Neural Transm Park Dis Dement Sect 1977; 40:305.
27. Greathouse DG, Currier DP, Gilmore RL. Effects of clinical infrared laser on superficial radial nerve conduction. Phys Ther 1985; 65:1184.
28. Basford JR. Laser therapy: Scientific basis and clinical role Orthopedics 1993; 16:541–547.
29. Anderson RR, Parrish JA. The optics of human skin. J Invest Dermatol 1981; 77:13–19.
30. Kolari PJ. Penetration of unfocused laser light into the skin. Arch Dermatol Res 1985; 277:342–344.
31. England S, Farrell AJ, Coppock JS, Struthers G, Bacon PA. Low power laser therapy of shoulder tendonitis. Scand J Rheumatol 1989; 18:427–431.
32. Vecchio P, Cave M, King V, Adebajo AO, Smith M, Hazleman BL. A double-blind study of the effectiveness of low level laser treatment of rotator cuff tendinitis. Br J Rheumatol 1993; 32:740–742.
33. Colov HC, Palmgren N, Jensen GF, Kaa K, Windelin M. Convincing clinical improvement of rheumatoid arthritis by soft laser therapy (abstract). Lasers Surg Med 1987; 7:77.
34. Goldman JA, Chiapella J, Casey H, et al. Laser therapy in rheumatoid arthritis. Lasers Surg Med 1980; 1:93.
35. Bliddal H, Hellesen C, Ditlevsen P, Asselberghs J, Lyager L. Soft-laser therapy of rheumatoid arthritis. Scand J Rheumatol 1987; 16:225.
36. Walker JB, Akhanjee LJ, Cooney MM, Goldstein J, Tamayoshi S, Sgal-Gidan F. Laser therapy for pain of rheumatoid arthritis. Clin J Pain 1987; 3:54–59.

37. Soto JJM, Moller I. La lasertherapia como coadyuvante en el tratemiento de la AR (artritis reumatoidea). Boletin Centro Documentacion Laser 1987; 14:4.

38. Oyamada Y. Biostimulation effect for rheumatoid arthritis by low power He-Ne laser surgery. In: Joffe SN, Goldblatt NR, Atsumi K, eds. "Laser Surgery: Advanced Characterization, Therapeutics and Systems." Bellingham, WA: International Society for Optical Engineering, 1989, p 1066.

39. Gartner C. Low reactive level laser therapy (LLLT) in rheumatology: A review of the clinical experience in the author's laboratory. Laser Ther 1992; 4:107–115.

40. Basford JR, Hallman HO, Matsumoto JY, Moyer SK, Buss JM, Baxter GD. Effects of 830 nm continuous wave laser diode irradiation on median nerve function in normal subjects. Lasers Surg Med 1993; 13:597–604.

41. Baxter GD, Allen JM, Bell AJ, Ravey J, Diamanthopoulos C. Effect of laser (830 nm) upon conduction in the median nerve. American Society for Laser Medicine and Surgery Abstracts. Laser Surg Med Suppl 1991; 3:79.

42. Bork CE, Snyder-Mackler L. Effect of Helium-Neon laser irradiation on peripheral sensory nerve latency. J Am Phys Ther Assoc 1988; 68:223.

43. Walker JB, Akhanjee LK. Laser-induced somatosensory evoked potentials: evidence of photosensitivity in peripheral nerves. Brain Res 1985; 344:281.

44. Walker JB. Temporary suppression of clonus in human by brief photostimulation. Brain Res 1985; 340:109.

45. Basford JR, Daube JR, Hallman HO, Millard TL, Moyer SK. Does low-intensity helium-neon laser irradiation alter sensory nerve action potentials or distal latencies? Lasers Surg Med 1990; 10:35–39.

46. Wu W, Ponnudurai R, Katz J, Pott CB, Chilcoat R, Uncini A, Rapport S, Wade P, Mauro A. Failure to confirm report of light-evoked response of peripheral nerve to low power helium-neon laser light stimulus. Brain Res 1987; 401:407.

47. Rochkind S, Barrnea L, Razon N, Bartel A, Schwartz M. Stimulatory effect of He-Ne low dose laser on injured sciatic nerves of rats. Neurosurgery 1987; 20:843.

48. Schwartz M, Doron A, Erich M, Lavie V, Benbasat S, Belkin M, Rochkind S. Effects of low-energy He-Ne laser irradiation of posttraumatic degeneration of adult rabbit optic nerve. Lasers Surg Med 1987; 7:51.

49. Rochkind S, Alon M, Ouakine GE, Weiss S, Avram J, Rzon N, Doron A, Lubart R, Friedmann H. Intraoperative clinical use of LLLT followup surgical treatment of the tethered spinal cord. Laser Ther 1991; 3:113–118.

50. Walsh DM, Baxter GK, Allen JM. The effect of 820 nm laser upon nerve conduction in the superficial radial nerve. Abst in The Fifth Int Biotherapy Laser Assoc Meeting, London, 1991.

51. Takeda Y. Irradiation effect of low energy laer on alveolar bone after tooth extraction: Experimental study on rats. Int J Oral Maxillofac Surg 1988; 17:388.

52. Bezuur NJ, Habets LL, Hansson TL. The effect of therapeutic laser treatment in patients with craniomandibular disorders. J Craniomandib Disord 1988; 2:83.

53. Hansen HJ, Thoroe U. Low power laser biostimulation of chronic oro-facial pain: A double blind placebo controlled cross-over study in 40 patients. Pain 1990; 43:169.

54. Carrillo JS, Calatayud J, Manso FJ, Barberia E, Martinez JM, Donado M. A randomized double-blind clinical trial on the effectiveness of helium-neon laser in the pre-

55. Renton-Harper P, Midda M. NdYAG laser treatment of dentinal hypersensitivity. Br Dent J 1992; 172:13–16.

56. Taube S, Piioren J, Ylipaavalniemi P. Helium-neon laser therapy in the prevention of post-operative swelling and pain after wisdom tooth extraction. Proceedings of the Finnish Dental Society 1990; 86:23.

57. Walker J. Relief from chronic pain by low power laser irradiation. Neurosci Lett 1983; 43:339–344.

58. Fernando S, Hill CM, Walker R. A randomised double blind comparative study of low level laser therapy following surgical extraction of lower third molar teeth. Br J Oral Maxillofac Surg 1993; 31:170–172.

59. Masse JF, Landry RG, Rochette C, Dufour L, Morency R, D'Aoust P. Effectiveness of soft laser treatment in periodontal surgery. Int Dent J 1993; 43:121–127.

60. In de Braekt MMH, Van Alphen FAM, Kuijpers-Jagtman AM, Maltha JC. The effect of low-level laser treatment on maxillary arch dimensions after palatal surgery on beagle dogs. J Dent Res 1991; 70:1467–1470.

61. Basford JR. Low-energy laser treatment of pain and wounds: Hype, hope, or hokum? Mayo Clin Proc 1986; 61:671.

62. Noble PB, Shields ED, Blecher PDM, Bentley KC. Locomotory characteristics of fibroblasts within a three-dimensional collagen lattice: Modulation by a helium/neon soft laser. Lasers Surg Med 1992; 12:669–674.

63. Kana JS, Hutschenreiter G, Haina D, Waidelich W. Effect of low-power density laser radiation on healing of open skin wounds in rats. Arch Surg 1981; 116:293.

64. Brunner R, Haina D, Landthaler M, Waidelich W, Braun-Falco O. Application of laser light of low power density: Experimental and clinical investigations. Curr Probl. Dermatol 1986; 15:111.

65. Ribari O: The stimulating effect of low power laser rays: Experimental examinations in otorhinolaryngology. Rev Laryngol Otol Rhinol (Bord) 1981; 102:531–533.

66. Surinchak JS, Alago ML, Bellamy RF, Stuck BE, Belkin M: Effects of low-level energy lasers on the healing of full-thickness skin defects. Lsaers Surg Med 1983; 2:267–274.

67. Bal HS. The skin. In Senson MJ, ed: "Dukes' Physiology of Domestic Animals," 9th ed. Ithaca, NY: Cornell University Press, 1977, pp 493–503.

68. Marcarian HQ, Calhoun ML. Microscopic anatomy of the integument of adult swine. Am J Vet Res 1966, 27:765–772.

69. Hunter J, Leonard L, Wilson R, Snider G, Dixon J. Effects of low energy laser on wound healing in a porcine model. Lasers Surg Med 1984; 3:285–290.

70. Basford JR, Hallman HO, Sheffield CG, Mackey GL. Comparison of the effects of cold quartz ultraviolet, low energy laser, and occlusion on wound healing in a swine model. Arch Phys Med Rehab 1986; 67:151–154.

71. Lundeberg T. Malm M. Low-power HeNe laser treatment of venous leg ulcers. Ann Plastic Surg 1991; 27:537–539.

72. Santoianni P, Monfrecola G, Martellotta D, Ayala F. Inadequate effect of helium-neon laser on venous leg ulcers. Photodermatology 1984; 1:245–249.

73. Ter Riet G, Van Houtem H, Knipschild P. Health-care professionals' views of the effectiveness of pressure ulcer treatments. Clin Exp Dermatol 1992; 17:328–331.

74. Klein RG, Eek BC. Low-energy laser treatment and ex-

ercise for chronic low back pain: double-blind controlled trial. Arch Phys Med Rehabil 1990; 71:34–37.

75. Rogvi-Hansen B, Ellitsgaard N, Funch M, Dall-Jensen M, Prieske J. Low level laser treatment of chondromalacia patellae. International Orthopaedics (SICOT) 1991; 15:359–361.

76. Lundeberg T, Haker E, Thomas M. Effects of laser versus placebo in tennis elbow. Scand J Rehabil Med 1987; 19: 135–138.

77. Haker E, Lundeberg T. Laser treatment applied to acupuncture points in lateral epicondylagic. Pain 1990; 43: 243–247.

78. Vasseljen O Jr, Hoeg N, Kjeldstad B, Johnsson A, Larsen S. Low level laser versus placebo in the treatment of tennis elbow. Scand J Rehab Med 1992; 24:37–42.

79. Snyder-Mackler L, Barry AJ, Perkins AI, Soucek MD. Effects of Helium-Neon laser irradiation on skin resistance and pain in patients with trigger points in the neck or back. Physical Therapy 1989; 69:336–341.

80. Olavi A, Pekka R, Pertti K. Effects of the infrared laser therapy at treated and non-treated trigger points. Acupuncture Electro-therapeutics Res. Int. J. 1989; 14:9–14.

81. Brockhaus A, Elger CE: Hypalgesic efficacy of acupuncture on experimental pain in man. Comparison of laser acupuncture and needle acupuncture. Pain 1990; 43:181–185.

82. King CE, Clelland JA, Knowles CJ, Jackson JR. Effect of helium-neon laser auriculotherapy on experimental pain threshold. Phys Ther 1990; 70:24–30.

83. McGuff PE, Bell EJ. The effect of laser energy radiation on bacteria. Med Biol III 1966; 16:191–194.

84. Macmillan JD, Maxwell WA, Chichester CO. Lethal photosensitization of microorganisms with light from a continuous-wave gas laser. Photochem Photobiol 1966; 5:555–565.

85. Okamoto H, Iwase T, Morioka T. Dye-mediated bactericidal effect of He-Ne laser irradiation on oral microorganisms. Lasers Surg Med 1992; 12:450–458.

86. Jarvis D, MacIver BM, Tanelian DL, Effects of He-Ne laser irradiation on corneal A-Delta and C-fiber nociceptor electrophysiology. Poster 105, S209, Supplement 5, 1990 (SPON:m.Lo). Department of Anesthesia, Stanford University Medical Center, Stanford, CA 94305.

87. Beckerman H, deBie RA, Bouter LM, De Cuyper HJ, Oostendorp RAB. The efficacy of laser therapy for musculoskeletal and skin disorders: A criteria-based meta-analysis of randomized clinical trials. Phys Ther 1992; 72: 483–491.

88. Gam AN, Thorsen H, Lonnberg F. The effect of low-level laser therapy on musculoskeletal pain: A meta-analysis. Pain 1993; 52:63–66.

Chapter 7

Lasers in Neurosurgery

Satish Krishnamurthy, MD, and Stephen K. Powers, MD

Milton S. Hershey Medical Center, Pennsylvania State University, Hershey

INTRODUCTION

The introduction of lasers into neurological surgery began in 1965 when Earle et al. [1] and Fine et al. [2] demonstrated that a single focused 20 joule or unfocused 100 joule pulse 1 msecond in duration from a ruby laser, applied to the cranium of mice, resulted in immediate death. Fox et al. [3] repeated these studies in guinea pigs and determined that death was due to apnea. The mechanism of brain injury was investigated further by directing laser energy at a series of animals that had been craniectomized on the side contralateral to the laser injury [4]. In another series [4], the laser energy from a ruby laser was directed onto the skull of decapitated animals. High-speed cinematography revealed that an explosive laser-skull interaction occurred, leading to recoil of the intracranial contents as a result of sudden tissue vaporization and rapid volume expansion with a concomitant sudden increase in intracranial pressure. However, when laser energy was directed at the surgically exposed cerebrum in craniectomized animals, some animals survived for several hours. Survival in these animals after laser energy delivery was postulated to occur because explosive expansion in the intracranial volume did not generate a rapid rise in intracranial pressure due to venting of gaseous products of vaporization into air and the provision of space for herniation of swollen heat-affected brain into the craniectomy defect. Thus the sudden rise in intracranial pressure that occurred when the laser was directed at the intact skull and led to brainstem compression causing apnea and animal death was circumvented by exposing the brain surface to direct application of the laser beam.

Stellar [5] investigated the effects of ruby laser pulses on the exposed brain, spinal cord, and peripheral nerves of cats. The laser pulses resulted in grossly visible wedge-shaped hemorrhagic lesions at the sites of impact. The effects on the spinal cord were similar to those in the brain, but the peripheral nerves demonstrated a greater resistance to ruby laser energy. Brown et al. [6] and Liss and Roppel [7] reported similar effects of ruby laser energy on neural tissue.

Rosomoff and Carroll [8] were the first to report the use of the laser in clinical neurosurgery. They focused pulsed ruby laser beams on brain tumors in an attempt to induce a selective tumor effect. Although areas of tumor necrosis were induced, the laser was not used to remove tumor tissue, and prolongation of survival was not documented. The thermal effects of ruby laser energy on neural tissues could not be controlled precisely because of its poor absorption by nonpigmented tissues. Neurosurgical interest in the pulsed ruby laser was also limited because of the uncontrolled photomechanical effects.

The introduction of continuous-wave lasers and improved delivery systems made lasers more applicable to neurosurgery. The harsh explosive effects on tissue were eliminated, and laser exposures and energies are more precise and controllable. Much of the initial work investigating the neurosurgical properties of the carbon dioxide (CO_2) laser was reported by Stellar and co-workers [9,10]. They confirmed that precise, hemostatic incisions could be made in the cat brain and spinal cord to depths controlled easily by the speed of movement of the laser beam. Histological studies demonstrated that the morphological alteration of tissue extended < 0.5 mm on either side of the incision. They also demonstrated the coagulative effect of defocused CO_2 laser energy on vessels up to 2 mm in diameter.

In 1969, Stellar and co-workers [11] used a carbon dioxide laser to subtotally vaporize a recurrent glioma. Although he recognized the advantages of no-touch cutting, Stellar used the laser only in patients with inoperable glioblastomas of the cerebrum with the goal of vaporizing tumor tissue. Since inoperable glioblastomas of the cerebrum are usually very large and well vascularized, the CO_2 laser had to be used at high power settings. Application of the laser to neurosurgical procedures seemed limited, and addition of the laser was very time-consuming. After a few publications and surgical failures, Stellar personally advised prominent neurosurgeons against using lasers at that time. However, the concept of the CO_2 laser as a no-touch and minimally traumatic cutting tool convinced some neurosurgeons to pursue its use in neurosurgery, although the laser

had not yet been adapted to neurosurgical purposes. Fox [12] summarized the problems of using the laser in neurosurgery at that time when he said, *"the massive probes used in other surgical fields prevented laser applications in neurosurgery. The reasons for this are simple. Once the decision has been made to use an invisible knife, then it would be illogical to surround the device by a material sheath or to decline the potential of aseptic technique by risking contact infection. And it would be especially illogical and defeat the purpose of the new instrument to further narrow the already limited neurosurgical field by again using a material probe."*

Due to these technical difficulties, the reported use of CO_2 lasers in neurosurgery remained anecdotal until Heppner [13], Ascher [14,15], Takizawa et al. [16], and Ascher and Cerullo [17] described individual experiences in large series of patients who had a variety of neurosurgical procedures performed with the CO_2 laser. From 1976 until 1979, Ascher [14,15] and Heppner [13] performed > 250 laser operations on the central nervous system, including 200 brain tumor operations and 13 spinal cord tumor operations. Many of these procedures were performed with a free-hand laser without the aid of an operating microscope [18]. The combination of the laser with the operating microscope for neurosurgical procedures was subsequently recognized by Ascher and Heppner, and they modified the carbon dioxide laser in two principal ways in 1976. The first was the addition of the helium laser to act as a pilot to help the surgeon direct the invisible CO_2 laser beam to the tissue target. This not only established use of the laser as a "contact-free" technique, as had been originally envisaged, but also enabled the operator to focus and defocus the laser treatment beam based upon focusing and defocusing the pilot beam without using a mechanical guiding instrument that might contact the tissue surface and/or obstruct the surgeon's view. The other modification was the coupling of the laser to the operating microscope in order to increase the precision of laser application to tissue. With these changes, the CO_2 laser became a powerful microsurgical tool that led to improved treatment of surgical lesions deep within the brain, in the brainstem and spinal cord and at the skull base.

The clinical experience of these pioneering neurosurgeons suggested that the microsurgical CO_2 laser could be used to particular advantage for the excision of critically located extra-axial tumors such as meningiomas, craniopharyngiomas, and acoustic schwannomas as well as small vascular lesions of brain and spinal cord. Subsequently, the advantages of CO_2 laser surgery for the excision of gliomas, especially recurrent gliomas, poorly accessible deep brain tumors, and fibrous calcified tumors involving the neuraxis were presented by investigators from several centers at the First American Congress on Lasers in Neurosurgery (1981).

The poor absorption and scattering of Nd:YAG laser energy by nonpigmented tissue in general results in extensive damage to neural tissues, and hence the Nd:YAG laser lacked the precision needed for use in most microneurosurgical and cerebral parenchymal surgery [10,19]. However, its application to neurovascular surgery, because of its selective absorption by blood, and thus blood vessels, was suggested in two reports. Yahr et al. [20,21] presented a technique for nonocclusive microanastomosis of vessels using the Nd:YAG laser. Later, Jain and Gorisch [22] demonstrated the ability to seal experimental lacerations in rat arteries and veins using intermittent pulses of Nd:YAG laser energy. Impressed by the ability of the Nd:YAG laser energy to occlude small vessels, Beck and associates [23] investigated the possibility of using this laser to supplement conventional neurosurgical techniques to limit hemorrhages. They compared the tissue effects of both CO_2 and the Nd:YAG laser on rabbit brains and found that although the Nd:YAG laser beam penetrates more deeply than the CO_2 laser, the depth of penetration using a defocused beam is predictable and the Nd:YAG laser beam has a more pronounced effect on highly vascularized tissue. On the basis of their studies, they began use of the Nd:YAG laser in clinical practice and reported their clinical experience [24] followed by Takeuchi et al. [25]. Both groups found the Nd:YAG laser was particularly useful for the excision of vascular meningiomas and arteriovenous malformations. Diffuse bleeding from the bone plate, dura, blood vessels under 2.5 mm in diameter, and the vascularized tumor capsule could easily be controlled. Tumor invading the cranial base and dural venous sinuses could be sterilized without resection, and the recurrence-free survival rate seemed to be increased over that for patients treated with conventional neurosurgical methods. In Beck's series [24], two patients who had died of other causes had no autopsy evidence of residual tumor within the laser-irradiated sagittal sinus. In all patients operated on with the Nd:YAG laser, blood loss was reduced compared to conventional techniques or to the CO_2 laser. The Nd:YAG laser was also found beneficial in softening fibrous or calcified tumors, and Takeuchi et al. [25] found it helpful in perforating thick sphenoid bones during transsphenoidal surgery.

The argon ion laser was utilized by ophthalmologists from the time of its introduction due to its transmissibility through water and clear media, very good hemostatic properties, and the available small laser beam spot size compared to the other lasers. Fox et al. [4] showed that brain and other tissues were easily vaporized by a nonfocused argon laser beam of low power density. Hobieka and Rockwell [26] introduced the argon laser into otolaryngology based on preclinical experience from laboratory. Maira et al. [27] photoradiated the walls of experimental saccular aneurysms and were able to thrombose the whole aneurysm in many cases. Even in aneurysms that were incompletely thrombosed, the aneurysmal walls were strengthened by the fibroblastic response to the thermal effect of argon laser photoradiation. Glasscock et al. [28] used argon laser to remove acoustic tumors and found it helpful despite the very low power available for vaporizing tumor tissue. Initially, the microscope adapter for the argon laser was very bulky and cumbersome to use and to sterilize, and the authors recommended some changes for using this laser with the microscope routinely. Fasano [29] reported the clinical use of this laser for the management of cerebral aneurysm and vascular malformations. Boggan et al. [30] compared the brain tissue response in rats to injury by argon and carbon dioxide lasers in an attempt to quantify the relative merits of each wavelength laser. They concluded that there was no significant difference in the overall brain tissue response to injury by the argon laser or the CO_2 laser, although the argon laser appeared to be more gentle.

Following this study, the same group used the argon laser in a large number of patients with a variety of neurosurgical lesions [31,32] and found it to be particularly helpful in the removal of small vascular tumors such as hemangioblastoma and small arteriovenous malformations, acoustic schwannomas, and small (< 2.5 mm diameter) extra- and intra-axial CNS tumors.

There are several new wavelength lasers that have been recently introduced into neurosurgery. The longer wavelengths neodymium:YAG lasers with wavelengths of 1.32 μm [33,34] and 1.44 μm [35] reportedly have comparable effects on nervous tissue to CO_2 laser. The potential advantages of these lasers are the increased absorption coefficient of water for wavelengths longer than 1.3 μm, thus likening the tissue effects of laser beam impact by these lasers to the carbon dioxide laser and the fact that these wavelength lasers can have the laser beam transmitted through quartz optical fibers, which increases the laser's maneuverability by the neurosurgeon.

The potassium titanyl phosphate (KTP) laser, also referred to as the frequency doubled Nd: YAG laser, has a wavelength of 532 nm. It was initially developed to be a second-generation laser to the argon ion laser. Preliminary clinical experience with the KTP laser is anecdotal. Gamache et al. [36] studied the histopathological findings of the KTP laser and the CO_2 laser-induced lesions on canine brain and spinal cord and found both the lasers comparable in terms of tissue penetration and tissue absorption. In addition, the KTP laser is more hemostatic than the CO_2 laser. Although the KTP laser was reported to have laser-tissue interactions similar to those of the argon laser [37], in the senior author's experience (unreported findings), the KTP laser, because of its longer wavelength, tends to be more scattered and less readily absorbed in myelinated nervous tissue, resulting in a larger volume of tissue injury than the argon laser for similar power and energy doses. It has been stated that the KTP laser is less pigment-dependent than the argon laser [36]; however, the opposite would be expected based upon wavelength characteristics of the two different lasers.

Experimental work is going on at some centers with the holmium-doped YAG laser, which has a wavelength of 2.15 μm. This wavelength laser has an intense water absorption peak and is being tested for laser discectomy since the nucleus pulposus is mainly comprised of water [38,39].

OPERATIVE TECHNIQUES

Because discrete volumes of tissue may be coagulated or vaporized without mechanical manipulation, damage to the surrounding normal tissues may be less when using lasers than with standard tissue removing techniques. When tumors are large or can be easily aspirated, the only advantage of laser use may be in obtaining hemostasis during or after tumor removal or in the removal of critically located tumor remnants, i.e., meningioma attached to and invading the dura propria of the optic nerve. Since the heat effect of the laser beam sterilizes as it vaporizes, it may be used advantageously in the removal and debridement of infected tissue [11,40].

Moist cottonoids are used to cover normal tissues surrounding the abnormal tissue to be irradiated with the laser. This precaution is taken to prevent (1) damage to normal structures due to reflection of the laser beam off instruments, (2) inadvertent irradiation, or (3) damage from hot gases created by vaporization of tissue. Evacuation of hot vapors by strong suction applied very near the area of active vaporization of tissue, and cooling of adjacent tissues by frequent irrigation, are two other methods of protecting normal tissue.

Extra Axial Lesions

Use of the laser for resection of extra-axial tumors entails a standard operative approach to the lesion, although exposure is usually limited to uncovering a "safe area" where tumor removal can be initiated. If significant retraction of normal tissue is not required, an arachnoidal plane is first developed and maintained with moist small cotton sponges to isolate the lesion from normal brain, spinal cord, nerves, and blood vessels. The tumor capsule is then coagulated using a low power density broad beam. This maneuver coagulates superficial feeding vessels and initiates tumor retraction from surrounding structures. Shrinkage of the laser-treated tissue occurs as a consequence of thermally induced tissue dehydration and contraction of heat-denatured proteins. After coagulation of the exposed tumor capsule, debulking of the tumor is performed by intracapsular vaporization of the tumor using a large spot size and high-power output, or by piecemeal removal of tumor using the focused laser to excise wedges of tumor (smallest laser spot size and a high power). Both techniques avoid significant manipulation of neural structures during tumor removal. Low power is used at first and then power is gradually increased as an appreciation of the tumor vascularity, consistency, and response to the laser energy is obtained.

During the vaporization of tumor, a suction device is the only other instrument necessary in the operative field. Thus visualization is improved and the need to retract delicate structures is decreased. The suction device is used to evacuate smoke and keep the field free of pooled blood. When tissue is removed by vaporization, the laser usually causes coagulation of bleeding vessels. After intracapsular debulking, a moderate power density beam in short pulses is used to shrink and ablate residual tumor capsule. Short pulses (<0.5 sec) tend to prevent significant intratissue spread of laser-induced heating or deep penetration of the laser beam and should be used when resecting tumor attached to important structures, located within the brainstem or spinal cord. With a focused laser beam, low continuous power output (1–3 watts), and short duration pulses (0.1–0.5 s), tumor can be sequentially shaved off individual nerve roots and vessels without thermal or traction injury that might interfere with their function. Residual attachments to or invasion of the dura can be thermally denatured by gentle application of low-power laser energy without destroying dural integrity. However, one must be careful if irradiating dura near foramina or that surrounds the cranial nerves. Extensions of meningiomas through venous sinus walls can be denatured with the Nd:YAG laser without opening the vessel wall. The rate of tumor recurrence with these techniques seems to be equal to that observed following radical removal of the dural attachment.

Meningioma

Roux et al. [41] reported on 17 meningiomas (13 supratentorial, 4 infratentorial) they removed using the combination of CO_2 and Nd:YAG laser. They found that the quality of hemostasis was associated with a very good vaporization and cutting effect when the combined laser was used, but they did not discuss outcome, especially long term. Lombard et al. [42] studied a series of 198 gliomas and 200 meningiomas operated upon either with a laser or with conventional techniques. The authors considered postoperative morbidity and the duration and quality of survival in their analysis. Concerning meningiomas, patients of both groups treated with and without the laser were clinically improved after operation, but meningiomas located in eloquent brain and operated with a laser had significantly better outcome. There is, however, no information available regarding the recurrence of these tumors over the long term. Desgeorges et al. [43] reported on 164 meningiomas treated over a 6-year period with the laser, of various intracranial and spinal locations. Eighty-two (50%) tumors were located in the posterior fossa and 36 were suprasellar or parasellar meningiomas. A CO_2 laser was used in 56 cases, a frequency doubled wavelength YAG laser in 101 cases, and simultaneous CO_2 and Nd:YAG combolaser in seven cases. Complete tumor removal was accomplished in 83% of cases and

overall mortality was 3%, leading the authors to conclude that microscope-guided laser techniques represent a significant advancement in the ability to remove deep seated meningiomas that might prove difficult to extirpate by conventional microsurgery. The obvious advantages of laser microsurgery for removal of meningiomas include: reduced brain retraction, ability to operate through narrower exposures, reduced amount of mechanical manipulation, vaporization and coagulation of the dural attachment of the tumor, improved operative precision, and decreased intraoperative blood loss.

Kopera et al. [44] reported the use of Nd:YAG laser in 63 cases of intracranial tumors, including 32 meningiomas. In 76.2% of cases, very good results were obtained. The Nd:YAG laser was found to be particularly helpful in the treatment of vascular meningiomas wherein the Nd:YAG laser was used to shrink and devascularize the tumors. The authors cited the reduction of mechanical trauma, reduction of blood loss, and more radical removal of tumor as the major advantages of the Nd:YAG laser. Again, long-term outcome was not mentioned in this report.

Conforti et al. [45] reviewed a series of 78 intracranial meningiomas, 68 suprasellar and 10 intraventricular, operated microsurgically. They opined that the mortality and morbidity in parasellar meningiomas are dependent upon the experience of the surgeon and are not influenced by the use of a laser or an ultrasonic aspirator. Naumann and Meixensberger [46] studied the factors affecting meningioma recurrence rate in a retrospective review of 23 recurrent meningiomas initially operated between 1983 and 1989. All tumors were removed microsurgically with the aid of the ultrasonic aspirator and the Nd:YAG laser. The authors found longer recurrence-free intervals after complete tumor removal (Simpson's grade I or II) than after subtotal tumor excision (Simpson's grade III or IV), but this tendency was not statistically significant. In this series, histomorphological criteria and grading of tumor extent at surgery did not correlate with predictions of the biological behavior of recurrent meningiomas. They concluded that laser use may help in obtaining a more complete removal and contribute to a longer recurrence-free interval.

Frontobasal meningiomas because of their location under the frontal lobes often grow to a large size (> 5 cm in diameter) before becoming symptomatic and diagnosed. These tumors are usually quite fibrous and vascularized and some are heavily calcified. In addition, as the meningioma grows into the suprasellar cistern, it may encase important structures such as the internal carotid, anterior and middle cerebral arteries and tiny perforating arteries to the hypothalamus, the optic nerves, and the optic chiasm.

Waidhauser et al. [47] studied the use of Nd:YAG laser in the microsurgery of frontobasal meningiomas. The goal of the study was to achieve a grade II resection of each meningioma by using the Nd:YAG laser in addition to bipolar coagulation. Forty-three patients with olfactory meningiomas removed microsurgically with the 1.32 μ Nd:YAG laser (histologically malignant meningiomas were excluded) were followed up for 5 years. A Simpson's grade II resection was achieved in 37 operations, grade IV in five, and grade V in one patient. Two patients died within a month of surgery, for an operative mortality of 4.6%. Average blood loss was reduced to a liter and less than two units were transfused per procedure due to the coagulation of the well-vascularized tumor surface and coagulation and closure of small vascular channels in dural and bony tumor attachment in the floor of the frontal fossa. There were no tumor recurrences during the 5 years of follow-up in the 37 patients with a grade II removal using the Nd:YAG laser to coagulate the tumor attachments. Tumor progression after grade IV resection was as frequent as reported by others. The authors concluded that 1.32 μ Nd:YAG laser radiation is the treatment of choice for dural and bony attachments of meningiomas, when these structures cannot be removed.

Acoustic Neuroma

Acoustic tumor surgery has evolved significantly with the advent of microsurgery. Given the reduced morbidity and mortality of surgery, the aim of surgery has focused on preservation of cranial nerve function especially facial nerve function. The CO_2, argon and KTP microsurgical lasers are extremely effective for removing acoustic neuromas, particularly vascular tumors [32,48, 49]. For avascular tumors, laser vaporization can be used to minimize blunt trauma from surgical manipulation when neoplasms are fibrous and noncystic. When a small remnant of infiltrating tumor is markedly adherent to facial nerve or brainstem, laser vaporization can help devascularize any residual tumor and reduce the risk of recurrence. Cool, intermittent irrigation with continuous suction of the laser plume is essential to reduce thermal injury to normal structures.

With intraoperative monitoring, early heating of the facial nerve can be identified by a widening of the EMG baseline as visualized on a monitor. Eiras et al. [50] compared their results following CO_2 microsurgical laser removal of 12 giant acoustic neurinomas with a historical control group of 12 similar cases operated on with only conventional microsurgical techniques. The authors used pre- and intraoperative evoked potentials. The parameters that were compared included mortality, facial nerve preservation, duration of surgery, hospitalization, and recovery. Although the duration of surgery was longer for patients whose tumors were removed with the aid of the CO_2 laser, all other parameters improved with the use of laser. On the contrary, others have found that the CO_2 laser is of limited benefit to them for removing acoustic neuromas [51]. However, most authors agree that CO_2 microsurgery is very helpful adjunct to removal of acoustic neuromas.

Roux et al. [41] reported operating on one patient with acoustic tumor and found the combolaser (CO_2 + 1.06 Nd:YAG) very helpful. Majchrzak et al. [52] have used Nd:YAG laser in a 13-year-old girl with a large, richly vascularized acoustic neurinoma. The application of Nd:YAG laser during the operation reduced bleeding and enabled radical removal of the tumor. However, in another report [44] by the same authors that reviewed the use of Nd:YAG laser in 63 intracranial tumors, of which there were eight acoustic neuromas, the Nd:YAG laser was not deemed helpful unless the tumor was vascular.

Transsphenoidal Laser Microsurgery

Although the morbidity of pituitary surgery has been reduced with conventional transsphenoidal microsurgery, the complete excision of macroadenomas is often not possible. Radiation has been helpful in delaying recurrent growth from residual tumors but has potential side effects. Surgical techniques that improve tumor removal and relieve hormonal hypersecretion are therefore needed in dealing with pituitary adenomas. The laser has been helpful in our experience in dealing with the recurrent, fibrotic, and previously irradiated tumors.

The typical soft or necrotic adenoma/microadenoma can be treated adequately by conventional techniques. However, the laser can vaporize tissue at the periphery of the tumor bed, which may contain residual tumor cells and may improve the cure rate for these lesions.

Oekler et al. [53] reported the use of Nd:YAG laser in 15 cases of pituitary adenomas approached transsphenoidally. The sellar floor was irradiated with the laser prior to opening it in order to arrest bleeding from the capsule. The adenoma was then removed using curettes in a conventional manner. Bleeding was then controlled with the laser irradiating "the basal capsule parts as well as the lateral walls" of the sella. The authors felt that they achieved a more radical removal and "inactivation" of tumor with improved hemostasis compared to that with conventional techniques. They reported no impairment in anterior pituitary functions compared to the preoperative condition and the same incidence of postoperative diabetes insipidus as with conventional surgery. There was an improvement in vision in six out of seven patients presenting with a chiasmal syndrome. The other patient's vision was unchanged. The absence of detectable damage to adjacent structures is remarkable because of the high degree of scattering upon impact of this laser with tissue.

Heiss et al. [54] have been reluctant to use the Nd:YAG laser in transsphenoidal surgery because of the several mm zone of thermal coagulation and necrosis that results from scattering. In addition, the laser radiation is transmitted through CSF, and hence the optic nerves and the chiasm are at a greater risk of being damaged by the transmitted laser energy. Excellent results were obtained by these authors as a result of the laser being used only in the beginning and in the end of the procedure. The amount of thermal injury is also limited by limiting the time of laser application. Another important factor was the use of the laser to treat only the basal capsule and the lateral aspects of the sella but not the suprasellar area. This reduces the risk of visual impairment.

Powers et al. [32] reported using the argon laser to resect a large recurrent fibrous prolactinoma with modest suprasellar extension that could not be aspirated; it was excised through a transsphenoidal approach. The argon laser was used to cut through the bone of the sellar floor, to open the dura, and to coagulate and vaporize the tumor. Complete removal was done without the use of multiple instruments, although this procedure could have been done with routine methods. The direct visualization of the laser beam with the argon laser makes it more precise than the CO_2 laser, which requires a separate aiming beam. Other advantages were smaller spot size and improved coagulative properties. Disadvantages were transmittance of the beam through CSF and a maximal power output of 20 watts. The argon laser was judged to be very helpful in two out of the three pituitary adenomas as the surgical result was better than what could be expected from standard microsurgical techniques. But in the tumor that was approached through the transsphenoidal route, the surgical result was judged to be the same as using the conventional technique. It is the authors' opinion that the role of microsurgical lasers for the removal of most pituitary tumors via a transsphenoidal approach is limited and that most tumors are best treated using conventional microsurgical technique.

Skull Base Tumors

The carbon dioxide laser used to play a critical role in the extirpation of benign tumors at the base of the brain, where deep exposures and location of critical neural and vascular structures rendered these lesions inaccessible, and removal with other methods had been associated with unacceptable morbidity and mortality. The laser has a role to play even after recent changes in our approach to the surgery of the skull base that emphasizes large surgical exposures and in some cases en bloc tumor removal. Tew and Tobler [55] reviewed their experience with 50 basal meningiomas and two chordomas that were operated using laser. They found that the primary benefits of the CO_2 laser are the availability of high power for tissue ablation, no-touch vaporization with less visual interference, minimal brain retraction or manipulation, excellent capillary hemostasis, and precise microscopic control.

Dural attachment was safely and completely vaporized with a low wattage defocussed beam (5–10 watts). Dural attachments at the entrance of the optic canal can be vaporized without damage to the optic nerves. One must clearly protect against spreading thermal damage, however, by using frequent irrigation and low powers. There is no clinical method to measure the potential or threshold of heat damage to nearby cranial nerves or brainstem by laser generated heat in a tumor bed. For a fibrotic or calcified lesion, carbon dioxide laser was found to be better than mechanical removal or with ultrasonic aspiration. Recognition of tumor encasement and proper identification of these vessels with microdissection are crucial. The risk of perforating an encased vessel with the laser can be sudden and devastating. This is clearly an added risk and vigilance is necessary to prevent vascular injury under these circumstances.

Intra-Axial Lesions

In the approach to intra-axial tumors, the surgeon can use the laser to make the corticotomy or myelotomy required to expose the lesion. Otherwise, standard microsurgery techniques and those outlined for the use of lasers on extra-axial tumors are employed. Taking advantage of the precise and relatively hemostatic ablation of tissue possible with the carbon dioxide laser, Kelly and colleagues [56–66] have incorporated it into a computer-assisted, three-dimensional stereotactic system for the resection of intra-axial neoplasms. This system allows the surgeon to make a stereotactic approach to deep-seated brain tumors and to resect them layer by layer with the aid of a computer-generated, two- dimensional reconstructed virtual image of the tumor that corresponds to the planar dimensions of the tumor perpendicular to the view line of the surgeon for the depth of focus for the operating microscope. The virtual image is projected back through the microscope eyepieces to the operator and aids the surgeon in defining the tumor boundaries for directing the laser beam.

Walker et al. [67] and others [32,68,69] vaporized tumors located in the brainstem as another example of the precise ablation of intra-axial neoplasms possible with the laser. Due to the biological aggressiveness and infiltrative characteristics of most glial neoplasms, which make up the majority of intra-axial neoplasms treated in practice, the overall long-term outcome results in these patients have not been significantly altered by the addition of lasers. In removing intra-axial lesions and obtaining postresection hemostasis in the tumor bed using lasers, the surgeon must take care not to leave heavily charred carbonaceous material. These charred tissue remnants may induce a inflammatory response that can cause postoperative edema or sterile abscess formation.

Intramedullary Tumor

The introduction of the operating microscope and refinement of the microsurgical techniques in the late 1960s and 1970s advanced surgery for intramedullary tumors, but aggressive removal of astrocytomas had to await the introduction of the ultrasonic surgical aspirator and the laser that allow tumor removal without undue traction or manipulation of the spinal cord. Radical removal of intramedullary spinal cord tumors has been accomplished with minimal morbidity to the patient by using carbon dioxide and argon lasers [15,31, 32,68,70–73]. A myelotomy is made with the laser using the smallest focused laser beam possible at a power of 3–5 watts in a continuous or intermittent mode. Lateral retraction applied to the edge of the myelotomy by means of pial retraction sutures minimizes damage to nerve fiber tracts that may result from heat damage along the incision edge due to their tendency to contract and migrate into the line of laser vaporization. After placing pial retraction sutures at the edges of the dorsal myelotomy, further manipulation of the cord is not necessary. Laser is used to vaporize and dissect the tumor by using the tumor edge coagulation technique. The CO_2 laser set at a low power, between 5 and 8 watts, has been valuable for removing the last remnants of obvious tumor. In patients with tumor that is subtotally resected, it is difficult to establish a tumor spinal cord interface either because of the infiltrative nature of the tumor or because the coagulation technique does not initiate formation of a tumor pseudocapsule. In these instances, excision is accomplished by vaporization alone. Somatosensory evoked potentials monitored during the operation on the intramedullary tumors have not shown amplitude or latency changes as a result of this technique. This is extremely important as it is known that in the immediate postoperative period following surgery for intramedullary tumor, most patients have worsened or new neurological deficits, particularly involving the posterior columns [74–76], may progress during the first 24 hours after surgery. Significant functional deterioration with gradual improvement is reported in 33% of cases [77]. Permanent refractory neurologic worsening is seen in < 5% of the patients [74]. Worsening may be due to direct surgical or vascular injury, the latter occurring especially with ependymomas, whose blood supply is derived from the anterior spinal artery.

Another important issue, particularly now that radical resection of intramedullary astrocytomas is feasible, is whether the extent of resection correlates with prognosis. A number of studies suggest that there is a survival advantage to more extensive resections compared with biopsy, whether or not adjuvant therapy is given [78–80]. Others, however, have indicated no such correlation [81]. The only large series of radical "gross total" resections of intramedullary astrocytomas during the era of laser microsurgery is that of Epstein [82], and the duration of follow-up is still relatively short. Recently, Epstein and Farmer [74] reported the long-term results in 73 patients with an average follow-up of 4 years. Progressive disease was seen in 10% of cases. Hence, use of lasers in intramedullary surgery helps the surgeon to resect the tumor radically with the least mechanical trauma to the already thinned out spinal cord and sets the stage for good prognosis.

Over the past 15 years, operative treatment for spinal lipomas and lipomyelomeningoceles has become standard due to accumulated experience in the literature with these difficult lesions [83–86]. In the case of lipomyelomeningocele, or a lipoma occurring as a part of occult spinal dysraphism, the goal of treatment is to release (untether) the conus medullaris from the mechanical constraint that the lipoma presents. Commonly, the lipoma has a substantial interface with the spinal cord and nerve roots of the cauda equina are intimately related to the mass. The interface between lipoma and conus is both extensive and poorly demarcated with gradual merging of neural and fibrolipomatous elements. In some cases of spinal lipoma, the large volume of fat may present a technical problem and it may produce neurologic deficits due to mass effect [87]. During operative dissection, it also obscures normal anatomic structures and represents an unacceptable bulk of tissue to be left in the spinal canal after untethering. The CO_2 laser is quite helpful for expeditious removal of fat. Maira et al. [88] used CO_2 laser to radically remove large spinal lipomas in two adult patients without any additional neural damage or complications. These patients were previously operated on by the same surgeon with conventional microsurgical techniques for partial excision. After CO_2 laser surgery both patients had significant improvement in neurological function at last follow-up at 24 and 36 months, respectively. McLone and Naidich [73] assessed the value of laser resection in 50 consecutive cases of pediatric spinal lipoma. There was no mortality or an increase in neurological or urological deficit. Use of the CO_2 laser reduced the length of operation, the intraoperative blood loss, and the degree of manipulation of the spinal cord and nerve roots. Most of the fat could be removed successfully from the liponeural junction, permitting more nearly anatomical removal of the intramedullary component of the lesion and greater ease in replacing the cord into a reconstructed arachnoid-dural canal. Postoperatively, 8 of 20 (40%) patients with prior motor deficit had substantially improved motor function. Two of 17 (12%) previously incontinent patients became continent of urine. One must use the laser with caution when there are functionally important neural elements within the fatty mass. This can occur with lipomas where the conus-lipoma interface is sufficiently rostral, i.e., above the lumbosacral junction [89]. A less radical resection is not a concern in intramedullary lipomas as improvement of neurological function has been noted with spinal cord decompression alone [87,90].

Arteriovenous Malformations—Cranial and Spinal

In the operative management of arteriovenous malformations (AVMs), all three lasers may be helpful in defining the plane between the malformation and normal brain, but the Nd:YAG laser is superior for coagulating delicate feeders, for coagulating dural components, and for achieving hemostasis. Beam power densities of 350–2,000 watts/cm² delivered by intermittent <5-s exposures are most helpful. The Nd:YAG laser was first used as an adjunct in the treatment of AVMs by Beck in 1980, when he successfully coagulated feeding vessels [24]. Fasano et al. [29,72,91] reported three AVMs completely extirpated with Nd:YAG laser and concluded that the laser allows extirpation of AVM with reduced blood loss and minimal manipulation of normal brain. Wharen et al. [92] reported ten AVMs that were resected with the Nd:YAG laser as an adjunct and concluded that the use of laser in AVM surgery has significant limitations. Van Loveren et al. [93] used the Nd:YAG laser to remove 14 thalamic AVMs with an overall morbidity of 15% and no mortality. There was no complication attributable to the use of laser.

Zuccarello et al. [94] excised ten arteriovenous malformations safely with no morbidity or increased neurological deficits attributable to the laser technique. Histological examination of the specimens after treatment with the Nd:YAG laser revealed that the most prominent effect of the laser was shrinkage of the collagen of the vessels of the AVM, which led to laser-induced narrowing of blood vessels.

Powers et al. [32] used argon laser for removing two arteriovenous malformations. They found that the argon laser was helpful in low-flow AVM that was composed of small-caliber blood vessels, but it was not helpful in the removal of a large, high-flow AVM. They concluded that this may be due to the transfer of heat away from the site of coagulation by the high blood flow. Roux et al. [33] reported similar findings with the use of 1.32 μm YAG laser for excising a large temporal AVM and had to use electric coagulation and 1.06 μm YAG laser to achieve hemostasis.

Spinal dural arteriovenous malformations (AVMs) are the most common type of AVM involving the spinal cord in adults. Direct obliteration of the fistula nidus located in the dura either by endovascular embolization or surgery is the preferred method of treatment. Strugar and Chyatte [95] reported five cases of spinal dural AVM treated by open surgical exposure, microsurgical disconnection of the dural nidus from the coronal venous plexus, and in situ obliteration of the nidus using the Nd:YAG laser. All patients improved neurologically following surgery, and complete obliteration of all lesions was verified by delayed angiography. There were no permanent complications related to either the surgical exposure or the use of the Nd:YAG laser. Open surgical treatment of spinal dural AVMs using the Nd:YAG laser appears to be a safe, effective, and durable alternative to extensive dural resections and its associated problems.

LASER INTERSTITIAL THERMOTHERAPY

From ancient times to the present, those in medicine have dreamed of utilizing hyperthermia or elevated temperature in the treatment of malignant tumors. The quest for a safe and efficient thermotherapy system was given great impetus by the anecdotal reports of nineteenth-century physicians who observed spontaneous regression of tumors in the wake of systemic fever or infection [96]. This desire has been consistently frustrated by technological limitations on our ability to deliver heat deep within the body in such a way that normal surrounding structures remain unharmed.

Heat is a physical agent, and its biological effects are related to both the intensity and the duration of application. The minimal amount of time required to produce irreversible cell damage at a given temperature has been termed the "thermal death time." A wide variety of neoplasms have been shown to be sensitive to damage from temperatures in excess of 40°C given over variable periods of time. In a number of naturally occurring human tumors and in a variety of transplantable rabbit and rodent tumors, approximately the same biological effect is achieved by halving the exposure time for each additional degree of temperature elevation above 42°C. Above 44°C, the thermal sensitivity of normal cells rapidly approaches that of neoplastic cells,

hence the need either to restrict the field of thermal irradiation to abnormal tissues only or to use temperatures in the range of 42–43°C. As the antineoplastic effect of hyperthermia becomes manifest at 42°C and metabolic damage to hepatocytes and neurons is well documented at 43°C, the therapeutic index of hyperthermia is quite narrow. In both normal and neoplastic cells, the deoxyribonucleic acid synthetic portion of the cell cycle (S phase) seems to be relatively more selectively heat-sensitive, whereas just the opposite is true for ionizing radiation [97].

In addition to the cellular effects, hyperthermia affects the electrical activity and the metabolic status. There is evidence that the damage occurs at the mitochondrial level, where inhibition of electron transport, loss of respiratory control, and uncoupling of phosphorylation between temperatures of 41°C–44°C. Indirect metabolic effects of hyperthermia on the brain are possible via an alteration in the blood–brain barrier. The effects are not immediately apparent to the eye but rather usually require at least 24 hours to develop into necrosis. The thermal energy causes denaturation and irreversible aggregation of macromolecules within the cell, which affects the metabolic machinery. Consequently, there is eventual cell death. The alterations in the electrical activity can be monitored during the application of hyperthermia to the tissue by means of EEG or evoked potentials. To provide a basis for the underlying tissue alterations, Schrober et al. [98] have analyzed the spatial and temporal patterns of interstitial hyperthermia lesions in the normal rat brain by histological, immunohistochemical, and electron microscopical methods. The acute changes corresponded to the temperature gradient surrounding the laser probe and showed a distinct zonal architecture. Membrane destruction on a cellular and subcellular level appears to be of major significance in the pathogenesis of the laser lesion. The tissue reaction followed the course known for coagulation necrosis and resulted in a well-defined defect. These results, although limited by the choice of the experimental model, may be helpful in the interpretation of images obtained in future applications of interstitial thermotherapy.

Glioblastoma multiforme is an inhomogenous tumor composed of multiple cellular compartments in which a distribution of diverse metabolic, kinetic, vascular, and genetic properties coexist. The greater part of the tumor mass is comprised of relatively undervascularized, under-oxygenated, metabolically quiescent, and resting G_0 cells (tissue conditions that are inimical to the efficacy of ionizing radiation and chemotherapy). As already discussed, the cellular and anti-neoplastic effects of hyperthermia are relatively independent of cell cycle and metabolic consider-ations. Furthermore, these effects of hyperther-mia are potentiated by hypoxia and inadequate tissue cooling because blood flow within the tu-mor is slower than in surrounding normal tissues as a rule, thereby creating a "heat-sink" of poorly dissipated energy. Hence there is a great poten-tial for hyperthermia as a component in the over-all treatment of glioblastoma. Unlike other treat-ment modalities, there does not seem to be any cumulative toxicity from hyperthermia, and its use on a repetitive basis, throughout the course of the disease and especially later when the tumor is relatively small, can be easily envisioned [97].

Potentiation between hyperthermia and che-motherapy has been well demonstrated in model tumors and possibly in humans. The safety and feasibility of both small and large field heating in the human brain has been demonstrated by at least three different techniques. Due to technolog-ical limitations on our ability to deliver heat safely and selectively to the brain, this theoretical rationale remains supported by relatively little experimental and clinical data.

Hyperthermia has been produced by several different means, which include immersion of the tumorous area into a hot water bath, perfusion of tumor-bearing tissues with heated solutions, fo-cused ultrasound, internal, or external micro-wave antennae, and electromagnetic heat gener-ators. The Nd:YAG laser has been used recently as a thermal source for hyperthermic treatment of intracerebral tumors [99–101]. It is necessary to restrict high thermal elevations (over 44°C) to the central tumor nidus and to limit the temperature elevations between 42°C and 43°C in the adjacent tumor-invaded brain. Conical-shaped, sapphire-tipped optical fibers have been designed to pro-duce a point source of emission for Nd:YAG laser energy when implanted into tissue. These can be positioned at different targets within the tumor tissue using stereotactic techniques [100]. There is an exponential falloff of temperature with dis-tance from the optical fiber tip in tissue that is similar to that seen with other point source forms of tissue heating [102]. Hyperthermia is an at-tractive technique if the extent of thermal dam-age of tumor and surrounding brain can be con-trolled. However, the physician is committed to

heating a geometric volume of tissue that may contain normal and abnormal tissue as well as varying degrees of necrotic central tissue (making uniform intratumoral heating difficult) and yet may not contain an extension of tumor tissue be-yond the volume of heating.

Real-time thermal analysis of the treated tissue volume is needed to better control and op-timize thermal surgery. One of the solutions to the central problem in thermal surgery of inter-active control of the heat zone might be the use of using image guidance. Jolesz [101] from Boston has reported that temperature changes can be fol-lowed as signal changes on magnetic resonance imaging (MRI). Fan et al. [103] studied the tem-perature distribution of interstitial laser thermo-therapy (ILTT) using implanted optical fibers in human cadaver brains to provide the necessary data for clinical application of ILTT and to find the correlation between the temperature and MRI signal intensity and explore the possibility of us-ing MRI as a noninvasive temperature-monitor-ing method. The authors have determined the re-lationship between the MRI signal intensity and real temperature according to the relationship be-tween T_1 and the temperature from their experi-ments, which is useful for the clinical application of ILTT. However, they found one major problem. MR imaging can reveal absolute temperature only in special cases (e.g., in a sample that is iso-thermal, is in a steady state, and has a known composition). There is a presence of hysteresis in the T_1 or T_2 weighted signals versus temperature in complex tissue. Furthermore, the relationship between T_1, and the temperature is complicated, mainly due to the multifactional nature of T_1, and accurate measurements of T_1 are not easy to make because of a high environmental sensitiv-ity, dominated by the effects of radiofrequency field inhomogeneities in the imaged volume. So, the applicability of this technique may be limited because a 1% change must be measured in order to detect a 1°C change in temperature.

Wyman et al. [104] have conducted a study to determine the accuracy and reliability of pro-ton spin-echo MR images of ILTT lesions in nor-mal brain. Both T_1 weighted and T_2 weighted im-ages of ILTT lesions induced by a continuous wave Nd:YAG laser in normal cat brain were cor-related with the actual lesions assessed histo-pathologically at 2, 5, and 14 days post-ILTT. An enhancing halo on gadolinium enhanced T_1 weighted images acquired immediately post-ILTT corresponded to the boundary of the total lesion at

48 hours. The results suggested that MR images acquired during ILTT can underestimate greatly the actual resulting necrotic lesion. The authors concluded that before fast MR imaging is used to monitor ILTT in the treatment of brain tumors, a study similar to the one described here should be conducted. All these studies are based on 2D heat flow calculated numerically to predict the temperature for a radially symmetric heat source. However, the 3D heat flow is required to estimate the lesion shape. Cline et al. [105] have developed a 3D thermal model to control thermal surgery that uses an elongated elliptical Gaussian heat source. Focused ultrasound heating of gel phantoms, bovine muscle, and in vivo rabbit were monitored with MRI imaging to give temperature profiles needed for thermal surgery. Determination of the temperature distribution using MRI molecular diffusion image sequences has recently been proposed and is undergoing investigation, because there is a direct relationship between temperature and molecular diffusion, which is more sensitive than using T_1-weighted MR images.

Clinical application of laser interstitial thermotherapy had to await the development of contact probes for tissue heating purposes, the use of MR to monitor temperature changes and adaptation of the instruments to make them MR compatible. So far, clinical use has been limited to a few specific cases, and reports of this technique are anecdotal.

Ascher et al. [106] treated so-called inoperable low-grade gliomas in the brainstem by stereotactic puncture, introduction of a laser fiber into the center of the tumor, and then delivering heat energy from a Nd:YAG laser to the tumor under real-time MRI control. They found that the cell structure is mostly preserved; low grade gliomas are converted to gliosis, whereas high grade gliomas tend to liquify. There is no mention of the length of follow-up or biopsy of the lesion or results of thermal surgery. Sugiyama et al. [100] studied laser hyperthermia using Nd:YAG laser both experimentally and clinically to treat deepseated brain tumors. In the clinical study, five patients with brain tumors were treated with laser hyperthermia using a computerized tomography-stereotactic technique. All tumors disappeared on computed tomography, and at the time of reporting three of the five patients were still alive without recurrence. It was possible to make an optimal lesion and to have accurate peripheral temperature control by using the combination of the Komai stereotactic method and the Nd:YAG

laser system. They concluded that interstitial laser hyperthermia using this method is easy and safe to use and is beneficial in the treatment of deep-seated brain tumors.

Bettag et al. [107] performed experimental studies on rat brains and found typical laser-tissue effects with central necrosis and a sharply demarcated zone of edema extending out into the normal brain. The size of the lesion depended upon the energy and exposure time applied. In a pilot series, they treated five patients with malignant cerebral gliomas (WHO grade II-III) in functionally important regions and monitored the therapeutic effects by MR imaging and position emission tomography (PET) scan. Early postoperative results showed irreversible edematous changes at the tumor margin. The PET scans showed sharply circumscribed activity defects consistent with tissue necrosis after laser-induced thermotherapy. This suggested that PET scanning during ILTT could serve as a cross-check method to interpret the MRI data.

Roux et al. [108] reported on their experience with six patients of which four had low grade gliomas in the region of the third ventricle, one had metastatic melanoma, and one a recurrent pituitary adenoma. Laser heat effects were monitored with MRI controls (5 hours, 24 hours, 8 days, then monthly). There was no mortality. One patient worsened transiently, and all remained in the same neurological state. Currently, ILTT remains experimental and its role in the treatment of brain tumors is purely speculative.

LASER TISSUE WELDING

Suturing works quite well for tissue joining in most surgical applications. Nonetheless, sutures are at the root of many complications in closure and anastomosis. Scarring, stenosis, aneurysm formation, and fluid leakage are all attributable to the trauma of suturing and the foreign body response to suture material. Alternatives to sutures include staples, mechanical coupling devices, glues—biological and nonbiological (cyanoacrylates), and laser tissue welding.

Laser-assisted microvascular anastomosis (LAVA) and laser-assisted nerve repair (LANA) have been achieved with all commonly available medical lasers [22,109,110]. Advantages of laser welding for microvascular anastomosis or nerve repair include greater ease and speed, faster healing, less myointimal hyperplasia, less scarring and foreign body reaction, and the ability of the repair to grow. Disadvantages include much lower initial tensile and bursting pressure strength, thermal injury to the tissues, aneurysmal development at the site of anastomosis, and the cost and complexity of the laser itself. Stay sutures to acquire precise coaptation obviate potential advantages of the laser welding. For these reasons the clinical application of laser welding has been minimal.

For laser welding to become a reasonable alternative to suture technique, the initial bond strength must be strong enough to prevent disruption under normal stresses, excessive thermal damage should be avoided, and reliance on stay sutures should be abandoned. Laser welding was originally performed using hand-held application of laser energy with a clinically observable endpoint, tissue shrinkage. The crude nature of the technique was responsible for many of the disadvantages observed. By more carefully defining the necessary conditions for the welding process to occur, and by more precisely controlling the delivery of laser energy, laser welding has been improved. Some of the improvements are noted below.

Computer control. One approach is to use a computer to control the laser settings. A database is generated for each tissue type and thickness based on experimentation correlating weld strength and tissue injury with power density and exposure duration. Optimum power densities are selected for each tissue type and thickness.

One such system uses a 1.32 nm Nd:YAG laser for its relatively deep tissue penetration, which allows uniform tissue exposure at thicknesses clinically encountered and regardless of a wet or bloody operative field [111]. In this way the surgeon can never damage the tissue by exposure to too high a power density or too long a pulse. The surgeon must still ensure that the entire repair is complete without gapping, which might create leaks. Issues of coaptation and cost remain.

Laser soldering. An approach to improve the weld strength involves the application of a tissue solder to the anastomotic site prior to laser exposure. Such "laser soldering" has the potential to enhance weld strength significantly while reducing thermal injury since the solder acts as a heat sink. Demands for precise coaptation are also somewhat reduced. Early animal studies in microvascular anastomosis showed that the burst strengths comparable to suture repair could be obtained (Fig. 1) [112]. Additional studies demon-

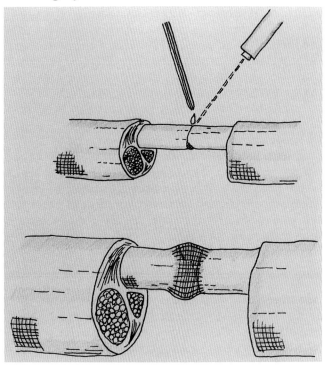

Fig. 1. Schematic illustration of interfascicular laser nerve repair using blood as a soldering agent.

strated that leakage pressure after laser soldering often exceeded that of suture repair [113]. This watertight nature of the laser weld can be used to reinforce suture repairs where water tightness would be critical to the success of the anastomosis.

Early solders included fibrinogen and egg albumin. These fell out of favor for the following reasons: handling properties were not ideal, short shelf life, risk of blood-borne pathogens as fibrinogen is prepared from pooled human blood, difficulty in applying and keeping it in weld site during the welding process.

Several multicomponent solders have been developed that provide the advantages of long shelf life, increased weld strength, and no risk of infection [114,115]. The viscosity of the solders can be adjusted as needed for different applications.

Mechanical welding devices. Computer control of laser welding still requires the surgeon to target the laser and assess the end-point of welding. The Exoscope™ system [116] (Laser-Surge, Rochester, NY) has been developed to overcome these limitations for intestinal anastomosis. The intestinal ends are apposed using a dissolvable intraluminal stent that exposes the entire circumference of the anastomosis to a uniform power density simultaneously allowing a reproducible creation of welds with a minimum of thermal injury and immediate weld strengths that exceed suture repairs. Anastomotic time is extremely short (just several seconds) [116,117].

Photoenhancement. Unwanted thermal injury to the tissue occurs in two ways: (1) nontarget tissue is exposed to laser light, and (2) heat produced in target tissue diffuses into adjacent tissue. A chromophore can be applied to target tissue that has a high absorption of the laser wavelength selected. If a wavelength can be chosen that is poorly absorbed by the target tissue, then heat will be generated only at the site of chromophore application and not in adjacent tissues. Diffusion can be limited by pulsing the laser light. An added advantage of this is that the incident power densities can be quite low. This reduces the risk of eye injury by personnel in the operating room and allows for the purchase of a smaller, lower cost laser. An example is the use of indocyanine green dye (absorption peak of 805 nm) matched with a gallium-aluminium-arsenide diode laser (810 nm) [118].

Preclinical Experience

Laser-assisted nerve repair. In an attempt to obviate the need for foreign material in a neurorrhaphy bed (either permanent, in the form of fine suture, or absorbable, in the form of various biologic tubes or glues) several authors [119–121] have used the milliwatt carbon dioxide laser in nerve repair. Although in theory potential benefits can be understood, in practice the thermal damage to the nerve appears to supersede any benefit gained by the absence of foreign material.

Some authors claim results with laser neurorrhaphy that are comparable with those with suture repair. However, Maragh et al. [119] reported that 10-0 nylon epineurial repair is superior to carbon dioxide laser repairs (200 μm, 90–95 mW, with 2-ms bursts) with respect to tensile strength, behavioral studies (toe spread), and compound action potential in the rodent sciatic nerve. No mention was made of the time required for each type of repair.

In a similarly designed study, Bailes et al. [120] compared the carbon dioxide laser (150 μm, 80–100 mW, continuous mode) with 9-0 nylon perineurial neurorrhaphy in a primate sural to peroneal nerve graft model. They found comparable results in the two groups when examining nerve conduction velocity and axon density.

In a less well designed study, Seifert and Stolke [121] compared the carbon dioxide laser (150 μm, 80–90 mW) with either fibrin glue or no repair of the cat oculomotor nerve. Although the laser yielded better results than the other two groups, no conclusions can be drawn until comparison is made with an accepted standard of repair (e.g., fine nylon suturing of the epineurium).

Campion et al. [122] compared functional and histological recovery following reconstruction of peripheral nerves using either epineurial nylon sutures or argon laser. The terminal branch of the peroneal nerve to the extensor digitorum longus in New Zealand White rabbits served as the experimental model. Histology and neuromuscular function were evaluated at 1, 2, and 6 months after repair. Nerves that had been repaired with the laser closely resembled the control group when diameters of the axons and the morphology distal to the site of repair were evaluated. However, laser-repaired nerves showed less foreign body reaction and axonal outgrowth compared to controls. Functional recovery paralleled histological findings and at 6 months postoperatively, laser-repaired nerves had consistently better neuromuscular function than those that had been repaired by epineurial suture.

Huang et al. [23] compared nerve regeneration following microsuture and CO_2 laser repair of transected sciatic nerves in rats in terms of morphology, electrophysiology, and function. Histologic studies revealed no difference in the size and number of regenerated axons, although there was less scar tissue formation at the anastomotic site with the laser repair. Recovery in terms of electrophysiology and function was identical for suture and laser repaired nerves. Laser-repaired nerves did have a higher dehiscence rate, although the authors felt that this could be prevented by splinting the rats postoperatively. The authors concluded that laser repair of peripheral nerves is possible with results comparable to conventional microsuture neurorrhaphy.

Korff et al. [124] studied the effect of laser irradiation on nerve regeneration and anastomotic strength on the rat sciatic nerve following laser nerve repair. Although they found similar numbers of regenerating axons when compared to suture controls 2 months following repair, problems with insufficient anastomosis strength and a consequently high rate of dehiscence left them recommending further preliminary investigation.

Finally, there is apparent interest in the use

of the carbon dioxide laser for freshening the edges of nerves prior to repair, with the expectation that this might be superior to a scalpel blade. Unfortunately, the only study examining the use of the laser is poorly conceived [125], as is discussed in the invited commentary of the article [126]. Summarizing the available data, Terris and Fee [127] concluded that although the objective of eliminating the need for foreign material in a nerve repair wound is a worthwhile pursuit, the use of a thermal burn to establish continuity likely results in tissue damage that is sufficient to outweigh the benefits. Given the conflicting results achieved thus far, further work is warranted in an animal model. We agree with the conclusions of Shapiro et al. [128] that it is probably not unreasonable to consider human application of laser-assisted nerve repair to small peripheral nerves that are difficult to suture, and in our experience LANA has been useful for neurorrhaphy of cranial nerves during the resection of some skull base tumors (cavernous sinus meningiomas and acoustic schwannomas).

Laser-assisted vascular anastomosis (LAVA). The original work with laser-assisted vascular anastomoses was reported in 1964 by Yahr et al. [20,21], and since then, LAVA has been evaluated not only in the microvascular system (i.e., 0.7–2.0 mm vessel diameter), but also in medium size and large vessels (i.e., 3–8 mm vessel diameter). Investigations of LAVA have included the creation of arteriovenous fistulae, venous and arterial bypass grafts, and end-to-end and end-to-side anastomoses.

The mechanism of vessel bonding in LAVA is not completely understood. It has been evaluated most extensively with CO_2 and argon lasers, and the mechanisms of welding with these two lasers appear to differ. The CO_2 laser welds by forming a coagulum of denatured collagen in the media and adventitia of the vessel wall that is subsequently replaced by fibrous tissue and smooth muscle cells [109,129]. In contrast, argon laser energy is thought to cause welding by cross linking collagen-collagen bonds in addition to the elastin-collagen [130]. This is valid only for medium-sized vessels as smaller vessels anastomosed using argon laser have been shown to have the same mechanism of damage as described for CO_2 laser welds [131].

It is important that in all LAVA that there be adequate tissue–tissue apposition; otherwise, a coagulum of platelet and fibrin forms that is not strong enough to support the anastomosis. If direct apposition of the vessel wall edges does not occur, disruption of the anastomosis is likely, and subsequent attempts at laser welding will be unsuccessful [132].

The results of LAVA can be best analyzed by differentiating microvascular anastomoses from anastomoses in medium- and large-sized vessels. In general, laser-assisted microvascular anastomoses have a higher rate of aneurysm formation, intimal hyperplasia, and thrombosis, whereas anastomoses in medium-sized and large vessels have a relatively high patency and a low incidence of aneurysm formation [130,133–138].

The potential applications of LAVA are not yet defined. For medium-sized and large arteries and veins, the technique has not produced patency rates significantly superior to those of sutured anastomoses, and it is more expensive. In addition, traction sutures at frequent intervals of 0.5 cm are required to provide close apposition of the vessel wall edges; otherwise, anastomoses are largely unsuccessful because of low initial tensile strength [139]. This may mean that much, if not most, of the actual strength of LAVA is related to the stay sutures rather than to tissue welding.

Poor success rates with LAVA may be due to difficulty in controlling the many variables involved in performing the technique. The variables that require a high degree of precision include close vessel wall apposition, maintaining a narrow temperature range (40°–50°C) during welding, maintaining a constant laser fiber distance from the vessel wall, and constant movement of the laser along vessel edges (1 cm/s) to maintain the appropriate depth of beam penetration. In addition, differences in vessel thickness and size, such as with anastomoses between vein and artery, or differences in the geometry of the anastomosis, such as end-to-side, can affect the outcome. In addition, with LAVA of calcified vessels, tissue apposition and temperature control can be dramatically altered, resulting in a lower success rate of fusion [140].

Venous laser-assisted vascular anastomoses may be more effective than arterial procedures, because the vein wall is thinner and requires lower energy for fusion and the anastomosis is subjected to a lower intraluminal pressure. Perhaps the most promising use of LAVA is for microvessels; the potential for growth of anastomoses has its greatest application in the pediatric population and may permit higher patency rates [141].

PHOTODYNAMIC THERAPY

Current techniques of treating locally invasive malignant tumors such as gliomas include surgery, radiation therapy, chemotherapy, and immunotherapy. Except for immunotherapy, none of these offers the possibility of selective destruction of tumor without injury to normal tissue. Photochemotherapy, also termed photodynamic therapy (PDT), is a relatively new technique for treating malignant tumors that depends on the light activation of a photoreactive drug, called a photosensitizer, that is selectively taken up or retained by the neoplasm. Assuming that the photosensitizer preferentially bonds to all tumor cells, PDT not only offers the possibility of selective killing of rapidly proliferating cells but is potentially effective against tumor cells in any phase of the cell cycle. Several criteria regarding the photosensitizer must be met for PDT to be effective: (1) selectivity for tumor tissue, (2) absence of systemic toxic reaction at doses required for photosensitization, (3) capacity to absorb wavelengths of light that are readily transmitted through the tissue being treated, and (4) ability to destroy malignant tissue efficiently when photoactivated.

The effectiveness of a photosensitizer will depend on the degree of localization of the drug in the tumor, which in turn is related to its solubility and partition and transport characteristics and to the biochemical and biophysical properties of the normal and tumor tissues. Also, the effectiveness of the photosensitizer will depend on the photophysical parameters of the sensitizer, which include the quantum yield, the lifetimes and energies of the excited singlet and triplet states of the photosensitizer, as well as consideration of tumor geometry in assessing light delivery.

Several chemical compounds are capable of photosensitizing malignant brain tumor cells. Those that have been studied include hematoporphyrin, hematoporphyrin derivative, rhodamine 123, acridine orange, pyrylium derivatives, and phthalocyanines. From among this group, HPD has been the most widely studied photosensitizer to date. Hematoporphyrin derivative is a mixture of porphyrins (tetrapyrrolic pigments) that is formed by the acetic acid-sulfuric acid treatment of hematoporphyrin. The resultant porphyrin mixture, now commercially known as Photofrin, contains hematoporphyrin and dihematoporphyrin ether (DHE), which appears to be the principal component of HPD responsible for in vivo pho-

tosensitization [142]. Because of the instability of DHE in solution, there is serious question regarding the actual purity of DHE in Photofrin and the active photosensitizer(s) are actually a mixture of polyporphyrins.

Hematoporphyrin derivative can sensitize the photo-oxidation of many kinds of biologically important molecules. Since the photoactive spectrum usually corresponds to the absorption spectrum of the photosensitizer, HPD can be activated by most visible light owing to its broad range of light absorption. When illuminated, HPD will absorb light energy and be transformed to an excited singlet state. Red fluorescence is seen with radiative decay from the excited singlet state. Transformation of the excited singlet-state HPD to the excited triplet state can occur by so-called intersystem crossover. Triplet-state lifetimes range over several hundred microseconds. During this time, triplet state porphyrins can transfer energy to ground state oxygen (which is in the triplet state) to produce excited singlet-state oxygen, which is chemically reactive. This is called a type II photo-oxidation process. A type I oxidative process may occur instead if the triplet-state porphyrin transfers an electron to a molecule of oxygen to yield a superoxide (O_2-) radical. In addition, the triplet-state porphyrin may react directly with certain biomolecules to initiate other free-radical processes. The ability to generate excited singlet oxygen is directly related to the length of porphyrin's triplet lifetime [143].

It is unclear at present how HPD and other porphyrins enter mammalian cells. It is assumed that HPD diffuses into cells, although it is recognized that active and passive transport processes as well as pinocytosis and phagocytosis may be involved. Porphyrin migration within cells as a function of incubation time has been demonstrated by the variable sites of intracellular damage following photoradiation for different periods between incubation and illumination [144]. The relative affinity of the various porphyrins of subcellular structures depends on their lipid solubility [145].

In vitro studies show that the plasma membrane is the main site of porphyrin-sensitized photodamage [146–152]. Photoinduced alterations in the cell membrane include inactivation of membrane enzymes, cross-linking of membrane proteins, alterations in membrane permeability, damage to transport systems, and cell lysis. With longer incubation times, porphyrins will localize to the mitochondria, microsomes, and lysosomes and sensitize photodamage in those areas [153,154]. Occasionally structural changes are produced [155]. Oxygen-dependent and hypoxic cells are extremely resistant to the lethal effects of HPD and light [156,157]. This suggests that hypoxic areas in tumor may limit HPD phototherapy.

Why HPD preferentially localizes to tumors is still largely unknown. Evidence supports the concept that differences in the extracellular environment between neoplastic and normal tissue, such as vascular permeability, lack of adequate lymphatic drainage, and nonspecific binding of proteins to stromal elements, are responsible for the selective uptake or retention of HPD and other porphyrins within the tumor [149,158]. Because of its large size and protein binding, HPD does not cross the blood brain barrier (BBB) [159,160]. It diffuses into tumor areas where the BBB may be altered and areas of the brain that are devoid of the BBB, such as the pituitary, area postrema, pineal gland, choroid plexus, and meninges [161–164]. Hematoporphyrin derivative thus leaks out into the intercellular space in areas of capillary permeability and is taken up or retained by both tumor and normal cells in the area. Tumor cells that are removed by distance from the BBB defect would not be expected to incorporate HPD and thus would not be expected to incorporate HPD and thus would not be photosensitive. In addition, the unselective staining of normal brain tissue by HPD in the region of BBB defect adjacent to the tumor mass could lead to injury of these cells during photoillumination.

Survival and quality of life in patients with supratentorial malignant astrocytoma has been shown to improve with a more extensive surgical resection [165,166]. However, the majority of these tumors do not have a distinct boundary, making complete resection difficult or impossible even with the use of intraoperative ultrasonography [167]. Although intraoperative computerized tomography has been advocated to enhance tumor resection [168], this is available only in a few centers. The clearance of the hematoporphyrin derivative from normal tissue is more rapid than from the tumor and hence it acts as a tumor-localizing dye during the resection of a malignant glioma. The exposed brain when examined under ultraviolet light can delineate and localize the tumor margin as red fluorescence. However, such visual detection schemes are limited by interference from the autofluorescence of the normal brain (400–600 nm) and maximum sensitivity would require examination in a nearly dark environment by dark adapted eyes.

Recently, Poon et al. [169] have studied the ability of laser-induced fluorescence spectroscopy using chloro-aluminium phthalocyanine tetrasulfonate (C1A1PcS$_4$) to delineate tumor margins intraoperatively in a rat intracerebral glioma model. The phthalocyanines have several advantages over HPD for laser-induced fluorescence localization of tumors. Their quantum yield for fluorescence is significantly greater and their fluorescence peak lies at 680 nm, a level at which background due to tissue autofluorescence is very low. With sensitive charge coupled device cameras used in connection with computer-aided image processing techniques, they found contrast ratios of up to 40:1 for glioma:normal brain fluorescence interface. Spatially resolved spectra were acquired in ~ 5 seconds using a fiberoptic probe. The animals that underwent laser-induced fluorescence guided microscopic resection had a significantly lower residual volume of tumor as compared with the animals that underwent resection with visual assessment alone.

Photochemotherapy with HPD does not affect tumor cell clonogenecity even at doses that produce macroscopic tumor destruction [170]. It is currently believed that tumor destruction by HPD and light is not cell specific and instead results from damage to the tumor circulation and treatment induced changes in tumor physiology [170–173]. Further concern with the use of HPD has arisen from reports that the nonfluorescing, intact, nontumor-bearing brain tissue from HPD-treated mice and rats may be injured following nonthermal levels of light exposure [174,175].

The most efficient excitation wavelength is that which corresponds to the maximum absorption wavelength of the photosensitizer. For HPD, maximum light absorption is seen with a wavelength between 400–410 nm; however, because of the poor brain tissue penetrability at shorter wavelengths, a wavelength of ~ 630 nm (red light) is used to excite the drug [176]. In vitro and in vivo studies indicate that the photosensitizing efficiency of HPD photodynamic therapy is not affected by nonthermal variations in dose rates of delivered light [177]. Photochemotherapeutic activity thus depends on the total dose of light that is delivered (total energy) and not the light fluency. Similar findings were reported with rhodamine 123, which demonstrated time-dependent tumoricidal activity in the presence of blue-green laser light that was independent of the rate of light delivery [178]. Continuous light delivery appears to be necessary for phototoxicity in that pulsed laser light is ineffective in activating HPD in vivo [179].

Lasers are used currently to produce high-intensity monochromatic light that is transmitted via a quartz fiberoptic cable to the tumor for treatment. The argon pumped dye laser with rhodamine 590 (kiton red, or DCM) produces red light with a wavelength of ~ 630 nm that is used to activate HPD. Newer systems have a maximum output of 2.0–5.0 W of red light. The gold vapor laser, which reportedly is capable of 5–10 W of red light output, is also under investigation [180].

Several techniques have been employed for light delivery of the laser light to the tumor. After gross tumor resection, laser light can be applied to the surface of the tumor cavity with either a divergent bare-tipped fiber [181] or micro lens assembly. Special diffusing media have also been employed to help scatter the laser light to illuminate the tumor cavity more thoroughly with a single laser application. A diffusion medium-filled balloon system into which the laser fiberoptic is placed has been devised by Muller and Wilson (Fig. 2a) [182]. Smaller centrencephalic tumors are best treated by the stereotaxic interstitial placement of spherical or cylindrical emitting laser fibertips.

The rate of light delivery will be limited by nonspecific thermal effects of the laser that are associated with higher fluencies. Duration of light exposure will depend on the penetrability of the light, the depth of tissue that is to be treated, and the light fluency, assuming that phototoxicity is a function of total light energy delivered.

Thermal Considerations

Hematoporphyrin derivative phototherapy as previously reported by most clinicians has had at least a partially hyperthermic effect [183,184]. It is known that only mild temperature elevations (41–42°C) for a sustained time are selectively cytotoxic to cancer cells [185,186]. Increases in temperature are correlated with increases in light fluency, that is, the rate of light delivery. During light delivery at a constant power setting, the temperature will rapidly rise during the first 4 minutes of exposure to an equilibrium temperature [183]. Temperature rise is more significant during interstitial laser light application through an implanted fiberoptic. Our laboratory has studied the thermal rise in normal rat brain in re-

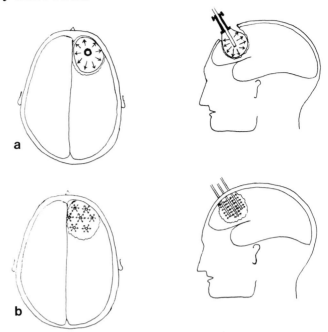

Fig. 2. Light delivery systems for photodynamic therapy. (**a**) Intracavitary balloon filled with a diffusing medium with the laser fiber in the center of the balloon to deliver light to the walls of tumor resection cavity. (**b**) Multiple stereotactically implanted cylindrical diffusing fibers that can deliver light directly into the solid tumor mass and the brain adjacent to tumor.

sponse to interstitial laser irradiation from both a bare-tipped and a diffusing sapphire-tipped quartz fiberoptic for both argon laser light (454–514.5 nm) and red light (630 nm) from an argon pumped dye laser with DCM dye. There is a much greater rise in tissue temperature, particularly near the fiberoptic tip for the bare-tipped fiber; this undoubtedly reflects the extremely high power density present at the tip of the bare fiber due to the smaller surface area of emission.

A synergistic interaction exists between PDT with HPD and hyperthermia (40.5–45°C) [187,188]. The sensitizing effect of hyperthermia varies both with temperature and the sequence of heat treatment and PDT treatment. The greatest potentiation of PDT with HPD occurs when hyperthermia is administered immediately after PDT [187–189]. It has been suggested that hyperthermia inhibits repair of PDT-induced damage. The temperatures generated during standard PDT surface irradiation with 100–200 mW/cm^2 do not appear to be high enough or long enough in duration to offer hyperthermic potentiation of PDT with HPD [187]. At longer exposure times or higher power densities, there may be hyperthermic interaction present. Certainly based on the temperature data obtained from interstitial laser light delivery, hyperthermia would be expected to play some role in the tissue changes following PDT.

Clinical Experience

Several medical centers are currently treating malignant brain tumors with PDT using HPD and red light. In the United States these are pilot clinical research projects designed to study the feasibility and potential efficacy of this form of treatment. At present, HPD is not commercially available for use in neurosurgical patients. Due to the lack of controls and the fact that PDT was performed in addition to surgical decompression or removal of tumor along with postoperative radiation therapy in many cases, it is impossible to determine the actual benefit derived from PDT in patients treated prior to 1985.

Laws and Wharen [190] reported a total clinical experience of 22 patients with malignant brain tumors (17 malignant gliomas, 2 metastases, 2 medulloblastomas, 1 rhabdomyosarcoma) in 1984. They were treating deep, surgically inaccessible solid or cystic tumors by stereotaxic implantation of a laser fiberoptic probe and irradiation without tumor removal 24 hours after intravenous administration of HPD. Other tumors were treated by tumor removal followed by irradiation of the tumor bed with either a high-intensity filtered white light source or broad-beam fiberoptic. Based on laboratory studies, they assumed a maximum depth or radius of tumor-cell kill of 8 mm using a power density of 25 mW/cm^2 and total dose of 160 J. In their series there were three postoperative infections, no deaths, and two instances of postoperative cerebral edema related to the therapy. Hematoporphyrin derivative was present in all of the tumor specimens removed, but the concentration varied.

Muller and Wilson [182] reported on eight patients with malignant primary brain tumors treated with PDT using HPD$_1$ and tumor cavity photoillumination with an inflatable balloon filled with a scattering medium into which was placed a fiberoptic coupled to an argon pumped dye laser. The total light energy delivered ranged from 8–68 J/cm^2. They had no adverse photosensitivity skin reactions and no cases of acute postoperative deterioration due to edema. Two patients developed wound infections; one required removal of infected bone flap.

McCulloch et al. [80] reported on 16 patients with malignant tumors (9 glioblastomas, 2 oligodendrogliomas, 1 grade 2/3 astrocytoma, 4 metastases) treated with red light 48 hours after intravenous HPD 5 mg/kg. Patients underwent standard neurosurgical treatment with craniotomy and radical tumor excision. Early in the series, red light was administered from either an argon pumped dye laser with rhodamine dye or from a special filtered incandescent lamp that was capable of a total output of 24 W in the spectral range between 620–720 nm. Recently, a gold vapor laser with an output of 1.5 W at 627.8 nm has been used. All patients with malignant gliomas were also treated with 5,000 rads of whole brain irradiation. Cerebral edema was present in nearly all cases after treatment. Mannitol and steroids were necessary to treat many of these cases. Of three patients with limited tumor resection, two had an increase in their postoperative neurologic deficit and one died of severe cerebral edema. Photosensitivity of the skin was seen in some patients, in whom precautionary measures were inadequate.

The earliest report using HPD PDT was by Perria et al. [191] in 1980. They treated nine patients with various types of malignant brain tumors using a dose of HPD between 2.5 and 10.0 mg/kg body weight and a light dosage of 9 J/cm^2 from a helium-neon laser. They, like every other investigator to date, were unable to demonstrate any real benefit from the treatment.

Powers et al. [192] treated patients with recurrent malignant gliomas and metastatic melanoma using purified HPD and stereotactic intratumorally implanted optical laser fibers. Tumor response to PDT was evaluated by recording changes in the volume and pattern of tumor enhancement between computed tomographic and magnetic resonance imaging scans done before and after PDT, metabolic changes in tumor tissue by ^{31}P MR spectroscopy, and patient outcome. Steroids were witheld to evaluate the toxicity of interstitial PDT in brain. Toxicity of PDT was evaluated by recording changes in the patients' neurological examinations and correlated with changes in brain adjacent to tumor seen on postoperative imaging studies. Dramatic tumor responses to PDT were seen in all gliomas, but no response of tumor to treatment was seen with melanoma. Transient signs and symptoms of increased peritumoral cerebral edema caused by PDT were seen in all patients. Two patients suffered permanent neurological sequalae, monocular blindness, and a partial visual field defect as a result of treatment. Two patients with recurrent anaplastic astrocytomas had remission for 45 and 35 weeks after PDT at the time of publication. They concluded that intratumoral photoradiation therapy of hematoporphyrin derivative-photosensitized malignant gliomas effectively produces necrosis of the solid component of malignant gliomas; however, intratumoral photoradiation may not reach the portion of tumor that invades normal brain.

Kostron [193] reported the results of 40 patients with primary or recurrent malignant brain tumors treated 51 times by photodynamic therapy after sensitization with Photofrin I, II or Photosan 3 24–48 hours prior to surgical removal of tumor mass. The sensitizer was activated by a conventional light source (energies ranging from 15–120 J/cm^2) or an argon dye pumped laser (energy flux between 150–500 mW/s; total dose 60–360 J/cm^2). Ten patients treated for a primary glioblastoma also recieved 60 Gy of radiation therapy. The median survival time of this group of patients was 19 months (0.5–29 months). The median time to recurrence was 13 months (2–17 months). Patients treated with one or multiple recurrences lived in the median 8 months (4–14 months) and recurred in the median 6 months after PDT. Whereas the first generation of the sensitizer (HPD, Photofrin I) caused severe skin sensitization, there were few side effects from the newer generation (Photosan 3). The histological investigation of the tumor immediately after treatment demonstrated in all the investigated cases tumor necrosis. When those biopsies are taken into tissue culture, almost no tumor cell growth was observed. Despite this immediate effect, tumors still recurred locally. The authors hypothesized that the recurrence might be due to exclusion of the photosensitizer in the most peripheral part of the tumor. The PDT was well tolerated by the patients, except one patient who experienced a transient diencephalic symptom during photoradiation. No brain edema was observed in patients even at the dose of light of 360 J/cm^2.

Origitano et al. [194] studied the photosensitizer uptake and distribution using indium-111 Photofrin-II SPECT scans in humans with intracranial neoplasms. Sixteen patients had malignant glial tumors, two had metastatic deposits, one had a chordoma, and one had a meningioma. Anatomical-spatial data correlated well between the SPECT images and contrast-enhanced CT/MR images. Regions of focal uptake on SPECT images correlated with the surgical histopathological findings of the neoplasm. They also found that there was a significantly greater uptake of isotope in glioblastomas, as compared to malignant astrocytomas. The study data showed that PDT may be tailored for each patient by correlating SPECT images with anatomical data produced by CT/MRI. The authors are currently using an image-based, computer-assisted, treatment-planning protocol to study the treatment variables leading to optimizing photodynamic therapy for intracranial neoplasms [195]. However, the resolution of SPECT studies is not sufficient to demonstrate photosensitizers in the infiltrating cells around the tumor margin, which are responsible for tumor recurrences. It is essential that PDT effectively treats these tumor cells for the therapy to be of any value [196].

The senior author is currently conducting a trial with the use of Photofrin and the implantation of multiple cylinder shaped, diffusion-tipped optical fibers stereotactically into the tumor and into the BAT to determine the optimal light dose for use in PDT of malignant gliomas (Figs. 2b, 3). Therefore, eight patients have been treated with the first six receiving a total light dose of 4,000 joules and an intravenous dose of 2 mg/kg Photofrin 24 hours prior to photoradiation. The last two patients have received a higher light 5,500 joules and have shown extensive post-PDT necrosis of tumor with greater extension of damage into the BAT resulting in some permanent neurological sequalae.

Better definition of the tumor volume with the use of MRI- and CT-based 3D stereotactic planning software should improve upon the precision of light delivery to tumor-involved brain and limit unnecessary PDT-induced injury of normal nontumor-involved brain.

The most common complication of PDT with HPD is skin sensitivity to sunlight or intense artificial light. In patients who are exposed to bright light, pain, swelling, and rash may result for up to 4 weeks after the injection of HPD. As a consequence, these patients must be kept isolated from potentially harmful light exposure. In addition, the scalp and meninges, since they contain high levels of HPD, must be protected from light exposure during the irradiation process in PDT.

As mentioned above, cerebral edema is commonly seen after PDT with HPD and can lead to secondary brain injury. Ji et al. [197] confirmed the histological evidence that brain injury, BBB disruption, and brain edema in-

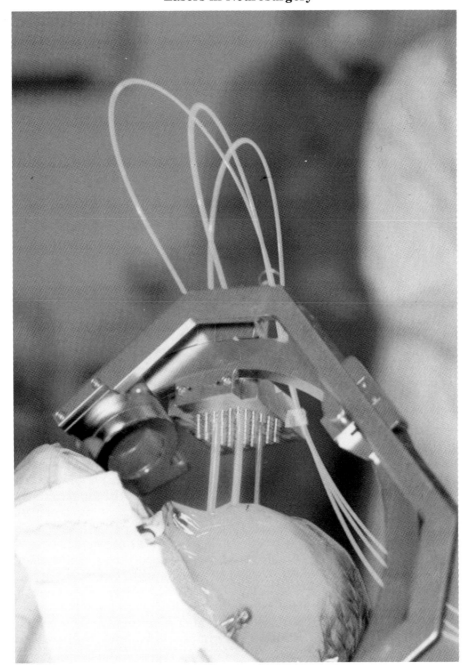

Fig. 3. Stereotactic implantation of optical fibers through transparent silicone catheters for uniform light delivery in photodynamic therapy of malignant glioma. This is done with the aid of a gridblock that is fixed to a stereotactic frame. See insert for color representation.

crease proportionally with increasing levels of interstitial laser irradiation in the rat brain tumor model. It is suggested that brain injury occurs from diminished or nonexistent blood supply to the laser irradiation area (LIA) that may be induced by arterial occlusion, capillary blockage due to local pressure increase, and stasis resulting from venous occlusion by laser injury to bordering tissue [6,198]. The authors found that the cortical mantle, which is rich in neurons, is more sensitive to laser irradiation than white matter, and histopathological changes were observed only at higher levels of output. Hence, the higher the laser power delivered through a single fiberoptic, the greater the risk of potential radiation injury.

In addition to the damage that occurs from laser irradiation alone, photodynamic therapy also produces scattered hemorrhages and vessel thromboses in brain adjacent to tumor tissue (BAT) [199] due to the preferential localization of HPD around the leaky capillaries of tumor-involved brain. Photoactivation of the HPD produces vascular toxicity, resulting in a further increase in BBB permeability, erythrocyte extravasation, and intravascular thrombosis. Recently, using the same experimental model, it was shown that the BBB permeability change following PDT is directly related to the dose of Photofrin administered [200]. Obviously, ischemia, secondary to vascular thromboses caused by PDT, is one of the mechanisms by which PDT kills the tumor cells. Steroids appear to offer protection against the development of edema following PDT.

Unfortunately, severe brain edema and other side effects related to ischemic damage of BAT may limit the therapeutic potential of this modality of glioma therapy. Jiang et al. [201] used ^{1}H Magnetic resonance imaging (MRI) to study the effects of photodynamic therapy (PDT) on normal rat brain using T_1-, T_2-, diffusion-, and proton density-weighted images. Rats received intraperitoneal injections of 12.5 mg/kg of Photofrin II, and 48 hours later the dural area over the frontal cortex was treated with 35 J/cm^2 of light. The T_1-, T_2-, and diffusion-weighted images revealed an evolving high contrast region of brain that corresponded to the PDT-treated area. Lesioned brain exhibited significant increases in T_1 and T_2 relaxation times at 1 day ($P < 0.01$) and 3 days (T_1, $P = 0.018$; T_2, $P < 0.01$) after treatment, compared with the contralateral equivalent volume of nonlesioned brain. Water proton diffusion coefficient (DW) in the lesioned area decreased at 1 day ($P = 0.026$) and increased at 3 days ($P = 0.012$) compared with nonlesioned brain. An increase in the proton density ratio from PDT versus nonlesioned side was found 3 days after PDT treatment ($P = 0.03$). The data indicated that the biophysical parameters obtained from magnetic resonance imaging scans, T_1, T_2, DW, and proton density can be used to monitor changes in an evolving photochemically induced lesion.

STEREOTAXY AND LASERS

CT- and MRI-based stereotactic biopsy for the diagnosis of intracranial tumors is common.

Several teaching medical centers have developed computer-interactive stereotactic systems that guide laser resection of deep-seated, intra-axial brain tumors defined by either stereotactic CT or MRI. Complete removal of the contrast-enhancing lesion defined by CT or MRI scans can be accomplished with minimal morbidity and risk of producing further neurologic injury. Although there is controversy regarding the indications for radical or gross total removal of higher grade lesions such as anaplastic astrocytomas and glioblastomas that tend to infiltrate a considerable distance into the noncontrast-enhancing brain surrounding the solid contrast-enhancing tumor mass, improved survival has been documented, particularly in young patients, after radical surgical extirpation of low grade astrocytomas.

Computer-assisted stereotactic laser systems help the surgeon with tumor removal by identifying tumor margins that may not be visibly clear due to edematous brain tissue at the periphery and/or the complex geometry of these lesions. The carbon dioxide laser enables precise removal of the tumor with minimal thermal effect on the bordering and often functional brain. The Nd:YAG laser has been used for coagulation and shrinkage of tumor and has been particularly helpful in the removal of more vascularized lesions.

The technique involves obtaining a stereotactic CT and/or MRI scan with the patient's head fixed in a CT or MRI compatible stereotactic head holder. Stereotactic stereoscopic digital angiography may also be performed, especially when planning to operate on vascular tumors or tumors adjacent to important blood vessels that must be preserved during the course of the resection. The surgeon then defines the tumor margin on each slice of the imaging study by tracing around the region of abnormality seen on the scan. This information is fed directly into the computer, which then interpolates tumor dimensions for intermediate slices and recreates a three-dimensional tumor volume based upon the digitized data obtained from the imaging studies (Fig. 4). The stereotactic positions of important neural and vascular structures in relation to the tumor are identified and the surgical approach is designed to avoid these.

A small craniotomy is centered around the calculated line of approach. Reference markers such as small radioopaque metallic balls (0.5 mm diameter) can be placed into the tumor prior to craniotomy in order to monitor possible movements of the tumor, especially cystic tumors, dur-

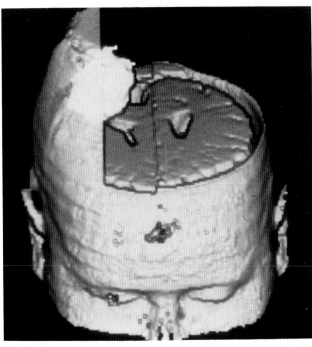

Fig. 4. Three-dimensional reconstruction of MRI to facilitate tumor treatment planning in stereotaxy.

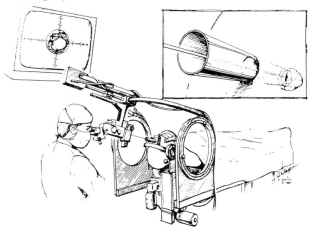

Fig. 5. Computerized stereotactic volumetric resection of an intraaxial tumor using carbon dioxide laser. Note the "heads up" display showing the tumor in relation to the end of the retractor. Inset shows the trajectory used to resect the tumor. (Courtesy Dr. Patrick Kelly; modified with permission from Kelly PJ, Mayo Clinic Proc 1988; 63:1186–1198.)

ing tumor exposure. A cortical incision is made and deepened down to the surface of the tumor using the CO_2 laser. A stereotactic retractor(s) is (are) placed to maintain exposure and a channel for passing surgical instruments and allowing access of the laser(s) to the tumor. The position of the laser and the retractor in relation to reformatted planar tumor boundaries on a graphics monitor in the operating room is continuously checked by the surgeon as deeper advances are made with tumor resection. The display may be viewed either on a standard television display monitor or by means of a "heads up" display unit that mounts directly on the operating microscope. The latter display allows the surgeon to see a virtual image of the tumor superimposed on the operative field (Fig. 5). The tumor is vaporized with the carbon dioxide laser slice by slice as depicted on the graphics monitor. Resection at each level begins laterally at the calculated margin of the tumor. Resection of the outer margins of the tumor first to establish a boundary helps to avoid the problem of altering the tumor borders that can occur by inward movement of the peripheral portions of tumor during central decompression.

Kelly and colleagues [63] reported their clinical experience in 500 consecutive cases in the resection of various lesions from specific anatom-

ical areas. Total overall morbidity was 7% and mortality 1%. This procedure is of most benefit in deep-seated circumscribed lesions and of less benefit in infiltrating tumors such as high grade gliomas and in fibrillary astrocytomas located in essential brain areas. In patients harboring glial tumors in eloquent brain areas, stereotactic resection is appropriate for the tumor tissue component only.

Lyons and Kelly [65] reported on 23 cases of pathologically verified thalamic pilocytic astrocytomas that underwent computer-assisted stereotactic volumetric laser resection/biopsy. Postoperative imaging demonstrated no residual contrast-enhancing tumor in 14 patients and a small amount of contrast-enhancing tumor (< 5% of the original tumor volume) in five patients. There was one postoperative death in a patient with tumor extending into the midbrain. The remaining 22 patients are alive and well after a follow-up of 27 months (range 6–69 months). Improvement in neurological function occurred in 12 patients with gross total resection and two patients with subtotal resection. The other five patients had stabilization of their preoperative deficits.

Morita and Kelly [66] performed 60 computer-assisted volumetric stereotactic resection procedures in 58 patients with intraventricular tumors (30 patients with third ventricular tumors and 28 patients with lateral ventricular tumors). The pathological findings of the tumors were as follows: colloid cyst in 27, giant cell astrocytoma in 5, central neurocytoma in 4, pilocytic astrocytoma in 4, meningioma in 3, subependymoma in 3, metastatic tumor in 3, oligodendroglioma in 2, ependymoma in 2, and miscellaneous tumors in 5 patients. All third ventricular tumors were approached via a frontal trajectory, and lateral ventricular tumors were approached according to the site and shape of the lesion. Total resection was achieved in 55 procedures. Overall outcome was excellent in 45 cases, good (some deficit but independent) in 5, and poor (dependent) in 3 (memory impairment, 2 patients; visual field cut, 1 patient). Two patients (3.4%) died postoperatively (one had a postoperative thalamic hemorrhage and pulmonary embolus; one had a subdural hygroma). In follow-up, three patients died from the extension of a malignant tumor or from primary cancer. Permanent morbidity was seen in three cases (5%).

A potential disadvantage of Kelly's system is the fact that a transparenchymal trajectory is used each time, and this results in greater neural injury than might be possible using a subdural, subarachnoid, intrasulcal, or intrafissural route.

ENDOSCOPY AND LASERS

Goodale et al. [202] in 1970 were one of the first groups to use CO_2 laser with a rigid endoscope to coagulate bleeding gastric ulcers and demonstrated its utility. Nath et al. [203] reported the use of a 6-watt argon laser through the biopsy channel of a conventional fiberoptic endoscope for the first time. They used a special quartz fiberoptic transmission system with a single 150 μ diameter optical fiber. Despite the introduction of endoscopes into neurosurgery early in this century, it is only during the last 15 years that some success has been achieved in the treatment of hydrocephalus by third ventriculostomy using endoscopes [204]. Also, endoscopic surgery is used for the treatment of multiloculated hydrocephalus [205,206], biopsy/resection of intraventricular lesions [207–211], and evacuation of spontaneous intracerebral hematomas [212–216]. The other area where endoscopes are felt to be very helpful is in stereotactic surgery where they provides real-time visual control and, when coupled with a laser, serve as a method of achieving hemostasis [217–226].

Carbon dioxide laser can be used only with rigid endoscopes and not with flexible endoscopes. This is because development of flexible fibers with a sufficient power durability at 10.6 μm is in its infancy. Argon, Nd:YAG, and KTP lasers can be used with either rigid or flexible endoscopes [227].

The most common indication for ventriculoscopy currently in neurosurgery is for the treatment of obstructive hydrocephalus, and specifically for opening multiloculated cysts within the ventricular system. The endoscope lends itself ideally for this procedure. Ventricular cysts can be communicated with each other and into one of the ventricular cavities in order to minimize the number of shunts required. The senior author reported his initial experience with two infants with hydrocephalus and compartmentalization of the lateral ventricles due to cerebrospinal fluid (CSF) infection, which were treated by fenestration of the ventricular cysts using the argon laser through a steerable flexible endoscope [205]. Postoperative scans showed arrested hydrocephalus in both cases, and they remained symptom-free for more than 6 months. Five out of seven patients with various CSF containing intraventricular cysts were successfully decompressed with the endoscope alone. Craniotomy was required in two patients in order to complete cyst fenestration [206]. The cysts tend to remain open once the communication has been achieved [204–206,208]. It is our opinion that laser-assisted ventriculoscopy with steerable flexible endoscopes is an alternative and sometimes a superior method of treating CSF containing cysts within the lateral ventricles of hydrocephalic patients.

Another form of CSF communication using endoscopic methods is that of third ventriculostomy. The advantages of endoneurosurgical management for obstructive hydrocephalus over those of the extracranial shunts are as follows: mechanical problems of equipment malfunction, such as breakage, deterioration, and migration do not exist; foreign body reactions do not occur; artificially low pressure syndromes do not develop; the ventriculostomy is never outgrown; and the morbidity associated with chronic and multiple shunt revisions is eliminated. There is also the cosmetic advantage because only one skin incision in the scalp is needed.

Third ventriculostomy can be done by open technique, percutaneous freehand technique, stereotactic technique, or endoscopic technique with or without stereotactic assistance (Fig. 6). Although the methods of bypassing the obstructed third ventricle are numerous, the technique with the lowest morbidity and mortality and highest success rate appears to be endoscopically guided

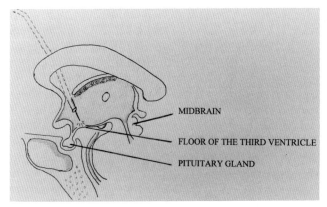

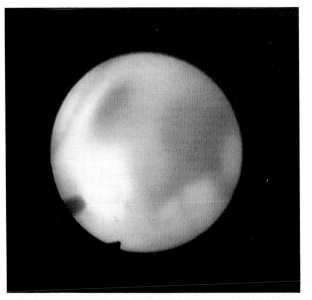

Fig. 6. Schematic illustration of endoscopic third ventriculostomy using flexible endoscope with a laser fiber.

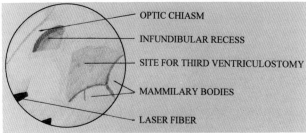

Fig. 7. Photograph of the details of the floor of the third ventricle as seen through the endoscope upon entering the third ventricle through the foramen of Monro. Note the laser fiber with a pilot light. Schematic illustration of the photograph shows the site for performing the third ventriculostomy. See insert for color representation.

third ventriculostomy with the option of streotactic assistance [223,228,229]. The selection of patients for third ventriculostomy is related to the overall results of the procedure. In all series, patients with aqueductal stenosis have fared the best [228]. It is also shown to be a preferred choice in children with aqueductal stenosis in the hands of a skilled surgeon [230]. These patients are good candidates for endoscopic ventriculostomy because they are at high risk from shunting procedures that may cause subdural hematoma due to overdrainage of ventricular CSF. Third ventriculostomy has been used successfully to treat intractable shunt infections [223,224,228] and even slit ventricles [231] in patients with shunts who have aqueductal stenosis. Patients with tumors may also be good candidates in selected cases, e.g., in tectal plate (midbrain) gliomas, patients with intraventricular tumors that can be biopsied at the same time, and patients with pineal region tumors that can be biopsied and then treated with radiotherapy [232].

The technique has been well described in a recent review by Drake [233], which the reader is encouraged to consult. Third ventriculoscopy via direct vision allows the surgeon to make vital intraoperative decisions regarding the placement of fenestration (Fig. 7), the avoidance of vital structures, and most importantly, the ability to discern when scarring and/or adhesions in the floor of the third ventricle makes the performance of the procedure unwise. The patency of the third ventriculostomy is assessed by special sequence MRI, which can demonstrate CSF flow through the opening. Improperly positioned ventricular catheters may become occluded with choroid plexus or ependyma. The risk of intraventricular hemor-

rhage associated with vigorous removal of catheters adherent to the choroid plexus often necessitates abandoning catheter removal. The senior author has used a steerable endoscope with argon laser to retrieve and free adherent ventricular catheters from their attachments to choroid plexus and intraventricular adhesions. Crone [234] has used KTP laser fiber to free the catheter. If there is intraventricular hemorrhage, endoscopy offers an excellent oppurtunity to clear the blood of the ventricles under direct vision. A new catheter can be introduced using the endoscope and placed under direct vision. Using a peel-away catheter for ventricular puncture, through which the ventriculoscope is inserted, there is no need for a second pass through the brain parenchyma in order to achieve appropriate catheter placement.

Although choroid plexectomy has proved to

be a failure for the treatment of the majority of patients with hydrocephalus, it may be of some benefit to a small subset of the group. There are some patients who, in the absence of a discrete tumor of the choroid plexus, produce unusually large amounts of CSF. Although it has not been demonstrated definitively, it is possible that in these cases the bulk of CSF produced can overwhelm the available absorptive mechanisms. Griffith [211] started performing this procedure in 1972 using a rigid endoscope that was inserted through a cylindrical guiding cannula. The initial report [211] of treating 71 patients with infantile hydrocephalus had very good results with only one mortality. Isotope studies using radiohippuran instilled into the ventricles before and after choroid plexus coagulation in many of these 70 patients demonstrated that ~ 50% of the choroid plexus had been destroyed by coagulation. With these encouraging results, 23 patients were treated with bilateral endoscopic choroid plexus coagulation, using postoperative perfusion with artificial CSF for 72 hours after endoscopic surgery in order to prevent blood and protein released at surgery from damaging the absorbing mechanism. This time, the success rate was 52%, which meant that there was no need for shunt placement, and there were no postoperative complications [235].

Buccholz and Pittman [236] reported a patient in whom choroid plexus was coagulated using Nd:YAG laser through an endoscope. This was a 29-month-old hydrocephalic infant with a ventriculoperitoneal shunt who had ascites. They used a rigid endoscope under stereotactic conditions with laser adjusted to a 7 W power constant mode. The authors have used a rigid endoscope that is passed under stereotactic conditions and fixed to a stereotactic frame. They then use a flexible endoscope to take advantage of the maneuverability of the flexible system while minimizing parenchymal damage at the entry site. Overall, the results of choroid plexectomy for the treatment of hydrocephalus have been poor. The mortality for the operation ranges between 5% to 15%. Significant morbidity is associated with the procedure. CSF leak, seizures, infection, secondary obstructive hydrocephalus, and cerebral collapse have been well documented, although the risks are not quantitated clearly [237]. Scarff [238] has obtained the best results performing the procedure with a 5-year survival rate of 80% for those patients operated on later in his career.

Auer et al. [212–216] described an ultra-sound-guided, laser-assisted endoscopic technique that was used for evacuation of 77 spontaneous intracerebral hematomas (30 lobar,11 putaminal,10 thalamic, 8 traumatic intracerebral hematomas, 13 ventricular hematomas, 8 cerebellar hematomas, and 1 brainstem hematoma). They used a rigid endoscope guided by means of an ultrasound through a burr hole in conjunction with Nd:YAG laser. Total or subtotal evacuation was achieved in 33% of intracerebral hematomas, and removal of more than 50% of the clot was achieved in 55%. The authors generally found that the clots were easier to evacuate before the third day than between the third and seventh days. In the case of cerebellar hematomas, additional blood could be removed from the third ventricle by gentle irrigation and suction through the aqueduct so that the patients did not require a ventricular shunt. Intraoperative bleeding was not a problem in any of the patients. Coagulation of the bleeding vessels in the wall of the hematoma cavity was necessary only in two patients. Postoperative rebleeding occurred in two patients following an interval of several hours. One patient died as a consequence of repeated hemorrhage 10 days after surgery. Two of the 51 patients died. The authors felt that this technique involves less surgical trauma and a shorter operative time as compared to surgery. Although there were only eight patients with traumatic intracerebral hematoma (and the authors do not mention the length of each procedure), they feel that this technique might be useful in expediting the removal of traumatic hematomas. They also conclude that this technique allows a better clearance of blood from the ventricular system and hence is better for treating intraventricular and cerebellar hemorrhages extending into the fourth ventricle.

Although experience is limited regarding tumor resection with the ventriculoscope, there is no question that this is the direction in which neurosurgery is headed with the use of this instrument. In order to overcome the limitations of the conventional stereotactic technique (i.e., lack of intraoperative visualization and direct monitoring of procedures and changes of intracranial coordinates after decompression of cystic lesions or aspiration of CSF in the management of intraventricular lesions), Zamorano et al. [239,240] used rigid-flexible endoscopy and Nd:YAG laser in association with image-guided stereotactic procedures. The major advantages of endoscopic laser stereotaxis includes intraoperative visualization, hemostasis, evacuation or resection assessment, and wide exploration of intracranial cavities or ventricles. The technique allows safe aspiration, biopsy, and resection or internal decompression of deep and subcortical lesions. Indications have been mainly cystic intra-axial (tumors, hematomas, benign cysts, abscesses, etc.) and some intraventricular lesions. Operative mortality was seen in one patient.

Otzuki et al. [241,242] described a new approach for stereotactic laser surgery of deep-seated brain tumors using open-system endoscopy, i.e., employing a stereotactic guiding tube and fine endoscopes. They treated 22 intra-axial lesions in which ten small (3–26 mm) tumors were totally removed, whereas partial resection and biopsy were performed on 8 larger (> 40 mm) lesions without significant complications. Accurate resection of intra-axial brain lesions with efficient hemostasis, according to the authors, could be achieved with CO_2 and Nd:YAG laser irradiation under computed tomographic and MRI imaging. Contact YAG laser tips were particularly effective for tissue vaporization, whereas noncontact tips were useful for coagulation and hemostasis. The merits of this method include precise resection of pathological tissues by stereotaxis and minimal damage to the normal brain.

Caemaert and Abdullah [243] described the multipurpose cerebral endoscope and their technique. Macrocystic tumors or tumors with liquid necrotic centers can occasionally be biopsied from inside, but care should be taken not to collect only necrotic material. Neuroepithelial cysts, colloid cysts of the foramen of Monro, and epidermoid cysts can be treated by opening the wall widely and partial or total evacuation of the contents. Treatment of the arachnoid cysts is very rewarding using this technique. In cases of obstructive hydrocephalus where preoperative assessment demonstrated good resorptive capacities, a perforation of the floor of the third ventricle is possible with enlargement of the hole by a Fogarthy catheter. Caemaert and Abdullah [243] also say that for larger and longer interventions general anesthesia is mandatory since under local anesthesia the constant changes of pressure in the ventricle cause vomiting, which is very disturbing for both patient and surgeon. A simple biopsy within the third ventricle can easily be done under local anesthesia. In their experience, one patient with colloid cyst was transiently unconscious for 3 days following surgery presumably due to manipula-

tion of the structures of the third ventricle through the endoscope.

Auer et al. [244] used endoscopes to biopsy parenchymal cystic tumors but could achieve only a partial excision. This was due to collapse of the cystic tumor upon entry into it. The authors have tried to circumvent this by maintaining irrigation pressure above 15 cm water. Minor but clinically silent bleeding into the cystic cavity occurred in one patient; all others remained completely uneventful. The authors felt that although evacuation of the cyst and biopsy could be obtained, the technique needs improvement to take out the solid part of the tumor.

Others have used rigid and/or flexible endoscopes with CO_2 laser [245] or Nd:YAG laser [208,220,246] to biopsy or attempt resection of tumors in or abutting the ventricles. The future of endoscopy is undoubtedly intimately associated with the development of frameless stereotaxy and appropriate guidance systems. One of the significant limitations of using endoscopes alone at the present time is not knowing the exact position of the tip of the intracranial portion of the endoscope. Using frameless stereotaxy with continuous computer updates regarding ventriculoscopic position will obviously increase the surgeons' confidence in the use of endoscopy. Improvement in instrumentation would allow endoscopes, probably a combination of rigid and flexible, to utilize the extracerebral routes as in microneurosurgery and minimize the damage to the neural structures.

LASER FOR NEUROABLATIVE PROCEDURES

Lasers have been used in functional neurosurgery to perform commissural myelotomies, to make dorsal root entry zone lesions in the spinal cord, for ablation of the descending tract of the trigeminal nerve, and for spinothalamic tractotomy [70,247–249]. The dorsal horn of the spinal cord plays an important role in processing nociceptive information, but its anatomy and physiology are still incompletely understood. The exact mechanism for pain relief with DREZ lesions is unclear, but it has been postulated that pathologically deafferented cells in the dorsal horn may become hyperactive and send impulses to supraspinal pain centers. DREZ lesions would destroy these hyperactive neurons and/or the cells of origin of the spinothalamic tract within laminae I and V [250]. Ablation of the dorsal root entry zone of the spinal cord, popularized by Nashold [251], may be performed using lasers [248,249,252,253].

In an initial series of 21 patients with various denervation pain syndromes, 19 of whom were treated with DREZ lesions made with argon laser and two with CO_2 laser, it was found that the lesions made with the laser could be done more safely and faster than with the radiofrequency technique [249].

Making precise lesions requires anesthesia incorporating neuromuscular paralysis and ventilatory control in order to minimize respiratory-related movements of neural structures during the laser application. After the DREZ has been identified, the beam is directed from a micromanipulator onto the spinal cord at an angle of 15–30° inclined from the midline in order to align the vaporization cavity with the dorsal horn. Occasionally it is necessary to section the dentate ligament, place pial retraction sutures, and rotate and/or suspend the spinal cord to ensure proper alignment of the laser beam with the dorsal horn. In patients who have root avulsions, the laminectomy is extended cephalad and caudad to identify normal dorsal roots.

The most frequent and most effective indication for DREZ lesioning has been pain caused by brachial plexus or cervical root avulsion [254–256]. Nashold and Bullitt [251] have also noted good success rates using DREZ lesions for patients with central pain caused by injuries to the thoracic spinal cord or cauda equina. Individuals with pain at the segmental level of injury and extending a variable distance caudally were characterized as having "end zone" pain. In 31 such patients, DREZ lesions produced satisfactory pain control in 80%. Patients with diffuse pain involving the entire body, the sacral dermatomes, or the legs below the level of the injury were much less likely to improve. Of the 25 patients in this group, pain was relieved in only 32%. Powers et al. [249] and Young [256] have reported comparable success rates for patients with "end zone" pain and relatively low success rates for patients with pain in dermatomes remote from the injury level.

DREZ lesions have been performed for postherpetic neuralgia, phantom limb, or postamputation stump pain, and pain from lumbar arachnoiditis or failed low back operations. The number of reported cases in each of these categories is small, and the likelihood of long-term success is unknown [257–259].

Laser has been used to remove or incise the epileptic lesion immediately adjacent to eloquent areas such as speech or motor areas, using the nontouch vaporization technique without mechanical trauma to the surrounding brain.

During AVM resections, Yeh et al. [260] utilized the CO_2 laser in 27 patients to remove adjacent epileptogenic foci. At the end of 2 years, 78% of them were seizure-free (recurrence rate = 22%). The authors opined that injury caused by the laser as a surgical instrument is less epileptogenic as compared to injury caused by conventional instruments; hence, use of the laser reduces the incidence of postoperative seizures after removal of structural lesions presenting with epilepsy [26]. Cascino et al. [262] reported that 40% of 15 patients who underwent stereotactic excision of lesions associated with epilepsy using CO_2 laser without resection or vaporization of surrounding glial tissue had recurrence of seizures by the end of 2 years. This difference probably represents the fact that more patients are seizure-free at 2-year follow-up after "seizure surgery" with removal of perilesional reactive gliosis than after simple excision of the lesion alone, which is in agreement with the conclusions of the meta-analysis conducted by Weber et al. [263].

Bebin et al. [264] reported nine patients with tuberous sclerosis who underwent stereotactic lesionectomy using the CO_2 laser. Surgical procedures performed included cortical resection (n = 2) and stereotaxic lesionectomy (n = 7). Neuropathologic diagnoses were cortical tubers (n = 7) and glioneural hamartomas (n = 2). Three of nine patients had multifocal interictal scalp epileptiform EEG activity; however, ictal recordings identified the focus of seizure activity, which in all cases corresponded to a prominent neuroimaging abnormality. Four patients are seizure-free with medication, two are seizure-free without medication, two had > 80% reduction in seizure frequency, and one experienced only an initial temporary reduction in seizure frequency after 10–72 months (mean 35 months) following surgery. Postoperative EEG recordings showed absence of epileptiform abnormalities in the five patients who are seizure-free; the other four patients continue to have multifocal abnormalities. These data suggest that focal resection may be beneficial in selected patients with tuberous sclerosis despite multifocal EEG and neuroimaging abnormalities.

Kelly et al. [265] have reported 18 patients with medically intractable complex partial seizures of temporal lobe origin who underwent stereotactic amygdalohippocampectomy using the carbon dioxide laser. The target structures can be accurately identified and completely resected, and all patients experienced a cessation or dramatic reduction in frequency of seizure activity. However, because of the trajectory used, the inferior optic radiations are disrupted resulting in partial visual loss. In addition, two of the patients who underwent surgery on the left side had transient speech problems.

In summary, although microsurgical lasers are capable of producing precise lesions, and probably less scarring, they do not appear to provide any additional benefit when compared to the use of conventional instruments in the surgery for epilepsy.

LASER DISCECTOMY

The surgical treatment of lumbar disc herniation constitutes a substantial proportion of spine operations and has been improved by the development of less invasive techniques [266–272]. However, reducing lumbar disc surgery to a mere "nerve root decompression procedure" falls short of the standards set by modern surgical philosophy, since failure not only arises from anatomical and biomechanical disturbances caused by the surgical approach itself [273–277], but lumbar disc herniation can lead to nerve root compression within the spinal canal (extradural), within the intervertebral foramen (intraforaminal), or outside the spinal canal (extraforaminal). The location determines the surgical approach. In all but the extraforaminal cases, disc herniations are removed by the "standard" interlaminar transspinal approach.

It has been demonstrated that surgical results are worse in patients with mere disc protrusions as compared to those with a sequestered disc [278–280]. The surgical procedure itself eliminates the influence of the initial stage of disc degeneration on the subsequent course of the disease by converting an "operated disc" into a new and mostly uniform pathological condition. This might contribute to the 2–17% recurrence rate reported in the literature irrespective of the technique used ("conventional" or microdiscectomy), whereas the outcome itself (excellent and good results) could be slightly improved by microsurgical techniques. Nevertheless, a great number of failures following lumbar discectomy are related directly or indirectly to the surgical approach to the disc space through the spinal canal [281].

In an attempt to avoid the extensive damage to the surrounding structures and achieve a disc

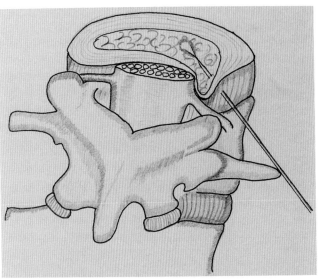

Fig. 8. Schematic illustration of ablation of a focal disc prolapse stretching the ipsilateral nerve root by laser transmitted through the optical fiber that is introduced percutaneously.

excision through a minimally invasive procedure, percutaneous nucleotomy was developed initially by Hijikata et al. [282] in 1975 and later on modified by others [283–286]. There are basically two different percutaneous discectomy procedures that involve the use of lasers. One system uses a laser fiber inserted through a thin gauge needle [38,287–290] (Fig. 8), and the other uses an endoscope to visualize the procedure of laser discectomy [291]. Percutaneous procedures can only address the problem of focal disc herniation with an intact annulus or at best a small "noncontained" lumbar disk herniation. Patients with severe motor deficits, conus or cauda equina syndrome, or rapidly progressing neurological symptoms cannot be treated by percutaneous methods. The same is true of patients with signs of segmental instability or previous surgery at the same site, pregnant women, and all patients with large noncontained discs, sequestered discs, spinal stenosis, or spondylolisthesis.

Percutaneous laser discectomy was first reported by Choy et al. [287], who performed this procedure in 12 patients employing the Nd:YAG laser introduced through an 18-gauge needle. This report also mentioned the use of Nd:YAG laser down an optical fiber through a 14-gauge needle was used for performing 33 disc ablations in 13 dogs. Subsequently, a number of reports have been published on laser discectomy both experimental as well as clinical. A variety of different lasers—CO_2 [292], Nd:YAG (1.32 μm, 1.06 μm) [293,294], KTP [289], Er:YAG [293], Ho:YAG [38,295], and XeCl [296,297]—have all been used on human cadaver and animal discs experimentally. A major difficulty faced by the investigators in the laser discectomy field has been the lack of an experimental model by which to compare different wavelengths and delivery systems with regard to the efficacy of disc removal and thermal effects of lasers on neural structures adjacent to the disc [298].

Quigley et al. [299] have developed a technique of intradiscal elastance (pressure/volume) that directly related the mass of disc removed after various intradiscal treatments with changes in the slope of the pressure curve generated by infusing saline into the disc through a large bore needle. Although it offers an objective criterion to refine and compare various treatment techniques in the laboratory, the relationship between the observed pressure alterations and clinical response in humans remains speculative. The only study that addressed this point was by Maroon et al. [300], who analyzed 1,054 automated suction device discectomy cases and found the average weight of disc removed in successful procedures did not vary significantly compared to failures.

Quigley et al. [38,298] and Vorwerk et al. [295] noted that laser disc destruction is affected by the absorption of energy by water, and hence the laser wavelength employed for percutaneous laser discectomy ought to be selected by matching the wavelengths of available laser systems to the known absorption bands of water. Employing this logic, the Ho:YAG laser (2.1 μm wavelength) would be a promising candidate because it closely approximates the 2.0 μm absorption band of water. Poor absorption is manifested by inefficient tissue vaporization and generalized disc space heating. Whereas the Er:YAG 2.94 μm and the recently developed Th:YAG 2.0 μm lasers do exhibit greater absorption efficiency compared with Ho:YAG, formidable technical problems will delay the development of convenient fiber optic delivery systems for these lasers [298].

Of the 12 patients reported by Choy et al. [287], nine of them initially improved, but five of these required open operations, leaving four pain-free at 7–16 months. In a follow-up communication [288], Choy later reported on a total of 333 patients having been treated in an outpatient setting. The longest follow-up was 62 months, with a mean of 26 months. According to the Macnab criteria, there was a good-to-fair response in 261 pa-

tients (78.4%), and a poor response in 72 (21.6%); 166 patients experienced relief of pain during the procedure. One-third of repeat magnetic resonance imaging scans at 4–6 months postlaser treatment showed modest to moderate decrease of disc herniation. The Nd:YAG employed was 1.32 μm as opposed to 1.06 μm device.

Davis et al. [289] reported using KTP laser through a 14-gauge needle introducer. Of the 40 cases, 85% were a "success," defined as "minimal residual discomfort to none" and "return to gainful employment"; follow-up interval is not detailed. Two of six patients required an open conventional L4–5 discectomy; four refused additional surgery. These failures are considered probably secondary to a subligamentous location of disc. Mayer et al. [291] described a technique that used rigid endoscope with flexible Nd:YAG laser fiber to perform discectomy in six patients. Immediate results were reported as good to excellent in five out of six patients, but long-term follow-up is not available.

It is obvious that none of the clinical trials was prospective and randomized, nor did they compare percutaneous laser discectomy with a "standard" treatment for a contained disc herniation, which should include microdiscectomy and, according to some, "vigorous conservative management" [301]. The comparison of percutaneous and open surgical techniques poses some problems. On the one hand, there are virtually no prospective or retrospective studies that compare and selectively analyze patients with a "contained" or slight subligamentous disc herniation. On the other hand, criteria for defining "success" or "failure" are inhomogenous and prevent exact comparison [298]. The place of percutaneous laser discectomy in the future practice of lumbar disc disease awaits the results of carefully designed experimental and clinical trials in the future.

A summary of the main uses of various types of lasers is presented in Table 1.

FUTURE APPLICATIONS

Although lasers have been available for many years, their use in neurosurgery has not reached its full potential. Compared with the number of surgical laser options formerly available, the present situation is much more complex. Future use of lasers in neurosurgery lies in tailoring the wavelength and delivery parameters to meet the actual clinical needs and not adapting a fixed wavelength laser to suit the various needs

TABLE 1. Main Uses of Various Types of Lasers in Clinical Neurosurgery

CO_2	Microneurosurgery (tissue ablation for tumor removal, epilepsy, pain surgery).
Nd:YAG (1.06 μm)	Volume coagulation of vascular lesions (AVMs, vascular meningiomas). Endoscopy for coagulation. Hyperthermia.
Nd:YAG (1.32 μm, 1.44 μm)	Microneurosurgery. Tissue ablation for percutaneous discectomy.
Argon;KTP	Microneurosurgery (precise microscopic lesions of spinal cord and brainstem). Endoscopy for coagulation. Percutaneous discectomy (KTP only).
Ho:YAG; Er:YAG	Percutaneous discectomy.
Gold vapor laser, Argon pumped or KTP pumped dye laser	Photodynamic therapy.

that is unattainable. We examine a number of interesting properties of newer laser technologies and their application to neurosurgery.

Tissue Ablation

The ultimate precision of laser cutting is never realized because of the optical and physical limitations of the surgeon and the energy delivery system. Probably, the full realization of the potential of laser tissue cutting will come only when there is integration of such cutting (the "efferent limb") with real-time techniques for recognizing and measuring very detailed tissue effects (the "afferent limb") [302]. Nonetheless, there have been advances in laser tissue cutting that are remarkable and point the way to the future of neurosurgery. The advantages of lasers for tissue ablation include greater precision and selectivity and compatibility with flexible or rigid endoscopic delivery systems.

One way to achieve precision is to select a wavelength that is intensely absorbed by the initial layers of the target tissue and the energy is therefore expended in heating up and vaporizing the initially impacted tissue layers, with relatively little energy left over to penetrate deeply and coagulate surrounding tissues. Thus, collateral damage is minimized. An excellent example of these concepts is the growing use of midinfrared lasers [303] such as THC:YAG, Ho:YAG, Er:YAG, and longer wavelengths of Nd:YAG, which radiate in the spectral region of ~ 2–3 μm. These lasers take advantage of certain fairly large absorption peaks of water for infrared energy in these wavelengths. Because water is a substantial and ubiquitous constituent of tissues, the ab-

sorption characteristics of a tissue exposed to a midinfrared laser are strongly dominated by the water absorption.

The term "excimer" refers to ultraviolet laser action based on a medium of rare gas halides. These lasers are pulsed, with durations from the nanosecond to the microsecond range. Owing to the short wavelengths, it is possible to focus the excimer laser beam to < 1 μm and thus obtain extremely precise tissue cutting. The mechanism of tissue cutting by the 193 nm excimer laser is nonthermal and involves direct breakage of covalent bonds by energy coupled to the bond by individual high-energy photons of ultraviolet light (photochemical process). Another characteristic of ultraviolet radiation is its high tissue absorption coefficient, leading to shallow penetration, independent of water content. The combination of pulsed delivery, limited tissue penetration, and nonthermal mechanism of tissue interaction is ideally suited for extremely precise, layer-by-layer ablation of tissues [304,305]. Excimer laser energy may be delivered by optical fibers or articulated-arm mirror systems. Besides direct tissue effects, excimer lasers are efficient sources for excitation of organic dyes in dye lasers [306]. Excimer lasers are relatively large machines and there is a potential problem from the release of toxic gases into the operating room environment, but these may be avoided by appropriate design.

It has been known for some time that if the pulse duration of the laser energy is sufficiently short, collateral thermal damage can be minimized. If the pulse is so short that no significant amount of energy can escape from the irradiated volume during the pulse time, the heat produced by the laser tissue interaction will tend to be used to vaporize tissue instead of coagulation. The critical time duration before which the irradiated energy does not diffuse beyond the field to which it is applied is called the thermal relaxation time. It has been shown that for pulses shorter than the thermal relaxation time, the collateral damage zone is approximately the optical penetration depth, and the rate of crater production or ablation rate depends on the energy applied per unit area or fluence [302]. There are some beneficial corollaries of the above considerations. A pulsed system that is operating on a time basis shorter than the thermal relaxation time can achieve reasonable rates of cutting without the high average powers required by a continuous-wave approach. Another advantage of pulsing is that it can make it easier for the surgeon to regulate the amount of tissue effect. If the repetition rate of the laser can be controlled and made very slow (i.e., just a few pulses per second) or a single shot, the surgeon can parcel out the energy in very small increments and produce gradual stepwise ablation of the tissue. A corollary of the existence of a definite thermal relaxation time is that if one applies the pulses more rapidly than the heat can be dissipated, one can obtain a thermal build-up that will expand the zone of collateral coagulation damage. By varying the repetition rate, it might be possible to provide both "cut" and "coag" modes that could be dialed in by these pulse-agile lasers, depending on clinical need [302].

The ultimate in variable wavelength, pulse-agile lasers is the free-electron laser (FEL). This type uses a beam of electrons that are energized by a linear accelerator and then "wiggled" by electromagnetic fields to produce coherent radiation. Other lasers use solid crystals or gases as the lasing medium, and the coherent radiation is limited to discrete wavelengths determined by the atomic or molecular energy levels of the medium. However, the FEL's lasing medium is the accelerated electron beam, and the radiation produced is a function of how the beam is wiggled. The production of coherent radiation in this fashion is flexible over a wide continuous range of wavelengths at variable pulse widths and pulse energies. Unfortunately, the FEL is a large machine, requiring an industrial-size room and a great deal of technical support. It is not intended to be used as a frontline clinical laser. The clinical value of the FEL is that it may point the way to the selection of discrete wavelengths and pulse parameters that can be implemented in far simpler and cheaper systems [302].

The future of laser in tissue ablation and tissue fusion will probably depend upon the availability of more compact, less power hungry, more reliable, and cheaper laser systems. Diode lasers are close to ideal in terms of size and they offer the potential of being as cheap as other mass-produced semiconductor devices. At the present time, diode units cannot develop enough power to take over the tissue cutting tasks. Advances in diode laser technology are occurring steadily, however, and eventually cheap, reliable, multiwatt diode units will be readily available [302].

Tissue Fusion

The various trends in improving the process of tissue fusion have already been discussed under laser tissue welding. Progress in automated welding techniques, refinement and development of better glues and solders, and availability of logistically simple diode lasers should eventually overcome the obstacles that face tissue fusion using lasers. To transcend the limitations of the human surgeon's senses, reflexes, and judgment, there are three areas that will come into play: sensors, computers, and robots. Optical sensing systems have been developed that can measure in real-time physical quantities such as temperature and spectroscopic data that help distinguish between normal and abnormal tissues [307]. It is possible to use a single fiber for both laser energy delivery and optical sensing of tissue features [308]. Other forms of sensing such as catheter-delivered miniaturized ultrasound probes can be coupled with the laser delivery device to obtain a precise luminal level view of what the laser is doing [309]. Real-time computer analysis of this information will be an advantage in supplementing clinical judgment and observation in order to obtain optimum control of laser exposure and tissue effect. Although substantial issues remain to be settled in terms of safety, the use of semi-independent active robots in the operating room will enable the surgeon to achieve tissue effects that are simply beyond the capability of human precision.

Hyperthermia

The central issue in the application of hyperthermia is to contain heat to the geometric volume of tumor tissue and prevent the spread of heat into the normal brain in order to have a good therapeutic ratio. This would mean development of durable and cheap probes with varying diffusivity to distribute heat evenly within the volume of a given tumor. A computer would then calculate the position and diffusivity of each of these probes in order to heat only the tumor volume and not the adjacent brain, based on the true extent of the tumor as shown by preoperative imaging. The probes would then be inserted stereotactically into the tumor and the entire process would then be monitored real time by means of imaging—either a 3D MRI [105] or 3D PET scan. As a way of further improvization, a simultaneous "cooling" of normal tissue (although purely hypothetical at this time) may help minimize the damage to normal tissues.

Minimally Invasive Neurosurgery

The attitude of minimizing the surgical trauma due to the particular susceptibility of the brain culminates in the concept of "keyhole neurosurgery." This imposes some prerequisites: (1) precision of reaching the target, (2) narrowness of approach, and (3) precise ablation of target, e.g., tumor.

The first requisite has been addressed for several years by such methods as stereotaxy, which has evolved into the development of "neuronavigators" [310]. These are echatronic arms that can help bridge the gap between three-dimensional multimodality (structural and functional) imaging data and the imaged object via interactive computer programs. In principle, neuronavigators add recent advances in electronics and image graphics to the mechanics used in conventional stereotactic frames. The movement of the neuronavigator is controlled by sensors at each joint of the arm. With the latest advances in computer speed and memory, sensor precision, and instrumentation, neuronavigators can provide stereotactic accuracy and real-time interaction with the surgical object (Fig. 9). Also, preoperative planning and simulation of the procedure are possible, as well as the transfer of simulation results to the actual operation to lessen the operating time and possibly even allow the neurosurgeon to operate remotely!

The issue of narrowness of approach involves the use of endoscopes (rigid and/or flexible) or a system of endoscopes utilizing different approaches to a large tumor. This can happen only if endoscopes can be used in routes currently used in microneurosurgery to remove the tumors. The problem of guiding the endoscope to the target is already being looked at by means of

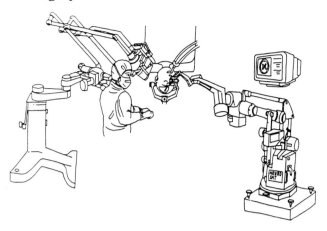

Fig. 9. Isocentric three-dimensional digitizer for neurosurgery devised by Dr. T. Takizawa. This comprises a frameless isocentric stereotactic mechanism and a three-dimensional digitizer for intraoperative spatial monitoring. The digitizer's multiarticulated arm has three joints related to the Cartesian co-ordinates, two quadrant arcs forming an isocenter system, a microdrive, and a probe holder. Any region selected by directing the probe tip can be displayed three-dimensionally. This is useful for open stereotaxy or CT/MRI guided stereotaxy. (Courtesy Dr. T. Takizawa, from Isocentric stereotactic three-dimensional digitizer for neurosurgery in Stereotact Funct Neurosurg, 1993; 60:182, with permission.)

intraoperative real-time magnetic guidance system for intracranial localization [311]. The ultrathin catheter-guided ultrasound probes may also be utilized to obtain real-time information [309].

Precise ablation of the target tissue with preservation of normal brain tissue calls for robotization of neurosurgical procedures. The increased dexterity provided by robotization will make possible what is today considered utopian. Related fields such as engineering, optics, biomaterials, artificial vision, and miniaturization will contribute to the conception and realization of flexible robots holding sensors (ultrasonic, barometric, or visual) capable of driving themselves along curved (and winding) trajectories amid deep and fragile anatomical landscapes, such as the sylvian fissure, the basilar cisterns, and the ventricular cavities, toward deep-seated, small-size, or even moving targets [312].

REFERENCES

1. Earle KM, Carpenter S, Roessman U, Ross MA, Hayes JR, Zettler EH. Central nervous system effects of laser radiation. Fed Proc 1965; 24:S–129.
2. Fine S, Klein E, Nowak W, Scott RE, Laor Y, Simpson L, Crissey J, Donaghue J, Dehr UE. Interaction of laser

radiation with biologic systems: I. Studies on interaction with tissues. Fed Proc 1965; 24:S–35.

3. Fox JL, Hayes JR, Stein MN. The effects of laser radiation on intracranial structures. First Annual Biomedical Laser Conference of the Laser Medical Research Foundation. Boston, MA, 1965.

4. Fox JL, Hayes JR, Stein MN, Green RC, Paanen R. Experimental cranial and vascular studies of the effects of pulsed and continuous wave laser radiation. J Neurosurg 1967; 27:126–137.

5. Stellar S. A study of the effects of laser light on nervous tissue. In: Proceedings of the Third International Congress of Neurological Surgery. Series No. 110. Copenhagen, 1965:542–551.

6. Brown TE, True C, McLaurin RL, Hornby P, Rockwell RJ Jr. Laser radiation: I. Acute effects on cerebral cortex. Neurology 1966; 16:730–737.

7. Liss L, Roppel R. Histopathology of laser-produced lesions in cat brains. Neurology 1966; 16:783–790.

8. Rosomoff HL, Carroll F. Reaction of neoplasm and brain to laser. Arch Neurol 1966; 14:143–148.

9. Stellar S, Polayni TA, Bredemeier HC. Experimental studies with the carbon dioxide laser as a neurosurgical instrument. Med Biol Eng 1970; 8:549.

10. Stellar S, Polayni TA, Bredemeier HC. Lasers in surgery. In: Wolbarsht ML, ed. "Laser Application in Biology and Medicine," Vol 1. New York: Plenum, 1971.

11. Stellar S, Polayni TA, Bredemeier HC. Lasers in surgery. In: Wolbarsht ML, ed. "Laser Application in Biology and Medicine," Vol 2. New York: Plenum 1974, pp 241–293.

12. Ascher PW. Lasers in neurosurgery. In: Spinelli P, Dal Fante M, Marchesini R, eds. "Photodynamic Therapy and Biomedical Lasers." Excerpta Medica, 1992, pp 93–96.

13. Heppner F. The laser scalpel on the nervous system. In: Kaplan I, ed. "Laser Surgery II." Jerusalem: Jerusalem Academic Press, 1978, pp 79–80.

14. Ascher PW. The use of CO_2 in neurosurgery. In: Kaplan I, ed. "Laser Surgery II." Jerusalem: Jerusalem Academic Press, 1978, pp 28–30.

15. Ascher PW. Neurosurgery. In: Andrews AH Jr, Polanyi TG, eds. "Microscopic and Endoscopic Surgery with the CO_2 Laser." Boston: John Wright-PSG, 1982, pp 298–314.

16. Takizawa T, Yamazaki T, Miura N, et al. Laser surgery of basal, orbital, and ventricular meningiomas which are difficult to extirpate by conventional methods. Neurol Med Chir 1980; 20:729–737.

17. Ascher PW, Cerullo LJ. Laser use in neurosurgery. In: Dixon J, ed. "Surgical Applications of Lasers." Chicago: Year Book Medical Publishers, 1983, pp 163–174.

18. Robertson JH, Clark WC. Carbon dioxide laser in neurosurgery. Contemporary Neurosurgery 1984; 5(12): 1–6.

19. Ognev BV, Vishnevskii AA Jr, Troitskii RA, Timokhina NI. Changes in the brain and eyes produced by lasers. Bull Biol Med 1972; 73:205.

20. Yahr WZ, Strully KJ, Hurwitt ES. Non-occlusive small arterial anastomosis with a neodymium laser. Surg Forum 1964; 15:224.

21. Yahr WZ, Strully KJ. Blood vessel anastomosis by laser and other biomedical applications. J Assoc Adv Med Intrum 1966; 1:28–31.

22. Jain KK, Gorisch W. Repair of small blood vessels with the neodymium-YAG laser: A preliminary report. Surgery 1979; 85:684.

23. Beck OJ, Wilske J, Schonberger JL, Gorisch W. Tissue changes following application of laser to the rabbit brain. Neurosurg Rev 1979; 1:31–36.

24. Beck OJ. The use of the Nd:YAG and the carbon dioxide laser in neurosurgery. Neurosurg Rev 1980; 3:261–266.

25. Takeuchi J, Handa H, Taki W, et al. The Nd:YAG laser in neurological surgery. Surg Neurol 1982; 18:140–142.

26. Hobieka CP, Rockwell RJ Jr. Argon laser microsurgery: Its advantages and applications in otolaryngology. Laryngoscope 1973: 960–965.

27. Maira G, Mohr G, Panisset A, et al. Laser photocoagulation for treatment of experimental aneurysms. J Microsurg 1979; 1:137–147.

28. Glasscock ME, Jackson CG, Whitaker SR. The argon laser in acoustic tumor surgery. Laryngoscope 1981; 41(9):1405–1416.

29. Fasano VA. The treatment of vascular malformation of the brain with laser source. Lasers Surg Med 1981; 1:347–356.

30. Boggan JE, Edwards MSB, Davis RL, et al. Comparison of the brain tissue response in rats to injury by argon and carbon dioxide lasers. Neurosurgery 1982; 11:609–616.

31. Edwards MSB, Boggan JE, Fuller TA. Review article: The laser in neurological surgery. J Neurosurg 1983; 59:555–566.

32. Powers SK, Edwards MSB, Boggan JE, et al. Use of the argon surgical laser in neurosurgery. J Neurosurg 1984; 60:523–530.

33. Roux FX, Devaux B, Merienne L, Cioloca C, Chodkiewicz JP. 1.32 μm Nd:YAG laser during neurosurgical procedures: Experience with about 70 patients operated on with the MC 2100 unit. Acta Neurochir (Wein) 1990; 107:161–166.

34. Roux FX, Mordon S, Fallet-Bianco C, Merienne L, Devaux BC, Chodkiewicz JP. Effects of 1.32 μm Nd:YAG laser on brain thermal and histological experimental data. Surg Neurol 1990; 34:402–407.

35. Martiniuk R, Bauer JA, McKean JDS, Tulip J, Mielke BW. New long wavelength Nd:YAG laser at 1.44 μm: Effect on brain. J Neurosurg 1989; 70:249–256.

36. Gamache FW Jr, Morgello S. The histopathological effects of the CO_2 versus the KTP laser on the brain and spinal cord: A canine model. Neurosurgery 1993; 32(1): 100–104.

37. Gamache FW Jr, Patterson RH Jr. The use of the potassium titanyl phosphate (KTP) laser in neurosurgery. Neurosurgery 1990; 26(6):1010–1013.

38. Quigley MR, Shih T, Elrifai A, Maroon JC, Lesiecki ML. Percutaneous laser discectomy with the Ho:YAG laser. Lasers Surg Med 1992; 12:621–624.

39. Gottlob C, Kopchok GE, Peng SK, Tabbara M, Cavaye D, White RA. Holmium:YAG laser ablation of human intervertebral disc: Preliminary evaluation. Lasers Surg Med 1992; 12(1):86–91.

40. Wilberger JE Jr, Abla A, Kennerdell J, et al. Mucocele of the pterygoid recess treated by laser. J Neurosurg 1985; 63:970–972.

41. Roux FX, Leriche B, Cioloca C, Devaux B, Turak B, Nohra G. Combined CO_2 and Nd-YAG laser in neurosurgical practice: A 1st experience apropos of 40 intra-

cranial procedures. [French] Neurochirurgie 1992; 38(4): 235–237.

42. Lombard GF, Luparello V, Peretta P. Statistical comparison of surgical results with or without laser in neurosurgery. (French). Neurochirurgie 1992; 38(4):226–228.

43. Desgeorges M, Sterkers O, Ducolombier A, Pernot P, Hor F, Rosseau G, Yedeas M, Elabaddi N, Le Bars M. Laser microsurgery of meningioma: An analysis of a continuous series of 164 cases treated surgically by using different lasers. (French). Neurochirurgie 1992; 38(4):217–225.

44. Kopera M, Majchrzak H, Idzik M. Use of the Nd:YAG laser in surgical treatment of intracranial tumors. (Polish). Neurol Neurochir Pol 1992; Suppl 1:237–242.

45. Conforti P, Moraci A, Albanese V, Rotondo M, Parlato C. Microsurgical management of suprasellar and intraventricular meningiomas. Neurochirurgie 1991; 34(3): 85–89.

46. Naumann M, Meixensberger J. Factors influencing meningioma recurrence rate. Acta Neurochir (Wien) 1990; 107(3–4):108–111.

47. Waidhauser E, Beck OJ, Oeckler RCT. Nd:YAG laser in the microsurgery of frontobasal meningiomas. Lasers Surg Med 1990; 10:544–550.

48. Cerullo LJ, Burke LP. Use of the laser in neurosurgery. Surg Clin North Am 1984; 64:995–1000.

49. Kartush JM, Lundy LB. Facial nerve outcome in acoustic neuroma surgery. Otolaryngol Clin North Am 1992; 25(3):623–647.

50. Eiras J, Alberdi J, Gomez J. The CO_2 laser in acoustic nerve tumors surgery. Neurochirurgie 1993; 39:16–23.

51. Deruty R, Pellissou-Guyotat I, Mottolese C, Amat D. Routine use of the CO_2 laser technique for resection of cerebral tumors. Acta Neurochir (Wien) 1993; 123:43–45.

52. Majchrzak H, Kopera M, Bierzynska-Macyszyn G, Dragan T, Idzik M. A case of acoustic neurinoma in a girl aged 13 (Polish). Neurol Neurochir Pol 1993; 27(1): 123–126.

53. Oekler RTC, Beck HC, Frank F. Surgery of the sellar region with the Nd:YAG laser. Fortschr Med 1984; 9:218–220.

54. Heiss JD, Tew JM. Transsphenoidal laser microsurgery. Neurosurgery: State of the Art Reviews 1987; 2(2):411–425.

55. Tew JM, Tobler WD. The role of the carbon dioxide laser in skull base tumors. Neurosurgery: State of the Art Reviews 1987; 2(2):397–409.

56. Kall BA, Kelly PJ, Goerss SJ. Interactive stereotactic surgical system for the removal of intracranial tumors utilizing the CO_2 laser and CT-derived database. IEEE Trans Biomed Eng 1985; 32(2):112–116.

57. Kelly PJ, Kall BA, Goerss S, Cascino TL. Results of computer-assisted stereotactic laser resection of deep-seated intracranial lesions. Mayo Clin Proc 1986; 61(1): 20–27.

58. Kelly PJ, Kall BA, Goerss S, Earnest F 4th. Computer-assisted stereotaxic laser resection of intra-axial brain neoplasms. J Neurosurg 1986; 64(3):427–439.

59. Kelly PJ, Kall BA, Goerss SJ. Computer-interactive stereotactic resection of deep-seated and centrally located intraaxial brain lesions. Appl Neurophysiol 1987; 50(1–6):107–113.

60. Abernathey CD, Davis DH, Kelly PJ. Treatment of colloid cysts of the third ventricle by stereotaxic microsurgical laser craniotomy. J Neurosurg 1989; 70(4):525–529.

61. Kelly PJ. Image-directed tumor resection. Neurosurg Clin N Am 1990; 1(1):81–95.

62. Kelly PJ. Stereotactic craniotomy. Neurosurg Clin N Am 1990; 1(4):781–799.

63. Kelly PJ. Computer assisted volumetric stereotactic resection of superficial and deep seated intra-axial brain mass lesions. Acta Neurochir Suppl (Wien) 1991; 52:26–29.

64. Camacho A, Kelly PJ. Volumetric stereotactic resection of superficial and deep seated intraaxial brain lesions. Acta Neurochir Suppl (Wien) 1992; 54:83–88.

65. Lyons MK, Kelly PJ. Computer-assisted stereotactic biopsy and volumetric resection of thalamic pilocytic astrocytomas: Report of 23 cases. Stereotact Funct Neurosurg 1992; 59(1–4):100–104.

66. Morita A, Kelly PJ. Resection of intraventricular tumors via a computer-assisted volumetric stereotactic approach. Neurosurgery 1993; 32(6):920–926.

67. Walker ML, Storrs BB, Goodman SG. Use of the carbon dioxide laser for excision of primary brain tumors in children: A 1 year experience. In: Raimondi AJ, ed. "Concepts in Neurosurgery 3." Basel: Karger, 1983, pp 207–215.

68. Edwards MSB, Boggan JE. Argon laser surgery of pediatric neural neoplasms. Child's Brain 1984; 11:171–175.

69. Tobler WD, Sawaya R, Tew JM. Successful laser-assisted excision of a metastatic midbrain tumor. Neurosurgery 1986; 18:795–797.

70. Ascher PW, Heppner F. Carbon dioxide laser in neurosurgery. Neurosurg Rev 1984; 7:123–133.

71. Cerullo LJ, Burke LP. Use of the laser in neurosurgery. Surg Clin North Am 1984; 64:995–1000.

72. Fasano VA. Observations on the use of three laser sources in sequence (CO_2-argon-Nd:YAG) in neurosurgery. Lasers Surg Med 1983; 2:199–203.

73. McLone DG, Naidich TP. Laser resection of 50 spinal lipomas. Neurosurgery 1986; 18:611–615.

74. Epstein FJ, Farmer J. Pediatric spinal cord tumor surgery. Neurosurg Clin N Am 1990; 1:569–590.

75. Greenwood J Jr. Surgical removal of intramedullary tumors. J Neurosurg 1967; 26:276–282.

76. McCormick PC, Torres R, Post DK, et al. Intramedullary ependymoma of the spinal cord. J Neurosurg 1990; 72:523–532.

77. Yasui T, Hakuba A, Katsuyama J, et al. Microsurgical removal of intramedullary tumors: Report of 22 cases. Acta Neurochir Suppl (Wein) 1988; 43:9–12.

78. Guidetti B, Mercuri S, Vagnozzi R. Long-term results of the surgical treatment of 129 intramedullary spinal gliomas. J Neurosurg 1981; 54:323–330.

79. Reimer R, Onofrio BM. Astrocytomas of spinal cord in children and adolescents. J Neurosurg 1985; 63:669–675.

80. Rossitch E, Zeidman SM, Burger PC, et al. Clinical and pathological analysis of spinal cord astrocytomas in children. Neurosurgery 1990; 27:193–196.

81. Hardison HH, Packer RJ, Rorke LB, et al. Outcome of children with intramedullary spinal cord tumors. Childs Nerv Syst 1987; 3:89–92.

82. Epstein F. Surgical treatment of intramedullary spinal

cord tumors in children. In: Pascual-Castroveijo I, ed. "Spinal Tumors in Children and Adolescents." New York: Raven Press, 1990:51–70.

83. Hoffman HJ, Taecholarn C, Hendrick EB, Humphreys RP. Management of lipomyelomeningoceles: Experience at the Hospital for Sick Children, Toronto. J Neurosurg 1985; 62(1):1–8.

84. Pierre-Kahn A, Lacombe J, Pichon J, Giudicelli Y, Renier D, Sainte-Rose C, Perrigot M, Hirsch JF. Intraspinal lipomas with spina bifida: Prognosis and treatment in 73 cases. J Neurosurg 1986; 65(6):756–761.

85. Kanev PM, Lemire RJ, Loeser JD, Berger MS. Management and long-term follow-up review of children with lipomyelomeningocele, 1952–1987. J Neurosurg 1990; 73(1):48–52.

86. Herman JM, McLone DG, Storrs BB, Dauser RC. Analysis of 153 patients with myelomeningocele or spinal lipoma reoperated upon for a tethered cord: Presentation, management and outcome. Pediatr Neurosurg 1993; 19(5):243–249.

87. Sathi S, Madsen JR, Bauer S, Scott RM. Effect of surgical repair on the neurologic function in infants with lipomeningocele. Pediatr Neurosurg 1993; 19(5):256–259.

88. Maira G, Fernandez E, Pallini R, Puca A. Total excision of spinal lipomas using CO_2 laser at low power: Experimental and clinical observations. Neurol Res 1986; 8(4):225–230.

89. Chapman PH, Davis KR. Surgical treatment of spinal lipomas in childhood. Pediatr Neurosurg 1993; 19(5):267–275.

90. Steinbok P, Cochrane DD, Poskitt K. Intramedullary spinal cord tumors in children. Neurosurg Clin N Am 1992; 3(4):931–945.

91. Fasano VA, Urciuoli R, Ponzio M. Photocoagulation of cerebral arteriovenous malformations and arterial aneurysms with the neodymium:yttrium-aluminium-garnet or argon laser: Preliminary results in twelve patients. Neurosurgery 1982; 11:754–760.

92. Wharen RE, Anderson RE, Sundt TM Jr. The Nd:YAG laser in neurosurgery. II. Clinical studies: An adjunctive measure for hemostasis in resection of arteriovenous malformations. J Neurosurg 1984; 60:540–547.

93. Van Loveren HR, Weil SM, Tew JM Jr. Complete excision of thalamic arteriovenous malformations with neodymium:YAG laser. In: Sawaya R, Tew JM Jr, eds. "Laser Applications in Neurosurgery." Philadelphia: Hanley and Belfus, 1987, pp 447–457.

94. Zuccarello M, Mandybur TI, Tew JM Jr, Tobler WD. Acute effect of the Nd:YAG laser on the cerebral arteriovenous malformation: a histological study. Neurosurgery 1989; 24(3):328–333.

95. Strugar J, Chyatte D. In situ photocoagulation of spinal dural arteriovenous malformations using the Nd:YAG laser. J Neurosurg 1992; 77(4):571–574.

96. Samaras GM, Cheung AY. Microwave hyperthermia for cancer therapy. CRC Crit Rev Bioeng 1981; 5:123–184.

97. Salcman M, Samaras GM. Hyperthermia for brain tumors: Biophysical rationale. Neurosurgery 1991; 9:327–335.

98. Schrober R, Bettag M, Sabel M, Ulrich F, Hessel S. Fine structure of zonal changes in experimental Nd:YAG laser-induced interstitial hyperthermia. Lasers Surg Med 1993; 13(2):234–241.

99. Nowak G, Rentzch O, Terzis AJA, Arnold H. Induced hyperthermia in brain tissue: Comparison between contact Nd:YAG laser system and automatically controlled high-frequency current. Acta Neurochir (Wein) 1990; 102:76–81.

100. Sugiyama K, Sakai T, Fujishima I, Ryu H, Uemera K, Yokoyama T. Stereotactic interstitial laser-hyperthermia using Nd:YAG laser. Stereotact Funct Neurosurg 1990; 54–55:501–505.

101. Jolesz FA, Bleier AR, Jakab P, Ryenzel PW, Huttl K, Jako GJ. MR imaging of laser tissue interactions. Radiology 1988; 168:249–253.

102. Elias Z, Powers SK, Atstupenas E, Brown JT. Hyperthermia from interstitial laser irradiation in normal rat brain. Lasers Surg Med 1987; 7:370–375.

103. Fan M, Ascher PW, Germann RH, Ebner F. Temperature profiles of interstitial 1.06 Nd:YAG laserthermia in human cadaver brain. In: Spinelli P, Dal Fante M, Marchesini R, eds. "Photodynamic Therapy and Biomedical Lasers." Excerpta Medica, 1992, pp 349–353.

104. Wyman DR, Tracz RA, Schatz SW, Little PB, Towner RA, Stewart WA, Wilson BC. Interpreting magnetic resonance images of interstitial laser photocoagulation in brain. Lasers Surg Med 1992; Suppl 4:38–39.

105. Cline HE, Schenck JF, Watkins RD, Hynynen K, Jolesz FA. Magnetic resonance-guided thermal surgery. MRM 1993; 30:98–106.

106. Ascher PW, Fan M, Schrottner O. A new less invasive method of treating central brain tumors (preliminary report). In: Spinelli P, Dal Fante M, Marchesini R., eds. "Photodynamic Therapy and Biomedical Lasers." Excerpta Medica, 1992, pp 354–357.

107. Bettag M, Ulrich F, Schober R, Furst G, Langen KJ, Sabel M, Kiwit JC. Stereotactic laser therapy in cerebral gliomas. Acta Neurochir Suppl (Wein) 1991; 52:81–83.

108. Roux FX, Merienne L, Fallet-Bianco C, Beuvon F, Devaux B, Leriche B, Cioloca C. Stereotactic laser interstitial thermotherapy: A new alternative in the therapeutic management of some brain tumors. (French). Neurochirurgie 1992; 38(4):238–244.

109. Frazier OH, Painvin GA, Morris JR, Thomsen S, Neblett CR. Laser-assisted microvascular anastomoses: Angiographic and anatomopathologic studies in growing microvascular anastomoses: Preliminary report. Surgery 1985; 97:585–590.

110. Quigley MR, Bailes JE, Kwaan HC, Cerullo LJ, Block S. Comparison of myointimal hyperplasia in laser assisted and suture anastomosed arteries: A preliminary report. J Vasc Surg 1986; 4:217–219.

111. Dew DK. Review and status report on laser tissue sealing. Proc SPIE 1990; 1200:38.

112. Grubbs PE, Wang S, Marini C, et al. Enhancement of CO_2 laser microvascular anastomoses by fibrin glue. J Surg Res 1988; 45:112–119.

113. Oz MC, Bass LS, Chuck RS, et al. Urokinase modulation of weld strength in laser vascular anastomosis. Lasers Surg Med 1990; 10:393–395.

114. Bass LS, Oz MC, Auteri JS, et al. Laparoscopic applications of laser-activated tissue glues. Proc SPIE 1991; 1421:164–168.

115. Oz MC, Bass LS, Williams MR, et al. Initial clinical experience with laser assisted solder bonding of human vascular tissue. Proc SPIE 1991; 1422:147–151.

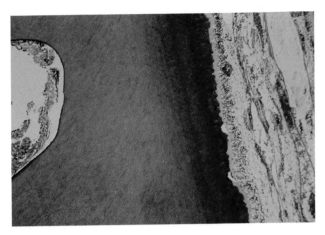

Fig. 21 (Ch. 2). Light photomicrograph showing tooth and pulpal tissue of an Er:YAG laser defect in a canine tooth. H&E (×100). See p. 47 for text discussion.

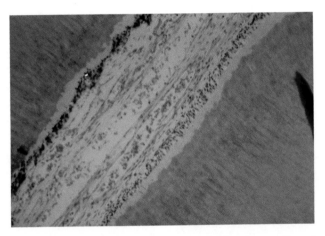

Fig. 22 (Ch. 2). Light photomicrograph showing tooth and pulpal tissue of a tooth with a defect created by a slow speed handpiece. H&E (×100). See p. 47 for text discussion.

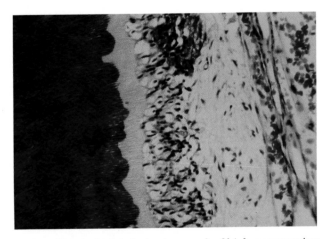

Fig. 23 (Ch. 2). Light photomicrograph of higher power view of the pulp in the tooth treated with the Er:YAG laser. H&E (×400). See p. 47 for text discussion.

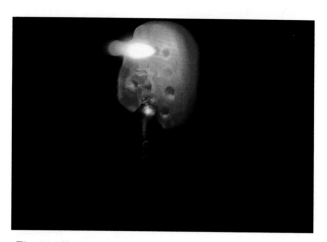

Fig. 28 (Ch. 2). Laser plume from a Er:YAG laser impact on tooth. See p. 49 for text discussion.

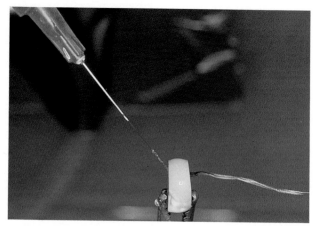

Fig. 29 (Ch. 2). Photograph of the scientific setup with the laser beam coming from the left. See p. 49 for text discussion.

Fig. 3 (Ch. 3). Patchwork hypopigmentation remains at the site of a large port wine stain following treatment with the argon laser. See p. 68 for text discussion.

Fig. 4 (Ch. 3). (a) Diffuse telangiectases are present on the cheek prior to treatment. (b) Nearly complete resolution without textural or pigmentary changes or scarring is seen 6 weeks after laser photocoagulation. See p. 68 for text discussion.

Fig. 5 (Ch. 3). (a) Large channel, high flow telangiectases are present on the nasal ala prior to laser treatment. (b) Excellent, but incomplete lightening is seen 6 weeks after laser photocoagulation performed at intervals along the length of each individual blood vessel. See p. 68 for text discussion.

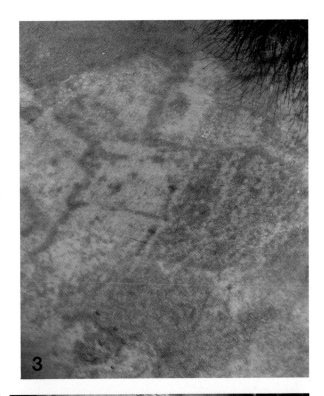

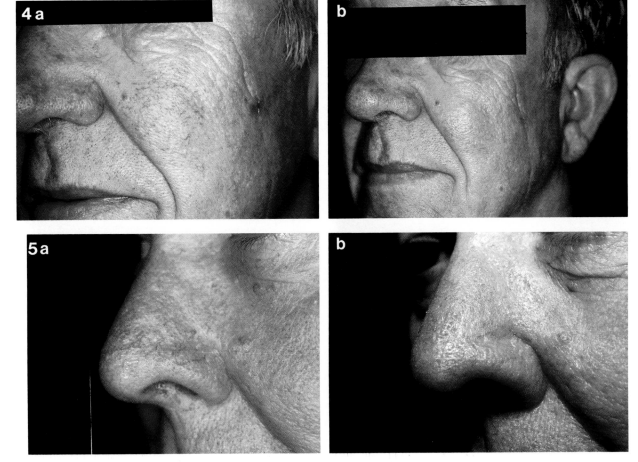

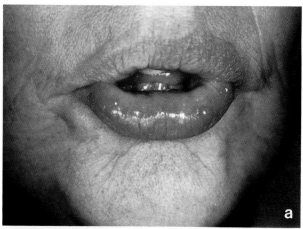

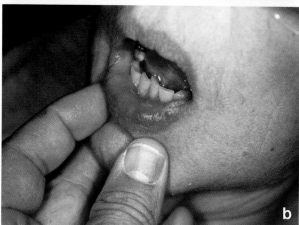

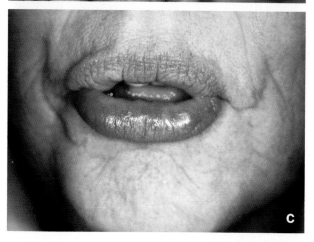

Fig. 9 (Ch. 3). **(a)** Two venous lakes are present on the lower lip prior to treatment. **(b)** Immediate whitening has occurred following photocoagulation with green laser light. **(c)** Complete disappearance of both lesions has occurred 6 weeks after one treatment without scarring or textural changes. See p. 76 for text discussion.

Fig. 11 (Ch. 5). Ratio of target (oxyhemoglobin) to background (melanin) absorption. Of the three oxyhemoglobin peaks, the second (532 nm) corresponds to KTP light (not shown) and the third (578 nm) corresponds to SPTL-1 dye laser light. By contrast, the two argon bands fall within one of the oxyhemoglobin absorption troughs. (Illustration courtesy Candela Lasers, Wayland, MA.) See p. 104 for text discussion.

Fig. 14 (Ch. 5). Hexascan. **c:** A large port wine stain of the left forearm, prior to treatment. **d:** The same patient, after initial hexascan photothermolysis. (Illustrations courtesy Lihtan Technologies, San Rafael, CA.) See page 104 for text discussion.

Fig. 20 (Ch. 5). Vascular rebound at the site of a vestibulectomy incision. See p. 104 for text discussion.

Fig. 21 (Ch. 5). **a:** Incapacitating hypervascularity and failure to re-epithelialize of the right side of a vestibulectomy incision, 6 months postsurgery. **b:** Appearances 2 months later, showing re-epithelialization and early shrinkage of the rebound vessels. Subsequently, all redness faded, and the patient was able to return to work and resume coitus. See p. 104 for text discussion.

Fig. 22 (Ch. 5). **a:** FEDL pulse captured on camera. **b:** Extreme vestibulitis, prior to FEDL photothermolysis. **c:** Intraoperative view showing immediate bruising at sites of impact. **d:** Successful outcome, 4 months after FEDL treatment. See p. 104 for text discussion.

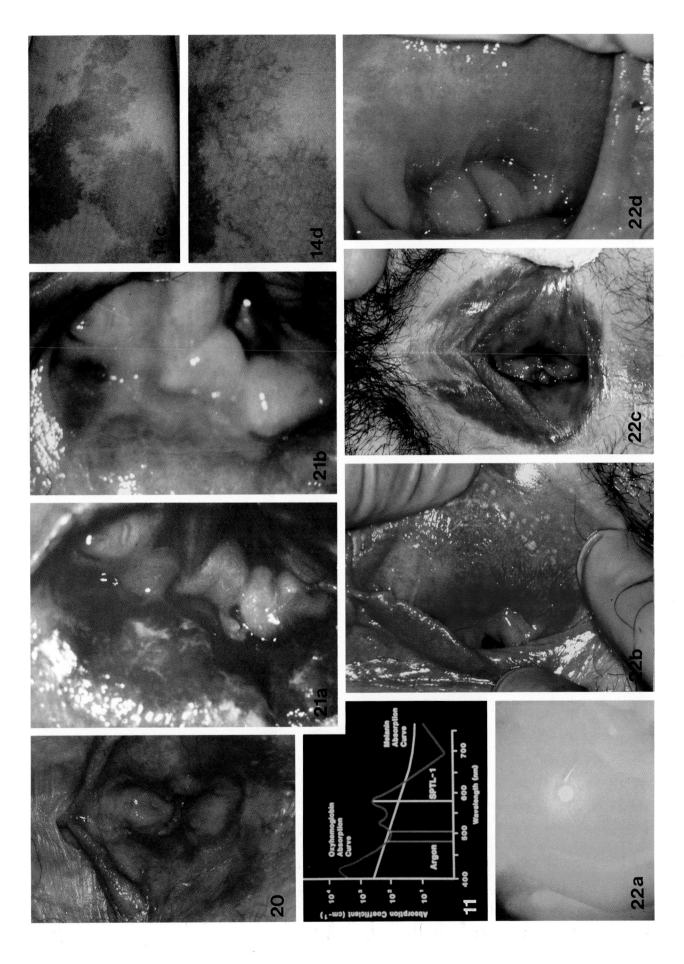

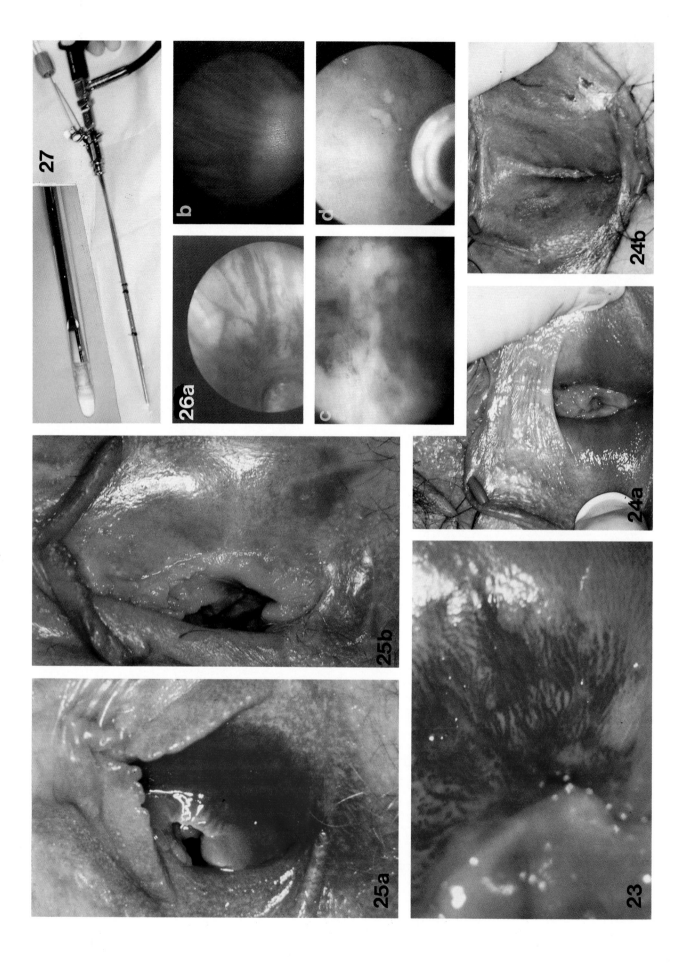

Fig. 23 (Ch. 5). Refractory pain loop, located deep within the right Bartholin's gland. See p. 115 for text discussion.

Fig. 24 (Ch. 5). **a:** Extreme vestibulitis, immediately prior to treatment with the hexascan adapted argon laser. **b:** Intraoperative view, showing some epithelial edema but no ecchymosis (contrast with Fig. 22c). See p. 115 for text discussion.

Fig. 25 (Ch. 5). **a:** Incapacitating surface vestibulitis, concentrated principally around the hymenal edge. **b:** Same patient after serial FEDL. Photothermolysis disappearance of the hypervascularity is almost always associated with resolution of symptoms. See p. 115 for text discussion.

Fig. 26 (Ch. 5). **a:** Extreme hypervascularity of the urethral mucosa, showing dilated, hyperemic, branching vessels of variable caliber. **b:** Laser beam in position to fire. **c:** Effect of cytoscopically directed argon laser, producing ecchymosis and vascular occulation with minimal epithelial damage. **d:** Long-term result, after healing, showing a pale, non-irritated mucosa. See p. 115 for text discussion.

Fig. 27 (Ch. 5). Standard cystoscope, modified by passing the angled delivery device *below* the lens, allowing the emitted KTP beam to diverge en route to its target on the opposite side of the urethral lumen. See p. 115 for text discussion.

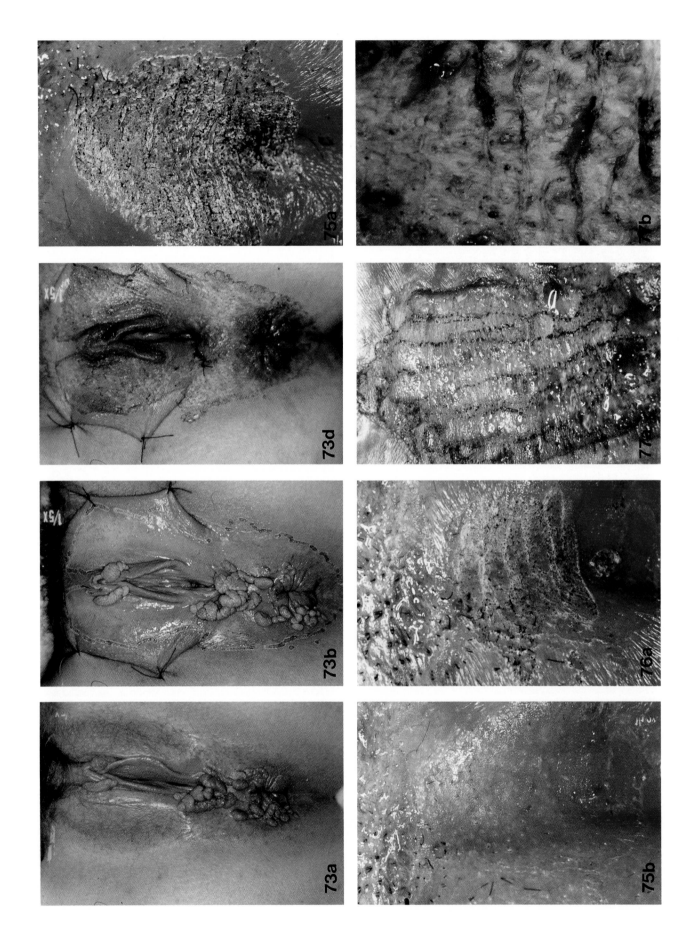

Fig. 73 (Ch. 5). **a:** Extensive vulvar condyloma before vinegar soaking. **b:** View of the same patient after a 3-minute soak with 4.5% acetic acid, showing extensive subclinical HPV infection of the intervening skin. Biopsy samples from this area showed prominent histologic features of active albeit subclinical viral expression. **d:** Extent of surgical destruction. Because healing occurs by epithelial regeneration from underlying skin appendages, healing time and postoperative discomfort are the same as that after local destruction of the exophytic condylomata alone. (From Reid et al. [28], reproduced with permission.) See p. 159 for text discussion.

Fig. 75 (Ch. 5). First surgical plane. **a:** View through the operating microscope after initial brushing with the laser. Beneath the charred remains of the surface squames can be seen the refractile remnants of plump keratinocytes within the proliferating zone of the epidermis. **b:** After wiping, the anatomically intact dermal surface is exposed. A small area of third plane penetration is shown at top. (From Reid [132], reprinted with permission.) See p. 159 for text discussion.

Fig. 76 (Ch. 5). Second surgical plane. **a:** The exposed papillary dermis has been gently released, sufficient to scorch (but not cut) the dermal surface. At top, there is an area of third plane (white) and at bottom an area of first plane (pink). (From Reid [132], reprinted with permission.) See p. 159 for text discussion.

Fig. 77 (Ch. 5). Third surgical plane. **a:** Slower, more deliberate movement of the laser beam has vaporized the upper half of the dermis, revealing barely visible fibrous grain, representing the coarse reticular dermis collagen obscured by a thin layer of surface eschar. **b:** Different patient, after rinsing the surface eschar. The stark white color of the reticular collagen and the arcuate vascular arcades are characteristic of this depth. (From Reid et al. [107], reproduced with permission. See p. 159 for text discussion.

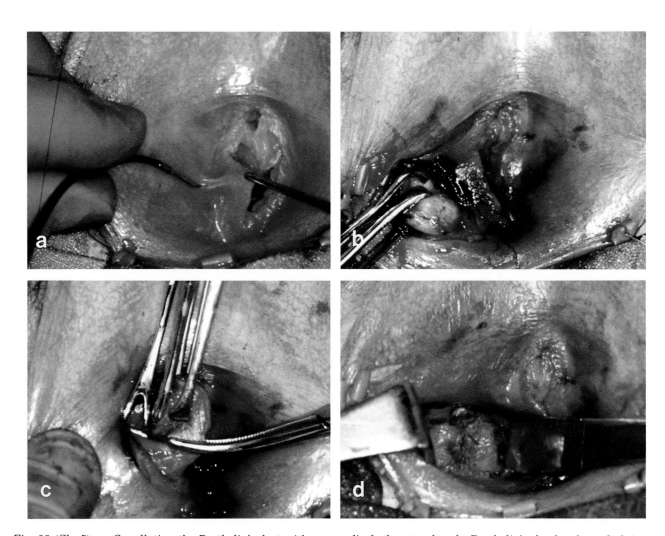

Fig. 93 (Ch. 5). **a:** Canullating the Bartholin's duct with a Sialogram canulla. **b:** Medial and lateral planes have been developed, and the Bartholin's gland is being elevated by a pair of baby Allis forceps. **c:** Clamping the deep (vascular) pedicule that attaches the Bartholin's gland to the underlying urogenital diaphragm. **d:** The cleaned-out Bartholin's fossa, showing pubococcygeus on the deep medial margin. See p. 176 for text discussion.

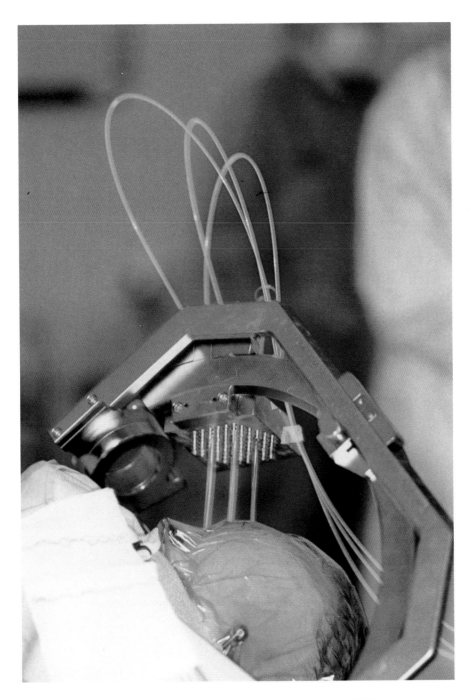

Fig. 3 (Ch. 7). Stereotactic implantation of optical fibers through transparent silicone catheters for uniform light delivery in photodynamic therapy of malignant glioma. This is done with the aid of a gridblock that is fixed to a stereotactic frame. See p. 227 for text discussion.

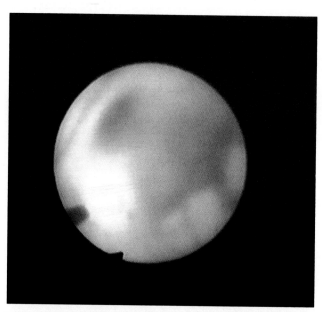

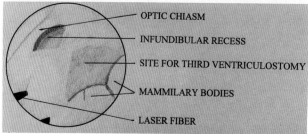

OPTIC CHIASM

INFUNDIBULAR RECESS

SITE FOR THIRD VENTRICULOSTOMY

MAMMILARY BODIES

LASER FIBER

Fig. 7 (Ch. 7). Photograph of the details of the floor of the third ventricle as seen through the endoscope upon entering the third ventricle through the foramen of Monro. Note the laser fiber with a pilot light. Schematic illustration of the photograph shows the site for performing the third ventriculostomy. See p. 231 for text discussion.

Fig. 3 (Ch. 8). Relative absorption vs. wavelength for various intraocular chromophores. The figure shows that: (1) macular xanthophyll has greater absorption for argon blue light than for other laser wavelengths, (2) hemoglobin has excellent blue, green, and yellow light absorption but much poorer red light absorption, (3) light absorption maxima for oxyhemoglobin are located at 542 nm (green) and 577 nm (yellow), (4) reduced (venous) hemoglobin has better krypton red light absorption than does oxygenated (arterial) hemoglobin, and (5) deoxyhemoglobin has roughly the same extinction coefficient for krypton red light as xanthophyll does for argon blue light. (Courtesy of Coherent, Palo Alto, CA.) See p. 253 for text discussion.

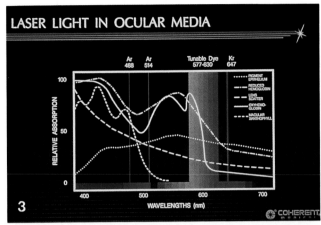

Fig. 25 (Ch. 8). False-color OCT tomograph obtained through the macula and optic disk of a human eye. See p. 288 for text discussion.

Fig. 26 (Ch. 8). OCT image of a neurosensory retinal detachment in a patient with a diagnosis of central serous chorioretinopathy. See p. 288 for text discussion.

Fig. 27 (Ch. 8). OCT image of the anterior human eye. See p. 288 for text discussion.

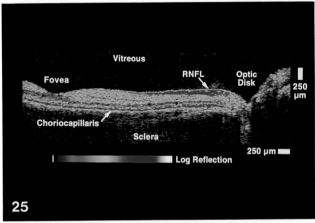

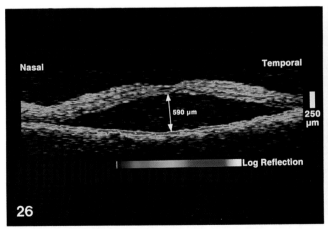

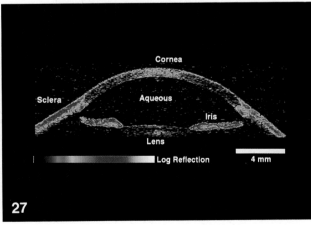

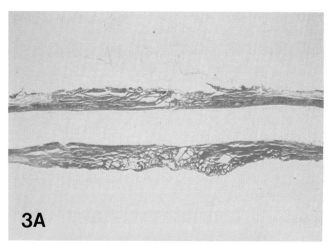

3A

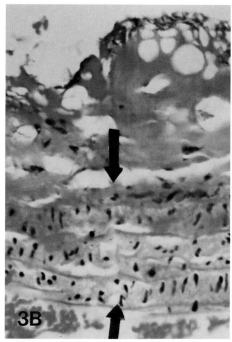

3B

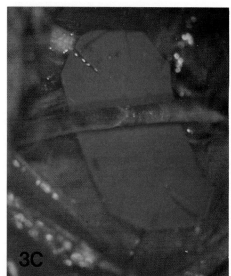

3C

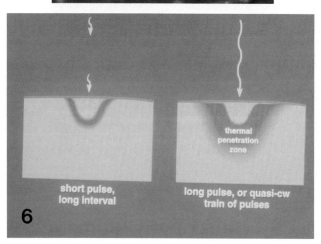

3D

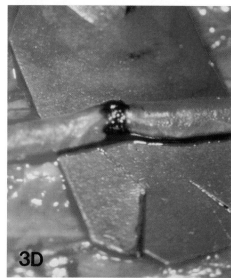

short pulse,
long interval

thermal
penetration
zone

long pulse, or quasi-cw
train of pulses

6

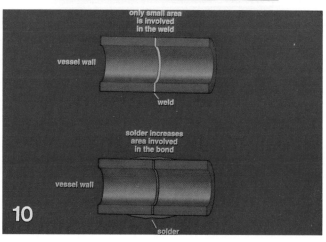

only small area
is involved
in the weld

vessel wall

weld

solder increases
area involved
in the bond

vessel wall

solder

10

Fig. 3 (Ch. 12). (**a**) Longitudinal section of the THC:YAG laser anastomosis 1 hour after creation. There is uniform transmural heating to weld the entire thickness of the vessel together (hematoxylin, phloxine, saffron stain, × 25). From Bass LS, Treat MR, Dzakonski C, Trokel SL. Sutureless microvascular anastomosis using the THC:YAG laser: A preliminary report. Microsurg 1989; 10:189–193. Reprinted with permission. (**b**) Longitudinal section at 1 hour of rat carotid artery end-to-end anastomosis, which was laser-soldered using the 810 nm gallium-aluminum-arsenide diode laser and indocyanine green-protein solder. Even though the solder shows extensive thermal damage including evidence suggestive of water boiling, the underlying vessel wall is essentially normal. The welded line, indicated by arrows, is barely discernable (hematoxylin, phloxine, and saffron, × 250). (**c**) Immediate postoperative view of an end-to-end rat carotid artery anastomosis produced with the 2.15-μm thulium-holmium-chromium:YAG laser. No charring or distortion is seen. The clinical endpoint of welding is a slight tanning and drying of tissue, as shown in this THC:YAG welded microvessel. See (a) for reference. (**d**) Immediate postoperative view of a rat carotid artery end-to-end anastomosis produced with an 810 nm diode laser and indocyanine green-protein solder. The band of solder acts as a "biological band-aid" to hold the vessel ends together without charring or significant thermal injury to the vessel. See p. 387 for text discussion.

Fig. 6 (Ch. 12). When the pulse is shorter than the thermal relaxation time of the tissue and the interval between pulses is long, relative spatial confinement of heat from that pulse occurs. If the pulse is longer than the thermal relaxation time, or if the tissue experiences a quasi-CW train of pulses, then local thermal build-up occurs, resulting in a larger zone of thermal injury. See p. 387 for text discussion.

Fig. 10 (Ch. 12). Solder increases lasered bond strength by increasing the percentage of edge to edge surface contact as well as greatly increasing the overall area involved in the bond (sleeve effect). See p. 387 for text discussion.

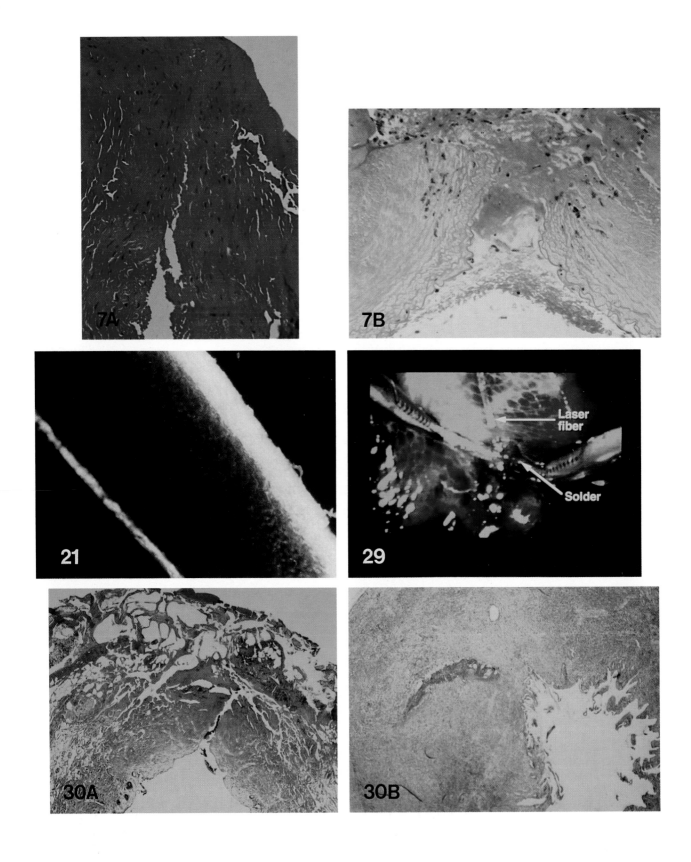

Fig. 7 (Ch. 12). (**a**) Transverse section at postop day 7 of a longitudinal rabbit aortotomy, which was welded using an argon laser without solder. Note the eosinophilic hyalinization throughout the media, which is representative of extensive thermal damage (hematoxylin, phloxine, and saffron stain, × 20). (**b**) Transverse section at postop day 7 of a longitudinal rabbit aortotomy which was laser-soldered using an argon laser and fluorescein isothiocyanate-protein solder. Note that the eosinophilic change indicative of thermal damage is essentially limited to the solder and that the vessel media is unaltered. Also, the solder has filled a slight gap caused by imperfect coaptation of the vessel edges (hematoxylin, phloxine, and saffron stain, × 20). See p. 391 for text discussion.

Fig. 21 (Ch. 12). Porcine femoral articular cartilage shows good penetration of the photochemical cross-linking dye following 30 minutes of exposure to a 0.98 mM concentration in 20% Cremophor EL. Courtesy of M.M. Judy. See p. 391 for text discussion.

Fig. 29 (Ch. 12). A longitudinal choledochotomy in the miniswine as viewed through the laparoscope. The cut edges are being apposed in preparation for laser soldering. Welding can be performed endoscopically with relative ease compared with suturing. See p. 391 for text discussion.

Fig. 30 (Ch. 12). Laser-soldered canine common bile duct at postoperative day 2 (**a**) exhibits significant thermal changes in the solder on the surface of the bile duct. There is little distortion of bile duct contour and only superficial thermal changes in the duct itself. On postoperative day 7 (**b**), mucosal resurfacing is complete. Solder is nearly resorbed and inflammatory response is minimal. Hematoxylin and eosin stain, × 25. From Bass LS, Libutti SK, Oz MC, Rosen J, Williams MR, Nowygrod R, Treat MR. Canine choledochotomy closure with diode laser-activated fibrinogen solder. Surgery 1994; 115(3): 398–401. Reprinted with permission. See p. 391 for text discussion.

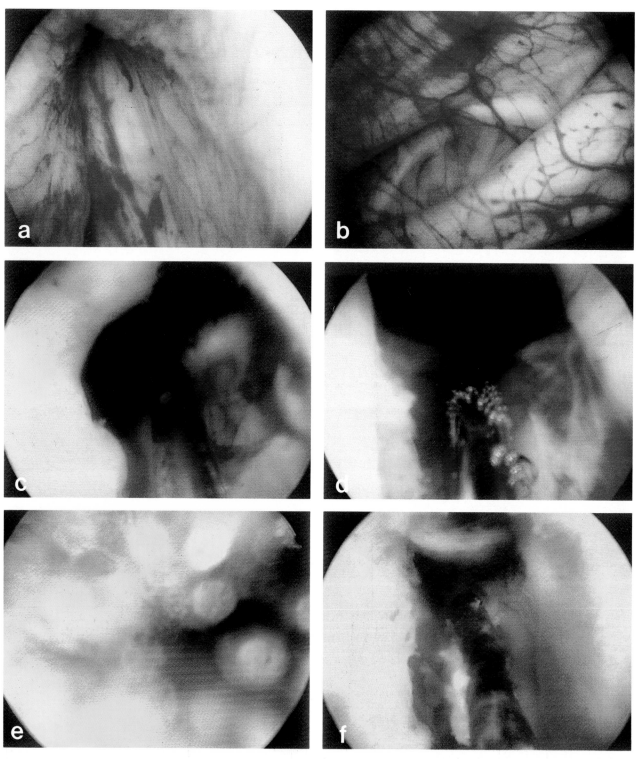

Fig. 2 (Ch. 13). Sequence of events during a typical laser ablation procedure for BPH with an ADD (Laserscope) using 60 watts of Nd:YAG lasing for 60 seconds in four quadrants. **a** shows the prostate gland; **b** shows trabeculations and pseudodiverticula of the bladder; **c** shows ADD with a helium neon beam ready to ablate that side; the other side has been ablated; **d** shows microbubbles on the probe tip during laser ablation; **e** shows blurring of view that is not uncommon; **f** shows a nearly burnt out probe. Good flow of irrigation in our experience was crucial for preventing the probe burn and for good visualization. See p. 427 for text discussion.

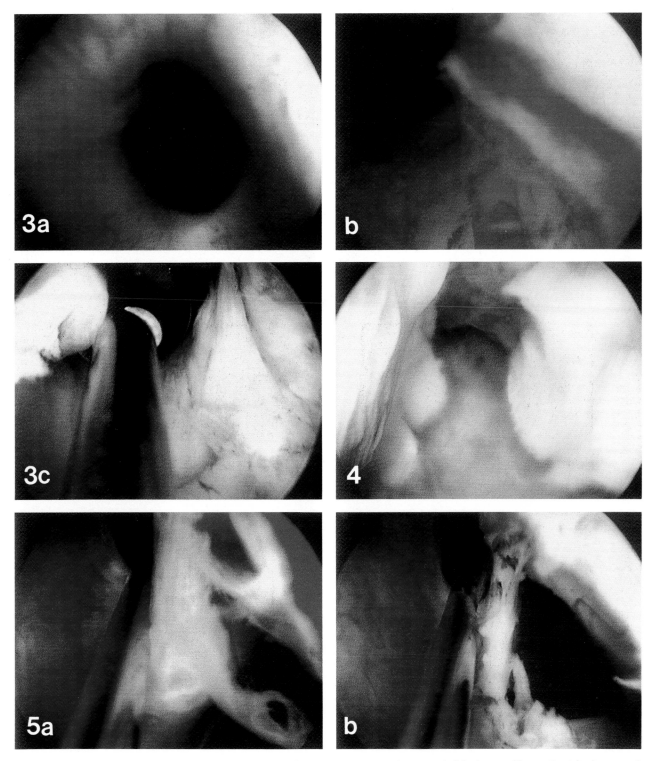

Fig. 3 (Ch. 13). **a:** An endoscopic view of a bladder neck stenosis following a TURP procedure in the past. **b:** 1 mm laser fiber delivering 30 watts of 1000 mm wavelength Phototome diode laser (Cynosure Inc.) power for incising a bladder neck stenosis. **c:** 3.5 mm Ball tip laser delivery fiber for contact prostatectomy using 30 watts of diode laser power in this case. See p. 428 for text discussion.

Fig. 4 (Ch. 13). Typical prostatic cavity 6 months after initial VLAP procedure. There is necrotic tissue seen attached to both sides of the prostatic fossa. Histologic examination confirmed it to be necrotic tissue. The bladder neck in this case

appears to be remarkably intact. The patient had concomitant papillary transitional cell carcinoma of bladder which allowed us to monitor his prostatic fossa at the time of his check cystoscopies. See p. 428 for text discussion.

Fig. 5 (Ch. 13). **a:** Interprostatic bridge following a previous TURP several years earlier causing irritative symptoms to the patient. **b:** The bridge was dealt with by contact laser cutting with the ADD fiber (Laserscope) with full irrigation and then resection of the remaining tissue with electrocautery loop. Note the presence of a passage above and below the bridge. See p. 428 for text discussion.

116. Sauer JS, Hinshaw JR. A fiber optic exoscope for laser tissue welding. Lasers Surg Med 1986; 6:219.

117. Sauer JS, Hinshaw JR, McGuire KP. The first sutureless, laser welded, end-to-end bowel anastomosis. Lasers Surg Med 1989; 9:70–73.

118. Oz MC, Chuck RS, Johnson JP, et al. Indocyanine green dye enhanced vascular welding with the near infrared diode laser. Vasc Surg 1990; 24:564–570.

119. Maragh H, Hawn R, Gould JD, Terzis JK. Is laser nerve repair comparable to microsuture coaptation? J Reconstr Microsurg 1988; 4:189–195.

120. Bailes JE, Cozzens JW, Hudson AR, et al. Laser assisted nerve repair in primates. J Neurosurg 1989; 71:266–272.

121. Seifert V, Stolke D. Laser-assisted reconstruction of the oculomotor nerve: Experimental study on the feasibility of cranial nerve repair. Neurosurgery 1989; 25:579–582.

122. Campion ER, Bynum DK, Powers SK. Repair of peripheral nerves with the argon laser: A functional and histological evaluation. J Bone Joint Surg Am 1990; 72(5):715–?

123. Huang TC, Blanks RH, Berns MW, Crumley RL. Laser vs. suture nerve anastomosis. Otolaryngol Head Neck Surg 1992; 107(1):14–20.

124. Korff M, Bent SW, Havig MT, Schwaber MK, Ossoff RH, Zealer DL. An investigation of the potential for laser nerve welding. Otolaryngol Head Neck Surg 1992; 106:345–350.

125. De la Torre JC, Karaca M, Merali Z, Fortin T, Richard M. Laser or razor? A novel experimental peripheral nerve repair technique. Neurosurgery 1988; 22:531–538.

126. Kline DG. Comment. Neurosurgery 1988; 22:538–539.

127. Terris DJ, Fee WE. Current issues in nerve repair. Arch Otolarngol Head Neck Surg 1993; 119:725–731.

128. Shapiro SA, Sartorius CJ, Campbell RL. The laser in vascular and neural welding. Neurosurgery: State of the Art Reviews 1987; 2(2):475–493.

129. Servre A, Withero EH, Thomsen S, et al. Comparison of carbon dioxide laser-assisted microvascular anastomosis and conventional microvascular sutured anastomosis. Surg Forum 1983; 34:634–636.

130. White RA, Kopchok GE, Donayre CE, et al. Mechanism of tissue fusion in argon laser-welded vein-artery anastomoses. Lasers Surg Med 1988; 8:83–89.

131. Pribil S, Powers SK. Carotid artery end-to-end anastomosis in the rat using the argon laser. J Neurosurg 1985; 63:771–775.

132. Quigley MR, Bailes JE, Kwaan HC, et al. Microvascular laser-assisted anastomosis: Results at one year. Lasers Surg Med 1986; 6:179.

133. Ashworth EM, Dalsing MC, Olson JF, et al. Large-artery welding with a milliwatt carbon dioxide laser. Arch Surg 1987; 122:673–677.

134. Frazier OH, Shehab SA, Zirl R, et al. Anastomosis of bypass grafts using a low-powered CO_2 laser. Lasers Surg Med 1989; 9:30–36.

135. McCarthy WJ, LoCicero J, Hartz RS, et al. Patency of laser-assisted anastomoses in small vessels: One year follow up. Surgery 1987; 102:319–326.

136. Quigley MR, Bailes JE, Kwaan HC, et al. Microvascular anastomosis using ten milliwatt CO_2 laser. Lasers Surg Med 1985; 5:357–365.

137. Quigley MR, Bailes JE, Kwaan HC, et al. Aneurysm formation after low power CO_2 laser-assisted vascular anastomosis. Neurosurgery 1986; 18:292–299.

138. White RA, Kopchok GE, Donayre CE, et al. Comparison of laser-welded and sutured arteriotomies. Arch Surg 1986; 121:1133–1135.

139. White RA, Kopchok GE, Donayre CE, et al. Large vessel sealing with the argon laser. Lasers Surg Med 1987; 7:229–235.

140. Lawrence PF, Li K, Merrel SW, et al. A comparison of absorbable suture and argon laser welding for lateral repair of arteries. J Vasc Surg 1991; 14:183–189.

141. Faught WE, Lawrence PF. Vascular applications of lasers. Surg Clin North Am 1992; 72(3):681–704.

142. Dougherty TJ, Boyle DG, Weishaupt KR, et al. Photoradiation therapy: Clinical and drug advances, In: Kessel D, Dougherty TJ, eds. "Porphyrin Photosensitization." New York: Plenum Press, 1983, p 3.

143. Spikes JD. Photobiology of porphyrins. In: Doiron DR, Gomer CJ, eds. "Porphyrin Localization and Treatment of Tumors." New York: Alan R Liss, 1984, pp 19–39.

144. Kessel D. Hematoporphyrin and HpD: Photophysics, photochemistry and phototherapy. Photochem Photobiol 1984; 39:851–859.

145. Sandberg S, Romslo I, Hovding G, et al. Porphyrin-induced photodamage as related to the subcellular localization of porphyrins. Acta Dermatol Suppl 1982; 100:75–80.

146. Girotti AW. Photodynamic action of protoporphyrin IX on human erythrocytes: Cross-linking of membrane proteins. Biochem Biophys Res Commun 1976; 72:1367–1374.

147. Dubbelman TMAR, DeGoeij AFPM, Van Steveninck J. Protoporphyrin-induced photodynamic effects on transport processes across the membrane of human erythrocytes. Acta Biochim Biophys Acad Sci Hung 1980; 595:133–139.

148. Kochevar IE. Phototoxicity mechanisms: Chlorpromazine photosensitized damage to DNA and cell membranes. J Invest Dermatol 1981; 76:59–64.

149. Moan J, Steen HB, Feren K, et al. Uptake of hematoporphyrin derivative and sensitized photoinactivation of C3H cells with different oncogenic potential. Cancer Lett 1981; 14:291–296.

150. Salzberg S, Lejbkowics F, Ehrenberg B, et al. Protective effect of cholesterol on Friend leukemic cells against photosensitization by hematoporphyrin derivative. Cancer Res 1985; 45:3305–3310.

151. Denstman SC, Dillehay LE, Williams JR. Enhanced susceptibility of HpD-sensitized phototoxicity and correlated resistance to trypsin detachment in SV40 transformed IMR-90 cells. Photochem Photobiol 1986; 43:145–147.

152. Shulok JR, Kluanig JE, Selman SH, et al. Cellular effects of hematoporphyrin derivative photodynamic therapy on normal and neoplastic rat bladder cells. Am J Pathol 1986; 122:277–283.

153. Sandberg S. Protoporphyrin induced photodamage to mitochondria and lysosomes from rat liver. Clin Chem Acta 1981; 111:55.

154. Hull DS, Green K, Hampstead D. Effect of hematoporphyrin derivative on rabbit corneal epithelial cell function and ultrastructure. Invest Ophthalmol Vis Sci 1985; 26:1465–1474.

155. Evensen JF, Moan J. Photodynamic actions and chromosomal damage: A comparison of hematoporphyrin derivative (HpD) and light. Br J Cancer 1982; 45:456.

156. See KL, Forbes IJ, Betts WH. Oxygen dependency of photocytotoxicity with hematoporphyrin derivative. Photochem Photobiol 1984; 39:631.

157. Mitchell JB, McPherson S, Degraff W, et al. Oxygen dependence of hematoporphyrin derivative-induced photoinactivation of Chinese hamster cells. Cancer Res 1981; 41:2008–2011.

158. Berns MW, Dhalman A, Johnson FM, et al. In vitro cellular effects of hematoporphyrin derivative. Cancer Res 1982; 42:2325–2329.

159. Winkelman J, Rasmussen-Taxdal DS. Quantitative determination of porphyrin uptake by tumor tissue following parenteral administration. Bull Johns Hopkins Hosp 1960; 107:228–233.

160. Wise BL, Taxdal DR. Studies of blood-brain barrier utilizing hematoporphyrin. Brain Res 1967; 4:387–389.

161. Wharen RE, Anderson RE, Laws ER. Quantitation of hematoporphyrin derivative in human gliomas, experimental central nervous system tumors, and normal tissues. Neurosurgery 1983; 12:446–450.

162. Boisvert DPJ, McKean JDS, Tulip J, et al. Penetration of hematoporphyrin derivative into rat brain and intracerebral 9L glioma tissue. J Neurooncol 1985; 3:113–118.

163. Boggan JE, Bolger S, Edwards MSB. Effect of hematoporphyrin derivative photoradiation therapy on survival in the rat 9L gliosarcoma brain tumor model. J Neurosurg 1985; 63:917–921.

164. Kaye AH, Mortsyn G, Ashcraft RG. Uptake and retention of hematoporphyrin derivative in an in vivo/ in vitro model of cerebral glioma. Neurosurgery 1985; 17:883–890.

165. Ammirati M, Vick N, Liao Y, et al. Effect of the extent of resection on survival and quality of life in patients with supratentorial glioblastoma and anaplastic astrocytomas. Neurosurgery 1987; 21:201–206.

166. MRC (Medical Research Council) Brain Tumor Working Party. Prognostic factors for high grade malignant glioma: Development of a prognostic index. J Neurooncol 1990; 9:47–55.

167. LeRoux PD, Berger MS, Ojemann GA, Wang K, Mack LA. Correlation of intraoperative ultrasound tumor volumes and margins with preoperative computerized tomography scans: An intraoperative method to enhance tumor resection. J Neurosurg 1989; 71:691–698.

168. Cofey RJ, Lunsford RD, Taylor FH. Survival after sterotactic of malignant gliomas. Neurosurgery 1988; 22:465–473.

169. Poon WS, Schomacker KT, Deutsch TF, Martuza RL. Laser-induced fluorescence: Experimental introperative delineation of tumor resection margins. J Neurosurg 1992; 76:679–686.

170. Henderson BW, Waldwow SM, Marg TS, et al. Tumor destruction and kinetics of tumor cell death in two experimental mouse tumors following photodynamic therapy. Cancer Res 1985; 45:572–576.

171. Bugelski PJ, Porter CW, Dougherty TJ. Autoradiographic distribution of hematoporphyrin derivative in normal and tumor tissue of the mouse. Cancer Res 1981; 41:4606–4612.

172. Boggan JE, Walter R, Edwards MSB, et al. Distribution of hematoporphyrin derivative in the rat 9L gliosarcoma brain tumor analyzed by digital video fluorescence microscopy. J Neurosurg 1984; 61:1113–1119.

173. Boggan JE, Edwards MSB, Berns MW, et al. Hematoporphyrin derivative photoradiation therapy of the rat 9L gliosarcoma brain tumor model. Lasers Surg Med 1984; 4:99–105.

174. Cheng MK, McKean J, Boivert D, et al. Effects of photoradiation therapy on normal rat brain. Neurosurgery 1984; 15:804–810.

175. Rounds DE, Doiron DR, Jacques DB, et al. Phototoxicity of brain tissue in hematoporphyrin derivative treated mice. In: Doiron DR, Gomer CJ, eds. "Porphyrin Localization and Treatment of Tumors." New York: Alan R Liss, 1984, pp 613–623.

176. Van Gemert JC, Berenbaum MC, Gijsbers GHM. Wavelength and light-dose dependence in tumor phototherapy with hematoporphyrin derivative. Br J Cancer 1985; 52:43–49.

177. Gomer CJ, Rucker N, Razum NJ et al. In vitro and in vivo light dose rates effects related to hematoporphyrin derivative phototherapy. Cancer Res 1985; 45:1973–1977.

178. Powers SK, Pribil S, Gillespie GY, et al. Laser photochemotherapy of rhodamine 123 sensitized human glioma cells in vitro. J Neurosurg 1986; 64:918–923.

179. Bellnier DA, Lin CW, Parrish JA, et al. Hematoporphyrin derivative and pulse laser irradiation. In: Doiron DR, Gomer CJ, eds. "Porphyrin Localization and Treatment of Tumors." New York: Alan R Liss, 1984, pp 533–540.

180. McCulloch GAJ, Forbes IJ, See KL, et al. Phototherapy in malignant brain tumors. In: Doiron DR, Gomer CJ, eds. "Porphyrin Localization and Treatment of Tumors." New York: Alan R Liss, 1984, pp 709–717.

181. Laws ER, Cortese DA, Kinsey JH, et al. Photoradiation therapy in the treatment of malignant brain tumors: A phase I feasibility study. Neurosurgery 1981; 9:672–678.

182. Muller PJ, Wilson BC. Photodynamic therapy: Cavitary photoillumination of malignant cerebral tumors using a laser coupled inflatable balloon. Can J Neurol Sci 1985; 12:371–373.

183. Kinsey JH, Cortese DA, Neel HB. Thermal considerations in murine tumor killing using hematoporphyrin derivative phototherapy. Cancer Res 1983; 43:1562–1567.

184. Svaasand LO, Doiron DR, Dougherty TJ. Temperature rise during photoradiation therapy of malignant tumors. Med Phys 1983; 10:10.

185. Mondovi B, Stom R, Rotilio G, et al. The biochemical mechanism of selective heat sensitivity of cancer cells: I. Studies on cellular respiration. Cancer 1969; 5:129–136.

186. Turano C, Ferraro A, Strom R, et al. The biochemical mechanism of selective heat sensitivity of cancer cells: III. Studies of lysosomes. Cancer 1970; 6:67–72.

187. Christensen T, Wahl A, Smedshammer L. Effects of hematoporphyrin derivative and light in combination with hyperthermia on cells in culture. Br J Cancer 1984; 50: 85–89.

188. Mang TS, Dougherty TJ. Time and sequence dependent influence of in vitro photodynamic therapy (PDT) survival by hyperthermia. Photochem Photobiol 1985; 42: 533–540.

189. Waldow SM, Henderson BW, Dougherty TJ. Potentiation of photodynamic therapy by heat: Effect of sequence and time interval between treatment in vivo. Lasers Surg Med 1985; 5:83–94.

190. Laws ER, Wharen RE. Comment effects of photoradiation therapy on normal rat brain. Neurosurgery 1984; 15:808–809.

191. Perria C, Capuzzo T, Cavagnaro G, et al. First attempts at the photodynamic treatment of human gliomas. J Neurol Sci 1980; 24:119–129.

192. Powers SK, Cush SS, Walstad DL, Kwock L. Stereotactic intratumoral photodynamic therapy for recurrent malignant brain tumors. Neurosurgery 1991; 29:688–696.

193. Kostron H. Photodynamic treatment of malignant brain tumors. In: Spinelli P, Dal Fante M, Marchesini R, eds. "Photodynamic Therapy and Biomedical Lasers." Excerpta Medica, 1992, pp 386–390.

194. Origitano TC, Karesh SM, Henkin RE, Halama JR, Reichman OH. Photodynamic therapy for intracranial neoplasms: Investigations of photosensitizer uptake and distribution using indium-111 Photofrin-II single photon emission computed tomography scans in humans with intracranial neoplasms. Neurosurgery 1993; 32:357–364.

195. Origitano TC, Reichman OH. Photodynamic therapy for intracranial neoplasms: development of an image-based computer-assisted protocol for photodynamic therapy of intracranial neoplasms. Neurosurgery 1993; 32(4):587–595.

196. Kaye AH. Comments. Neurosurgery 1993; 32:363.

197. Ji Y, Walstad D, Brown JT, Powers SK. Interstitial photoradiation injury of normal brain. Lasers Surg Med 1992; 12(4):425–431.

198. Toya S, Kawase T, Iisaka Y, Iwata T, Aki T, Nakamura T. Acute effect of carbon dioxide laser on the epicerebral microcirculation. J Neurosurg 1980; 53:193–197.

199. Ji Y, Walstad D, Brown JT, Powers SK. Improved survival from intracavitary photodynamic therapy of rat glioma. Photochem Photobiol 1992; 56(3):385–390.

200. Ji Y, Powers SK, Brown JT, Walstad D, Maliner L. Toxicity of photodynamic therapy with photofrin in the normal rat brain. Lasers Surg Med 1994; 14:219–228.

201. Jiang Q, Knight RA, Chopp M, Helpern JA, Ordidge RJ, Qing ZX, Hetzel FW. ^{1}H magnetic resonance imaging of normal brain tissue response to photodynamic therapy. Neurosurgery 1991; 29:538–543.

202. Goodale R, et al. Rapid endoscopic control of bleeding gastric erosions by laser radiation. Arch Surg 1970; 101:211.

203. Nath G, Gorisch W, Kiefhaber P. First laser endoscopy via a fiberoptic transmission system. Endoscopy 1973; 5:208–213.

204. Walker ML, Mac Donald J, Wright LC. The history of ventriculoscopy: Where do we go from here? Pediatr Neurosurg 1992; 18:218–223.

205. Powers SK. Fenestration of intraventricular cysts using a flexible, steerable endoscope and the argon laser. Neurosurgery 1986; 18:637–641.

206. Powers SK. Fenestration of intraventricular cysts using a flexible, steerable endoscope. Acta Neurochir Suppl (Wein), 1992; 54:42–46.

207. Cohen AR, Heilman CB. Endoscopic ventricular surgery. (abstract). Annual Meeting Section of Pediatric Neurological Surgery, American Association of Neurological Surgeons, San Diego, December 1990.

208. Cohen AR. Endoscopic ventricular surgery. Pediatr Neurosurg 1993; 19:127–134.

209. Fukushima T. Endoscopic biopsy of intraventricular tumours with the use of ventriculofiberscope. Neurosurgery 1978; 2:110–113.

210. Griffith HB. Technique of fontanelle and persutural ventriculoscopy and endoscopic ventricular surgery in infants. Child's Brain 1975; 1:359–363.

211. Griffith HB. Endoneurosurgery: Endoscopic intracranial surgery. In: Symon. L. et al., eds. "Advances and Technical Standards in Neurosurgery," Vol. 14 New York: Springer, 1987, pp 2–24.

212. Auer LM, Deinsberger W, Niederkorn K, Gell G, Kleinert R, Schneider G, Holzer P, Bone G, Mokry M, Korner E, Kleinert G, Hanusch S. Endoscopic surgery versus medical treatment for spontaneous intracerebral hematoma: A randomized study. J Neurosurg 1989; 70:530–535.

213. Auer LM, Ascher PW, Heppner F, Ladurner G, Lechner H, Tolly E, Gell G. Does acute endoscopic evacuation improve the outcome of patients with spontaneous intracerebral hemorrhage? Proceedings of the 5th South-East-European Conference for Neurology and Psychiatry, Graz, 1983.

214. Auer LM. Endoscopic evacuation of intracerebral hemorrhage. Acta Neurochir (Wein) 1985; 74:124–128.

215. Auer LM, Ascher PW, Heppner F, Ladurner G, Bone G, Lechner H, Tolly E. Does endoscopic evacuation improve the outcome in patients with spontaneous intracranial hemorrhage. Eur Neurol 1985; 24:254–261.

216. Auer LM. Endoscopic evacuation of intracerebral hemorrhage: High tec surgical treatment—a new approach to the problem? Acta Neurochir (Wein) 1985; 74:124–128.

217. Hellwig D, Eggers F, Bauer BL, Likoyiannis A. Endoscopic stereotaxis: Preliminary results. Stereotact Funct Neurosurg 1990; 54+55:418.

218. Hellwig D, Bauer BL. Endoscopic procedures in stereotactic neurosurgery. Acta Neurochir Suppl (Wein) 1991; 52:30–32.

219. Hellwig D, Bauer BL, List-Hellwig E, Mennel HD. Stereotactic-endoscopical procedures on processes of the cranial midline. Acta Neurochir Suppl (Wein), 1991; 53:23–32.

220. Hor F, DesGeorges M, Rosseau GL. Tumour resection by stereotactic laser endoscopy. Acta Neurochir Suppl (Wein), 1992; 54:77–82.

221. Iizuka J. Development of a stereotaxic endoscopy of the ventricular system. Confin Neurol 1975; 37:141–149.

222. Jacques S, Shelden CH, Lutes HR. Computerized microstereotactic neurosurgical endoscopy under direct three dimensional vision. In: Lunsford LD, ed. "Modern Stereotactic Neurosurgery." Boston: Martinus Nijhoff, 1988, pp 185–194.

223. Jones RFC, Stening WA, Brydon M. Endoscopic third ventriculostomy. Neurosurgery 1990; 26:86–92.

224. Jones RFC, Stening WA, Kwok BCT, Sands TM. Third ventriculostomy for shunt infections in children. Neurosurgery 1993; 32:855–860.

225. Jones RFC. Neuroendoscopic third ventriculostomy. (Abstract) Childs Nerv Syst 1991; 7:277.

226. Jones RFC. Third ventriculostomy versus shunts: A

comparison of risks. (Abstract) Childs Nerv Syst 1992; 8:175.

227. Reidenbach HD. Technological fundamentals of endoscopic hemostasis. Acta Neurochir Suppl (Wein), 1992; 54:26–33.

228. Kelly PJ. Stereotactic third ventriculostomy in patients with non-tumoral adolescent/adult onset aqueductal stenosis and symptomatic hydrocephalus. J Neurosurg 1991; 75:865–873.

229. Sainte-Rose C. Third ventriculostomy. In: Manwaring KH, Crone KR, eds. "Neuroendoscopy," Vol 1. New York: Mary Ann Leibert, 1992:47–62.

230. Hirsch JF, Hirsch E, Sainte-Rose C. Stenosis of aqueduct of Sylvius: Etiology and treatment. J Neurosurg Sci 1986; 30:29–39.

231. Reddy K, Fewer HD, West M, et al. Slit ventricular syndrome with aqueduct stenosis: Third ventriculostomy as a definitive treatment. Neurosurgery 1988; 23:756–759.

232. Drake JM. Neuroendoscopy tumor biopsy. In: Manwaring KH, Crone KR, eds. "Neuroendoscopy," Vol 1. New York: Mary Ann Leibert, 1992:103–107.

233. Drake JM. Ventriculostomy for treatment of hydrocephalus. Neurosurg Clin N Am 1993; 4(4):657–666.

234. Crone KR. Endoscopic technique for removal of adherent ventricular catheters. In: Manwaring KH, Crone KR, eds. "Neuroendoscopy," Vol 1. New York: Mary Ann Leibert, 1992:41–46.

235. Griffith HB, Jamjoom AB. The treatment of childhood hydrocephalus by choroid plexus coagulation and artificial cerebrospinal fluid perfusion. BJN 1990; 4:95–100.

236. Buchholz RD, Pittman MD. Endoscopic coagulation of the choroid plexus using the Nd:YAG laser: Initial experience and proposal for management. Neurosurgery 1991; 28(3):421–427.

237. Pittman T, Buchholz RD. Endoscopic choroid plexectomy. In: Manwaring KH, Crone KR, eds. "Neuroendoscopy," Vol 1. New York: Mary Ann Leibert, 1992:97–102.

238. Scarff JE. Treatment of non-obstructive (obstructive) hydrocephalus by endoscopic cauterization of choroid plexus. J Neurosurg 1979; 33:1–18.

239. Zamorano L, Chavantes C, Dujovny M, Malik G, Ausman J. Stereotactic endoscopic interventions in cystic and intraventricular brain lesions. Acta Neurochir Suppl (Wein) 1992; 54:69–74.

240. Zamorano L, Chavantes C, Dujovny M, Malik G, Ausman J. Image-guided endoscopic laser stereotaxis (ELS). Stereotact Funct Neurosurg 1990; 54+55:421.

241. Otzuki T, Jokura H, Yoshimoto T. Stereotactic guiding tube for open system endoscopy: A new approach for the stereotactic endoscopic resection of intra-axial brain tumours. Neurosurgery 1990; 27(2):326–330.

242. Otzuki T, Jokura H, Yoshimoto T, Saso S. Stereotactic endoscopic resection of intraaxial and intraventricular brain tumors using high-power lasers. Stereotact Funct Neurosurg 1992; 59:148.

243. Caemaert J, Abdullah J. Diagnostic and therapeutic stereotactic cerebral endoscopy. Acta Neurochir (Wein) 1993; 124:11–13.

244. Auer LM, Holzer P, Ascher PW, Heppner F. Endoscopic neurosurgery. Acta Neurochir (Wein) 1988; 90:1–14.

245. Ajuria JE, Vinas JA. Endoscopic treatment of intracranial lesions: Report on 8 cases. Neurochirurgie 1991; 37:278–283.

246. Merienne L, Leriche B, Roux FX, Devaux B. Nd:YAG laser with cerebral endoscopy: Preliminary experience in stereotactic conditions. Neurochirurgie 1992; 38:245–247.

247. Fink RA. Neurosurgical treatment of nonmalignant intractable rectal pain: Microsurgical commissural myelotomy with carbon dioxide laser. Neurosurgery 1984; 14:64–65.

248. Levy WJ, Nutkiewicz A, Ditmore QM, et al. Laser induced dorsal root entry zone lesions for pain control: Report of three cases. J Neurosurg 1983; 59:884–886.

249. Powers SK, Adams JE, Edwards MSB, et al. Pain relief from dorsal root entry zone lesions made with argon and carbon dioxide microsurgical lasers. J Neurosurg 1984; 61:841–847.

250. Shetter AG. Pain surgery techniques for specialty neurosurgical practice. Clin Neurosurg 1993; 40:197–209.

251. Nashold BS Jr, Bullitt E. Dorsal root entry zone lesions to control central pain in paraplegics. J Neurosurg 1981; 55:414–419.

252. Levy WJ, Gallo C, Watts C. Comparison of laser and radiofrequency dorsal root entry zone lesions in cats. Neurosurgery 1985; 16:327–330.

253. Nashold BS Jr, Walker JS. Laser effect on spinal cord (letter to the editor). Neurosurgery 1984; 60:870.

254. Freidman AH, Nashold BS Jr, Bronec PR. Dorsal root entry zone lesions for the treatment of brachial plexus avulsion injuries: A follow up study. Neurosurgery 1988; 22:369–373.

255. Thomas DGT, Jones SJ. Dorsal root entry zone lesions (Nashold's procedure) in brachial plexus avulsion. Neurosurgery 1984; 15:966–968.

256. Young RF. Clinical experience with radiofrequency and laser DREZ lesions. J Neurosurg 1990; 72:715–720.

257. Freidman AH, Bullitt E. Dorsal root entry zone lesions in the treatment of pain following brachial plexus avulsion, spinal cord injury and herpes zoster. Appl Neurophysiol 1988; 51:164–169.

258. Saris SC, Iacono RP, Nashold BS Jr. Dorsal root entry zone lesions for post-amputation pain. J Neurosurg 1985; 62:72–76.

259. Saris SC, Veiera JFS, Nashold BS Jr. Dorsal root entry zone lesions coagulation for intractable sciatica. Appl Neurophysiol 1988; 51:206–211.

260. Yeh HS, Kashiwagi S, Tew JM, et al. Surgical management of epilepsy associated with cerebral arteriovenous malformations. J Neurosurg 1990; 72:216.

261. Yeh HS. Use of the CO_2 laser in epilepsy surgery. In: Sawaya R, Tew JM Jr, eds. "Laser Applications in Neurosurgery." Philadelphia: Hanley and Belfus, 1987:509–513.

262. Cascino GD, Kelly PJ, Hirschorn KA, Marsh WR, Sharbrough FW. Stereotactic resection of intra-axial cerebral lesions in partial epilepsy. Mayo Clin Proc 1990; 65(8):1053–1060.

263. Weber JP, Silbergeld DL, Winn HR. Surgical resection of epileptogenic cortex associated with structural lesions. Neurosurg Clin N Am 1993; 4(2):327–336.

264. Bebin EM, Kelly PJ, Gomez MR. Surgical treatment for epilepsy in cerebral tuberous sclerosis. Epilepsia 1993; 34(4):651–657.

265. Kelly PJ, Sharbrough FW, Kall BA, Goerss SJ. Magnetic resonance imaging-based computer-assisted stereotactic resection of the hippocampus and amygdala in

patients with temporal lobe epilepsy. Mayo Clin Proc 1987; 62(2):103–108.

266. Caspar W, Campbell B, Barbier DD, et al. The Caspar microsurgical discectomy and comparison with a conventional standard lumbar disc procedure. Neurosurgery 1991; 28:78–87.

267. Ebeling U, Reichenberg W, Reulen HJ. Results of microsurgical lumbar discectomy. Review of 485 patients. Acta Neurochir (Wein) 1986; 81:45–52.

268. Harbaugh RE. Microsurgical lumbar disc excision. In: Schmidek HH, Sweet WH, eds. "Operative Neurosurgical Techniques," Vol. 2. Orlando: Grune & Stratton, 1988, pp 1395–1397.

269. Williams RW. Microlumbar discectomy: A conservative surgical approach to the virgin herniated lumbar disc. Spine 1978; 3:175–182.

270. Wilson DH, Harbaugh RE. Lumbar discectomy: A comparative study of microsurgical and standard techniques. In: Hardy RW, ed. "Lumbar Disc Disease." New York: Raven Press, 1982, pp 147–156.

271. Wilson DH, Kenning J. Microsurgical lumbar discectomy: Preliminary report of 83 consecutive cases. Neurosurgery 1979; 4:137–140.

272. Yasargil MG. Microsurgical operation of herniated lumbar disc. Adv Neurosurg 1977; 4:81–82.

273. Burton VC. How to avoid the failed back surgery syndrome. In: Cauthen JC, ed. "Lumbar Spine Surgery Indications, Techniques, and Alternatives." Baltimore: Williams & Wilkins, 1983, pp 204–215.

274. Finneson BE. Lumbar disc excision. In: Schmidek HH, Sweet WH, eds. "Operative Neurosurgical Techniques," Vol. 2. Orlando: Grune & Stratton, 1988, pp 1375–1392.

275. Hardy RW (ed): "Lumbar Disc disease: Seminars in Neurological Surgery." New York: Raven Press, 1982, pp 147–156.

276. Haughten VM, Eldevik OP, Magnaes B, et al. A prospective comparison of computed tomography and myelography in the diagnosis of herniated lumbar disks. Radiology 1982; 142:103–110.

277. Spangfort EV. The lumbar disc herniation: A computer-aided analysis of 2054 operations. Acta Orthop Scand Suppl 1972; 142:1–95.

278. Kusswetter W, Cording R. Langzeitergebnisse nach lumbaler Nukleotomie, In: Schollner D, ed. "Rezidive nach lumbalen Bandscheibenoperationen." Uelzen: Medizin Literatur Verlagsgesellsschaft, 1980, pp 12–15.

279. Neithardt FU. Das Pseudorezidiv nach Nukleotomien. In: Schollner D, ed. "Rezidive nach lumbalen Bandscheibenoperationen." Uelzen: Medizin Literatur Verlagsgesellsschaft, 1980, pp 28–31.

280. Loew F, Jochheim KA, Kivelitz R. Klinik und Behandlung der lumbalen Bandscheibenschaden. In: Olivecrona H, Tonnis W, eds. "Handbuch der Neurochirurgie." Berlin: Springer-Verlag, 1969:164–237.

281. Mayer HM, Brock M. Percutaneous endoscopic discectomy: Surgical technique and preliminary results compared to microsurgical discectomy. J Neurosurg 1993; 78:216–225.

282. Hijikata S. Percutaneous nucleotomy: A new concept technique and 12 years experience. Clin Orthop 1989; 238:9–23.

283. Suezawa Y, Ruttimann B. Indikation, Methodik and Ergebnisse der perkutanen Nukleotlmie bei lumbaler Diakushernie. Z Orthop 1983; 121:25–29.

284. Suezawa Y, Schreiber A. Komplexe Indikationen in der Chirurgie des lumbalen Spinalkanals. Z Orthop 1987; 125:308–319.

285. Schreiber A, Suezawa Y. Transdiscoscopic percutaneous nucleotomy in disk herniation. Orthop Rev 1986; 15:75–78.

286. Schreiber A, Suezawa Y, Leu H. Does percutaneous nucleotomy with discoscopy replace conventional discectomy? Clin Orthop 1989; 238:35–42.

287. Choy DSJ, Case RB, Fielding W, Hughes J, Liebler W, Ascher PW. Percutaneous laser nucleolysis of lumbar discs. N Engl J Med 1987; 317:771–772.

288. Choy DS, Ascher PW, Ranu HS, Saddekni S, Alkaitis D, Liebler W, Hughes J, Diwan S, Altman P. Percutaneous laser disc decompression: A new therapeutic modality. Spine 1992; 17(8):949–956.

289. Davis JK. Early experience with laser disc decompression: A percutaneous method. J Fla Med Assoc 1992; 79(1):37–39.

290. Sherk HH, Black J, Rhodes A, Lane G, Prodoehl J. Laser discectomy. Clin Sports Med 1993; 12(3):569–577.

291. Mayer HM, Brock M, Berlien HP, Weber B. Percutaneous endoscopic laser discectomy (PELD): A new surgical technique for non-sequestrated lumbar discs. Acta Neurochir Suppl (Wien) 1992; 54:53–58.

292. Kolarik J, Nadvornik P, Rozhold O. Photonucleolysis of intervertebral disc and its herniation: Preparation to percutaneous laser discectomy. Zentralbl Neurochir 1990; 51(2):69–71.

293. Mayer HM, Brock M, Stern E, Muller G. Percutaneous endoscopic laser discectomy: experimental results. In: Mayer HM, Brock M, eds. "Percutaneous Lumbar Discectomy," 1st ed. Heidelberg: Springer-Verlag, 1989, pp 187–196.

294. Yonezawa T, Onomura T, Kosaka R, Miyaji Y, Tanaka S, Watanabe H, Abe Y, Imachi K, Atumi K, Chinzei T, et al. The system and procedures of percutaneous intradiscal laser nucleotomy. Spine 1990; 15(11):1175–1185.

295. Vorwerk D, Husemann T, Blazek V, Zolotas G, Gunther RW. Laser ablation of the nucleus pulposus: optical properties of degenerated intervertebral disk tissue in the wavelength range 200 to 2200 nm. [German] Rofo Fortschr Geb Rontgenstr Neuen Bildgeb Verfahr 1989; 151(6):725–728.

296. Wolgin M, Finkenberg J, Papaioannou T, Segil C, Soma C, Grundfest W. Excimer ablation of human intervertebral disc at 308 nanometers. Lasers Surg Med 1989; 9(2):124–131.

297. Buchelt M, Katterschafka T, Horvat R, Kutschera HP, Kickinger W, Laufer G. Fluorescence guided excimer laser ablation of intervertebral discs in vitro. Lasers Surg Med. 1991; 11(3):280–286.

298. Quigley MR, Maroon JC. Laser discectomy: A review. Spine 1994; 19(1):53–56.

299. Quigley MR, Maroon JC, Shih T, Elrifai A, Lesiecki ML. Laser discectomy: Comparison of systems. Spine 1994; 19(3):319–322.

300. Maroon JC, Allen RC. A retrospective study of 1054 APLD cases: A twenty month clinical follow up at 35 US centers. J Neurol Orthop Med Surg 1989; 10:335–337.

301. Dunsker SB. Point of view. Spine 1994; 19(1):56.

302. Treat MR, Oz MC, Bass LS. New technologies and fu-

ture applications of surgical lasers: The right tool for the right job. Surg Clin North Am 1992; 72(3):705–742.

303. Treat MR, Trokel SL, DeFillippi VJ, et al. Mid-infrared lasers for endoscopic surgery: A new class of surgical lasers. Am Surg 1989; 55:81–84.

304. Grundfest WS, Litvack IF, Goldenberg T, et al. Pulsed ultraviolet lasers and the potential for safe laser angioplasty. Am J Surg 1985; 150:220–226.

305. Linsker R, Srinivasan R, Wynne JJ, et al. Far ultraviolet laser ablation for atheroscleortic lesions. Lasers Surg Med 1984; 4:201–206.

306. Pokora LJ. Excimer and excimer-dye laser systems for medical applications. Proc SPIE 1990; 1200:499–506.

307. Deckelbaum LI, Lam JK, Cabin HS, et al. Discrimination of normal and atherosclerotic aorta by laser induced fluorescence. Lasers Surg Med 1987; 7:330–335.

308. Garrand TJ, Stetz ML, O'Brein KM, et al. Design and evaluation of a fiberoptic fluorescence guided laser recanalization system. Lasers Surg Med 1991; 11:106–116.

309. White RA, Kopchok GE, Tabara MR, et al. Intravascular ultrasound guided holmium:YAG laser recanalization of occluded arteries. Lasers Surg Med. 1992; 12(3):239–245.

310. Koivukangas J, Louhislami Y, Alakuijala J, Oikarinen J. Ultrasound-controlled neuronavigator-guided brain surgery. J Neurosurg 1993; 79:36–42.

311. Manwaring KH. Intraoperative real-time magnetic field guidance system for intracranial localization. Childs Nerv Syst 1991; 7:284.

312. Benabid AL, Lavallee S, Hoffman D, Cinquin P, Demongeot J, Danel F. Potential use of robots in endoscopic neurosurgery. Acta Neurochir Suppl (Wein) 1992; 54:93–97.

Chapter 8

Lasers in Ophthalmology

Joel M. Krauss, MD and Carmen A. Puliafito, MD

*New England Eye Center, Tufts University School of Medicine,
Boston, Massachusetts*

INTRODUCTION

Ophthalmologists have been at the forefront of developing medical uses for new laser technology since the report of the first laser in 1960 [1]. Photocoagulation was the earliest therapeutic laser procedure and remains the most widely employed. There are myriad ocular applications, which have dramatically changed the treatment of eye diseases ranging from diabetic retinopathy to glaucoma. Photodisruption was introduced in the early 1980s. First used to treat secondary cataracts noninvasively, it also has seen an increasing number of applications.

Few recent advances in medical technology have garnered as much public interest as corneal ablation, which may revolutionize the treatment of the most common ocular disease: refractive error. Even as the excimer laser is in the final stages of clinical trials, work continues on the next generation of ablation lasers. The precise tissue removal afforded by these devices also may be applicable to other eye disorders. Less prominent and ubiquitous than their therapeutic counterparts, diagnostic lasers have served an important role in ophthalmic practice, often permitting more accurate and timely treatment with lasers or other modalities.

New instruments and techniques are continually being developed, and few go untested for potential ophthalmic use. Whereas the last decade has seen photodisruption, and increasingly ablation, join photocoagulation as established procedures, there is good reason to believe that the field of ophthalmic lasers is far from mature.

LASER–TISSUE INTERACTIONS

The effect of laser radiation on a particular target depends on the properties of both the laser and the target. The most important laser output parameters are wavelength, duration, and power. Wavelength is a function of the laser cavity's excited medium, which is a gas in argon, krypton, and excimer lasers, a liquid in dye lasers, and a semiconductor in diode lasers. According to the principle of wave-particle duality, radiation is propagated in the form of both waves and discrete quanta, or photons. As such, radiation of a given wavelength is associated with photons of a corresponding energy, such that $E = h\nu = hc/\lambda$, where h = Planck's constant, ν = frequency, c = speed of light, and λ = wavelength. Thus frequency and energy increase as wavelength decreases. The visible spectrum extends approximately from 380 to 760 nm. The first law of photochemistry (Grotthus-Draper) states that photons must be absorbed by a target in order to initiate a chemical reaction [2]. A chromophore is a molecule, or a portion thereof, that absorbs a photon of a particular energy. Depending on the photon's energy, a chromophore can undergo bond-breaking, ionization, or various types of molecular excitation.

The ability of a target, which may or may not be of a homogeneous composition, to absorb radiation is measured by the attenuation in incident radiation after a certain length of the material has been traversed. The absorbance, A, of a material is defined as $A(d) = \log[I_0/I(d)] = \varepsilon cd$, where I_0 = initial intensity, $I(d)$ = intensity at distance d, ε = absorptivity of the material, and c = molarity of the material. Transmission is that fraction of the incident energy that is not absorbed after traversing a particular target thickness. It is usually written in the form of Beer's law, $T(d) = 10^{-A(d)} = e^{-\alpha d}$, where $\alpha d = 2.3A$ defines the absorption coefficient α. α is generally given in units of cm^{-1} and represents the fraction of incident energy that is absorbed per unit length of target material. Absorption length is defined as α^{-1}, or that distance at which $e^{-1} = 0.368$ of incident energy is transmitted, corresponding to 63.2% absorption. The thermal susceptibility of the irradiated tissue is denoted by the thermal relaxation time, τ, which gives an indication of the time required for the irradiated tissue to carry away heat energy from the target site. It is wavelength-dependent and is proportional to $1/4\alpha^2\kappa$, where κ measures the tissue diffusivity in cm^2/s.

The absorption maximum of a compound is that wavelength in a given portion of the spectrum that has the highest probability of absorption. A plot of absorption vs. wavelength yields an absorption spectrum that is characteristic of the chemical composition of that compound. Quantum yield is a measure of the efficiency with which absorbed radiation produces chemical changes, whereas an action spectrum is a plot of the relative efficiency of the photoreaction vs. wavelength.

PHOTOCOAGULATION
Non-laser Photocoagulation

The ocular effects of radiant energy have been recognized since at least the time of Socrates, who described solar retinitis after direct observation of an eclipse. Meyer-Schwickerath, following an eclipse in 1945, noted the similarity between damage to the macula (Fig. 1) in viewers and that produced by diathermy and began to study radiation sources and delivery systems for intentional therapeutic photocoagulation [3]. He constructed a device that focused sunlight on the retina, but despite some clinical success, the difficulty in regulating exposure—not to mention the frequent occurrence of cloudy days—made this approach impractical. In 1956, Meyer-Schwickerath settled on the xenon arc, which soon gained widespread acceptance. Although primarily for technical reasons this instrument has been largely replaced by lasers, it is often equally efficacious [4] and remains in use in many areas around the world where lasers are unavailable. Xenon emission consists of all wavelengths between 400 and 1,600 nm, so that a full-thickness burn is achieved without the ability for selective targeting of ocular tissue. The exposures last several seconds, requiring retrobulbar anesthesia to reduce pain and eye movement.

Laser Photocoagulation

In contrast to incandescent sources, a laser emits one or several discrete wavelengths. A high degree of collimation (low divergence) permits focusing to very small spot sizes. The ruby laser produces 694.3 nm radiation in pulse durations in the hundreds of μs and was the subject of early clinical investigation. Although this device was of negligible value for direct vascular treatment, it was effective in controlling proliferative diabetic retinopathy (PDR, see Diabetic retinopathy) [5]. L'Esperance introduced the ophthalmic argon laser in 1968 [6], and it was not until the value of that instrument was fully realized in the early 1970s that laser photocoagulation became an established procedure. Over the past two decades, several other photocoagulation lasers—especially the krypton laser in 1972, tunable dye laser in 1981, and most recently, the diode laser—have found their way from the lab to the clinic. Many applications have been based on empirical observation, but as laser technology and photobiology advance, selective therapeutic approaches achieve desirable biochemical, cellu-

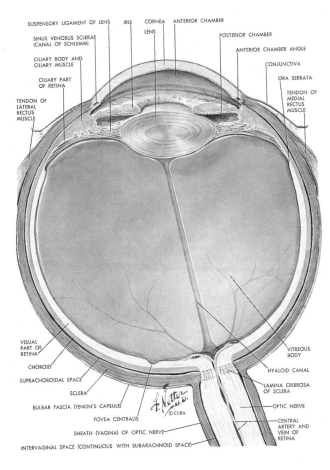

Fig. 1. Cross section of the eye. (© Copyright 1989. CIBA-GEIGY Corporation. Reprinted with permission from *Atlas of Human Anatomy*, illustrated by Frank H. Netter, M.D. All rights reserved.)

TABLE 1. Principal Wavelengths of Common Photocoagulation Lasers

Laser	Wavelength (nm)
Argon (blue-green)	488.0
Argon (green)	514.5
Frequency doubled Nd:YAG	532.0
Krypton (yellow)	568.2
Krypton (red)	647.1
Tunable Dye	Variable (most 570–630 nm), depending on dye
Diode	Variable (most 780–850 nm), depending on diode
Nd:YAG	1,064.0

lar, and tissue effects to the exclusion of unwanted damage.

Laser principles. Principal wavelengths for common photocoagulation lasers are listed in Table 1. (The carbon dioxide [CO_2] laser, with emission at 10.6 μm in the mid-infrared [IR], also has coagulative effects, but since it is used primarily to induce vaporization due to its high absorption by water, it is discussed in the section on ablation.) Most such lasers run in a continuous or quasi-continuous mode, so that exposure is controlled by an external shutter. Photocoagulation is generally performed at durations of 100–200 ms, increasing to ~ 500 ms in cases of ocular media opacity. This should be distinguished from the Q-switched neodymium-yttrium aluminum garnet (Nd:YAG) and other ultra-short pulsed lasers, in which the laser actually produces only very

brief bursts of radiation, with resulting average and peak (rather than constant) powers. Thus, whereas output for photodisruption and ablation lasers is listed in units of energy (joules), that of photocoagulation lasers is given in units of power (watts). For a given amount of power, the shorter the time over which it is delivered, the greater the risk of tissue rupture and hemorrhage. Several hundred mW generally suffices for most purposes, although up to 1 W may be necessary. Irradiance is measured in W/cm^2 and increases as the spot size, to which the laser output is focused, decreases. Spot sizes as small as 50 μm diameter are used to target individual vessels or in the presence of opacity, whereas those of 200 μm and 500 μm are generally employed for photocoagulation of the macula and peripheral retina, respectively. Smaller spots are more affected by dissipation of heat to surrounding tissue, and hence require higher irradiance to achieve the same central effect as larger spots.

Photocoagulation lasers, as the name implies, exploit tissue absorption and heating [7]. Sophisticated theoretical models have been developed to explain and predict laser-induced thermal damage in the retina [8–11], which is proportional to the magnitude and duration of the temperature increase (represented by the Arrhenius integral) [12]. The temperature rise produced by laser irradiation is a function of time, laser energy, and wavelength, and the optical and thermal properties of the absorber. Modest increases of 10–20 °C induce alteration of the genetic apparatus of cells, inactivation of enzymes, and denaturation of proteins and nucleic acids, which lead to necrosis, hemostasis, and coagulation [13]. Immediate effects are visible ophthalmoscopically because of focal increases in necrotic cells and a mechanical disruption of the adjacent neurosensory retina that interferes with its normal transparency [14]. Delayed effects result from inflammation and repair processes. Water vaporization and gas bubble formation, with their attendant secondary mechanical effects, may be seen with greater temperature increases. A moderate increase in temperature under 100°C is associated with breakage of hydrogen bonds and van der Waal's forces, which stabilize the conformation of biologic macromolecules such as proteins, resulting in loss of biologic or structural activity [15].

Argon and krypton lasers. Intraocular applications require the transmission of radiation, which occurs to different extents between ~ 380 and 1,400 nm. Except for the long-pulsed Nd: YAG and now the diode laser, photocoagulation lasers employ radiation in the visible portion of the electromagnetic spectrum. In this range, important chromophores are melanin, in the retinal pigment epithelium (RPE) [Fig. 2] and iris pigment epithelium, uvea, and trabecular meshwork, hemoglobin in blood vessels, and xanthophyll in the inner and outer plexiform layers in the macula, as well as in certain cataracts. Figure 3 demonstrates how the absorption by those chromophores varies in the region relevant for photocoagulation. Melanin absorption is relatively constant between 400 and 700 nm, although the gradual decrease in absorption at longer wavelengths results in deeper retinal burns. Argon green light, at 514.5 nm, is minimally absorbed by xanthophyll, but strongly absorbed by both hemogloblin and melanin. Except in the presence of a large retinal vessel, it typically produces a cone-shape lesion, which spares the inner retina [16] and is appropriate for direct coagulation of retinal vessels, but not for treatment through hemorrhage [17]. Collagen shrinkage in and around vessel walls and hemoglobin heating sufficient to cause thrombi are thought to be the mechanisms by which photocoagulation seals arteries [18]. Xanthophyll absorbs blue light strongly, but green and especially red and yellow much less so. Photocoagulation at 488 nm thus may damage the retinal nerve fiber layer (RNFL) [19] and is inappropriate for most macular applications [16,20]. There is also concern that use of blue laser light over an extended period may decrease color discrimination in ophthalmologists in a tritan color-confusion axis [21].

Hemoglobin has strong absorption for all colors with wavelengths shorter than that of red. Red light is thus effective in the presence of vitreous or retinal hemorrhage, through which the light readily passes, whereas shorter wavelengths are useful for blood vessel closure. Red light is

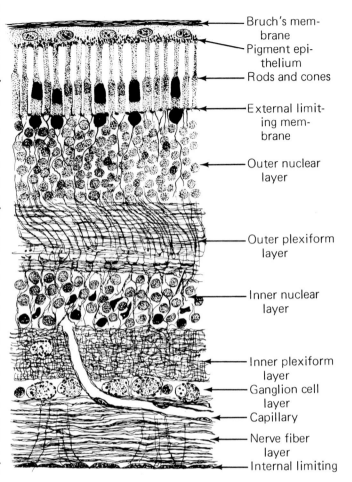

Fig. 2. Cross section of the retina. (Reprinted from Wolff et al. [534] with permission of Chapman & Hall.)

Labels on figure:
- Bruch's membrane
- Pigment epithelium
- Rods and cones
- External limiting membrane
- Outer nuclear layer
- Outer plexiform layer
- Inner nuclear layer
- Inner plexiform layer
- Ganglion cell layer
- Capillary
- Nerve fiber layer
- Internal limiting

appropriate for macular applications, but unlike green and yellow is unable directly to coagulate vessels in the event of inadvertent hemorrhage, so that it is not useful for vascular pathology. Krypton red's primary absorption is in the RPE and choroid, and it has also proven useful in panretinal photocoagulation (PRP) for proliferative diabetic retinopathy (PDR) [20]. Disadvantages of this wavelength include increased patient discomfort and risk of choroidal hemorrhage or disruption of Bruch's membrane due to the deeper penetration, and the lower efficiency and greater complexity of krypton lasers compared with argon lasers. If the temperature increase is too great, heat conduction can spread damage to the inner retina [14].

Yellow light is attractive for retinal photocoagulation, since it is poorly absorbed by xanthophyll, is scattered less than argon wavelengths, is

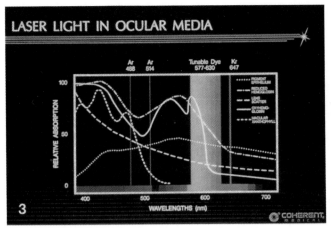

Fig. 3. Relative absorption vs. wavelength for various intraocular chromophores. The figure shows that: (1) macular xanthophyll has greater absorption for argon blue light than for other laser wavelengths, (2) hemoglobin has excellent blue, green, and yellow light absorption but much poorer red light absorption, (3) light absorption maxima for oxyhemoglobin are located at 542 nm (green) and 577 nm (yellow), (4) reduced (venous) hemoglobin has better krypton red light absorption than does oxygenated (arterial) hemoglobin, and (5) deoxyhemoglobin has roughly the same extinction coefficient for krypton red light as xanthophyll does for argon blue light. (Courtesy of Coherent, Palo Alto, CA.) See insert for color representation.

at the peak of oxyhemoglobin absorption, and has the highest oxyhemoglobin to melanin absorption ratio, as well as a high oxyhemoglobin to deoxyhemoglobin absorption ratio [14]. Retinal damage caused by krypton red light is mostly limited to the area near the RPE, whereas krypton yellow light causes less RPE damage, but does result in RNFL and ganglion cell edema and coagulation at the border between the outer plexiform and nuclear layers [22].

Nd:YAG laser. Radiation at 1,064 nm is much less absorbed by melanin than is visible light, so that it penetrates much deeper than the output of other photocoagulation lasers. Nd:YAG lasers can be configured so that their output is continuous or long-pulsed (up to 20 ms), with predominantly thermal effects. Peyman and associates [23,24] showed that a continuous wave Nd:YAG laser produced retinal lesions that were similar in histologic appearance to those created with a krypton red laser, although because of the lower absorption by melanin of the IR wavelength and greater absorption (30%) by the ocular media, some 5–10 times more energy was required with the Nd:YAG. The ratio of oxyhemoglobin absorption to that of deoxyhemoglobin is almost six times greater at 1,064 than at 647 nm, and com-

bined with the IR wavelength's overall lower absorption by hemoglobin, should allow Nd:YAG radiation to maximally penetrate subretinal hemorrhage and treat vascular structures at threshold irradiances [14]. Fankhauser [25] employed 10 ms Nd:YAG pulses for experimental retinal photocoagulation and laser trabeculoplasty (LTP, see Glaucoma, under Clinical Applications), although the former resulted in fibroblast proliferation that penetrated Bruch's membrane and invaded the retina [26].

A potassium-titanium-phosphate (KTP) crystal has been used to double the frequency, and thus halve the wavelength, of the Nd:YAG laser. Quasicontinuous output is typically achieved by high repetition (10 kHz) of 1 μs pulses. The resulting "pea-green" output, at 532 nm, is more highly absorbed by the RPE and hemoglobin than is argon green light. As it is nearer to absorption peaks of oxyhemoglobin and deoxyhemoglobin than are other common laser wavelengths, this light requires less power to achieve similar occlusive or obliterative effects on vessels.

Tunable dye laser. Dye lasers, themselves pumped by other lasers, employ one or more dyes to produce emissions over a wide range of wavelengths [27]. Tunable dye lasers allow the operator to select the desired wavelength within the range of the dye in use. This offers at least the theoretical potential for perfect matching of laser output with tissue absorption. Most photocoagulation needs would be met by a tunable dye laser capable of emitting between 560 and 640 nm, as well as at the standard wavelengths of an argon laser pump [22]. Melanin and hemoglobin would be best targeted with output in the 560–580 nm range. Selective treatment of RPE and choroidal melanin could be achieved between 610 and 640 nm. Orange light at 580–610 nm would allow partial absorption by the RPE and any underlying neovascularization while permitting sufficient energy to penetrate to the choroid to coagulate any feeder vessels. Oxyhemoglobin absorption decreases dramatically from 590 to 600 nm, enabling highly efficient treatment of vascular abnormalities by suitable wavelength selection in this region. Thus, whereas red light would be preferable in the treatment of subretinal neovascularization (SRNV) in cases of at least normal RPE and choroidal melanin concentration, orange light should be superior for hypopigmented individuals. Orange light is also appropriate for treatment of retinal or vascular tumors, as it achieves strong penetration and coagulation. Treatment may be further customized by employ-

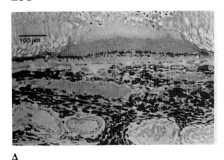
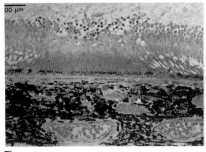
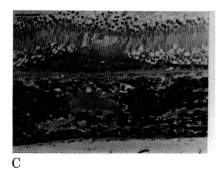

A   B   C

Fig. 4. Lesions produced at 100 mW using **(A)** 577 nm (yellow) light, **(B)** 590 nm (orange) light, and **(C)** 630 nm (red) light. Each lesion shows damage to the RPE, choroid, and photoreceptor nuclei and outer segments. (Reprinted from Romanelli [29] with permission of International Ophthalmology Clinics.)

ing multiple wavelengths, such as irradiation with red light to obliterate deep feeder vessels, followed by yellow or orange light to directly target SRNV. It should be noted, however, that white lesions appear such because of light scattering and that once such a lesion develops, it shields underlying tissues from subsequent irradiation [28].

Romanelli and Puliafito [29] performed a histologic and metabolic comparison of retinal effects in monkeys of a tunable dye laser at 577, 590, and 630 nm. All exposures were performed at 0.1 s and with a 100-μm spot size. Lightly visible white lesions were produced with 100 mW, whereas more intense ones were created with 200 mW. All lesions were morphologically similar, with the 200 mW lesions displaying more inner retinal damage than the 100 mW ones, regardless of wavelength (Fig. 4).

Diode laser. Diode lasers emit radiation with exceptional electrical-to-optical efficiency (~ 50%). They are much smaller, less expensive, and more portable than traditional ophthalmic lasers, requiring only a standard electrical outlet to achieve clinically necessary power levels. Such devices are constructed by joining n- and p-type semiconductors, which serve as electron donors and acceptors, respectively, creating a recombination region at their junction. The size of the band gap, across which photons jump and which thus establishes the emission wavelength, is determined by the addition (doping) of other atoms. The band gap in gallium arsenide (GaAs) semiconductors is particularly well suited to producing radiation, with the application of an external electrical potential across the p-n junction creating an electron population inversion and the parallel GaAs crystal faces serving as semitransparent mirrors. Internally reflected light then stimulates further photon emission in the recombination region, ultimately resulting in output that is coherent and monochromatic, albeit very divergent (in contrast to the collimated output of the argon and many other lasers). Laser power is increased by constructing arrays of many diodes, with coupling between active zones making the total output spatially coherent.

Most diode lasers studied for ophthalmic use contain GaAs crystals doped with aluminum (GaAlAs) and emit between 780 and 850 nm (commercial versions are now generally 810 nm), although any given laser has only a single emission line and is not tunable. Radiation in this range is readily transmitted by the ocular media, and in contrast to some shorter wavelengths, much less energy incident on the retina is absorbed by the RPE or choroid. However, this lower absorption requires higher laser power, whose achievement prevented the diode laser's introduction into clinical use until recently.

Puliafito and associates [30] reported the first therapeutically useful diode laser lesions. Their endophotocoagulation system produced lesions in rabbit retinas that were similar to argon, krypton, and Nd:YAG laser ones on the basis of ophthalmoscopy and fluorescein angiography, but with histologic damage limited to the outer retina. Brancato and Pratesi [31] achieved similar early experimental results, and also reported the first transpupillary diode laser photocoagulation. Using a diode laser endophotocoagulation system in rabbits, Smiddy and Hernandez [32] demonstrated that retinal cell disruption was confined primarily to the outer nuclear layer in mild burns, involved the inner nuclear layer in moderate burns, and involved ganglion cell loss in severe burns. Brancato et al. [33] first coupled a diode laser to a slit-lamp biomicroscope, achieving retinal photocoagulation in rabbits; they subsequently tested this system on a human eye scheduled for enucleation [34].

Brancato and colleagues [35] conducted a histologic comparison of diode and argon retinal lesions in rabbits. Diode lesions had zones of coagulation necrosis and vacuolation in the RPE, whereas sensory retina damage was confined to photoreceptor cells and nuclei of the inner nuclear layer. The ganglion cell layer contained many intercellular lacunae, but no alterations were observed in the inner limiting membrane. These changes varied somewhat from those produced by the argon green laser, where some damage occurs in all retinal layers. McHugh and associates [36] demonstrated that, as might be expected, diode laser lesions are histologically most similar to those produced with the krypton red light of 647 nm. Wallow et al. [37] found that moderate diode laser lesions in monkey retinas were comparable to argon ones, but more intense diode laser lesions involved scarring of ciliary nerves in the choroid or sclera, with macrophage invasion and loss of myelin sheaths and axis cylinders.

Radiation at 810 nm readily traverses the sclera, and Jennings et al. [38] successfully performed experimental transscleral retinal photocoagulation in rabbits, transmitting the laser output via a fiber optic. Treatment at 200 mW produced lesions after exposures of 5–10 s, reflecting a variability experienced with other transscleral wavelengths. The sclera overlying the chorioretinal lesions remained intact, and there was substantially less disruption of the blood-retinal barrier than is seen with cryotherapy (see Retinopathy of Prematurity), which may be important in reducing the incidence of proliferative vitreoretinopathy following retinal detachment surgery. It has been suggested that the lesion variability may be overcome by gradually titrating exposure power and duration to achieve clinically desirable levels, with an endpoint of gray or gray-white, rather than white, spots [39]. More recent work indicates that altering the diode laser output to bursts of microsecond pulses contained within millisecond envelopes allows more selective and reproducible retinal photocoagulation [40].

Clinical Applications

It is instructive to consider some currently employed photocoagulation procedures, as well as the mechanisms by which they achieve their effects. Only the more common techniques are dis-

cussed here in detail, but because the number of laser-treatable diseases is far greater than the number of fundamentally unique laser modalities and since many of the diseases have common pathologic components, these will serve as paradigms for those entities, e.g., retinal neovascularization associated with angioid streaks [41] and histoplasmosis [42], not mentioned here.

Diabetic retinopathy. Most diabetics eventually develop retinopathy, which ranges from background (nonproliferative), with microaneurysms and macular edema, to proliferative, with neovascularization and hemorrhages that may obscure the retina and/or lead to detachment. Early laser therapy of proliferative diabetic retinopathy (PDR) relied on direct and intense targeting of neovascular elements [6], which often actually exacerbated the problem. It is now accepted that PRP, in which usually several thousand argon blue-green or krypton red burns are placed in the peripheral retina (Fig. 5), indirectly improves PDR by reducing the stimulus for neovascularization [43–45]. This follows from destruction of hypoxic retina, especially photoreceptors with their high oxygen requirement [46], creating tighter adhesions to the choriocapillaris and resulting in decreased vasoproliferative tendencies and better oxygen perfusion to the remaining viable retina [44,47]. Retinal pigment epithelium (RPE) cells produce a substance that inhibits neovascularization, which PRP may release [48]. If PRP relies on improved oxygen diffusion from the choroid, the deeper penetration of krypton red light would likely be counterproductive [49]. Considering the amount of tissue damage induced by the laser, it is reasonable to expect that not all the effects are salutary, and complications ranging from transient macular edema and elevated intraocular pressure (IOP) to the development of optic atrophy many years later have been attributed to PRP [50]. Peripheral vision is generally somewhat compromised both qualitatively and quantitatively, with the goals of preventing further deterioration and preserving central vision [51].

Macular edema is the most common manifestation of diabetic retinopathy, and the localized and diffuse forms are generally treated with focal and grid laser application, respectively [52]. Focal treatment may reduce edema by preventing fluid passage from the subretinal space through the RPE and directly sealing leaking microaneurysms or capillaries. Damage by grid photocoagulation occurs principally in the RPE, with some effect on the photoreceptors and the underlying

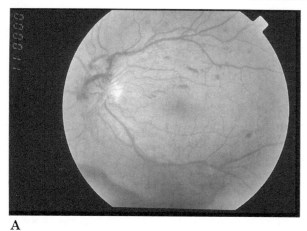

A

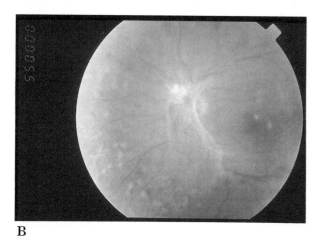

B

Fig. 5. Diabetic neovascularization extending from the optic nerve before (**A**), and after (**B**) panretinal photocoagulation.

choriocapillaris [53]. It is unclear exactly how this improves macular edema, but possibilities include reduction of blood flow, increase of inner retinal oxygen, replacement of coagulated RPE cells with new ones [54], and proliferation of endothelial cells in capillaries and venules overlying the lesions, capable of reinforcing the outer and inner blood-retinal barriers, respectively [55]. The inner retinal effects are believed to result indirectly from targeting of the outer retina; this may explain the superior results sometimes realized with the krypton red, rather than the argon blue-green, laser [56], although other studies have shown no such difference [57]. Orange dye laser light has not demonstrated any benefit over argon blue-green and may be associated with more patient discomfort [58].

Retinal vein occlusion. Treatment of branch (BRVO) or central (CRVO) retinal vein occlusion consists of two main approaches: treat-

ing the ocular symptoms or trying directly to address any underlying systemic pathology. Earlier work with diabetic retinopathy showed that laser irradiation can selectively destroy parts of the retina, thus reducing metabolic requirements and the stimulus for retinal or iris neovascularization. Although there is a theoretical risk of hemorrhage or other intraocular damage, usually the only side effects experienced by the patient are small, gradually resolving peripheral scotomata. Initial studies on laser treatment of BRVO (Fig. 6) offered often conflicting recommendations. Michels et al. [59] suggested observing patients for at least 1 year before considering laser, Gutman [60] recommended laser only after at least 6 months, and Zweng et al. [61] advised early intervention to forestall complications. Kelley and associates [62] could document no benefit of laser treatment for BRVO with macular edema.

More recently, landmark reports based on extensive multicenter trials have established widely recognized guidelines. The Branch Vein Occlusion Study Group has recommended that since approximately one-third of macular edema cases spontaneously resolve, and considering the frequent early presence of preretinal hemorrhage, which can prevent proper laser treatment and which often resorbs, patients should be carefully followed without treatment for 3–6 months [63]. Recommended laser parameters for grid photocoagulation of macular edema call for making numerous medium white burns of 100 μm diameter surrounding the macula, using argon blue-green light. Although another, smaller study reported that BRVO patients' macular edema did not significantly improve following laser therapy [64], the Study Group found that the two-thirds of BRVO patients whose macular edema does not spontaneously resolve experience significantly improved visual acuity. The Study Group only examined BRVO/macular edema patients with acuity ≤ 20/40, and it did not prescribe an optimum time for laser use. A later study suggests that krypton red light may be preferable to argon blue-green for such purposes, given the absorption properties detailed above [65].

In 1986, the Study Group [66] published guidelines for treating BRVO complicated by retinal neovascularization, which was present in 36% of patients with large areas of retinal nonperfusion. Employing scatter or panretinal photocoagulation on those patients with ≥ 5 disc diameters of nonperfusion, they showed decreases of 50% in both retinal neovascularization and vitre-

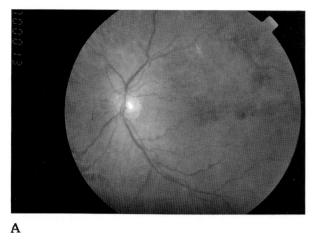

A

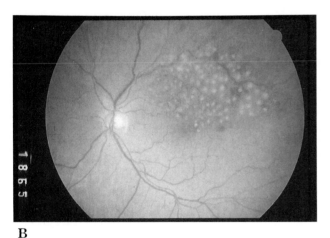

B

Fig. 6. Branch retinal vein occlusion, with dilated tortuous veins, flame-shaped, and blot-like hemorrhages before (A) and after (B) grid photocoagulation with the argon green laser. (Reprinted from Margolis with permission of Ophthalmic Practice [535].)

ous hemorrhage if neovascularization already existed, compared with untreated patients (40% of whom will develop retinal neovascularization, of whom 60% will eventually sustain vitreous hemorrhage). Their recommendation is to not treat retinal neovascularization, since treatment after it develops—but before the serious complication of vitreous hemorrhage occurs—was found to be equally effective.

No comparable studies have been completed on laser treatment of CRVO. Macular edema in CRVO can be caused by either macular capillary leakage or nonperfusion; in the former case, no treatment exists and vision is irreversibly lost, whereas in the latter, approximately one-third each will spontaneously recover, remain stable, and have decreased acuity [67,68]. Laser therapy may be useful in such instances but is more likely

to play a role in preventing the devastating effects of neovascular glaucoma. Magargal and colleagues [69], in a non-randomized, uncontrolled study, found that whereas some 20% of all CRVO patients and 60% of those with extensive ischemia tend to develop neovascular glaucoma, none of those treated prophylactically with panretinal argon laser photocoagulation experienced neovascular glaucoma. Three other studies, using the criterion of ≥ 10 disc diameters of ischemia, also reported the efficacy of preemptive laser treatment for prevention of neovascular glaucoma in severely ischemic CRVO [70–72], yet at least one investigator still questions the need for such therapy [67,73]. In a 10-year prospective study, Hayreh et al. [73] found that PRP reduced the incidence of iris neovascularization and peripheral visual field loss, but only if treatment was performed within 90 days of the CRVO, and in no case did the laser affect angle neovascularization, neovascular glaucoma, retinal or optic disc neovascularization, vitreous hemorrhage, or acuity. A multicenter CRVO study, similar to the BRVO one, is currently in progress to establish the best therapeutic approach to CRVO [74].

Macular degeneration. SRNV associated with age-related macular degeneration (AMD) is the most common cause of blindness in the United States and other developed countries. Central, color vision is gradually lost or distorted, especially affecting reading and other tasks requiring fine vision (Fig. 7). Laser treatment is likely successful because of heat-induced closure of the new vessels [75]. As is the case with diabetic neovascularization, laser treatment may cause the release of angiogenesis-inhibiting factors, cauterize vessels in the choriocapillaris, and seal breaks in Bruch's membrane that are thought to engender SRNV [76]. Early guidelines for treating SRNV associated with AMD, calling for laser treatment at least 200 μm from the foveal avascular zone (FAZ), were based on photocoagulation with argon blue-green light [77]. Five-year follow-up has shown that laser treatment decreases by a third the risk of losing six or more lines of visual acuity within 5 years [78].

It was initially felt that SRNV within the FAZ is not amenable to laser therapy and that attempts at photocoagulation in that region would jeopardize central vision [79]. Krypton red light transmission through blood and xanthophyll and vessel destruction at the level of the choriocapillaris makes it an excellent choice for treatment of juxtafoveal SRNV, assuming there is suf-

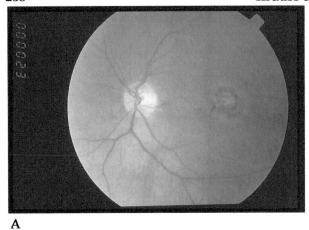

A

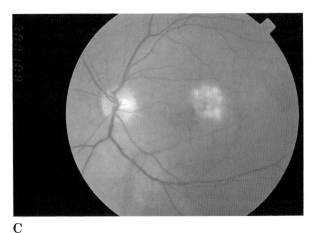

B

C

Fig. 7. Subretinal neovascularization associated with AMD. Fundus photograph (**A**) and fluorescein angiogram (**B**) before treatment, and fundus photograph (**C**) after treatment.

only from 58% to 49% [80]. At 5 years, untreated patients without systemic hypertension with juxtafoveal neovascularization had a risk of 1.82 relative to laser-treated patients of losing at least six lines of acuity, whereas hypertensive patients with AMD realized no benefit from photocoagulation [81].

Reports by the Macular Photocoagulation Study Group [82,83] indicate that patients meeting specific criteria tend to benefit from photocoagulation of subfoveal neovascular lesions, but there is no apparent difference between argon green and krypton red wavelengths (although the latter may be associated with a higher rate of persistence of all AMD-related lesions) [84]. Whereas laser treatment causes an immediate decrease of six or more lines of acuity in 20% of patients, at 2-year follow-up untreated patients are almost twice as likely to have such a decrease. However, the most recent recommendations take initial acuity and lesion size into consideration; patients with small lesions and moderate or poor acuity or medium lesions and poor acuity respond best to laser treatment, whereas those with large lesions and moderate or good acuity respond worst and achieve no discernible benefit from laser therapy through 4-year follow-up [85].

The high incidence of neovascular recurrence [86,87], although such recurrent membranes may themselves be treated with laser photocoagulation [88], reflects the inadequacy of current laser therapy in achieving long-term success. Whereas the underlying disease process is certainly a factor, it clearly would be advantageous to enhance absorption of laser energy within the entire membrane. The proximity of the SRNV to the RPE makes it difficult to determine the relative importance of the vessels' absorption, but it is likely that enhancement of direct laser absorption by the neovascular membranes would increase the destruction of the abnormal vessels (see Selective absorption).

Diode laser. In early clinical trials, McHugh et al. [89] and Balles et al. [90] demonstrated the potential efficacy of diode laser transpupillary photocoagulation, via a slit-lamp biomicroscope, for the treatment of retinal vascular diseases. The McHugh group encountered no side effects, such as lenticular or corneal opacities, RPE tears, or choroidal hemorrhage. RPE photocoagulation was achieved even through a layer of blood ~ 150 μm thick. Neovascularization had regressed 6 weeks following treatment of diabetic retinopathy, with visual acuity changes

ficient surrounding melanin [17]. Krypton red laser treatment of SRNV with a proximal edge 1–199 μm from the center of the FAZ decreases the 3-year loss of six or more lines of acuity, but similar to those associated with other lasers. Follow-up of all patients as late as 9 months demonstrated the potential success of diode laser photocoagulation for these conditions.

The Balles group found that 4.5 times more energy, 2.5 times more power, and 1.8 times more irradiance and exposure duration were required to produce diode laser lesions that were clinically comparable to those achieved with the argon laser, all consistent with the much lower absorption by the RPE of the longer wavelength. The deeper diode penetration, even greater than for krypton red light, necessitated retrobulbar anesthesia, but resulted in only four cases of Bruch's membrane rupture or subretinal hemorrhage out of a total of > 9,000 treatment exposures. There was excellent penetration through macular edema and serous retinal thickening [91]; transmission through cataracts and hemorrhages was much greater than for shorter wavelength lasers, with less light scattering. It was also noted that since the diode radiation is invisible, there were no complaints of bright flashes. Moreover, the permanent filter blocking the diode wavelength both permits continuous viewing throughout the procedure and eliminates the clicks typically associated with movable shutters, which may startle some patients. However, the diode laser's greater beam divergence did require a larger intraocular focusing cone angle, which limited peripheral treatment. Ulbig et al. [92] used a diode laser to close membranes in seven of nine eyes with parafoveal choroidal neovascularization secondary to AMD or angioid streaks, although four lesions required repeat treatment.

Given the experimental evidence that the diode laser can effectively produce chorioretinal adhesions, with less blood-retinal barrier destruction than either cryotherapy or the argon laser [93], Haller et al. [94] performed transscleral diode laser retinopexy in conjunction with scleral buckling in a series of patients with rhegmatogenous retinal detachment. Minor complications included a scleral thermal effect and presumed ruptures in Bruch's membrane in 30% of the patients, the latter accompanied by audible "pops." However, these problems were not encountered once the researchers used smaller, gray lesions as their endpoint. Nine of ten retinas were successfully attached at 6 months, whereas the tenth redetached at 6 weeks secondary to proliferative vitreoretinopathy but responded to reattachment. A multicenter trial is currently under way to evaluate this modality more precisely. It remains to be seen whether the average of 520 J used by the Haller team is necessary to create retinopexy and whether such high energy will not cause some hemorrhages in a larger study group.

Endoprobe. As clinical experience with the diode laser accumulates, there has been concomitant progress in refining both the laser itself and the means for delivering its output to the eye. This laser's compactness makes it particularly well suited to use with the endoprobe and indirect ophthalmoscope (Fig. 8). Numerous applications have been developed for endophotocoagulation since the technique was first introduced in the early 1980s [95]. Recent uses have included treatment of a choroidal bleed in a patient following evacuation of a subretinal clot [96] and ablation of experimental choroidal melanomas in rabbits with high-power argon radiation [97]. Building on early work in animals [30,32,98], Smiddy [99] reported the first clinical use of diode endolaser photocoagulation, treating patients with PDR, proliferative vitreoretinopathy, complex retinal detachments, and retinal breaks. Exposure parameters were dictated by the particular pathology, always avoiding reaching the whitish lesions typically desired with the argon laser, which with the diode laser has been associated with iatrogenic choroidal folds [100]. It was felt that endophotocoagulation with the diode laser is as clinically efficacious as with the argon laser, but the former offers significant logistic and ergonomic advantages.

In the past few years, considerable advances have been made in probe technology, especially in conjunction with the diode laser, all aimed at maximizing the functions that can be performed by a single probe. Peyman et al. [101,102] developed a couple of such 20-gauge devices, combining fiber optic diode or argon lasers and aspiration and infusion capabilities, with one also including fiber optic illumination. These instruments can be used to both drain subretinal fluid and photocoagulate the retinotomy site, thereby obviating repeated forays into the eye with separate devices. Uram [103,104] also constructed a 20-gauge probe incorporating diode laser and illumination fiber optics, but rather than aspiration/infusion capability, his has a microendoscope with a 70° field of view and recording capability. Using this device, he was able to deliver precisely titrated laser exposures to a specific number of ciliary processes, potentially enabling more effective treatment of neovascular glaucoma. Vitreoretinal endophotocoagulation was similarly facilitated,

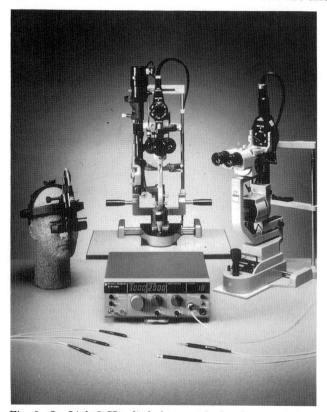

Fig. 8. OcuLight® SLx diode laser with the three means by which up to 2 W can be delivered to the eye: slit-lamp biomicroscope, endoprobe, and indirect ophthalmoscope. The laser console measures 10 cm × 30 cm × 30 cm, weighs 5.5 kg, and runs on either 115 or 230 V without requiring external air or water cooling. (Courtesy of Iris Medical Instruments, Mountain View, CA.)

with the probe providing a clear view even when more anterior structures would obscure the view through an operating microscope, and permitting post-treatment inspection for retinal breaks without resorting to indirect ophthalmoscopy.

Laser indirect ophthalmoscope. The laser indirect ophthalmoscope (LIO) is another instrument that has seen increasing use over the past decade. First described by Mizuno [105], this laser has all the advantages and disadvantages inherent in indirect ophthalmoscopy, but is indispensable for selected applications. Unlike with slit-lamp delivery, the spot size is impossible to standardize, as it depends on the power and position of the hand-held and headset lenses, and refractive power of the treated eye, and the presence of any intraocular gas. Macular work is not recommended given the inherent limitations in aiming. However, the field of view is greater than with other laser modalities, and in conjunction with scleral depression, this technique reduces

the laser power needed for photocoagulation, probably as a result of the stretched choroid's diminished ability to dissipate heat from the RPE [106]. The LIO is very useful in cases requiring far peripheral treatment, such as retinal tears or peripheral neovascularization, especially those with localized lens opacities or small pupils [107]. It is essential for pneumatic retinopexy reattachment [108] or laser treatment of retinopathy of prematurity (ROP, see following section), and has also been reported for treatment of retinoblastoma [109] and choroidal melanoma [110]. Complications include occasional choroidal hemorrhage from too intense exposures, superficial burns of the iris and cornea [111], and melted haptics (which keep artificial intraocular lenses (IOLs) in position) made of Prolene (which contains copper phthalocyanine dye) [112].

ROP, *retinopathy of prematurity,* is a potentially devastating condition affecting, to some extent, about two-thirds of infants with birthweight below 1,251 gm [113]. Cryotherapy has assumed an important role in treating ROP, cutting almost in half the rate of unfavorable outcomes. Nevertheless, it is often ineffective and has been associated with such complications as intraocular hemorrhage, retinal detachment, and scleral trauma [114], generally because of the pressure with which the probe is applied and the freezing process itself. This pressure, along with the intravenous sedation frequently employed, may also induce episodes of apnea, bradycardia, and oxygen desaturation [115].

Studies with the argon laser indicated that photocoagulation was at least as effective as cryotherapy, with less trauma to the eye [116–121]. Given its technical convenience, the diode laser has been the subject of most recent studies on photocoagulation of ROP [122,123]. McNamara et al. [124] and Hunter et al. [125] performed randomized trials comparing diode LIO photocoagulation and cryotherapy for the treatment of threshold ROP. In the McNamara study, exposure parameters were 120–600 mW and 0.3 s, with an average of 959 burns placed (Fig. 9). Transient vitreous hemorrhages were noted in 3.6% of the laser and 12.5% of the cryotherapy eyes. Lid edema, conjunctival hyperemia, and chemosis lasting 1–3 days were seen in all of the cryotherapy eyes, whereas one laser eye showed mild conjunctival hyperemia lasting only several hours. Pain was difficult to assess, but appeared to be comparable to treatment with an argon laser and less than with cryotherapy. In the laser group, 25 of 28 eyes

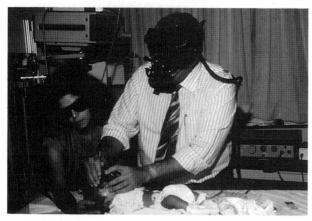

Fig. 9. Diode laser indirect ophthalmoscope photocoagulation for ROP. (Courtesy of Iris Medical Instruments, Mountain View, CA.)

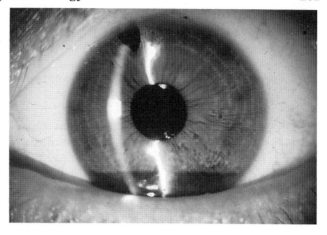

Fig. 10. Iridectomy in an eye with angle closure glaucoma. The opening in the iris, which reestablishes aqueous flow from the posterior chamber through the trabecular meshwork and out of the eye, is ordinarily hidden by the upper eyelid. (Courtesy of Roger Steinert, M.D.)

followed for 3 months and all seven of those followed for 1 year showed regression; the corresponding numbers for the cryotherapy group were 20 of 24 and all seven. Diode laser treatment thus appeared at least as efficacious as cryotherapy and has the advantage over the argon laser of portability, permitting treatment in neonatal units that might not have access to other lasers. Similar results were obtained by the Hunter group, which noted that treatment through hazy media was easier with the diode laser than with cryotherapy. There was also much less damage to the peripheral fundus. Considering that all preliminary studies have supported the efficacy of photocoagulation and its greater tolerance in the treatment of ROP, Tasman [126] has suggested that future multicenter trials concentrate on establishing the optimal threshold and parameters for laser treatment, rather than on randomized comparisons with cryotherapy.

Glaucoma. Angle closure glaucoma develops when the anterior iris presses against the posterior cornea. This prevents the usual drainage of aqueous humor through the trabecular meshwork and Schlemm's canal into the episcleral space (Fig. 1), causing a rise in IOP (22 mmHg is usually considered the maximum normal in humans). The mechanism of an iridectomy or iridotomy in an eye with angle closure is thus clear: producing a passageway (at least 50 μm in diameter [127]) for aqueous to reach the anterior chamber (Fig. 10). Given the pigmentation of most irises, photocoagulation offers an attractive alternative to invasive procedures; indeed, Meyer-Schwickerath [128] was able to perforate the tissue with the

xenon arc, albeit with considerable heat production and pigment dispersion. The argon laser minimized these complications and made surgical iridectomy virtually obsolete [129]. Although this approach allows simultaneous coagulation of any hemorrhaging vessels, it generally requires dozens of exposures, especially in lightly pigmented irises, and many clinicians now prefer the Q-switched Nd:YAG laser for iridectomy (see Iridectomy).

Jacobson and associates [130] created diode laser peripheral iridectomies in rabbits that were similar to argon blue-green iridectomies. These authors speculated that the greater transmission through the iris stroma and stronger absorption by the iris pigment epithelium at 810 nm may make the diode laser preferable for this procedure, especially in dark irises. This group [131] also reported the first human iridectomies produced with the diode laser.

Laser trabeculoplasty (LTP) was first reported by Wise and Witter [132] in 1979, and although it is often successful in controlling elevated intraocular pressure (IOP) in primary and other forms of open angle glaucoma, its precise mechanism of action remains to be determined. Typically, argon green or diode lasers are used to place circumferential 50 μm burns on the trabecular meshwork, usually ~ 90° or 180°, as 360° was found to be associated with more IOP spikes [100]. However, apraclonidine, an α_2-adrenergic agonist, has shown great promise in minimizing post-laser IOP rise, including following treatment of all 360°

[133]. There is no significant difference in facilitation of aqueous outflow between argon and krypton wavelengths [134], whereas the exact location of the laser burns [135], the percentage of treated trabecular meshwork [136], and even laser energy [137] are not correlated with clinical effect. It was initially believed that LTP works by shrinking the superficial collagen of the corneo-scleral meshwork, preventing closure of Schlemm's canal by anteriorly displacing the inner trabecular meshwork [135]. More recently, attention has focused on the biochemical effects of LTP [138], with observation of phagocytic action by trabecular meshwork cells and proliferation of the corneal endothelium onto the trabecular surface, possibly with stimulation of special Schwalbe line's cells capable of producing a phospholipid substance that facilitates aqueous egress through the trabecular meshwork [139]. In any event, it is now believed that mechanical effects of LTP are relatively minor and that some biochemical changes in and around the trabecular meshwork more likely explain the procedure's clinical efficacy [140]. Although LTP has traditionally been reserved for patients unresponsive to medical therapy alone, it rarely obviates it entirely. LTP has been found to adequately control IOP without surgery or further laser treatment in approximately three-quarters of patients after 1 year and one-half of patients by 5 years, with success rates at 10 years ranging from one-third [141] to one-half [142]. A new multicenter trial has compared outcomes among subjects randomized to initial treatment with either medication or LTP [143]. At 2-year follow-up, 44% of those eyes treated by LTP alone were controlled, whereas only 30% of those receiving only timolol had normal IOP. However, it has been noted that when all single medications were considered, the balance was in favor of medical treatment [144].

McHugh and coworkers [145] conducted a pilot clinical investigation of diode LTP. Employing parameters of 0.8–1.2 W, 0.2 s, and 100 μm, and placing 50 burns for 180°, they noted that the desired exposure endpoint was a mild blanching of the pigmented portion of the trabecular meshwork. IOP was lowered just as much as with the more established laser (9.6 mmHg at 6 months), with an even greater effect 2–4 weeks after the LTP, possibly as a result of the deeper penetration at 810 nm. There was no IOP spike immediately following treatment. These researchers [146] also showed that the trabecular meshwork damage is histologically similar whether LTP is performed with the diode or argon laser, further reflecting the procedure's independence of wavelength. Indeed, in a direct clinical comparison, Brancato et al. [147] showed that patients undergoing diode LTP retained the same lowering of IOP through 12 months as those individuals treated with argon LTP. Moriarty and associates [148] noted only a small decline in IOP, from 8.4 to 7.9 mmHg, between 12 and 24 months after diode LTP, without the peripheral anterior synechiae seen in some one-third of argon LTP cases [149].

In patients in whom medical therapy and laser or other surgical procedures designed to increase outflow fail to reduce IOP, cyclodestructive methods for partially destroying the aqueous-producing ciliary body may be necessary. There is a narrow therapeutic window; too much destruction is also not good, as the eye would become hypotonous from inadequate IOP. Cyclodestructive techniques have included diathermy and cryotherapy [150], the latter of which is still used. In the early 1970s, Lee and Pomerantzeff [151] proposed laser cyclophotocoagulation, but their transpupillary technique proved inadequate. Transscleral radiation with the xenon arc had been described as early as 1961 [152], with use of the ruby laser reported in 1972 [153]. Nd:YAG laser cyclophotocoagulation, first described by Wilensky et al. [154] in 1985, has now proved effective in numerous clinical studies and may become the cyclodestructive treatment of choice [155–158].

Schuman and colleagues [159] performed contact (via fiber optic) transscleral diode laser cyclophotocoagulation on rabbits and found IOP lowering and ultrastructural damage comparable to that achieved with the Nd:YAG laser. Work on human cadaver eyes revealed that only some 75% of the energy used with the Nd:YAG laser is needed for the diode laser procedure, consistent with melanin's greater absorption of the latter's wavelength (despite its somewhat lower transmission through the sclera) [160]. These findings were in contrast to those of Simmons et al. [161], who found that the diode laser produces most of its effect in the ciliary body stroma, rather than in the ciliary epithelium as is the case with the Nd-YAG laser, although the clinical significance of this difference is not clear. Initial clinical studies of contact diode laser cyclophotocoagulation by Gaasterland and associates [162] realized average IOP reductions from 36 mmHg pre-laser to 23 mmHg at 3-month follow-up, without any hypotony but with mild surface burns in 40% of patients.

Oculoplastic surgery. Although many of the oculoplastic procedures for which photocoagulation techniques have been attempted are probably better performed by non-laser methods, there are several applications for which lasers appear to offer distinct advantages. Trichiasis, in which eyelashes grow inward and abrade the ocular surface, has been treated with numerous procedures, most effectively with cryotherapy. However, this is often associated with such side effects as corneal ulceration and eyelid edema. As first proposed by Berry [163], argon laser treatment of trichiasis offers the potential for more selective, less traumatic lash removal. Nevertheless, increasing clinical experience suggests that it may not be applicable to severe cases, and at energy levels sufficiently low to avoid complications, multiple treatments may be necessary [164]. Since blue-green light is well absorbed by hemoglobin and melanin, the argon laser may be used to treat such vascular and pigmented lesions as capillary hemangioma, nevus flammeus, seborrheic keratosis, and telangiectasia [165]. Approximately three-quarters of dark nevi flammeus, known as port-wine stains, respond to argon laser therapy [166]. With its superior penetration, radiation from the Nd:YAG laser may be preferable to that from the argon laser for certain applications, particularly large lesions (Fig. 11) [167]. The copper vapor laser produces green light at 511 nm and yellow light at 577 nm [168]. The former is strongly absorbed by melanin and can lighten many pigmentary skin lesions, whereas the latter's absorption by hemoglobin permits eradication of vascular skin lesions. (Oculoplastic uses of the CO_2 and other ablation lasers are discussed in Ablation.)

Ophthalmic oncology. Surgery and radiation therapy remain the mainstays for treating eye tumors, but certain cases may be amenable to laser treatment. Retinoblastoma, the most common malignant intraocular tumor in children, often can be destroyed successfully with the argon laser (by eliminating the tumor's blood supply) if detected early [169], although about one-quarter require additional treatment with other methods. Similarly, small choroidal melanomas may be treated with argon or krypton laser photocoagulation, but the complexity of the protocol and the occasional development of side effects have resulted in a return to radiotherapy in most instances [170]. (Use of exogenous dyes for selective tumor destruction is discussed in the following section.)

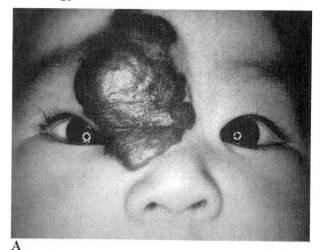

A

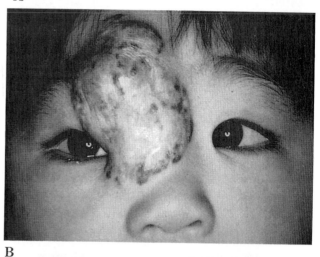

B

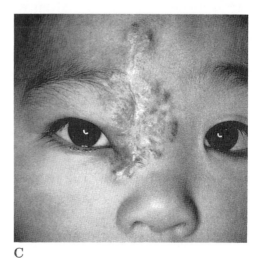

C

Fig. 11. **A.** Rapidly growing capillary/cavernous hemangioma of the forehead, upper eyelid, and nose. **B.** Three months after Nd:YAG laser photocoagulation and direct injection of steroids. **C.** Following Nd:YAG laser photocoagulation using a sapphire tip, showing good resection of the hemangioma, with improvement of color, contour, and symmetry. (Reprinted from Apfelberg et al. [167] with permission of Annals of Plastic Surgery.)

Investigational Techniques

Despite the theoretical appeal of highly precise targeting of ocular tissues by appropriate selection of wavelength, it has been suggested that differential absorption is essentially irrelevant beyond threshold lesions [171]. The specificity of laser wavelength and pulse selection greatly exceeds the absorption specificity of the target tissues. The greatest absorption of all photocoagulation wavelengths occurs in the RPE, and aside from the deeper penetration of longer wavelengths due to decreasing melanin absorption, most clinical lesions appear identically gray-white regardless of wavelength. A study of patients with pathologic myopia and SRNV treated with the tunable dye laser revealed no significant anatomic or clinical differences among 577, 590, and 620 nm, although the authors still recommended selection of a specific wavelength according to the precise pathology being treated [172]. Nevertheless, several new investigational approaches do unequivocally enhance the target specificity of ophthalmic laser surgery.

Selective absorption. Anderson and Parrish [173] proposed one method of enhanced absorption, selective photothermolysis, in which selective tissue damage is determined not by precise aiming of the laser beam but by the unique absorption properties of the intended target. If the target has an absorption coefficient at least twice that of the surrounding tissue at a given wavelength, preferential absorption will result in thermal damage localized to the target if the irradiation is performed at a duration similar to or less than the thermal diffusion constant. Brevity of the exposures is determined principally by the size of the target. They used this method to selectively damage blood vessels (3×10^{-7} s, 577 nm) and melanocytes (2×10^{-8} s, 351 nm), although selective photothermolysis is, in principal, applicable even at the subcellular level.

Krauss et al. [174] investigated localization of retinal thermal damage by employing an interferometric technique to project a fringe pattern at various exposure powers and durations. The periodicity of the fringe pattern could be adjusted from macroscopic dimensions to a scale of microns without the need for an imaging plane. Periodicity is more adjustable and unambiguously measurable than spot size, and comparison of tissue response with theoretical models is simplified because the sinusoidal fringe pattern is itself an eigenfunction of the thermal diffusion equation.

Tests in rabbits confirmed that exposures at 10 ms, comparable to the retinal relaxation time, resulted in localized damage, whereas those at 100 ms displayed diffusion that belied the fringe pattern of the irradiating beam. Although exposures too short may cause acoustic shock wave and mechanical damage, these findings suggest that, especially in the macula and near blood vessels, treatments at shorter exposure times might result in more localized and effective results. Roider and colleagues [175] employed argon laser 514.5 nm, 5 μs pulses in rabbits to selectively coagulate the RPE without creating ophthalmoscopically visible lesions and corresponding damage to the adjacent neural retina and choroid.

Dye enhancement. Intravenous injection of exogenous dyes can substantially increase the specificity and effectiveness of certain laser procedures. Hematoporphyrin derivative (HpD), with strong absorption between 625 and 635 nm, is preferentially taken up by neoplasms [176]. Production of singlet oxygen for selective tumor destruction can be induced with red laser light, such as from a dye laser using rhodamine 6G (which emits at 630 nm) or a gold vapor laser (which emits at 628 nm) [177]. Liposomal benzoporphyrin derivative (BPD), stimulated by a dye laser at 692 nm, has been used in animal models to treat SRNV [178] and choroidal melanoma [179].

Indocyanine green (ICG) is a tricarbocyanine dye with an absorption peak at 805 nm. It fluoresces at 835 nm, allowing transmission through overlying blood, exudate, and melanin, and recent advances in IR imaging and digital angiography have made it a powerful tool in defining SRNV [180,181]. The dye's predilection for choroidal neovascular membranes makes it a useful exogenous chromophore for diode laser selective photocoagulation and thermal enhancement of membrane closure [182]. In patients receiving ICG-enhanced diode laser photocoagulation of SRNV, minimal deep retinal whitening is noted acutely, followed by chorioretinal scar formation. Reichel and associates [183] reported a small study in which high resolution ICG digital angiography followed by ICG-enhanced diode laser photocoagulation successfully treated poorly defined SRNV, in most cases with minimal decrease in visual acuity (Fig. 12).

Chloro-aluminum sulfonated phthalocyanine (CASPc) is a photoactive dye that generates singlet oxygen upon irradiation at 675 nm and fluoresces at 680 nm [184]. Unlike HpD, it is easily prepared as a chemically pure compound and

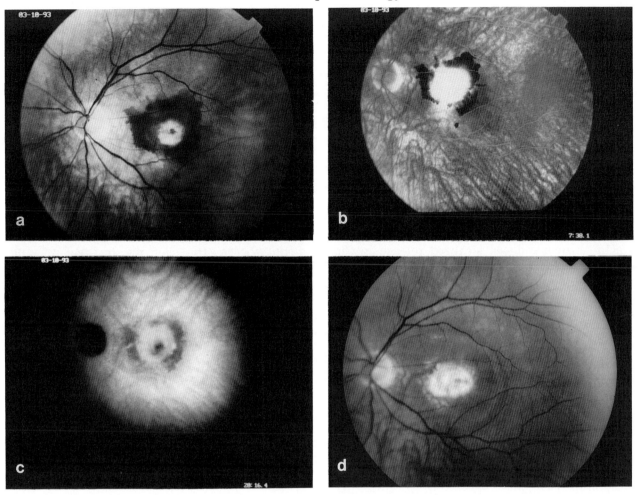

Fig. 12. ICG-diode laser treatment of choroidal neovascularization. (a) Fundus photograph of fibrovascular scar with surrounding subretinal fluid and hemorrhage. (b) Late phase fluorescein angiogram showing leakage of fluorescein from the choroidal neovascularization and surrounding ring of blocked fluorescence consistent with hemorrhage. (c) Late phase ICG angiogram showing a central area of hyperfluorescence consistent with CNVM. (d) Red-free photograph 4 months after treatment. The scar is centered on the fovea. (Reprinted from Reichel E and Puliafito CA [536] with permission of the New England Eye Center.)

is associated with minimal systemic toxicity and skin sensitization (although it is not now approved for human use) [185]. CASPc has been proposed as a possible photodynamic adjunct to tumor therapy and vessel closure, with less reliance on thermal mechanisms. Bauman et al. [186] demonstrated that dye laser 675 nm irradiation with CASPc, but not irradiation alone, of rabbits with experimental choroidal melanomas achieved significant vessel closure and tumor regression. Ozler et al. [187] found that such tumors regressed in response to CASPc and 675 nm light at 22–60 J/cm^2, only temporarily so at 15–22 J/cm^2, and not at all at < 15 J/cm^2. All eyes receiving > 15 J/cm^2 showed transient corneal edema and conjunctival hyperemia, whereas only those

treated with > 43 J/cm^2 experienced retinal hemorrhages. Kliman and associates [188,189] showed that CASPc localizes in experimental choroidal neovascular vessels, which can then be closed with irradiation at 675 nm, with minimal damage to the overlying retina compared with standard thermal techniques. Although CASPc work to date has been conducted with dye lasers, it is likely that diode lasers doped with other elements will soon provide sufficient output at that wavelength [190–192]. Although CASPc's 675 nm absorption peak is the longest among commercially available photosensitizers, allowing greater penetration of exciting light through tissues, pigment, fluid, and blood, it would be preferable to use an even longer wavelength, with still better penetration and at which diode lasers are currently capable of sufficient energy production. Silicon naphthalocyanines (SlNc) offer promise in this regard, as they have absorption maxima between 770 and 800 nm and a 20% quantum yield of singlet oxygen production [193]. Garrett et al. [194] achieved necrosis of experimental rabbit melanomas with SlNc stimulated by a solid state titanium-sapphire laser at 770 nm (see Future Developments).

Liposomes. Zeimer et al. [195] and Khoobehi et al. [196–198] have conducted a series of studies on the intravenous injection of liposomes containing drugs or dye. Low level irradiation with argon blue-green or dye yellow light is used to achieve heat-induced localized release in the retinal vasculature of those substances from the miniature phospholipid containers with a transition temperature of 41°C. Potential applications include measurement of blood flow and selective angiography. Work on the latter has shown that with a spot size of 1.5–2.0 mm centered on the optic disc and energy densities of 0.5–3.4 J/cm^2, it is possible to obtain multiple angiograms up to 3 hours following dye injection [198]. Potential advantages of this technique include reduction of choroidal fluorescence, which permits optimal viewing of the retinal microcirculation, and clear separation of arterial and venous fluorescence. Selective angiography of a suspected leaking vessel could be documented by specifically targeting it with the laser. Blood flow might be monitored during and after laser treatment of tumors and angiomas. Before any clinical use, however, more extensive tissue damage studies are needed, as are data on the potential toxicity of the liposomes and carboxyfluorescein dye.

Scleral buckling. Scleral buckling is the standard procedure for the treatment of rhegmatogenous retinal detachment, but is not without its complications. Looking for a method that would avoid episcleral sutures and large exoplants, Ren and co-workers [199] used the holmium:YAG laser on human cadaver eyes to induce tissue shrinkage and create a buckling effect. Five 250 μs pulses were applied via a fiber optic probe held some 5 mm from the sclera, to achieve a fluence of 11.3±1.2 J/cm^2, which affected only the outer two-thirds of the sclera; there was no damage to the remaining sclera or the underlying retina. Although their system was successful, they speculated that a continuous wave laser tunable over the 1.8–2.4 μm range would permit more controllable treatment, ad-

justable to the various absorption characteristics of pathologic sclera. They also suggested the possibility of combining this with laser retinopexy, whose early clinical results were promising [94].

Tissue welding. Using lasers to join tissue without the need for sutures has been an attractive but elusive goal and remains the subject of periodic studies. Burstein et al. [200] employed the continuous wave hydrogen fluoride (HF) laser to create seals of corneal incisions in porcine cadaver eyes. The welding spot of ~ 0.2 mm diameter was moved across the incision at a rate of 1 mm/min. The fundamental mode, with wavelength 2579 nm and power 30 mW, produced a weld some 100 μm deep, which failed at 14 mmHg, whereas the overtone at 1,340 nm and 320 mW created a weld 300 μm deep, which withstood pressures up to 34 mmHg. Scleral welding was found to be less successful. Considerably greater resistance was noted by Khadem and coworkers [201] in human cadaver eyes whose corneal incisions had been sealed with a fibrinogen mixture containing a photosensitive singlet oxygen generator, activated by an argon blue-green laser to cross-link a protein solder with stromal collagen. Wolf and associates [202] used the diode laser to convert ICG-enhanced fibrinogen to fibrin in rabbit retinas and speculated that this may provide a quick chorioretinal adhesion, assisting in the treatment of retinal breaks.

PHOTODISRUPTION

Photodisruption is the use of high peak-power ionizing laser pulses to disrupt tissue. Energy is concentrated in space and time to create optical breakdown, or ionization of the target medium, with formation of a plasma, seen as a spark. The use of optical radiation to produce a plasma became possible only after the development of lasers capable of emitting high power through very brief radiation pulses. Although the first lasers were too weak to achieve optical breakdown, in 1962, Hellwarth developed the method of Q-switching, which allowed the creation of very brief but large ruby laser pulses over 10–50 nanoseconds (ns, 10^{-9} s), with maximum powers in the tens of megawatts [203].

In 1972, Krasnov [204] reported the first use of clinically desirable intraocular photodisruption. To emphasize the relative importance of nonthermal acoustic mechanisms in creating these tissue effects, he used the term "cold laser," which ignores the fact that plasma formation causes very localized temperature increases greater than 10,000°C. Further work demonstrated that, because of the ruby laser's high-order mode structure (which limits the minimal spot size that can be achieved), it is not the ideal source for a clinically practical ophthalmic photodisruptor. However, the increasing popularity of extracapsular cataract extraction (ECCE, see Posterior capsulotomy) and the pioneering research of Aron-Rosa [205] and Fankhauser [206] with the Nd:YAG laser, combined to make this technique a reality.

Laser Principles

Laser power can be increased by either increasing energy or, more practically, decreasing the period over which the energy is delivered. The two principal means of compressing the laser output in time to achieve high-peak power are mode-locking and Q-switching. Mode-locking is comparable to the audible summation of musical tones with similar frequencies, known as beating, which is heard as a periodic surge in intensity. The phase relationships in lasers are synchronized by a shutter near one of the cavity mirrors. For ophthalmic applications, the most common shutter is a saturable dye, employed in a process known as passive mode-locking. The dye absorbs low-power radiation pulses, but becomes transparent on exposure to high-power ones.

The Q-switch is an intracavity shutter that requires an active medium that allows atoms to remain in the high-energy state for a relatively long time to create high-peak power. Solid-state media such as Nd:YAG are particularly well suited for this process. At the appropriate time, the Q-switch shutter is opened, exposing the mirror. Oscillation and stimulated emission follow quickly, with emission of a single brief high-power pulse. Methods of Q-switching include saturable dyes, rotating mirrors, and acousto-optic modulators. Pockel's cell, an electro-optic modulator that is the most common Q-switch, applies voltage across a crystal to vary polarization. Polarity can be rapidly changed by 90°, making the cell either opaque or transparent to the polarized laser beam. The "Q" refers to the quality factor of the laser cavity, which is defined as the energy stored in the cavity divided by the energy lost per cycle. Rapid extraction of high power is accomplished as the Q-switch changes the quality factor of the cavity from a high to a low Q.

Whereas typical mode-locked laser output consists of a train of seven to ten 25-picosecond (ps, 10^{-12} s) pulses, at intervals of 5 ns and contained within a 35–50 ns envelope, Q-switched laser output generally consists of a single 2–30 ns pulse. The total energy required for a single Q-switched pulse and a train of mode-locked pulses is the same, but the peak power necessary to cause avalanche ionization must be 100–1,000 times greater for mode-locked than Q-switched lasers [207,208]. Maximum outputs of most ophthalmic models are 10–30 mJ and 4.5 mJ for Q-switched and mode-locked lasers, respectively.

Optical breakdown and plasma formation. When a target is heated by absorbing radiant energy, the effect is linearly proportional to the cause. In contrast, nonlinear effects are sudden, all-or-nothing phenomena. Optical breakdown, a nonlinear reaction, occurs when the laser output is sufficiently condensed spatially and temporally to achieve high irradiance. It is manifested by a spark and accompanied by an audible snap, producing dramatic target damage. When focused to a small spot, typically < 50 μm in diameter, short-pulsed Nd:YAG lasers can produce enough irradiance, usually 10^{10}–10^{11} W/cm^2, to induce optical breakdown, dissociating electrons from their atoms and creating a plasma. Q-switched pulses cause ionization mainly by focal target heating in a process called thermionic emission, whereas mode-locked ones rely primarily on multiphoton absorption [209]. In either case, once the initial free electrons have been generated, plasma expands via electron avalanche or cascade if the irradiance is adequate to cause rapid ionization. Plasma absorbs and scatters incident radiation, thereby shielding underlying structures. Plasma radiation absorption and growth both occur through inverse bremsstrahlung, the process of photon absorption and electron acceleration in the presence of an atom or ion.

Mechanisms of damage. In biologic systems, thermal denaturation of protein and nucleic acids is theoretically confined to a radius of 0.1 mm for a 1 mJ pulse [210]. As such, although high local temperatures exist briefly, total heat energy is low, and significant clinical photocoagulation does not occur.

Several mechanisms combine to generate pressure waves radiating from the zone of optical breakdown, the foremost of which is the rapid plasma expansion that begins as a hypersonic wave [211,212]. A secondary source of hypersonic and sonic waves is stimulated Brillouin scattering, in which the laser light generates the pressure wave that scatters it [213]. The focal heating may lead to vaporization, melting, and thermal expansion, generating acoustic waves [214]. If sufficiently strong, the radiation's electric field will deform a target through electrostriction, which causes simple Brillouin scattering, and radiation pressure induced by momentum transfer from photons to atoms in inverse bremsstrahlung.

The shock wave begins immediately with plasma formation and expands at a hypersonic velocity of 4 km/s, falling to sonic velocity within 200 μm. The acoustic transient lasts 50 ns at a distance of 300 μm from the focal point, whereas the pressure falls from 1,000 to 100 atm within 1 mm [215]. The next process is cavitation, or vapor bubble formation. This begins within 50–150 ns after breakdown in water, expands rapidly for the first 20 μs, reaches a maximum size of ~ 0.6 mm at 300 μs, and collapses within 300–650 μs [211,212]. Cavity propagation velocity is ~ 20 m/s at 300 μm from the breakdown [216]. Many shock waves may be generated along the laser beam's path as impurities are encountered [217]. Damage zone size depends on the irradiance and total energy, the plasma's duration, and the mechanical properties (including density, mass, tensile strength, and elasticity) of the target tissue [218–221].

In recent years, most cataract operations have included the insertion of IOLs, which are generally made of polymethylmethacrylate (PMMA), although older ones may be of glass and newer ones may be of foldable silicone. These lenses can affect the intraocular use of lasers, especially posterior capsulotomy (see Clinical Applications) where damage may take the form of microcracks, melted voids, and large pulverized regions. Unlike the situation in liquids, optical breakdown in PMMA and glass may be associated with self-focusing and self-trapping with both ns and ps pulses [222]. The damage threshold for glass is ~ 100 times greater than that for PMMA, but once glass damage occurs, it tends to be more extensive [223]. As damage tends to be cumulative, IOLs may be damaged more by bursts of laser shots than by single pulses. Various IOL designs, including the use of spacers to increase the separation between the IOL and the posterior lens capsule, have been created in the attempt to minimize damage from photodisruption.

Since clinical applications of Nd:YAG photodisruption involve energies significantly above retinal damage thresholds, it is important to consider how the retina is protected during these laser procedures. Beam divergence is the angle formed by the cone of light converging on and

diverging from the laser system's focal point. The border of the laser beam is described as either the $1/e$ or $1/e^2$ points of the solid angle. Commercial ophthalmic Nd:YAG lasers usually broaden the laser beam with an inverse galilean telescope and then employ a large-diameter, high-power final focusing lens to achieve the desired combination of cone angle, minimal spot size, and comfortable working distance. As such, for retinal injury to occur during Nd:YAG laser posterior capsulotomy, 96 mJ, some 20 times the energy clinically used, would have to be incident on the cornea.

Plasma formation is a secondary factor in retinal protection during photodisruption in the pupillary plane. It absorbs and scatters incident radiation, thereby diminishing the transmission of radiant energy along the beam path. Plasma shielding assumes a more important role in retinal protection during vitreous photodisruption. Nevertheless, the pressure waves still propagate unattenuated, and may cause retinal or choroidal damage even in the absence of suprathreshold radiation levels.

Instrumentation

Although photodisruption is possible with other lasers and at other wavelengths, including some Nd:YAG harmonics, the fundamental Nd:YAG output at 1,064 nm is the only one used in commercial ophthalmic photodisruptors. Most clinical Nd:YAG lasers employ the fundamental TEM_{00} mode, so that the spot size, and consequently the energy required for optical breakdown, can be minimized. Beam divergence is generally 0.5–3.0 mrad. The lasers are cooled by ambient air or internally recirculated water and require only standard 110 V outlets. Whereas 5 mJ is sufficient for most applications, many ophthalmic Q-switched Nd:YAG lasers are capable of producing up to 30 mJ. Higher energies may be needed to cut very dense material and in cases of hazy media, such as corneal edema or blood in the anterior chamber. Mode-locked systems have a maximum output of ~ 5 mJ per pulse train, but because of the greater control and relative safety of the Q-switch, those models employing mode-locking have largely fallen out of favor.

An aiming beam is required to guide the pulsed, invisible Nd:YAG output. This is achieved with a continuous wave helium-neon (He-Ne) laser, which produces 632.8 nm output coaxial with the Nd:YAG's and below the retinal injury threshold. Since high-peak power pulses cannot be satisfactorily transmitted via fiber optics, oph-

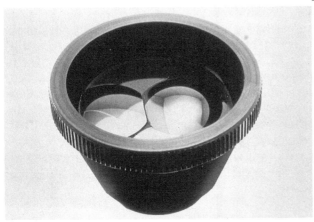

Fig. 13. Goldmann three-mirror contact lens, which permits selective targeting of intraocular structures. (Courtesy of Ocular Instruments, Bellevue, WA.)

thalmic Nd:YAG lasers employ fixed mirrors to guide the output to the patient, who is generally seated opposite the surgeon at a specially configured, slit-lamp biomicroscope. The larger the solid cone angle, the lower the energy required for optical breakdown and the risk of IOL or retinal damage, but the greater the chances of beam vignetting during some applications. The slit-lamp design limits the angle to ~ 20°, and most systems employ one of 16°.

Contact lenses are generally not required for simple posterior capsulotomy, but they may be helpful to stabilize the eye, prevent blinking, and maintain a regular optical surface. However, to treat the vitreous and some other intraocular structures effectively, specialized instruments with a variety of lenses and mirrors are required (Fig. 13).

Clinical Applications

Posterior capsulotomy. In the past decade, cataract surgery has largely changed from intracapsular cataract extraction (ICCE), in which the entire lens capsule is removed together with the opaque lens, to extracapsular cataract extraction (ECCE), in which the posterior lens capsule is left in place. This serves both to reduce the incidence of postoperative vitreoretinal complications, such as cystoid macular edema (CME), and to provide support for posterior chamber IOLs. Unfortunately, this membrane often also opacifies, forming a so-called secondary cataract [224]. Until the advent of photodisruption, this membrane was ruptured by introducing a needle into the eye with the patient seated at the slit-

lamp, with all the attendant risks of any invasive procedure. Laser-assisted removal of primary cataracts remains the subject of considerable research, but is not yet clinically feasible (see Future Developments). However, the Nd:YAG laser has proven so successful at sectioning opacified posterior lens capsules that it has completely replaced the traditional surgical approach for the often equally debilitating secondary cataracts.

Although secondary cataracts can substantially diminish vision, their removal does not guarantee normal vision. Especially in older patients, concomitant ocular pathology (such as macular degeneration or CME) may impair vision even after capsulotomy. Such instruments as the laser interferometer (see Diagnostic Lasers) and the potential acuity meter can be used to assess best potential acuity even through cataracts, preventing a possibly useless or even deleterious procedure.

Prior to laser capsulotomy, the pupil is dilated to provide the surgeon with maximum visibility of the membrane. Topical anesthesia is necessary only if a contact lens is employed. With most Nd:YAG lasers, a posterior capsule can be opened with pulses of 1–2 mJ. Shots are placed along tension lines, as indicated by capsular wrinkles, to create the most efficient opening (Fig. 14). This procedure, associated with a high degree of visual improvement, is not without occasional complications [225]. By far the most commonly encountered difficulty is a transient rise in IOP [226], likely caused by impaired aqueous outflow resulting from capsular debris, acute inflammatory cells, and heavy molecular weight protein [227]. IOP is typically checked for several hours following the procedure, with pressure-reducing agents given topically or systemically as needed [228]. Patients with preexisting glaucoma are more susceptible to this IOP elevation, but since it has been encountered in all types of patients, some clinicians advocate prophylactic treatment [229].

Iridectomy. Although argon laser iridectomy has largely supplanted the traditional surgical approach, many instances remain in which its use is problematic. The argon laser relies on coagulation, vaporization, and necrosis to cut through tissue, and light blue or gray irises may not absorb sufficient energy. Conversely, the strong absorption by dark brown irises may generate a char, which impedes further penetration. Since photodisruption does not depend on target pigmentation, the short-pulsed Nd:YAG laser

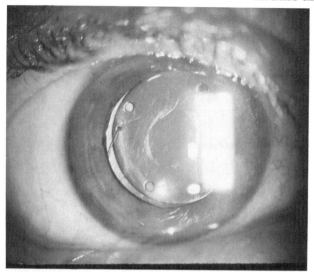

Fig. 14. Secondary cataract after Nd:YAG laser capsulotomy. The IOL edge and haptic are visible. (Courtesy of Roger Steinert, M.D.)

represents an attractive alternative for creating iridectomies. This was verified in clinical studies, which demonstrated that the Q-switched Nd:YAG laser can create openings in the iris, which unlike some openings created with the argon laser do not gradually close [230]. Small, self-limited hemorrhages are occasionally encountered with the Nd:YAG laser [231], but as with all photodisruption procedures, this laser would be unable to coagulate any significant bleeding that might occur. The loss of corneal endothelial cells overlying the treatment site can be minimized with proper technique [232]. To facilitate laser iridectomy, the iris is drawn taught by instilling miotic drops, which constrict the pupil. Openings are often achieved with only a single Nd:YAG laser shot of 4–8 mJ. Nd:YAG laser iridectomy has proved effective in cases in which the argon laser has failed [223], whereas use of the two lasers together on dark irises may allow less energy to be employed than with either laser alone [234].

Posterior segment. Although technically more demanding and potentially more dangerous, Nd:YAG laser photodisruption also may be applicable to pathology in the posterior segment. Vitreous membranes sometimes form and if adherent to the retina, may lead to that tissue's detachment. Experimental vitreous membranes in rabbits have been successfully sectioned with 4 mJ pulses as close as 4 mm to the retina, without retinal injury [235]. Since these membranes may be complex and fibrous, hundreds or thousands of pulses, often in multiple sessions, may be neces-

sary. Aside from the risk of retinal or choroidal hemorrhage, which rises exponentially with proximity to the retina, a lens (crystalline or IOL) also may be damaged if work is performed too close to its posterior surface. However, despite initial concern that photodisruption of the posterior lens capsule or vitreous may cause liquefaction and other vitreous disturbance, Krauss et al. [236] employed MRI and other techniques to demonstrate that this process does not significantly affect the structural integrity of the normal vitreous body.

ABLATION

The term "ablation" is often used casually to refer to many laser procedures, including photocoagulation. For present purposes, only those methods that involve actual removal of tissue are considered. These include many promising areas of current investigation, which offer hope for correction of ocular pathology ranging from refractive errors to epiretinal membranes.

The ophthalmic laser development with the most widespread potential applicability, and which has thus received the greatest public attention, is corneal ablation. Photorefractive keratectomy (PRK) with the excimer laser at 193 nm has become a successful clinical procedure some 10 years after the first experimental reports and will likely soon receive FDA approval. Nevertheless, the technology and techniques are still evolving, and there have been many reports of potential alternatives or successors to the excimer. Moreover, although the cornea remains the most common and suitable target for laser ablation, there is considerable interest in extending the process to intraocular structures.

Cornea

The human cornea consists of five main layers, starting anteriorly: epithelium, Bowman's membrane, stroma, Descemet's membrane, and endothelium (Fig. 15). Corneal thickness ranges from ~ 520 μm centrally to 650 μm peripherally. Water is the largest component of the cornea, representing ~ three-quarters of its wet weight [237]. The epithelium is ~ 50 μm thick; its basement layer, Bowman's membrane, is acellular and some 12 μm thick. The main solid components of the stroma, which constitutes ~ 90% of corneal thickness, are collagen, other proteins, and glycosaminoglycans. The endothelium, whose basement layer is Descemet's membrane, is a sin-

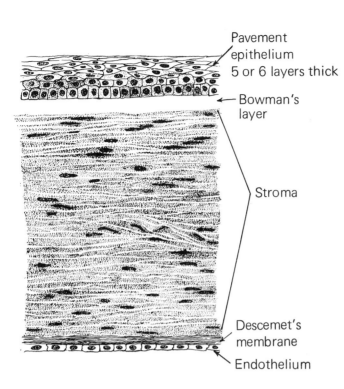

Pavement
epithelium
5 or 6 layers thick

Bowman's
layer

Stroma

Descemet's
membrane

Endothelium

Fig. 15. Cross section of the cornea. (Reprinted from Wolff [534] with permission of Chapman and Hall.)

gle layer of cells. These cells lack significant mitotic ability, and damage to them may alter corneal hydration and, potentially, clarity.

The cornea accounts for about two-thirds of the eye's refractive power. Whereas some refractive errors such as astigmatism (irregular curvature) or keratoconus (cone-shape deformity) are corneal irregularities per se, others such as myopia and hyperopia—most cases of which are secondary to too long and too short axial length, respectively—can be corrected by recontouring the cornea. This is the basis for keratorefractive surgery, which is discussed in Refractive keratoplasty.

Early ophthalmic laser applications, particularly retinal photocoagulation, relied on the transmission by the cornea of the (visible wavelength) light. Although use of the argon laser has been reported for the treatment of such corneal disorders as neovascularization, lipid keratopathy, and adhesions [238], the cornea had generally not been considered an appropriate target for laser therapy. However, work with the CO_2 laser, and more recently and extensively with the excimer and other new ablation lasers, has dramatically changed this notion.

Carbon dioxide laser. Ophthalmic investigation of the CO_2 laser followed soon after its development in 1964 [239]. The laser emits radiation with a much higher efficiency (some 15%) than argon or krypton lasers and at a mid-IR wavelength of 10.6 μm. That this radiation is strongly absorbed by water ($\alpha = 950$ cm^{-1}) makes the CO_2 laser of potential use in any water-containing tissue, and it is currently employed in many other medical fields. Heat diffusion away from the target area coagulates adjacent vessels and provides hemostasis, which is particularly useful in patients with bleeding diatheses. Along with the lymphostasis afforded by the CO_2 laser, this approach is valuable when treating malignant or severely infected tissues. Water is the most ubiquitous substance in the eye, and the CO_2 laser has been employed, either experimentally or clinically, to treat ophthalmic pathology ranging from the eyelids and adnexa to the vitreous [240–242]. The major disadvantage of the CO_2 laser is that current fiber optics are not capable of effectively transmitting at this wavelength, necessitating the use of less flexible articulated arms. Also, smoke and steam often develop and must be vented.

Figure 16 shows an incision in a bovine cornea produced with the CO_2 laser. There is considerable damage and disorganization to the surrounding tissue. Beckman et al. [243] suggested that the use of a pulsed (60–300 s^{-1}) CO_2 laser might significantly reduce thermal damage to surrounding tissue by allowing less time for heat conduction. This technique enabled them to achieve high peak powers to vaporize tissue rapidly, with relatively low average powers and minimal dissipation of heat. However, there was still a 0.12 mm zone of charred tissue around the incision site, and the edges were considered less sharp than they would have been with mechanical techniques. Keates et al. [244] proposed an even greater reduction in exposure duration, using a Q-switched CO_2 laser with 500 ns pulses to make experimental corneal incisions. This laser had a repetition rate of 7200 s^{-1}, and although the peak output reached 450 W, the average was only 1.6 W. This technique was found to produce more uniform and reproducible lesions than a 90-s^{-1}-pulsed mode, with less carbonization. Nevertheless, a study by Peyman et al. [245] in which CO_2 laser burns of various intensities, locations, and patterns were placed on rabbit corneas showed no significant alterations in corneal curvature. Whereas the notion of using the CO_2 laser

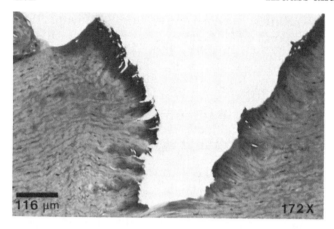

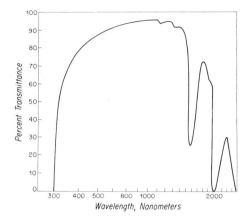

Fig. 16. Light micrograph of CO_2 laser (10.6 μm) ablation in a bovine cornea. Dosage parameters: 25 pulses, 0.2 Hz, 6 J/cm²/pulse; BaF_2 lens. (Reprinted from Krauss et al. [238] with permission of Survey of Ophthalmology.)

Fig. 17. Transmission of human cornea. (Reprinted from Boettner et al. [298] with permission of Investigative Ophthalmology and Visual Science.)

as a welding substitute for, or adjunct to, sutures may be alluring (see Tissue welding), Keates and his colleagues [246] were unable to achieve adherence with scleral or corneal eye bank tissue. A difficulty of the CO_2 laser remains the degree of tissue shrinkage and vaporization [244].

Excimer lasers. Ultraviolet radiation and the cornea. Two far-ultraviolet (UV) wavelengths, 193 and 248 nm, are the excimer emission lines that have been most extensively studied for potential laser surgery of the cornea. As indicated in Figure 17, corneal absorption rapidly increases below 300 nm [247]. Since water does not significantly absorb radiation between 193 and 293 nm [248], it must be the solid components of the cornea that are responsible for that tissue's absorption in this region and for the mediation of any photophthalmic changes.

The majority of corneal solids are proteins, particularly collagen, which comprises ∼ 70% of the stromal dry weight. Protein absorption maxima around 190 nm have been associated with absorption by the C-N peptide linkage [249–252]. To a first approximation, peptide bonds behave as isolated chromophores [250]. Nucleic acids in the cornea are largely restricted to the epithelium. They absorb strongly at 248 nm, due to a peak around 260 nm corresponding to absorption by the nucleotide bases [253]. Absorption at 193 nm is approximately twice as great as that at 248 nm [254]. The different types of glycosaminoglycans demonstrate absorption spectra that are comparable to one another, with absorption peaks around 190 nm and no significant absorption at 248 nm [255].

UV radiation has been shown to have numerous deleterious effects on cellular activity [256–258]. These are largely mediated by the radiation's effects on DNA, and whereas the most serious effect is cell killing, others include mutagenesis, carcinogenesis, interference with synthesis of DNA and protein, delay of cell division, and changes in permeability and motility [252]. The action spectrum for UV-radiation-induced mutations parallels the absorption spectrum for DNA [252], and almost all ultimate carcinogens have been shown to be mutagens [259]. It is well established that UV effects on the cornea are caused in part by absorption of radiation within the nucleoproteins [260]. Since it absorbs strongly and is the most anterior structure, the epithelium is the first corneal layer to be affected by UV radiation [261].

Early damage studies of the excimer laser indicate that the nucleic acid components of irradiated epithelial cells are the initial absorption sites in the cornea at 248 nm and that such damage may involve initial DNA lesions leading to suppressed protein synthesis [262]. However, the avascularity and low cell content of the stroma make it relatively resistant to UV damage [263]. As expected on the basis of their absorption spectra, glycosaminoglycans are very sensitive to UV radiation [264]. Stromal swelling following UV irradiation may be caused by a breakage of glycosaminoglycans, which interconnect adjacent fibers, or by destruction of the endothelium, which has been observed under certain conditions and which may disrupt normal corneal hydration [265]. Endothelial cells have shown a high rate of

TABLE 2. Principal Wavelengths of the Rare Gas Monohalide Excimer Laser

Gas fill	Wavelength (nm)
Argon fluoride (ArF)	193
Krypton chloride (KrCl)	222
Krypton fluoride (KrF)	248
Xenon chloride (XeCl)	308
Xenon fluoride (XeF)	351

unscheduled DNA synthesis when exposed to UV radiation, although the repair capacity is partially responsible for the unexpectedly strong resistance of the endothelium toward UV radiation damage [266].

Excimer laser surgery of the cornea.

Laser principles. Excimers, or excited dimers, are molecules with bound upper states and weakly bound ground states. The most common excited molecules exhibiting laser action are rare gas excimers, such as F_2 and Xe_2, which emit radiation at 157 and 170 nm, respectively. Such lasers, however, are impractical for clinical or most laboratory uses, not least because oxygen absorption below 190 nm precludes working in room air. The best performance has been demonstrated by excimers formed by the reaction of an excited rare gas atom with a halogen molecule, in which the rare gas atom acts as the corresponding alkali metal and becomes very reactive in the presence of halogen-containing molecules [267]. Such rare gas monohalides emit radiation as they decay from the bound upper state to the rapidly dissociating ground state. Lasers employing this principle were first developed in 1975 [268] and have been valuable sources of UV radiation for research in chemistry, spectroscopy, remote sensing, and dye laser pumping [269]. Different combinations of a rare gas and a halogen gas can be used as the active laser medium to generate a variety of UV wavelengths (Table 2).

Excimer lasers, emitting pulses of $\sim$ 10 ns duration, have been employed as a new means of materials processing. Since the early 1980s, excimer lasers have been used to precisely etch submicrometer patterns in a variety of polymer materials [270,271]. Srinivasan [272] has termed this controlled removal of material, in which molecules on the irradiated surface are broken into small volatile fragments, "ablative photodecomposition." Several theoretical models have been proposed to explain the results of this process [273–275]. UV photons are strong enough to di-

rectly break molecular bonds. The driving force for ablative photodecomposition is the energy of the photon in excess of that of the broken chemical bonds, which serves to excite the fragments and ultimately leads to their ablation from the surface [276]. Ablative photodecomposition is thus probably caused by a combination of the high absorption for far-UV radiation possessed by organic polymers, which limits the depth of the radiation's penetration, and the high quantum yield for bond breaking, which results in the formation of numerous fragments in a small volume near the surface [277]. Ablation is thought to result from the intense pressure build-up within this volume [272,276]. The relative photochemical and thermal contributions to excimer laser ablation have been debated, but it appears that there is an increasing thermal effect at longer wavelengths [278–280].

Excimer lasers offer an intriguing option for ablation and cutting of tissue [279]. They have been used to etch clean and precise patterns in hair and cartilage [281], arterial tissue [282], and skin [283] and are being considered for use in angioplasty and neurosurgery, among other surgical procedures [284].

Refractive keratoplasty. There are numerous surgical options for altering corneal curvature, but for present purposes it suffices to briefly describe the main procedures and examine some of the areas in which laser techniques may offer advantages. Radial keratotomy is a still widely practiced procedure in which radial incisions in the cornea reduce its curvature and counteract myopia. Its most serious shortcoming is the lack of reproducible incision depth and hence refractive accuracy [285]. With current techniques, incisions are made only one at a time, and it has been reported that corneal dehydration caused by operating microscope lights may thin the cornea up to 10% during the procedure [286]. The goal of maximal radial keratotomy is to bring the incisions as close as possible to Descemet's membrane, which increases the chances for endothelial damage or even perforation. Mean endothelial cell loss may be as high as 10% [287], whereas corneal perforation may occur in up to 20% of cases [288]. Although serious complications arising from perforation are uncommon, there have been cases of endophthalmitis following such inadvertent entries into the anterior chamber [289].

Keratomileusis, keratophakia, and epikeratophakia are all techniques of using a suitably lathed lenticule, obtained from either donor cornea or the patient's own cornea, to alter refractive power. With these procedures, freezing and unfreezing of the tissue is required, causing swelling of the central corneal stroma, shrinking of the diameter, and keratocyte death, often complicating prediction of final results and compromising visual recovery [290]. Although attempts have been made to incorporate these factors into the computer programs that control the cryolathing process, it would clearly be advantageous if the reshaping of the lenticule could be done at room temperature. Direct reprofiling of the whole cornea in situ, if feasible, would obviate lenticule use altogether.

Corneal ablation. In 1983, Trokel and co-workers [291] reported the first use of the excimer laser to achieve precise and controlled etching of the cornea. Using 193 nm radiation, they selectively ablated narrowly defined areas of bovine corneas by employing masks of various designs to restrict the laser energy. Tissue ablation to a depth of 1 μm was achieved with a total energy deposition of ~ 1 J/cm^2. Laser damage was localized to the zone of ablation, with no evidence of thermal effects. Edges of the laser incisions were parallel and straight, and no disorganization of the stromal lamellae or epithelial edge was apparent in the histologic sections.

Puliafito et al. [292] performed a comparative study of excimer laser ablation of the cornea at 193 and 248 nm. Slits of several thicknesses were made in the corneas of freshly enucleated human and bovine eyes, using either a mask or a cylindrical lens. The lowest per pulse fluences at which human corneal ablation was observed were 46 mJ/cm^2 at 193 nm and 58 mJ/cm^2 at 248 nm. Depending on the width of the corneal exposure, 193 nm ablations were either trough-like or slit-like (Fig. 18a). Transmission electron microscopy revealed a zone of damaged stroma approximately 0.1–0.3 μm thick on the edges of the ablation, with preservation of corneal fine structures beyond this region. Such edge effects were thought to represent a thin band of thermal denaturation or photoablated material which was not completely ejected and which adhered to the wall of the incision. Scanning electron microscopy gave further evidence of the sharp demarcation of the cuts (Fig. 18b). In contrast, ablation at 248 nm produced incisions with a region of adjacent stromal damage at least 2.5 μm wide (Fig. 19). In addition to the wider zone of damage at 248 nm, the stroma was also markedly disrupted. Residual thermal damage produced by 248 nm excimer la-

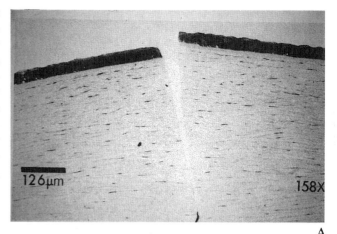

A

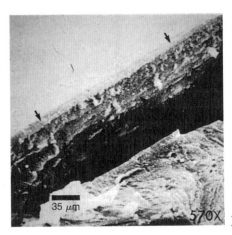

B

Fig. 18. Slit-like corneal ablation performed with excimer laser at 193 nm. Dosage parameters: 20,000 pulses, 50 Hz, 125 mJ/cm^2/pulse, 10 μm mask. **A.** Light micrograph. **B.** Scanning electron micrograph, showing sharp cleavage of the corneal epithelium (arrow) and stroma (arrowhead). (Reprinted from Puliafito et al. [292] with permission of Ophthalmology.)

ser pulses is similar to that produced by CO_2 laser pulses of 2 μs duration [293]. This is consistent with the respective absorption levels measured at the two wavelengths, α = 2700 cm^{-1} at 193 nm and α = 210 cm^{-1} at 248 nm. Kerr-Muir and associates [294] found that excimer laser ablation yields tissue at least ten times as smooth as does conventional diamond knife surgery and further described the pseudomembrane which seals laser-treated surfaces and appears to minimize postoperative scarring.

A number of factors may explain the minimal damage to adjacent tissue observed with 193 nm corneal ablation. The absorption length of 193 nm radiation in stroma is only 3.7 μm, so that incident energy is deposited in a relatively small

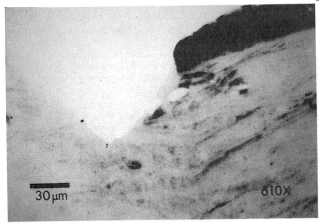

A

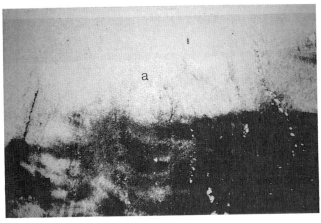

B

Fig. 19. Corneal ablation performed with excimer laser at 248 nm. Dosage parameters: 1,050 pulses, 50 Hz, 190 mJ/cm²/pulse, quartz lens. **A.** Light micrograph. Note irregular edge and disorganization of stromal collagen adjacent to the ablation. **B.** Transmission electron micrograph. The corneal stroma adjacent to the region of ablation (a) shows a broad zone of disorganization measuring at least 2.5 μm wide. (Reprinted from Puliafito et al. [292] with permission of Ophthalmology.)

volume of tissue. Moreover, the incident laser radiation is short pulsed (10–20 ns), so that heat diffusion beyond the irradiated region is minimized. Indeed, calorimetric studies suggest that these laser pulses have a much shorter penetration depth than the simple absorption coefficient would indicate, and that Beer's law may not hold for ablation [295]. As previously noted, other investigators have demonstrated decreased thermal effects at shorter exposure times using non-UV wavelengths. Non-CO_2 laser alternatives to the excimer are discussed below, but it is possible that ablative photodecomposition at 193 nm may

be fundamentally different from ablation using IR radiation. This may be related to differences in photon energy, and the type and location of target chromophores (i.e., tissue water at IR wavelengths vs. organic biomolecules at 193 nm). The photon energy of 6.4 eV for 193 nm radiation is more than sufficient to cleave peptide bonds (3.0 eV) or the adjacent carbon-carbon bonds (3.5 eV) of the polypeptide chains, especially collagen. It is possible that the high quantum yield for peptide bond cleavage at 193 nm, along with the high absorption of glycosaminoglycans, which are intertwined throughout the stromal collagen moiety, are responsible for the superior tissue removal and lower fluence requirement associated with 193 nm ablation.

Krueger and his associates [296, 297] further investigated some of the quantitative aspects of excimer laser ablation of the cornea. They found that plots of etch depth per pulse vs. fluence per pulse generate roughly sigmoidal curves in whose steep parts there is an approximately logarithmic relationship, as had already been observed in simpler polymer materials. Inflection points in these plots correspond to minima of graphs of fluence required to remove a given depth of tissue vs. fluence per pulse. These values—~ 200 mJ/cm² at 193 nm, 1,000 mJ/cm² at 248 nm, and 1,500 mJ/cm² at 308 nm—represent the per pulse fluences for the most efficient ablation, where the largest portion of incident energy is converted to tissue removal. Since corneal transmission is high at this wavelength [298] and can lead to damage of intraocular structures, 308 nm radiation is probably not useful for such work. A study by Peyman et al. [299] demonstrated that exposure of the cornea to 308 nm excimer laser radiation produced a combined ablative and coagulative effect, with corneal necrosis, stromal opacification, and endothelial cell damage. The tissue depths removed per excimer laser pulse were 0.45 μm and 6.25 μm at the above maximum efficiency levels for 193 and 248 nm radiation, respectively. Since 193 nm radiation removes considerably less tissue per pulse, control of etch depth is more precise at this wavelength. Energy in excess of these optimum values may produce undesired side effects such as heat or shock waves. Whether these levels produce the best clinical results, however, remained to be determined [300–302]. Recent clinical applications have employed fluences in the 160–180 mJ/cm²/pulse range, and Campos and coworkers [303] found that even lower fluences may prolong laser hardware lifetime, allow larger ablation zones (thereby minimizing duplex optical images [304]), and produce a thinner pseudomembrane, although the clinical ramifications of the last are uncertain.

Many issues remained to be resolved before excimer laser corneal ablation could be attempted clinically. Corneal smoothness also may be affected by the inherent inhomogeneity of the excimer beam, which as described in Photoretractive keratectomy requires elaborate techniques to minimize, and by the somewhat asymmetric distribution of the corneal components and variation with age of its UV absorption [298].

Dehm et al. [305] reported that 193 nm excimer laser incisions to 90% of corneal depth produce endothelial alterations similar to those seen underlying diamond knife incisions of comparable depth. These include minimal disruption of cell junctions, cellular edema, and a ridge that corresponds to the site of the incision. Stress waves generated during ablation were thought to be analogous to the mechanical injury associated with conventional surgery. No endothelial cell loss was observed with scanning electron microscopy for 193 nm ablation, whereas severe endothelial cell damage and loss were observed for 248 nm ablation performed at identical fluences. Differences in endothelial damage may be due to differences in absorption length, damage mechanisms, and recoil forces associated with ablation at these two wavelengths. Zabel et al. [306] found that although the pressure near the back of the cornea reaches ~ 100 atm during ablation of the superficial stroma, endothelial disruption occurs only after some 85–90% of the corneal thickness has been ablated.

Since the excimer laser employs UV radiation, possible mutagenesis and carcinogenesis are obvious concerns and were the subject of several early studies. Nuss et al. [307] found that unscheduled DNA synthesis, a measure of excision repair of pyrimidine dimers, was not increased in rabbit corneas following 193 nm irradiation at 400 mJ/cm^2/pulse, as compared with diamond knife controls. In contrast, 248 nm did produce a statistically significant increase in such repair. Kochevar [308] indicated that the fact that excimer laser radiation at 193 nm causes less cytotoxicity than predicted by the DNA absorption spectrum may be due to absorption at that wavelength by protein present between the cell surface and the nucleus, or to induction by photons reaching the nucleus of DNA photoproducts, which are either not cytotoxic or readily repaired by the cells. DNA-damaging effects resulting in cytotoxicity were least at 193 nm, greatest at 248 nm, and intermediate at 308 nm. It has also been shown that 193 nm irradiation of the cornea at a fluence of 60 mJ/cm^2/pulse causes a fluorescence emission between 295 and 425 nm [309]. Although this includes wavelengths known to be cataractogenic, the percentage of incident energy reaching the crystalline lens is only some 10^{-5} that incident on the cornea, and is thus clinically insignificant.

There are two principal categories of clinical application of excimer laser corneal ablation: PRK and phototherapeutic keratectomy (PTK). The goals and technical details differ, but they both rely on a comprehensive understanding of excimer laser-tissue interaction and corneal wound healing.

Photorefractive keratectomy. Preliminary experimental work on animal studies [310–329] preceded clinical trials [330–350] of excimer laser ablation. Several researchers performed radial keratotomies with the excimer laser [310,311,315,320], but most concentrated on wide area corneal ablation [238,312,318,325,326]. Radiation at 193 nm consistently yielded smoother surfaces than did that at 248 nm, and use of the longer wavelength was discontinued. Even at the shorter wavelength, however, wound healing was often associated with some degree of opacification and regression in refractive results, especially with deeper ablation. Moreover, there was visual and histologic variability in wound healing.

Unlike the emissions of many lasers, such as the argon and the krypton, that of the ordinary excimer laser is largely non-Gaussian and irregular. Modifications are necessary for ophthalmic applications if the beam's homogeneity is to be commensurate with the fundamentally precise laser-tissue ablation, allowing macroscopic as well as microscopic smoothness; L'Esperance [316] described one such technique using prisms to create a "top hat" beam configuration. With the exception of astigmatism, correction of refractive errors requires radially symmetric alteration of the corneal curvature. This is most commonly achieved with a computer-controlled iris diaphragm [325]. Ordinarily this would be useful only for myopic corrections, but a rotating diaphragm has been described that can create spherical negative and positive, as well as cylindrical, corrections, to treat myopia, hyperopia, and astigmatism, respectively [314].

Conventional radial keratotomy spares the

optical axis. Although refractive keratoplasty necessarily violates this region, only the stroma is actually lathed. However, for the excimer laser to realize its full potential for refractive surgery, the corneal curvature must be altered in situ. This means that for laser keratomileusis, not only must the optical axis be treated, but this must involve disruption, if not obliteration, of what has traditionally been viewed as the inviolable Bowman's membrane. However, one advantage of this greater invasiveness is the ability to correct much higher myopia than that treatable with radial keratotomy [329]. The pseudomembrane covering the ablation surface, which consists of a dense exterior part 20–100 nm wide and a less dense interior portion 60–200 nm wide, may act as a substitute for Bowman's membrane, by supporting the establishment of a regular basal epithelial layer until a true basement membrane, albeit slightly more undulating than the original, reappears [318].

Munnerlyn et al. [319] calculated the ablation diameters and depths necessary to correct spherical refractive errors, assuming that the epithelium will regrow with a uniform thickness and produce a new corneal curvature determined by the new stromal curvature. They showed that flattening to correct myopia is determined by the equation $t_0 \approx -S^2 D/8(n-1)$, where t_0 is the required ablation depth, $D = (n-1)/(1/R_2 - 1/R_1)$, n is the corneal index of refraction, 1.377, R_1 and R_2 are the initial and final corneal radii of curvature, respectively, and S is the diameter of the ablation zone. This is often approximated as $t_0 = $ dioptric correction $\times S^2/3$ and indicates that the required ablation depth per diopter increases with increasing optical zone, going, e.g., from 3.0 μm at 3 mm, to 5.3 μm at 4 mm, and to 8.3 μm at 5 mm. Hyperopic correction is achieved by sparing the visual axis and removing tissue peripherally, in an amount nearly equal to that required for the same magnitude of myopia.

A team led by L'Esperance and Taylor performed the first PRK trial on humans in the United States [330,331]. Initial FDA investigational device exemptions limited work to blind eyes or those scheduled for enucleation, and results were consistent with the preceding animal work. Using a delivery system with enlarging apertures for myopic correction, this group treated eyes with parameters of 10 Hz and 80–125 mJ/cm²/pulse, creating ablations 3–5 mm in diameter and 30–150 μm in depth. With the patient in the supine position, the eye to be treated was stabilized with a vacuum ring and retrobulbar injection of lidocaine. Prior to the start of ablation, the epithelium was mechanically debrided with a blade to ~ 1 mm beyond the intended ablation zone. Following the procedure, the eye was treated with balanced salt solution and antibiotic ointment, and then taped closed for 2–3 days. Patients reported either no or minimal postoperative pain, the latter relieved with oral analgesics. Reepithelialization occurred in all eyes within 3 days, with no subsequent erosions. All eyes not enucleated by 1 week showed some inflammatory response, albeit without any corneal leukocyte reaction; whether this resulted from the ablation per se, or was secondary to the suction ring or epithelium removal, could not be determined. The early inflammatory response was only partially responsive to local corticosteroids, and there was no apparent effect on the amount of clinical haze, but the study group was quite small (ten patients). As had been observed in animals, there was a gradual filling in of the ablation zone, with residual refractive change two-thirds that originally obtained. Slit-lamp exam initially revealed mild superficial edematous haze in the ablated area, which progressed after 2 weeks to a mild speckled interface haze between the epithelium and stroma. Specular microscopy at 3 months showed no loss of endothelial cells. Increased collagen and ground substance was observed at 4 months, and these researchers suggested that the use of pharmacologic means of maintaining the communication between the epithelium and the underlying keratocytes, in the absence of Bowman's membrane, may reduce new collagen formation and retain the initial ablation results. In a similar study, McDonald et al. [332] found that regression in refractive correction was proportional to the amount initially attempted and that, unlike many conventional keratorefractive procedures, excimer laser ablation did not cause any astigmatism.

Seiler and associates [333], working in Germany, published early results of PRK on both blind and sighted humans. Using parameters of 180 mJ/cm²/pulse and 10 Hz, and a computer-controlled diaphragm dilating in step widths of 5 μm, they ablated 4.5-mm-diameter discs for correction of up to −6 D, gradually decreasing to 3.5 mm discs for −10 D so as to avoid unnecessarily deep keratectomies. Postoperative treatment consisted of gradually tapered topical antibiotics and steroids. All patients reported considerable discomfort and foreign body sensation and were provided with systemic analgesics. Glare was common initially in the sighted eyes, but subsided after 2 weeks. There were no diurnal fluctuations in vision, although one patient complained of persistent halos at night (prompting these investigators to eschew 3.5 mm ablation zones in future work). Manifest refraction showed the typical initial overcorrection and subsequent mild reversal, and although there was a temporary reduction in best-corrected visual acuity, at 1 month it was back to the original level in most patients and was even increased by one line in a few subjects. That stromal remodeling is the likely cause of refractive regression was suggested by the relative stability in those eyes undergoing small corrections, in which Bowman's membrane was not completely ablated. IOP was unaffected in all but one patient, in whom reduction in steroid frequency lowered the pressure from a high of 21 mmHg to 18. After 3 months, 12 of 13 sighted eyes had corrections within 1 D of those intended, whereas at 6 months only ten did. Although transient subepithelial haze occurred in almost all eyes, it resolved to clinically insignificant levels after 6 months.

Brancato and colleagues [335] reported the results of > 1,000 myopic patients who underwent excimer laser PRK in an Italian multicenter study. Patients with at least 10 D of myopia were treated in a two-step process, in which the initial ablation attempted more correction in a smaller diameter than did the second one immediately following it, permitting shallower ablations than with the one-step method. All patients received topical corticosteroids, for a minimum of 2.5 months following the procedure. The percentage of eyes within 1 D of attempted correction at 12 months ranged from 71.2% for those with initial errors less than −6 D to 28.2% for those with initial errors between −10 and −25 D, with mean residual errors of −0.52 ± 1.04 D and −1.86 ± 3.47 D, respectively. There were no severe postoperative complications, but 2.4% of patients lost two or more lines of best-corrected visual acuity; at least half of these cases were attributable to other, concomitant ocular pathology. Recent reports of 2- [336] and 3-year [337] follow-ups of PRK patients suggest that minimal refractive changes occur after the first year.

In a Swedish study, Tengroth and coworkers [338] experienced residual refractive errors at 12 months of 0.31 ± 0.52 D and −0.42 ± 1.05 D in subjects with initial errors of −1.25 to −2.90 D and −5.00 to −7.50 D, respectively, confirming the greater tendency toward myopic shift at higher attempted corrections observed in other studies. All patients received steroids, with 12-month refractions of 0.17 ± 0.47 D and −0.09 ± 0.29 D in those treated for 3 months and 5 weeks, respectively, indicating that longer drug therapy reduces early regression in the refractive results. Subepithelial haze developed in all patients, peaking at 4–5 months postoperatively and declining to a mean of 0.75+ on a scale to 5+ by 1 year. Both myopic shift and haze could be diminished by later use of steroids, but longer treatment was required and less effect was achieved compared with earlier institution. Gartry et al. [339] found no significant difference in haze or refractive regression between patients treated with steroids for 3 months and those who received a placebo and recommended against routine pharmacologic intervention, although they did not follow patients beyond 6 months. Stevens et al. [340] found higher complication rates with no significant benefits in those patients receiving steroids for 6 months compared with those treated for only 3 weeks.

Liu and associates [341] analyzed numerous factors in blind and sighted humans potentially affecting the outcome of PRK. They found that the larger the attempted correction, the greater the residual myopia. Refraction after 1 month is not predictive of that at 3 or 6 months, whereas refraction at 2 and 3 months is highly correlated with results at 6 months. There was no correlation between patient age and either rate of healing or development of corneal haze, whereas there was some evidence that older patients tend to have more accurate refractive and visual results at 6 months. Some correlation may exist between corneal haze and ablation depth or diameter, but refractive and visual results were entirely unrelated to the rate of healing. Significant regression of refractive results occurred only for attempted corrections of greater than 5 D.

Seiler et al. [345] followed 193 PRK eyes for up to 2 years. In contrast to radial keratotomy, PRK resulted in less induced astigmatism and progressive hyperopia. Complications were rare in patients with less than −6 D of myopia, but higher myopes were much more likely to experience steroid-induced rises in IOP, scars, loss in glare vision, under- and overcorrection, and continued regression. These researchers suggested, however, that these effects might be mitigated by using larger ablation zones. Sher et al. [329] performed PRK on a series of highly myopic patients (up to -14.5 D), with ablation depths to 230 μm and diameters to 6 mm, and achieved mean refractions at 6 months of -0.90 ± 2.13 D, although the long-term effect on corneal mechanical stability of such deep ablation remains to be determined. Heitzmann and coworkers [346] employed a multi-zone (4-, 5-, and 6-mm) protocol for correction of myopia greater than -8 D, which allowed shallower ablations but still resulted in considerable regression and haze. They suggested that such patients might be better treated by multiple ablation sessions (as has also been recommended by Förster [347]) or by some combination of PRK and radial keratotomy.

Binder and coworkers [348] found decreases in eye bank eyes' central and peripheral endothelial cell counts from 2,035–3,051/mm^2 to 940–1,836/mm^2 following PRK. In contrast, Carones et al. [349] observed no such changes up to 12 months in a series of 76 eyes that underwent PRK. Only 18.4% of eyes had endothelial cell loss $> 5\%$, which was unrelated to ablation depth.

Central islands, or areas of localized steepening, probably caused by a combination of technical factors involving the laser beam and the corneal surface, have been noted in some patients [350]. Although they tend to improve with time, they may cause a decrease in best-corrected visual acuity. Loss of corneal sensation may complicate any refractive procedure, but Campos et al. [342] showed that postoperative recovery is less in those patients treated for high myopia, undoubtedly because of the larger ablation volume.

It has been shown that PRK yields a relatively small central area of uniform refractive power, surrounded by a large transition zone of linearly decreasing power [351]. Moreira et al. [352] have proposed deliberately attempting a multifocal refractive effect to compensate for presbyopia, although such an approach may be complicated by monocular diplopia or a decrease in image contrast.

Astigmatism. The large variety of surgical procedures developed for the correction of natural and postoperative astigmatism is testimony to the inability of any single approach to treat all patients effectively. The excimer laser may prove valuable in this effort as its output can be harnessed for a diversity of techniques. In 1988, Seiler et al. [353] used the excimer laser to produce linear corneal T-excisions for the correction of astigmatism in a series of blind and sighted patients in Germany. Radiation was directed at metal-foil-coated PMMA contact lenses containing tangential slits 4.5 mm $\times$ 150 μm, resulting in cylindrical corrections of up to 4.16 D. Postoperative care was as for this group's myopia work [333], although topical antibiotics and steroids were used for only 1 week after the procedure. Astigmatism initially fluctuated, but tended to stabilize within 2 weeks. Epithelial regrowth occurred within 3 days, but even after a month there was considerable variation in the extent to which the entire keratectomy was filled with an epithelial plug. Visual acuity was stable after 1 week, although some patients noted glare for up to 8 weeks.

One of the attractions of the excimer laser is that corneal excisions are not limited to patterns produced with conventional surgery, and McDonnell and coworkers [354] proposed the use of the excimer laser to create toric ablations for the correction of cylindrical errors. In contrast to the linear excision method, in which tissue removal ranged from 51% to 93% of corneal thickness [353], this approach allows more superficial areas to be ablated, using an expanding slit with flattening in the meridian of expansion, perpendicular to the slit itself. Preliminary tests were conducted on rabbits, and although there was good correlation with intended corrections, keratometry at 12 weeks revealed corrections only about half of those expected. Initial clinical use of this technique, including for the combined treatment of myopia and astigmatism, termed photoastigmatic refractive keratectomy (PARK), also showed significant regression [355,356]. Gibralter and Trokel [357] employed a combination of PRK and PTK ablation patterns to treat two patients with irregular astigmatism. Although there was some residual astigmatism and regression, topographic analysis did reveal a more regular and spherical corneal surface. Refinements of this technique might include using the topographic information to generate ablation algorithms, which could be incorporated into the laser controls.

Trephination. Of course, the greatest promise for the excimer laser is in situ reprofiling, but the technology may also prove useful for precise trephination, such as in obtaining tissue for transplants. Conventional trephination is often associated with significant residual astigmatism and requires suction or some other means of direct stabilization along with contact cutting, introducing further distortion. In 1987, Lieurance and associates [358] reported using the excimer laser to remove lenticules from human eye bank eyes, resulting in a normal epithelium, intact Bowman's membrane, normal stroma, and a smoother surface than is achieved with cryolathing. Serdarevic et al. [359] employed a rotating slit delivery system [317] for trephination of donor and recipient human eye bank and rabbit corneas. Fluence was 110 mJ/cm^2/pulse, and operating at a rate of 15–20 Hz, the laser required from 30 s to a few minutes to achieve perforation, depending on corneal thickness and eye stability. Trephination diameter ranged from 4 mm to 8 mm, according to the distance from the spherical lens in this configuration. Buttons and recipient beds produced with the excimer laser were freer of distortion and damage to adjacent tissue, including loss of fewer endothelial cells, when compared with those created by free-hand or suction trephines. Deposits at the wound edges never measured > 0.08 μm, minimizing the disparity between donor and recipient wound configuration. Healing through 3 months was comparable between the laser and mechanical trephination groups.

Lang et al. [360] proposed using the excimer laser with appropriate corneal masks for elliptical corneal transplants, conforming to the natural elliptical meniscus shape of the cornea, facilitating suture placement, and enhancing graft stability. Gabay and his associates [361] used the excimer laser to prepare plano donor lenticules for clinical use by placing a mechanically obtained lenticule in a special mold and ablating the excess tissue. Surface topography was superior to that of a hand-cut lenticule, and postoperative recovery was uneventful. The laser's cost is considerable, but the actual lenticule preparation was performed at a fraction of the expense of conventional techniques, and the group recommended using this method for processing optical power epikeratophakia tissue by providing a concave mold base for hyperopia and a convex one for myopia.

Phototherapeutic keratectomy. Although the great attention, both among researchers and the popular press, that the excimer laser has garnered in recent years is due to its potential for PRK, PTK is at least as efficacious. In 1985, Serdarevic et al. [362] reported that 193 nm excimer laser ablation, but not that at 248 nm, was successful in completely eliminating and sterilizing experimental *Candida albicans* corneal infections in rabbits. The underlying stroma was unaffected, although since removal of tissue may reduce tensile strength and alter refractive power, this was deemed advisable only in instances of antifungal therapy failure. Dausch and Schröder [363] used excimer laser ablation to treat patients with malignant melanomas of the conjunctiva, pterygia, recurrent erosions, persistent epithelial defects following keratoplasty, and herpes infection. Steinert and Puliafito [364] used the excimer laser to remove a 1 mm zone from a patient with longstanding keratoconus who developed an apical fibroblastic nodule. At 1 week the surface contour was smooth, albeit with minor subepithelial anterior stromal haze, and although visual acuity remained at 20/25, the patient reported a subjective sense of improved vision and increased contact lens tolerance.

Sher et al. [365] conducted a trial of PTK for such conditions as anterior stromal and superficial scarring following infection or trauma, anterior corneal dystrophy, recurrent erosion, and band keratopathy. Most patients received peribulbar anesthesia and underwent mechanical removal of the epithelium. Corneal scarring was reduced in most subjects, whereas approximately half had improved visual acuity. Reepithelialization occurred within 5 days, without significant scarring. Postoperative treatment consisted of application of a patch with or without a disposable contact lens and slowly tapered antibiotics and steroids. These researchers proposed a combination of myopic ablation followed by secondary hyperopic steepening to minimize the hyperopic shift encountered in about half the patients. Induced hyperopia, which increases with ablation depth, may also be lessened by shifting the ablation zone and employing different spot sizes to modify the transition zone [366]. They also concluded that removal of the epithelium is undesirable for PTK, as the intact tissue can serve as a modulator of ablation. In another series of PTK patients [367], these researchers treated a variety of corneal scars and found that at 6 months postoperatively, 49% of subjects had visual acuity improvement of at least two lines, 36% had change of less than two lines, and 15% had worsening of at least two lines.

Kornmehl et al. [368] compared several masking fluids intended to shield deeper tissues while exposing surface irregularities during PTK. Dextran 70, with high absorption at 193 nm and moderate viscosity, was found to produce the least surface irregularity, followed by carboxymethylcellulose and saline; corneas ablated without fluid had the greatest irregularity. Compared with surgical superficial keratectomy, PTK has the potential to result in considerably less astigmatism and more predictable corneal power [369].

Mid-infrared lasers. Although the vast majority of PRK research has been concentrated on the excimer laser at 193 nm, there have been periodic reports of attempts at employing other lasers and wavelengths to achieve the same precise ablation. Many of these studies have used IR lasers, motivated by early concern about the excimer laser's toxic gases and possible UV mutagenesis, the latter without any evidence, as well as the inability to transmit its output via fiber optics. In 1986, Loertscher and associates [370] created corneal incisions in eye bank eyes with a pulsed HF gas laser, which produced a combination of emissions from 2.74 to 2.96 μm and was operated at fluences of 0.7–2.3 J/cm^2/pulse and a rate of 10 Hz. Water has an absorption peak around 2.9 μm, which makes the HF laser theoretically superior to the CO_2 laser in limiting thermal damage to adjacent tissue. The 200 ns pulse duration is considerably shorter than the 1.7 μs relaxation time of HF-irradiated water, further reducing heat spread. However, whereas damage to deep portions of the HF incisions was limited to 1–2 μm, that in the shallow parts was some 10–15 μm wide and was similar to damage associated with the excimer laser operating at 248 nm [292]. It was believed that greater penetration by some of the shorter HF emission lines, along with difficulty in focusing the laser output on the cornea, may have contributed to the larger than expected thermal effects.

Similar results were reported by Thompson et al. [371], who compared HF, 193 nm excimer, and 2.94 μm solid-state erbium:YAG (Er:YAG) lasers in experimental corneal trephination. Excimer excisions were the sharpest, and although the mid-IR lasers required less time to penetrate the tissue, they also produced a 10–15 μm zone of adjacent stromal damage and wounds some 2.5 times larger than those made with metal scalpels. Peyman et al. [372] used an Er:YAG laser, emitting 200–μs pulses, to ablate 3.5 mm discs in rabbit corneas. Thermal damage extended up to 40 μm from the margins of the ablation zone, yet the endothelium was unchanged by ablations as deep as 320 μm. There was faint corneal light scattering in most animals, which progressively cleared. It was believed that the multimodal nature of that laser's output may have produced the less than optimal results. Tsubota [373] transmitted 400 μs Er:YAG pulses via a 200-μm-diameter fiber optic, achieving fluences of 636–954 mJ/cm^2/pulse. Ablation of the cornea and various intraocular structures yielded thermal damage results consistent with previous findings. Seiler et al. [374] found that Q-switched 80 μs Er:YAG pulses reduce thermal damage to 1–2 μm.

Stern et al. [375] studied corneal incisions produced by a Raman-shifted Nd:YAG laser, operating at 2.8 and 2.92 μm and emitting 8 ns pulses. At 2.8 μm, there was an ablation threshold of 250 mJ/cm^2/pulse, and etch depth per pulse increased sigmoidally from 0.15 μm at 390 mJ/cm^2/pulse to 3.8 μm at 2,200 mJ/cm^2/pulse. The considerable difference in ablation threshold and etch rate between the 193 nm excimer and this mid-IR laser undoubtedly reflects their fundamentally different mechanisms for tissue removal, i.e., photodecomposition and heating, respectively. In contrast to results with the excimer laser, thermal damage in this case was highly dependent on fluence, ranging from 1.5 μm at 600 mJ/cm^2/pulse to 10 μm at 2,200 mJ/cm^2/pulse, better than achieved with the HF laser but still inferior to the 0.3 μm zone of damage surrounding excimer ablations [292]. As with the HF laser, thermal damage surrounding the incisions decreased from top to bottom. It was expected that results at 2.92 μm should have been even better than those at 2.8 μm, and their similarity to those at the shorter wavelength was attributed to large pulse-to-pulse fluence variations at 2.92 μm.

Visible and non-excimer ultraviolet lasers. Another study by the Stern group [376] examined several short-pulsed lasers in the visible portion of the spectrum for production of corneal incisions in enucleated bovine eyes. They demonstrated that ablation threshold energy is proportional to the square root of the pulse duration, going from 2.5 μJ at 100 femtoseconds (fs, 10^{-15} s) with a colliding-pulse-mode-locked ring dye laser, to 500 μJ at 8 ns with a frequency-doubled, Q-switched Nd:YAG laser. Ablation with ns lasers at visible wavelengths proved impractical, as excision morphology and control of ablation depth were poor. Collagen denaturation and disorganization were severe at high energies with both the ps and fs lasers, but 30 ps pulses near the ablation threshold produced almost as little collateral damage as seen with 193 nm excimer excisions, with nearly identical precision of ablation depth. It is important to note that these were single ps pulses and that the mode-locked train common in some commercial ps Nd:YAG lasers would likely have a much higher ablation threshold and thus cause far greater collateral tissue damage. Similar results were achieved with the fs laser, although occasional shock-wave damage raised concerns about potential damage to the endothelium. It was believed that some nonlinear process aside from optical breakdown may account for the increased ablation efficiency of ps and shorter pulses. These researchers concluded that ultrashort-pulsed lasers at visible and near-IR wavelengths may be an alternative to the excimer laser for corneal surgery, but more likely, may offer unique advantages for vitreous surgery (see Vitreous and retina).

Laser thermokeratoplasty. Whereas excimer laser PRK for mild-to-moderate myopia is relatively predictable and successful, that for high myopia and especially hyperopia is less so. Thermokeratoplasty is an old idea that has been recently resurrected for the alteration of corneal curvature without removing any tissue. It was originally proposed as a treatment for keratoconus [377] and despite such early complications as transient refractive results, recurrent erosions, scars, and necrosis, Seiler et al. [378,379] used the pulsed solid-state holmium:YAG laser at 2.06 μm to create intrastromal, cone-shape coagulations to correct hyperopia. Patients reportedly have no complaints of pain with this technique, termed laser thermokeratoplasty, and the epithelium regrows in 24–48 hours. Although still in early clinical trials, at present this is the most widely accepted means of laser therapy for hyperopia [380]. At least one manufacturer currently offers a single unit containing both excimer and holmium lasers (Fig. 20). Holmium laser scleroplasty has been suggested as a means of reducing both axial myopia [381] and postoperative astigmatism [382]. There also has been a report of a micropulsed diode laser being employed to achieve 7 D of steepening in porcine cadaver corneas to whose surfaces ICG had been added [383].

Non-corneal Applications

Eyelids and adnexa. Disorders of the conjunctiva and ocular adnexa are especially well suited to treatment with the CO_2 laser. Clinical applications have included removal of neoplasms near the punctum [384], superficial lid margin tissue in tarsorrhaphy [385], plexiform neurofibromas of the lid and orbit [386], squamous conjunctival papillomas [387], and orbital lymphangiomas [388], and repair of ectropion [389]. In the treatment of nasolacrimal duct obstruction, Gonnering et al. [390] avoided cutaneous scars

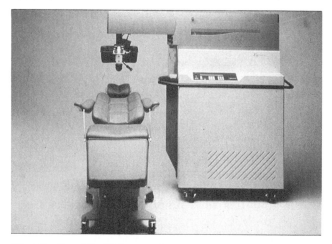

Fig. 20. OmniMed™ laser refractive workstation, combining excimer and holmium:YAG lasers for the correction of myopia and hyperopia, respectively. The manufacturer also offers the emphasis™ Erodible Mask for hyperopia correction using the excimer laser. (Courtesy of Summit Technology, Waltham, MA.)

and minimized recovery time and postoperative pain by performing dacryocystorhinostomies (DCRs) and conjunctivodacryocystorhinostomies with either CO_2 or frequency-doubled Nd:YAG lasers. Mittelman and Apfelberg [391] found no differences in pain, edema, or healing between the CO_2 laser and conventional techniques in blepharoplasty. More recently, Woog and associates [392] employed the holmium:YAG laser to perform endonasal DCRs, achieving excellent intraoperative hemostasis without medial canthal scarring. Long-term ostium patency was 82%. Troutman et al. [393] have suggested excimer or other ablation for precise transconjunctival weakening or strengthening of extraocular muscles.

Crystalline lens. After the cornea, the ocular structure that has attracted the most attention for possible ablation is the crystalline lens. In 1986, Nanevicz et al. [394] published a comprehensive report on parameters for bovine lens ablation using various excimer wavelengths. Using a rate of 20 Hz for 4 minutes and fluences up to 1,280 mJ/cm²/pulse, they found that the ablation thresholds were 110, 265, and 160 mJ/cm²/pulse at 193, 248, and 308 nm, respectively, while no ablation at 351 nm was achieved within the tested fluence range. Once the threshold was surpassed, the greatest ablation rate was observed for 248 nm. Ablation craters were smoothest at 193 nm, whereas those produced with 248 nm radiation showed vacuolation and greater disruption in the surrounding tissue and those at 308 nm were of intermediate smoothness. Absorption coefficients were calculated to be 1360, 410, 122, and 36 cm^{-1} at 193, 248, 308, and 351 nm, respectively. The fact that ablation at 308 nm was only slightly less than that seen at 193 nm, despite the tremendous difference in absorption coefficients, suggested that 308 nm radiation may produce UV-absorbing chromophores, enhancing ablation at that wavelength.

UV absorption by the lens is much more dependent on age than is that of the cornea; indeed, Bath and associates [395] showed that human cataractous lenses have lower ablation thresholds than those reported in normal bovine eyes. One of the main advantages of 308 over 193 nm for lens ablation is the ability of the former to be transmitted via fiber optics and the very high absorption of the latter by chloride ions in saline, which would complicate intraocular applications. However, Keates and his colleagues [396] found that exposure of the eye to 308 nm produces fluorescence that is potentially harmful to the retina and other intraocular structures, whereas absorption at 193 nm by chloride and saline is not sufficiently large to preclude that wavelength's use for photoablative cataract surgery if an appropriate delivery system can be devised.

Studies by Ross and Puliafito [397] and Gailitis et al. [398] showed that the Er:YAG laser may be useful for lens ablation, consistent with its high water absorption coefficient and corresponding short absorption length, although fiber optic technology at that wavelength is also not optimal.

Glaucoma. For any filtering procedure aimed at creating a fistula between the anterior chamber and the episcleral space, precise incision and minimization of trauma and wound healing are of paramount importance if patency is to be maintained. Procedures may be performed either endoscopically or gonioscopically through the anterior chamber (ab interno), or externally with or without conjunctival dissection (ab externo). In 1979, Beckman and Fuller [240] created scleral dissections and filters with the CO_2 laser in patients with neovascular and open and closed angle glaucoma. L'Esperance et al. [399] achieved considerable success in treating patients with neovascular glaucoma by performing CO_2 laser trabeculostomies and sclerotrabeculostomies. More recently, photoablative lasers have been considered as alternatives to the thermal lasers previously examined for sclerostomy [400]. Berlin et al. [401] coupled the 308 nm output of an excimer to

an optical fiber and reported scleral perforation in eye bank specimens using 80–100 pulses at 35 mJ/cm^2/pulse and 20 Hz. Seiler and co-workers [402] identified the juxtacanalicular portion of the trabecular meshwork as the primary site of outflow resistance by using the excimer laser at 193 nm to create partial trabeculectomies; increased aqueous outflow immediately stopped the ablation process. Although this approach obviates entering the anterior chamber, it does require prior episcleral dissection. Allan and associates [403] avoided dissection during 193 nm excimer laser sclerostomy by employing an open mask to plicate the conjunctiva before ablation. They suggested that this technique would avoid the secondary thermal and mechanical damage caused by contact endoscopic systems. An en face air jet to prevent aqueous outflow enabled ablation to continue until sufficiently large fistulas were created. Margolis et al. [404] created filtering blebs in bovine and eye bank sclera with both the Er:YAG (250 µs) and holmium:YAG (300–500 µs) lasers, coupled to optical fibers, without significant disruption of adjacent structures.

Based on preliminary eye bank studies, Eaton et al. [405] suggested that the thulium-holmium-chromium (THC)-doped YAG laser at 2.01 µm (Fig. 21) may be preferable to the holmium, since the former requires fewer pulses and less energy to create sclerostomies, presumably causing less collateral damage. Initial clinical work by Iwach and colleagues [406] with THC:YAG ab externo laser sclerostomy (requiring a total of 1.4–7.2 J) in patients with intractable glaucoma (in whom IOP in the low teens is often desirable) yielded a success rate of 66% at 12 months and 57% at 30 months. McAllister and co-workers [407] obtained similar results and suggested strategies for avoiding the most frequent complication, iris plugging of the sclerostomy. Employing this laser, Namazi et al. [408] found that the anti-metabolites 5-fluorouracil, and especially mitomycin C, significantly increase the duration of laser-created filtration channels.

Vitreous and retina. Although retinal photocoagulation was the first medical use of lasers, practical applications of ablation in the posterior segment have been far more elusive. The CO_2 laser at 10.6 µm has been employed in animals to cut vitreous bands [242] and drain subretinal fluid [409], but it cannot be used close to the retina, is large and inefficient, and requires an articulated arm. Experimental vitreous membranes in rabbits were cut with the excimer laser

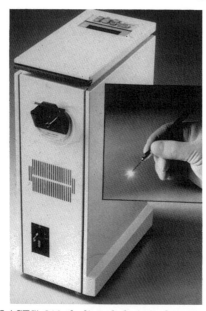

Fig. 21. gLASE™ 210 thulium holmium chromium-yttrium aluminum garnet (THC-YAG) laser, which produces 2.1 μm radiation at 5 Hz, 300 μs pulses, and up to 350 mJ, transmitted via the SUN-LITE™ probe (a 200-μm fiber optic in a casing with outer diameter of 712 μm [22 gauge]). It is currently employed for sclerostomies, but is under early investigation for thermokeratoplasty treatment of hyperopia. (Courtesy of Sunrise Technologies, Fremont, CA.)

at 308 nm [410], but no additional work in this area has been reported. Margolis et al. [411] used a fiber optic-coupled, 250-μs pulsed Er:YAG laser to cut experimental vitreous membranes in rabbits, at distances of 500–3,600 μm from the retina. All attempts at cutting the membranes were successful, although 53% resulted in some form of retinal lesion, either hemorrhages or non-hemorrhagic burns. Nevertheless, the 200–300 μm size of the latter was not considered a contraindication to clinical application of the technique if the membranes occurred in extramacular sites. Lin et al. [412] showed that the Er:YAG output creates a bubble at the tip of the fiber through which it is transmitted, which can cause thermal and mechanical tissue damage. To minimize the size and movement of this bubble and thus the resulting damage to the retina, they suggested reducing the pulse energy below 0.5 mJ and using a shielded tip. These steps may have their own adverse consequences, namely, requiring a higher repetition rate and decreasing some of the advantages of laser ablation over mechanical cutting for removal of membranes tightly adherent to the retinal surface, respectively; investigation of these issues is

ongoing. Use of pulses in the ps domain just above the ablation threshold may significantly reduce untoward thermal and mechanical effects, allowing safe cutting very near the retina. Indeed, another group led by Lin [413] showed that 100-ps Nd:YAG laser pulses achieved optical breakdown in vitreous with only 70 μJ of energy, almost two orders of magnitude less than that used in ns Nd:YAG lasers. Efficient cutting with the ps laser occurred at pulse rates of 50–200 Hz.

Borirakchanyavat et al. [414] attempted transection of experimental vitreous membranes using a 250-μs pulsed holmium:YAG laser at 2.12 μm. When an optical fiber was used alone, only thin membranes could be sectioned at energy levels or repetition rates that permitted work near the retina. This problem was solved by encasing the fiber in a retinal-shielding pick, which allowed almost three-quarters of membranes, as close as 0.5 mm to the retina, to be completely transected. The laser directly caused one non-hemorrhagic retinal burn, whereas the pick caused two retinal injuries, including one with a small hemorrhage. Cutting precision was histologically comparable to that of the CO_2 laser, but an order of magnitude less than that of the Er:YAG laser [411]. One technical advantage of holmium:YAG radiation is that it is much more easily transmitted by existing fiber optics.

Selective RPE damage has been reported with the Q-switched Nd:YAG [415] and micropulsed diode [416] and argon [417] lasers. A significant impediment to the intraocular use of 193 nm excimer laser radiation is the technical difficulty in transmitting it with the necessary accuracy. Lewis and co-workers [418] constructed a guide consisting of a fused silica lens of 1,000 mm focal length and a rapidly tapered stainless steel tube whose outer diameter was that of an 18-gauge needle, with an inner diameter of 120 μm. They used this instrument to ablate bovine cadaver retinas and rabbit retinas in vivo following lensectomy and vitrectomy, employing pulses of 0.5–1.2 J/cm^2 and 120 μm, at 30–100 Hz. Once a low pressure stream of air was used to displace the thin layer of adherent fluid from the area to be treated, they were able to achieve retinal ablation with the precision typically associated with the cornea. Possible applications include ablation of epiretinal membranes—as even a slight amount of underlying fluid would protect the retina—and the creation of precise retinal incisions.

DIAGNOSTIC LASERS

Scanning laser ophthalmoscope

As first described by Webb and colleagues [419,420], the scanning laser ophthalmoscope (SLO) produces video images of the retina. A low-power laser beam is scanned horizontally and vertically across the retina, creating a raster pattern that is used to map the retina or take highly localized measurements. The SLO also has excellent depth resolution and can produce tomographic images [421]. This is particularly valuable in creating three-dimensional images of the optic disc [422], since increased cupping is a frequent antecedent of visual field loss in glaucoma. Edema, scars, and macular holes are among other retinal conditions that have been assessed with this technique [423,424].

SLO image contrast can be further enhanced by employing confocal optics [425]. Figure 22a shows a confocal SLO specifically designed to analyze the RNFL. It uses a polarization detector to produce a thickness map of the RNFL, to document and follow glaucomatous changes. Normal RNFLs have a symmetric, hourglass-shape distribution, which is gradually eroded as glaucoma progresses (Fig. 22b). The thickness of the form birefringent RNFL determines the degree to which the low-power diode laser beam is polarized [426]. This device obtains readings in less than 1 s, does not require pupil dilation, may be used in patients with cataracts, and avoids the flashes associated with conventional fundus photography. Since the RNFL ordinarily does not exceed 150 μm in thickness, yet the optical depth resolution of the human eye is ~ 200 μm, the potential advantage of this method, with its resolution of 15–20 μm, over standard photographic techniques is apparent [427].

Figure 23 shows how a tomographic SLO is employed to perform topographic analysis of the retina. This device, which relies on specular reflection of laser light from the retina's internal limiting membrane, can be used to determine optic nerve head volume [428] and map the macula and tumors. It assesses contour, in contrast to the instrument described above, which measures thickness.

Visual evoked potentials can be measured more precisely with the SLO [429]. Visual function testing is performed by varying the SLO laser beam intensity to create patterns in the raster. The examiner sees the same pattern, localized to a specific portion of the retina, that the patient

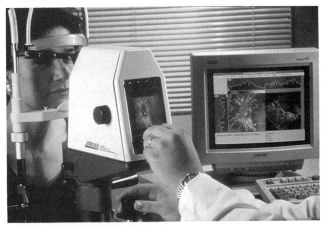

A

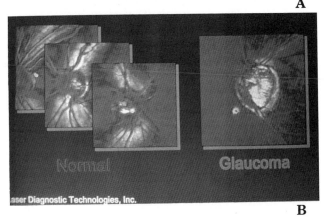

B

Fig. 22. **A.** Instrument head of the Nerve Fiber Layer Analyzer™. An integrated monitor allows the physician to simultaneously view the retina and maintain eye contact with the patient. **B.** At left are nerve fiber layer thickness maps of three normal eyes, with thick superior and inferior arcuate bundles. At right is a map of a glaucomatous eye, with thinning superior arcuate bundle and absent inferior arcuate bundle. (Courtesy of Laser Diagnostic Technologies, San Diego, CA.)

perceives, allowing the locus of fixation to be correlated with retinal pathology [430]. Angiography is another process that has been aided by the SLO. Less fluorescein than is required with conventional angiography is excited by an argon blue laser, yielding more and higher resolution images [431]. A method for stereoscopic video angiography has been described [432]. The SLO has been particularly important for ICG angiography (see Dye enhancement), in which the low fluorescence dye is excited by a diode laser to more precisely delineate SRNV membranes [433,434]. An alternative technique—combining slit-lamp and He-Ne 543 nm laser illumination—has been described to enhance visualization of fine vitreoretinal structures [435].

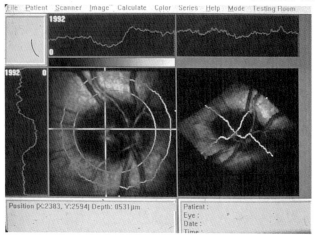

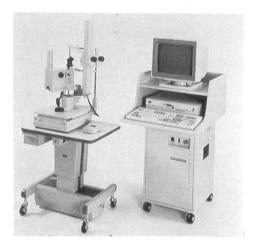

Fig. 23. Display screen of the Topographic Scanning System TopSS™. At left is an intensity image of an optic nerve head. Above and to the left of this image are horizontal and vertical cross sections, respectively, through the optic nerve head. To the right is a three-dimensional view of the same optic nerve head. The viewing angle can be adjusted by the physician. A peripapillary retinal contour of nerve fiber layer height along the circle superimposed around the optic nerve head is displayed in the screen's upper righthand corner. (Courtesy of Laser Diagnostic Technologies, San Diego, CA.)

Fig. 24. Kowa FC-1000 laser flare cell meter, showing slit-lamp-based system and computer. (Courtesy of Kowa Acculas, San Jose, CA.)

Laser flare and cell meter

Anterior segment inflammation, which may result from numerous types of intraocular pathology, causes breakdown of the blood-aqueous barrier and is manifested by increases in aqueous protein and cells. Fluorophotometry was the first method to quantify this process objectively but is relatively time-consuming and requires intravenous injection of dye [436,437]. In 1988, Sawa et al. [438] reported the development of a slit-lamp-based instrument that employs a low-power He-Ne or diode laser to detect the amount of protein—to which flare, produced by the Tyndall phenomenon, is linearly related over a wide range of protein concentrations—and the number of cells in the anterior chamber (Laser Flare Cell Meter [LFCM], Kowa Acculas, San Jose, CA) (Fig. 24). Flare measurements are corrected for background scatter, are reproducible to within some 8% [439], and take less than 1 s [440]. These readings may be converted directly to protein concentration if the latter's type is known, but not in cases of heterogeneous scatterers such as low-molecular weight albumin and high-molecular weight globulins. Studies have shown that flare has a diurnal variation [441] and tends to increase with age [442]. The LFCM has been used clinically to examine inflammation associated with uveitis of various etiologies [443], retinal detachment [444], cataract removal and IOL insertion [445], posterior capsulotomy [446], and LTP [447]. Cytomegalovirus (CMV) retinitis is a frequent complication in AIDS patients, and this instrument's ability to detect slight increases in aqueous flare before any retinal changes are visible allows earlier institution of treatment [448].

To count cells, the laser beam is repeatedly scanned over a 0.075 mm^3 volume, with peaks further analyzed so that only white blood cells are registered. Cell count is less reproducible than flare measurements, especially with relatively few particles, whereas a spurious cell count in the clinical absence of cells may be caused by agglutination of proteins in very high concentrations [449]. There is also less correlation with direct slit-lamp measurements, which are made over larger volumes and longer periods, so that the clinical value of this application is less certain than that for flare.

Laser Interferometer

The interference pattern produced with the laser interferometer is largely independent of the eye's various optical components. It offers the potential to assess visual acuity by projecting the pattern onto the retina and determining the greatest periodicity (corresponding to the closest fringe spacing) at which the subject is able to resolve discrete fringes [450]. To be of much practical value, the examiner must know the periodicity, which is estimated by using standard values for the refractive indices of the cornea and lens, and ultrasound to measure the eye's axial length. The laser interferometer has been used to determine potential visual acuity in patients undergoing cataract extraction [451], and therapy for amblyopia [452], and uveitis [453], especially in the presence of concomitant retinal or neurologic pathology. Laser interferometry has generally been found to be more accurate than previous techniques [454], although this may not be the case in the presence of maculopathy [455]. Although it has been suggested that this instrument may be employed even in the presence of dense cataracts or turbid media, these factors necessarily diminish the fringe pattern contrast. To avoid underestimating postoperative visual acuity, correction for any significant optical obstruction is necessary [456].

Recently, laser interferometric techniques have been described for precise depth measurements of the cornea, retina, and other ocular structures. Both Fabry Perot and Michelson systems have been developed and offer the promise of highly accurate one- and two-dimensional measurements [457–472].

Use of the laser Doppler principle allows considerably faster readings than are achievable by interpretation of static interferometric images. Selection of IOL refractive power is based largely on the eye's axial length, which the non-contact laser interferometric approach may determine more precisely and safely than the standard ultrasound method [473]. Although patient fixation is required with the laser, further technical enhancements should reduce scan time to under 1 s. The potential use of such systems in excimer laser surgery is described below.

Optical coherence tomography. A group of researchers from Tufts University and M.I.T. has developed a new technique for in vitro and in vivo imaging of ocular tissue employing an interferometer. Known as optical coherence tomography (OCT) [459–471] it is a two-dimensional extension of laser interferometric ranging techniques, which produces high-resolution, cross-sectional images of the eye [460,462]. OCT is similar to ultrasound B-mode imaging except that the use of light rather than sound allows much higher image resolution with a non-invasive and non-contact measurement. Distance information is extracted from the time-of-flight delay of light reflected from different structures within the eye using low-coherence interferometry. With this technique, interference fringes appear at a detector only when the path length of light reflected

from the eye matches a reference path length to within the coherence length of the light source. A short coherence-length superluminscent diode light source enables a longitudinal resolution of ~ 10 μm. The transverse resolution is determined by the probe beam spot size on the retina and can be made as small as a few μm. Optical heterodyne detection and the application of noise reduction techniques originally developed for optical communication achieve a high sensitivity to weakly reflected light.

The high resolution and sensitivity of OCT make it uniquely suited among existing ophthalmic imaging techniques for clinically relevant tomography of the human retina [466]. The available numerical aperture and ocular aberration limit the resolution at the retina of scanning confocal imaging devices, whereas acoustic attenuation makes the posterior segment unreachable by high frequency ultrasound. Figure 25 shows a false-color OCT tomograph obtained through the macula and optic disc of a human volunteer. Bright and dim colors correspond in the image to regions of high and low relative optical reflectivity, respectively. The cross-sectional anatomy of the fovea and disc are evident as is the layered structure of the retina. The posterior retina is bounded by a red layer corresponding to the choriocapillaris and retinal pigment epithelium. Significantly reduced reflectivity from the photoreceptors is observed just anterior to this layer. The retinal nerve fibers are visible as a brightly backscattering layer that increases in thickness toward the optic disc. OCT shows significant promise for the quantitative evaluation and monitoring of a variety of diseases of the macula and optic nerve head. Initial clinical studies [467–470] have shown that OCT is useful in staging macular holes, evaluating vitreous detachments and traction of the vitreous on the retina, quantifying retinal thickness in macular edema, monitoring detachments of the neurosensory retina and retinal pigment epithelium, and in measuring retinal nerve fiber layer degeneration in glaucoma. As an example, Figure 26 depicts an OCT image of a neurosensory retinal detachment taken in a patient with the diagnosis of central serous chorioretinopathy.

OCT also represents a new imaging modality for examination of the anterior eye [471]. The μm scale resolution permits accurate biometry of large-scale ocular structures as well as the evaluation of changes in cellular morphology associated with pathologies of the cornea, iris, and lens.

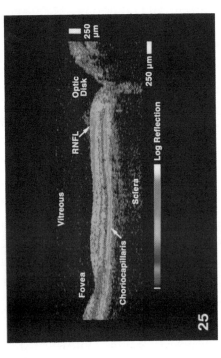

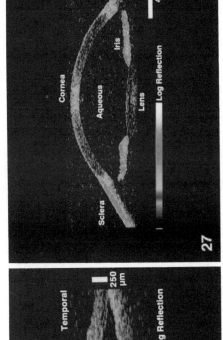

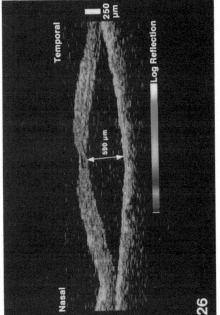

Fig. 25. False-color OCT tomograph obtained through the macula and optic disk of a human eye. See insert for color representation.

Fig. 26. OCT image of a neurosensory retinal detachment in a patient with a diagnosis of central serous chorioretinopathy. See insert for color representation.

Fig. 27. OCT image of the anterior human eye. See insert for color representation.

An OCT image of the anterior eye of a human volunteer appears in Figure 27. Reflected signals are evident within both nominally transparent structures such as the cornea and lens and throughout opaque ones such as the iris and sclera. Clinically relevant measurements may be directly extracted from the image, including anterior chamber depth and angle, corneal thickness and curvature, and refractive power.

Laser Doppler Velocimeter

The laser Doppler velocimeter (LDV) [474] was developed over 20 years ago but is probably the least common type of ophthalmic diagnostic laser; it has been used almost exclusively for research purposes. It typically combines a low-power He-Ne or diode laser with a fundus camera or slit-lamp biomicroscope, permitting simultaneous viewing and projection of an approximately 100-μm-diameter laser spot onto the desired vessel. Light of frequency v is scattered by red blood cells, and autodyne optical mixing spectroscopy is employed to measure the resulting frequency shift of Δv relative to the light scattered from the wall of the vessel containing the cells. Since there is a range of cell velocities, the LDV produces a spectrum indicating how many cells are moving at each velocity. This method measures only relative velocity, but absolute velocity can be determined by adding a second detector [475]. Readings can be taken in patients with poor fixation or those who require particularly long study by using rapid calculation algorithms or techniques to compensate for eye movement [476]. The LDV has shown normal retinal blood flow to be ~ 80 μl/min, which increases with anti-glaucoma medication [471], hyperglycemia [478], and transition from dark-adaptation to light [479], and decreases after treatment with insulin [480], in cases of optic atrophy [481], and in PDR [482].

FUTURE DEVELOPMENTS

The diode laser is revolutionary more for economic and ergonomic reasons than because it provides some fundamentally new laser-tissue interaction. Aided by advances in endoprobes and indirect ophthalmoscopy, it is already being used to treat a variety of vascular diseases and may become the treatment of choice for ROP. Its low cost and easy portability will permit treatment in remote areas, including many third world nations. Just as GaAlAs diode technology has improved in the past several years so that sufficient power is now available for many applications, the future holds the promise that with new materials, useful diode output will be achieved at visible wavelengths, perhaps supplanting the much bulkier and less efficient argon, krypton, and dye lasers. At present, diodes are beginning to replace flashlamps and other lasers as pumping sources for visible wavelengths [483]. If sufficient energy can be generated by Q-switched diode lasers, they might be used in place of Nd:YAG lasers for photodisruption. Lesion variability—with the diode or other lasers—is unavoidable, but early work with a dynamic confocal reflectometer offers the possibility of reproducible retinal photocoagulation independent of pigmentation, media opacities, or optical aberrations [484,485].

As phase III clinical trials proceed at numerous academic centers, excimer laser ablation algorithms are still being refined. Recent work suggests that aspheric PRK may yield better optical homogeneity than the standard spherical approach [486] (perhaps by minimizing the refractive transition zone at the ablation periphery) and that a series of several concentric ablations may allow shallower tissue removal to achieve greater corrections, similar to a Fresnel lens [487].

Erodible masks have been proposed as an alternative to the usual apertures or diaphragms, theoretically permitting correction of myopia, hyperopia, and astigmatism (including irregular forms), but initial animal work in this area has been successful primarily for myopia [488]. The unqualified success of PTK notwithstanding, the widespread acceptance and use of the excimer laser will likely depend on the successful correction of refractive errors. Individual variation in wound healing may be an insurmountable biologic reality, but overall control of wound healing appears necessary for maintenance of optimal refractive and visual results. Studies of corticosteroids and the anti-metabolite mitomycin C, [489,490] suggest that the former is more successful in safely modifying the results of PRK. Lohmann and associates [491] found that tear plasmin levels increase after ablation, so that inhibitors of plasmin and plasminogen activator, perhaps in conjunction with steroids, might be used to modify post-laser healing. Moreover, individuals with initially high plasmin levels experienced more regression and may not be candidates for PRK in its current form. Topical interferon-alpha 2b, alone or as an adjunct to steroid therapy, has also been identified as a potential agent in minimizing corneal haze [492], as have antioxidants [493] and inhibitors of glycosaminoglycan formation [494]. The topical NSAID diclofenac has been shown to significantly reduce pain in the 2–3 days following ablation [495].

It is also necessary to determine whether, if regression cannot be entirely controlled, repeat ablation is possible, as this is not allowed under current FDA investigational guidelines. Studies of patients undergoing repeat PRK because of initial undercorrection, scarring, or regression indicate that the additional laser treatment is successful [496,497], as is PRK following undercorrection with radial keratotomy [498]. Thompson et al. [499] proposed circumventing variable corneal wound healing following PRK by performing excimer laser ablation of (as yet unidentified) acellular synthetic epikeratoplasty lenticules, which would be attached to the cornea in a technique termed "laser adjustable synthetic epikeratoplasty" (LASE).

Even if standard excimer laser PRK proves unreliable for treatment of high myopia, this laser may still be employed for room temperature keratomileusis, preserving Bowman's membrane and permitting ablation based on the visual center even if such does not correspond to the center of the lenticule (a luxury not now afforded by the cryolathe). This could be done on the posterior stromal surface of the lenticule, or on the anterior surface of the exposed stromal bed, the latter termed "laser in situ keratomileusis (LASIK)" [500].

Correction of hyperopia needs to be more carefully studied, since although it is theoretically similar to that of myopia, in practice epithelium or stroma has tended to fill in the ablated annulus, negating the refractive effects. If it proves feasible, PRK for hyperopia might be combined with either conventional or laser cataract surgery. Various ablation strategies have been proposed [501], with at least one attempted—with moderate success at 3-month follow-up—on blind eyes in a phase I FDA study [502].

Clinical experience is insufficient to discount all potential side effects, but results to date are encouraging. There may be an early decrease in contrast sensitivity following PRK, but this has been found to resolve within a year of surgery [503]. There is also debate within the medical community about whether excimer laser ablation constitutes surgery, and some optometrists have been lobbying for the right to use the technique.

Whereas there are many engineering and treatment nuances among the major ophthalmic

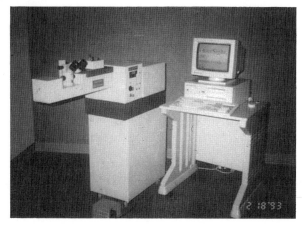

Fig. 28. Compak-200 "mini-excimer," (Courtesy of Laser-Sight, Orlando, FL.)

excimer lasers, the systems are much more alike than not. Significant technical hurdles had to be overcome before the excimer laser was ever used clinically, but recent enhancements and modifications have largely been variations on the same theme. Different strategies are continually being studied to optimize refractive outcome and minimize healing complications. A significant improvement would be the addition of real-time eye-tracking [504] and tissue depth monitoring; possible approaches to the latter include fs laser optical ranging [505] and optical coherence domain reflectometry [459,464]. However, clinical considerations aside, the excimer's considerable size, cost, and energy requirements represent significant impediments to its widespread use. There is also concern about exposure to fluorine gas. LaserSight (Orlando, FL) has introduced the "mini-excimer" (Fig. 28), which at some 70 kg weighs much less than conventional ophthalmic excimer lasers. It operates from a 110 V outlet, is air-cooled, and uses an excimer gas mixture containing only 0.19% fluorine. Since this device can generate sufficient fluences for ablation over spot sizes only 1.0–1.5 mm in diameter, it utilizes a computer-controlled scanning system to treat the cornea. Preliminary clinical trials for correction of myopia were conducted in China in early 1993, reportedly with good results, with phase I FDA studies scheduled for later. Studies on hyperopia correction are also planned.

Work on laser modification of corneal curvature is proceeding so rapidly that even before the excimer laser has received FDA approval, potential replacements are being studied. Early worries about possible mutagenesis appear to have subsided (except for radiation of ~ 248 nm, which has not been used clinically), and despite the achievement of IR laser ablation, researchers have not been able to duplicate the precision of the argon fluoride excimer laser. As such, several investigators are studying solid-state UV alternatives to the excimer. Researchers from the Bascom Palmer Eye Institute are collaborating with LaserSight on the use of the Nd:YAG fifth harmonic at 213 nm (achieved with a combination of cesium-dihydrogen-arsenate and barium borate crystals) [506], 250 mJ/cm^2, 10 ns, and 10 Hz for possible ablation [507]. Since sufficient energy for ablation can be achieved only with a small spot size, tissue removal is effected by scanning a 0.5–1.0 mm quasi-Gaussian beam across the cornea in a precise pattern to achieve the desired profile [508]. Although technically difficult, such scanning may permit more gradual and customized ablations. Preliminary results in cadaver and rabbit eyes revealed ablations comparable to those of the argon fluoride excimer laser, with damage areas < 1 μm wide, no step-like transition zones, and mild residual subepithelial haze at 3 months, but with poor correlation between intended and achieved refractive changes [509,510]. Although commercial availability is at least several years away, another goal of this group is the development of a laser capable of generating several harmonics at various pulse durations, potentially also permitting photocoagulation and photodisruption [511]. Researchers at Tufts University and Schwartz Electro-Optics (Concord, MA) are investigating ablation with the titanium-sapphire laser, using barium borate crystals to frequency-quadruple its 10 ns, 10 Hz output to 205–225 nm [512]. Although it is very inefficient, the free electron laser is capable of generating a wide range of IR wavelengths and allows independent variation of wavelength, energy, and pulse duration. Very preliminary studies achieved corneal ablation [513,514], including central steepening for hyperopia correction [515], but it remains to be seen whether this is preferable to any of the solid-state IR lasers.

Studies have shown the importance of the epithelium in moderating repair and reducing corneal haze and reversal of refractive changes following excimer ablation [323]. Although in conjunction with steroids or anti-metabolites the cornea appears to heal with little or no residual scarring, the long-term implications of this procedure remain to be determined. Some researchers have thus proposed selective intrastromal ablation without damage to the anterior layers as an alternative to excimer laser anterior ablation [393], although the best such laser remains to be determined.

Zysset et al. [516] provided early guidance for intrastromal ablation by demonstrating that for suprathreshold Nd:YAG laser corneal lesions, the damage zone radius is proportional to the cube root of the pulse energy. Although ps and ns pulses of equal energy cause approximately the same damage, since the former tend to be on the order of μJ and the latter on the order of mJ, in practice the use of low energy ps pulses can significantly reduce collateral tissue damage. In contrast to ns exposures, ps ones were not associated with significant shock wave propagation or cavitation bubble expansion in the primary interaction zone. However, given the low energy of individual ps pulses, they concluded that in order to achieve effective cutting or ablation, it would be necessary to employ many such exposures at moderate-to-high repetition rates.

At least two companies now produce short-pulsed lasers capable of intrastromal ablation and other applications. The Phoenix Model 2500 Ophthalmic Laser Workstation (Phoenix Laser Systems, Fremont, CA) employs a frequency-doubled, 532 nm Nd:YAG laser with 8 ns, 40–350 μJ pulses. It has a nominal spot size of 5 μm, with three-dimensional accuracy consistent with a 15–20 μm treatment area, and incorporates an eye-tracking system to eliminate effects of even subtle movements. Early attempts at intrastromal ablation (which the company terms "transepithelial stromal keratectomy") with this laser in enucleated cat eyes yielded vacuoles 30–80 μm in diameter, surrounded by compressed collagen anteriorly and edematous collagen posteriorly, without significant endothelial damage (Fig. 29) [517,518]. The vacuoles collapse as the fluid inside is absorbed, thereby altering corneal curvature. Work is ongoing to determine the ablation scanning patterns necessary for correction of various types of refractive error. The only procedure for which the laser has already been approved is posterior capsulotomy, but other applications in various stages of investigation, for which the laser's precision may provide unique advantages, include nuclear photofragmentation (see below), sclerostomy, PTK, radial keratotomy, iridectomy, and focal retinal ablation.

The Nd:YLF (yttrium lithium fluoride) Eye Laser System™ (Intelligent Surgical Lasers, San Diego, CA) produces 1,053 nm pulses of energy

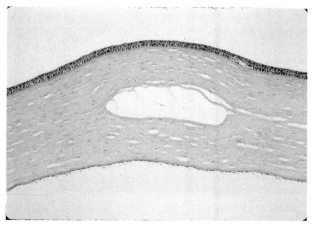

Fig. 29. Histologic view following intrastromal ablation of a porcine cornea with the Phoenix Model 2500 Ophthalmic Laser Workstation. (Courtesy of Phoenix Laser Systems, Fremont, CA.)

20–350 μJ, spot size ≤7 μm, duration ≤60 ps, and repetition rate 10–1,000 Hz. It consists of a stable, mode-locked oscillator laser operating at 80 MHz whose output is a continuous train of 1 nJ pulses, which a high-gain, Q-switched regenerative amplifier then converts to 1 mJ pulses [519]. Nd:YLF has a larger fluorescence bandwidth than Nd:YAG, which allows pulses of shorter duration to be generated. Using an earlier ISL model, Frueh and colleagues [520] created intrastromal transverse excisions in rabbit corneas, which initially induced ~ 5 D of flattening, without intrastromal scarring. Steroids were not employed and the changes regressed by 6 weeks. Remmel et al. [521] demonstrated that a continuous layer of stroma could be removed in human cadaver eyes. Also using this system in human cadaver eyes, at 80–140 μJ, 50 ps, and 1 kHz, Niemz et al. [522] scanned the laser beam in a spiral pattern to create intrastromal vacuoles some 40 μm in diameter and 20 μm deep, 100 μm below Bowman's membrane, without damaging it or the epithelium. It has also been demonstrated that this process causes no acute endothelial damage [523]. However, Brown and associates [524] found that ablation depth in human and rabbit cadaver corneas was related to energy but not to programmed depth. Collagen disorganization ranged from 3–8 μm with 100 μJ pulses, and 10–20 μm at 300 μJ. The ablation effect varied with the beam path direction and plasma threshold changes within the cornea. Moreover, there was ablation of tissue anterior to the desired target, lamellar separation by plasma/gas formation without ablation, and inconsistent ablation, indi-

cating the need for further studies and refinement of this technique. The Nd:YLF laser has also been used to create sclerectomies in human cadaver eyes [525], sclerostomies in rabbits [526], and iridotomies in patients [527], all with a high degree of precision. As of mid-1993 the ISL laser had received FDA clearance only for posterior capsulotomy, but was in phase I trials for vitreolysis and phase II for cataract fragmentation. There was an open iridotomy study while investigational device exemptions were filed for intrastromal ablation and internal and external sclerostomy.

Taboada and associates [528] described a technique they termed "intrastromal photokeratectomy," in which Q-switched Nd:YAG laser pulses at 100 ns and 500–2,000 Hz were applied to the cornea via a contact probe. This resulted in vacuoles ~ 100 μm in diameter, localizable within 20 μm, and with a transition zone between normal tissue of 0.5 μm. The track of vacuoles, which can be created in radial, wide area, or other patterns, optically disappeared within 2 days, as treated tissue dissolved into a diffusive liquid, yet the refractive effects in the rabbit and monkey eyes persisted for the 5-month duration of the study. There was no immediate or long-term damage to either the epithelium or endothelium. It remains to be seen whether intrastromal ablation with any laser can approach the precision of the excimer and whether Descemet's membrane is not more likely to push forward than Bowman's membrane backward, but potential advantages include increased patient comfort and no need to patch or instill antibiotics, due to retention of the epithelium, as well as lower cost and avoidance of any UV radiation.

Novatec Laser Systems (San Diego, CA) indicates that its LightBlade™ laser is capable of corneal surface, intrastromal, and intraocular ablation, and includes an eye-tracking system, but clinical trials of the as-yet-unspecified "deep UV solid-state" device have yet to begin.

Whereas laser removal of primary cataracts remains a popular misconception, reality may be catching up with myth. Photophacofragmentation is the process of employing pulsed laser energy to soften a cataractous lens, to facilitate aspiration at the time of surgery; studies employing the Nd:YAG laser have been reported [529,530]. It has been shown that the threshold for excimer laser ablation of the lens capsule is significantly higher than that for the nucleus and cortex [531]. This raises the possibility of ablation, such as with the excimer, or the Nd:YLF, the frequency-doubled Nd:YAG, or some other very-short-pulsed laser, through a tiny opening in the anterior capsule, via an anterior or pars plana approach. This could preserve the zonules and potentially allow the use of injectable polymers to reconstitute the lens following aspiration of the ablated remnants, perhaps even restoring accommodation [532].

REFERENCES

1. Maiman TH. Stimulated optical radiation in ruby. Nature 1960; 187:493–497.
2. Longsworth JW. Photophysics. In Regan JD, Parrish JA, eds. "The Science of Photomedicine." New York: Plenum, 1982, p 43.
3. Meyer-Schwickerath G. Koagulation der Netzhaut mit Sonnenlicht. Ber Deutsch Ophth Gesellsch 1949; 55:256–259.
4. Blankenship GW. Fifteen-year argon laser and xenon photocoagulation results of Bascom Palmer Eye Institute's patients participating in the diabetic retinopathy study. Ophthalmology 1991; 98:125–128.
5. Beetham WP, Aiello LM, Balodimos MC, et al. Ruby laser photocoagulation of early diabetic neovascular retinopathy. Arch Ophthalmol 1970; 83:261–272.
6. L'Esperance FA. An ophthalmic argon laser photocoagulation system: Design, construction, and laboratory investigations. Trans Am Ophthalmol Soc 1968; 66:827–904.
7. Mellerio J. The thermal nature of retinal laser photocoagulation. Exp Eye Res 1966; 5;242–248.
8. Clarke AM, Geeraets WJ, Ham WT. An equilibrium thermal model for retinal injury from optical sources. Applied Optics 1969; 8:1051–1054.
9. Mainster MA, White TJ, Allen RG. Spectral dependence of retinal damage produced by intense light sources. J Opt Soc Am 1970; 60:848–855.
10. Roulier A. Calculation of the thermal effect generated in the retina by photocoagulation. Graefe's Arch Clin Exp Ophthalmol 1971; 181:281–289.
11. Birngruber R, Hillenkamp F, Gabel VP. Theoretical investigations of laser thermal retinal injury. Health Phys 1985; 48:781.
12. Birngruber R. Thermal modeling in biologic tissues. In Hillenkamp F, Pratesi R, Sacchi CA, Eds. "Lasers in Biology and Medicine." New York: Plenum, 1980, pp 77–97.
13. Hillenkamp F. Interaction between radiation and biological systems. In Hillenkamp F, Pratesi R, Sacchi CA, eds. "Lasers in Biology and Medicine." New York: Plenum, 1980, pp 37–68.
14. Mainster MA. Wavelength selection in macular photocoagulation: tissue optics, thermal effects, and laser systems. Ophthalmology 1986; 93:952–958.
15. Lapanje S. "Physicochemical Aspects of Protein Denaturation." New York: Wiley & Sons, 1978.
16. Trempe CL, Mainster MA, Pomerantzeff O, et al.: Macular photocoagulation: Optimal wavelength selection. Ophthalmology 1982; 89:721–728.
17. Swartz M. Histology of macular photocoagulation. Ophthalmology 1986; 93:959–963.
18. Boergen K-P, Birngruber R, Hillenkamp F. Laser-induced endovascular thrombosis as a possibility of selective vessel closure. Ophthalmic Res 1981; 13:139–150.
19. Apple DJ, Wyhinny GJ, Goldberg MF, et al.: Experimental argon laser photocoagulation. I. effects of retinal nerve fiber layer. Arch Ophthalmol 1976; 94:137–144.
20. Marshall J, Bird AC. A comparative histopathological study of argon and krypton laser irradiations of the human retina. Br J Ophthalmol 1979; 63:657–668.
21. Arden GB, Berninger T, Hogg CR, et al.: A survey of color discrimination in German ophthalmologists: Changes associated with the use of lasers and operating microscopes. Ophthalmology 1991; 98:567–575.
22. Peyman GA, Raichand M, Zeimer RC. Ocular effects of various laser wavelengths. Surv Ophthalmol 1984; 28:391–404.
23. Peyman GA, Conway MD, House B. Transpupillary CW YAG laser coagulation: A comparison with argon green and krypton red lasers. Ophthalmology 1983; 90:992–1002.
24. Peyman GA, Larson B. Effects of the CW YAG laser on the human iris and retina. Ophthalmology 1984; 91:1034–1039.
25. Fankhauser F. The Q-switched laser: principles and clinical results. In Trokel S, ed. "YAG Laser Ophthalmic Microsurgery." Norwalk, CT: Appleton-Century-Crofts, 1983, pp 128–131.
26. Van der Zypen E, Fankhauser F, Loertscher HP. Retinal and choroidal repair following low power argon and Nd:YAG laser irradiation. Doc Ophthalmol Proc Ser 1984; 36:61–70.
27. L'Esperance FA. Trans-spectral organic dye laser photocoagulation. Trans Am Ophthalmol Soc 1985; 83:82–111.
28. Halldórsson T, Langerholc J, Senatori L. Thermal action of laser irradiation in biological material monitored by egg-white coagulation. Applied Optics 1981; 20:822–825.
29. Romanelli JF, Puliafito CA. Metabolic studies of dye laser retinal photocoagulation. Int Ophthalmol Clin 1990; 30:95–101.
30. Puliafito CA, Deutsch TF, Boll J, et al. Semiconductor laser endophotocoagulation of the retina. Arch Ophthalmol 1987; 105:424–427.
31. Brancato R, Pratesi R. Applications of diode lasers in ophthalmology. Lasers Ophthalmol 1987; 1:119–129.
32. Smiddy WE, Hernandez E. Histopathologic results of retinal diode laser photocoagulation in rabbit eyes. Arch Ophthalmol 1992; 110:693–698.
33. Brancato R, Pratesi R, Leoni G, et al. Retinal photocoagulation with diode laser operating from a slit lamp microscope. Lasers Light Ophthalmol 1988; 2:73–78.
34. Brancato R, Pratesi R, Leoni G, et al. Semiconductor diode laser photocoagulation of human malignant melanoma. Am J Ophthalmol 1989; 107:295–296.
35. Brancato R, Pratesi R, Leoni G, et al. Histopathology of diode and argon laser lesions in rabbit retina: a comparative study. Invest Ophthalmol Vis Sci 1989; 30:1504–1510.
36. McHugh JDA, Marshall J, Capon M, et al. Transpupillary photocoagulation in the eyes of rabbit and human using a diode laser. Lasers Light Ophthalmol 1988; 2:125–143.
37. Wallow IHL, Sponsel WE, Stevens TS. Clinicopathologic

correlation of diode laser burns in monkeys. Arch Ophthalmol 1991; 109:648–653.

38. Jennings T, Fuller T, Vukich JA, et al. Transscleral contact retinal photocoagulation with an 810-nm semiconductor diode laser. Ophthalmic Surg 1990; 21:492–496.

39. Fankhauser F, Kwasniewska S, Henchoz P-D, et al. Versatility of the cw-Nd:YAG and diode lasers in ocular surgery. Ophthalmic Surg 1993; 24:225–231.

40. Trokel S, Wapner F, Schubert H. Contact transscleral retinal photocoagulation using a micropulsed diode laser. Invest Ophthalmol Vis Sci 1992; 33(Suppl):1311.

41. Lim JI, Bressler NM, Marsh MJ, et al. Laser treatment of choroidal neovascularization in patients with angioid streaks. Am J Ophthalmol 1993; 116:414–423.

42. Macular Photocoagulation Study Group. Krypton laser photocoagulation for neovascular lesions of ocular histoplasmosis: Results of a randomized clinical trial. Arch Ophthalmol 1987; 105:1499–1507.

43. The Diabetic Retinopathy Study Research Group. Photocoagulation treatment of proliferative diabetic retinopathy: Clinical application of Diabetic Retinopathy Study (DRS) findings. DRS report number 8. Ophthalmology 1981; 88:583–600.

44. Early Treatment Diabetic Retinopathy Study Group: Results from the early treatment diabetic retinopathy study. Ophthalmology 1991; 98 (Suppl 5):739–840.

45. The Krypton Argon Regression Neovascularization Study Research Group. Randomized comparison of krypton versus argon scatter photocoagulation for diabetic disc neovascularization: The krypton argon regression neovascularization study report number 1. Ophthalmology 1993; 100:1655–1664.

46. Wolbarsht ML, Landers MB. The rationale of photocoagulation therapy for proliferative diabetic retinopathy: A review and a model. Ophthalmic Surg 1980; 11:235–245.

47. Weiter JJ, Zuckerman R. The influence of the photoreceptor-RPE complex on the inner retina: An explanation for the beneficial effects of photocoagulation. Ophthalmology 1980; 87:1133–1139.

48. Glaser BM, Campochiaro PA, Davis JL. Retinal pigment epithelial cells release an inhibitor of neovascularization. Arch Ophthalmol 1985; 103:1870–1875.

49. Singerman LJ. Red krypton laser therapy of macular and retinal vascular diseases. Retina 1982; 2:15–28.

50. Liang JC, Goldberg MF. Treatment of diabetic retinopathy. Diabetes 1980; 29:841–851.

51. Prendiville PL, McDonnell PJ. Complications of laser surgery. Int Ophthalmol Clin 1992; 32:179–204.

52. Early Treatment Diabetic Retinopathy Study Research Group: Photocoagulation for diabetic macular edema: Early treatment diabetic retinopathy study report number 1. Arch Ophthalmol 1985; 103:1796–1806.

53. Wilson DJ, Finkelstein D, Quigley HA, et al. Macular grid photocoagulation: An experimental study on the primate retina. Arch Ophthalmol 1988; 106:100–105.

54. Bresnick GH. Diabetic maculopathy: A critical review highlighting diffuse macular edema. Ophthalmology 1983; 90:1301–1317.

55. Okisaka S, Kuwabara T, Aiello LM. The effects of laser photocoagulation in the retinal capillaries. Am J Ophthalmol 1975; 80:591–601.

56. Clover GM. The effects of argon and krypton photocoagulation on the retina: Implications for the inner and outer blood retinal barriers. In Gitter KA, Schatz H, Yannuzzi LA, eds. "Laser Photocoagulation of Retinal Disease." San Francisco: Pacific Medical Press, 1988, pp 11–17.

57. Olk RJ. Argon-green (514 nm) versus krypton red (647 nm) modified grid laser photocoagulation for diffuse diabetic macular edema. Ophthalmology 1990; 97:1101–1113.

58. Seiberth V, Schatanek S, Alexandridis E. Panretinal photocoagulation in diabetic retinopathy: Argon versus dye laser coagulation. Graefe's Arch Clin Exp Ophthalmol 1993; 231:318–321.

59. Michels RG, Gass JDM: The natural course of retinal branch vein obstruction. Trans Am Acad Ophthalmol Otolaryngol 1974; 78:166–177.

60. Gutman FA: Macular edema in branch retinal vein occlusion: Prognosis and management. Trans Am Acad Ophthalmol Otolarygnol 1977; 83:488–493.

61. Zweng HCH, Fahrenbruch RC, Little HL. Argon laser photocoagulation in the treatment of retinal vein occlusions. Mod Probl Ophthalmol 1974; 12:261–270.

62. Kelley JS, Patz A, Schatz H. Management of retinal branch vein occlusion: the role of argon laser photocoagulation. Ann Ophthalmol 1974; 6:1123–1134.

63. Branch Vein Occlusion Study Group. Argon laser photocoagulation for macular edema in branch vein occlusion. Am J Ophthalmol 1984; 98:271–282.

64. Shilling JS, Jones CA. Retinal branch vein occlusion: A study of argon laser photocoagulation in the treatment of macular oedema. Br J Ophthalmol 1984; 68:196–198.

65. Kremer I, Hartman B, Siegel R, et al. Static and kinetic perimetry results of krypton red laser treatment for macular edema complicating branch vein occlusion. Ann Ophthalmol 1990; 22:193–197.

66. Branch Vein Occlusion Study Group. Argon laser scatter photocoagulation for prevention of neovascularization and vitreous hemorrhage in branch vein occlusion: A randomized clinical trial. Arch Ophthalmol 1986; 104:34–41.

67. Hayreh SS. Classification of central retinal vein occlusion. Ophthalmology 1983; 90:458–474.

68. Finkelstein D. Laser treatment of branch and central retinal vein occlusion. Int Ophthalmol Clin 1990; 30:84–88.

69. Magargal LE, Brown GC, Augsburger JJ, et al. Neovascular glaucoma following central retinal vein obstruction. Ophthalmology 1981; 88:1095–1101.

70. May DR, Klein ML, Peyman GA, et al. Xenon arc panretinal photocoagulation for central retinal vein occlusion: a randomised prospective study. Br J Ophthalmol 1979; 63:725–734.

71. Laaitkainen L, Kohner EM, Khoury D, et al. Panretinal photocoagulation in central retinal vein occlusion: A randomised controlled clinical study. Br J Ophthalmol 1977; 61:741–753.

72. Magargal LE, Brown GC, Augsburger JJ, et al. Efficacy of panretinal photocoagulation in preventing neovascular glaucoma following ischemic central retinal vein obstruction. Ophthalmology 1982; 89:780–784.

73. Hayreh SS, Klugman MR, Podhajsky P, et al. Argon laser photocoagulation in ischemic central retinal vein occlusion: A 10-year prospective study. Graefe's Arch Clin Exp Ophthalmol 1990; 228:281–296.

74. Clarkson JG. Photocoagulation for ischemic central retinal vein occlusion. Arch Ophthalmol 1991; 109:1218–1219.

75. Bird AC, Grey RHB. Photocoagulation of disciform macular lesions with krypton laser. Br J Ophthalmol 1979; 63:669–673.

76. McMeel JW, Avila MP, Jalkh AE. Subretinal neovascularization in senile macular degeneration. Trans New Orleans Acad Ophthalmol 1983; 291–298.

77. Macular Photocoagulation Study Group. Argon laser photocoagulation for neovascular maculopathy: three-year results from randomized clinical trials. Arch Ophthalmol 1986; 104:694–701.

78. Macular Photocoagulation Study Group. Argon laser photocoagulation for neovascular maculopathy: Five-year results from randomized clinical trials. Arch Ophthalmol 1991; 109:1109–1114.

79. Bressler SB, Bressler NM, Fine SL, et al. Natural course of choroidal neovascular membranes within the foveal avascular zone in senile macular degeneration. Am J Ophthalmol 1982; 93:157–163.

80. Macular Photocoagulation Study Group. Krypton laser photocoagulation for neovascular lesions of age-related macular degeneration: Results of a randomized clinical trial. Arch Ophthalmol 1990; 108:816–824.

81. Macular Photocoagulation Study Group. Laser photocoagulation for juxtafoveal choroidal neovascularization: Five-year results from randomized clinical trials. Arch Ophthalmol 1994; 112:500–509.

82. Macular Photocoagulation Study Group. Laser photocoagulation of subfoveal neovascular lesions in age-related macular degeneration: results of a randomized clinical trial. Arch Ophthalmol 1991; 109:1220–1231.

83. Macular Photocoagulation Study Group. Laser photocoagulation of subfoveal neovascular lesions of age-related macular degeneration: Updated findings from two clinical trials. Arch Ophthalmol 1993; 111:1200–1209.

84. Macular Photocoagulation Study Group. Persistent and recurrent neovascularization after krypton laser photocoagulation for neovascular lesions of age-related macular degeneration. Arch Ophthalmol 1990; 108:825–831.

85. Macular Photocoagulation Study Group. Visual outcome after laser photocoagulation for subfoveal choroidal neovascularization secondary to age-related macular degeneration: The influence of initial lesion size and initial visual acuity. Arch Ophthalmol 1994; 112:480–488.

86. Macular Photocoagulation Study Group. Recurrent choroidal neovascularization after argon laser photocoagulation for neovascular maculopathy. Arch Ophthalmol 1986; 104:503–512.

87. Macular Photocoagulation Study Group. Persistent and recurrent neovascularization after argon laser photocoagulation for subfoveal choroidal neovascularization of age-related macular degeneration. Arch Ophthalmol 1994; 112:489–499.

88. Macular Photocoagulation Study Group. Laser photocoagulation of subfoveal recurrent neovascular lesions in age-related macular degeneration: Results of a randomized clinical trial. Arch Ophthalmol 1991; 109:1232–1241.

89. McHugh JDA, Marshall J, ffytche TJ, et al. Initial clinical experience using a diode laser in the treatment of retinal vascular disease. Eye 1989; 3:516–527.

90. Balles MW, Puliafito CA, D'Amico DJ, et al. Semiconductor diode laser photocoagulation in retinal vascular disease. Ophthalmology 1990; 97:1553–1561.

91. Balles MW, Puliafito CA. Semiconductor diode lasers: A new laser light source in ophthalmology. Int Ophthalmol Clin 1990; 30:77–83.

92. Ulbig MW, McHugh DA, Hamilton AMP. Photocoagulation of choroidal neovascular membranes with a diode laser. Br J Ophthalmol 1993; 77:218–221.

93. Sato Y, Berkowitz BA, Wilson CA, et al. Blood-retinal barrier breakdown caused by diode vs argon laser endophotocoagulation. Arch Ophthalmol 1992; 110:277–281.

94. Haller JA, Lim JI, Goldberg MF. Pilot trial of transscleral diode laser retinopexy in retinal detachment surgery. Arch Ophthalmol 1993; 111:952–956.

95. Charles S. Endophotocoagulation. Retina 1981; 1:117–120.

96. Thomas MA, Halperin LS. Subretinal endolaser treatment of a choroidal bleeding site. Am J Ophthalmol 1990; 109:742–744.

97. Jaffe GJ, Mieler WF, Burke JM, et al. Photoablation of ocular melanoma with a high-powered argon endolaser. Arch Ophthalmol 1989; 107:113–118.

98. Duker JS, Federman JL, Schubert H, et al. Semiconductor diode laser endophotocoagulation. Ophthalmic Surg 1989; 20:717–719.

99. Smiddy WE: Diode laser photocoagulation. Arch Ophthalmol 1992; 110:1172–1174.

100. Diskin J, Maguire AM, Margherio RR. Choroidal folds induced with diode endolaser. Arch Ophthalmol 1992; 110:754.

101. Peyman GA, Lee KJ. Multifunction endolaser probe. Am J Ophthalmol 1992; 114:103–104.

102. Peyman GA, D'Amico DJ, Alturki WA. An endolaser probe with aspiration capability. Arch Ophthalmol 1992; 110:718.

103. Uram M. Ophthalmic laser microendoscope ciliary process ablation in the management of neovascular glaucoma. Ophthalmology 1992; 99:1823–1828.

104. Uram M. Ophthalmic laser microendoscope endophotocoagulation. Ophthalmology 1992; 99:1829–1832.

105. Mizuno K. Binocular indirect argon laser photocoagulator. Br J Ophthalmol 1981; 65:425–428.

106. Friberg TR. Principles of photocoagulation using binocular indirect ophthalmoscope laser delivery systems. Int Ophthalmol Clin 1990; 30:89–94.

107. Friberg TR. Clinical experience with a binocular indirect ophthalmoscope laser delivery system. Retina 1987; 7:28–31.

108. Friberg TR, Eller AW. Pneumatic repair of primary and secondary retinal detachments using a binocular indirect ophthalmoscope laser delivery system. Ophthalmology 1988; 95:187–193.

109. Augsburger JJ, Faulkner CB. Indirect ophthalmoscope argon laser treatment of retinoblastoma. Ophthalmic Surg 1992; 23:591–593.

110. Augsburger JJ, Mullen D, Kleineidam M. Planned combined I-125 plaque irradiation and indirect ophthalmoscope laser therapy for choroidal malignant melanoma. Ophthalmic Surg 1993; 24:76–81.

111. Irvine WD, Smiddy WE, Nicholson DH. Corneal and iris

burns with the laser indirect ophthalmoscope. Am J Ophthalmol 1990; 110:311–313.

112. Morley MG, Frederick AR. Melted haptic as a complication of the indirect ophthalmic laser delivery system. Am J Ophthalmol 1992; 113:584–586.

113. Palmer EA, Flynn JT, Hardy RJ, et al. Incidence and early course of retinopathy of prematurity. Ophthalmology 1991; 98:1628–1640.

114. Cryotherapy for Retinopathy of Prematurity Cooperative Group. Multicenter trial of cryotherapy for retinopathy of prematurity: One-year outcome—structure and function. Arch Ophthalmol 1990; 108:1408–1416.

115. Cryotherapy for Retinopathy of Prematurity Cooperative Group. Multicenter trial of cryotherapy for retinopathy of prematurity: preliminary results. Arch Ophthalmol 1988; 106:471–479.

116. Nagata M, Kanenari S, Fukuda T, et al. Photocoagulation for the treatment of retinopathy of prematurity. Jpn J Clin Ophthalmol 1968; 24:419–427.

117. Landers MB, Semple HC, Ruben JB, et al. Argon laser photocoagulation for advanced retinopathy of prematurity. Am J Ophthalmol 1990; 110:429–431.

118. Landers MB, Toth CA, Semple HC, et al. Treatment of retinopathy of prematurity with argon laser photocoagulation. Arch Ophthalmol 1991; 110:44–47.

119. Schechter RJ. Laser treatment of retinopathy of prematurity. Arch Ophthalmol 1993; 111:730–731.

120. Iverson DA, Trese MT, Orgel IK, et al. Laser photocoagulation for threshold retinopathy of prematurity. Arch Ophthalmol 1991; 109:1342–1343.

121. McNamara JA, Tasman W, Brown GC, et al. Laser photocoagulation for stage 3 + retinopathy of prematurity. Ophthalmology 1991; 98:576–580.

122. Fleming TN, Runge PE, Charles ST. Diode laser photocoagulation for prethreshold, posterior retinopathy of prematurity. Am J Ophthalmol 1992; 114:589–592.

123. Capone A, Diaz-Rohena R, Sternberg P, et al. Diode-laser photocoagulation for zone 1 threshold retinopathy of prematurity. Am J Ophthalmol 1993; 116:444–450.

124. McNamara JA, Tasman W, Vander JF, et al. Diode laser photocoagulation for retinopathy of prematurity: preliminary results. Arch Ophthalmol 1992; 110:1714–1716.

125. Hunter DG, Repka MX. Diode laser photocoagulation for threshold retinopathy of prematurity: a randomized study. Ophthalmology 1993; 100:238–244.

126. Tasman W. Threshold retinopathy of prematurity revisited. Arch Ophthalmol 1992; 110:623–624.

127. Fleck BW. How large must an iridotomy be? Br J Ophthalmol 1990; 74:583–588.

128. Meyer-Schwickerath G. Erfahrungen mit der Lichtkoagulation der Netzhaut und der Iris. Doc Ophthalmol 1956; 10:91–118.

129. Rodrigues MM, Streeten B, Spaeth GL, et al. Argon laser iridotomy on primary angle closure or pupillary block glaucoma. Arch Ophthalmol 1978; 96:2222–2230.

130. Jacobson JJ, Schuman JS, El Koumy H, et al. Diode laser peripheral iridectomy. Int Ophthalmol Clin 1990; 30:120–122.

131. Schuman JS, Puliafito CA, Jacobson JJ. Semiconductor diode laser peripheral iridotomy. Arch Ophthalmol 1990; 108:1207–1208.

132. Wise JB, Witter SL. Argon laser therapy for open angle glaucoma: A pilot study. Arch Ophthalmol 1979; 97:319–322.

133. Allf BE, Shields MB. Early intraocular pressure response to laser trabeculoplasty 180 degrees without apraclonidine versus 360 degrees with apraclonidine. Ophthalmic Surg 1991; 22:539–542.

134. Spurny RC, Lederer CM. Krypton laser trabeculoplasty: a clinical report. Arch Ophthalmol 1984; 102:1626–1628.

135. Wise JB. Glaucoma treatment by trabecular tightening with the argon laser. Int Ophthalmol Clin 1981; 21:69–78.

136. Schwartz LW, Spaeth GL, Traverso C, et al. Variation of techniques on the results of argon laser trabeculoplasty. Ophthalmology 1983; 90:781–784.

137. Rouhiainen HJ, Teräsvirta ME, Tuovinen EJ. Laser power and postoperative intraocular pressure increase in argon laser trabeculoplasty. Arch Ophthalmol 1987; 105:1352–1354.

138. Melamed S, Epstein DL. Alterations of aqueous humour outflow following argon laser trabeculoplasty in monkeys. Br J Ophthalmol 1987; 71:776–781.

139. Raviola G. Schwalbe line's cells: A new cell type in the trabecular meshwork of *Macaca mulatta*. Invest Ophthalmol Vis Sci 1982; 22:45–56.

140. Van Buskirk EM, Pond V, Rosenquist RC, et al. Argon laser trabeculoplasty: Studies of mechanism of action. Ophthalmology 1984; 91:1005–1010.

141. Shingleton BJ, Richter CU, Dharma SK, et al. Long-term efficacy of argon laser trabeculoplasty: A 10-year follow-up study. Ophthalmology 1993; 100:1324–1329.

142. Ticho U, Nesher R. Laser trabeculoplasty in glaucoma: Ten-year evaluation. Arch Ophthalmol 1989; 107:844–846.

143. The Glaucoma Laser Trial Research Group. The glaucoma laser trial (GLT): 2. Results of argon laser trabeculoplasty versus topical medicines. Ophthalmology 1990; 97:1403–1413.

144. Lichter PR. Practice implications of the glaucoma laser trial (editorial). Ophthalmology 1990; 97:1401–1402.

145. McHugh D, Marshall J, ffytche TJ, et al. Diode laser trabeculoplasty (DLT) for primary open-angle glaucoma and ocular hypertension. Br J Ophthalmol 1990; 74:743–747.

146. McHugh D, Marshall J, ffytche TJ, et al. Ultrastructural changes of human trabecular meshwork after photocoagulation with a diode laser. Invest Ophthalmol Vis Sci 1992; 33;2664–2671.

147. Brancato R, Carassa R, Trabucchi G. Diode laser compared with argon laser for trabeculoplasty. Am J Ophthalmol 1991; 112:50–55.

148. Moriarty AP, McHugh JDA, ffytche TJ, et al. Long-term follow-up of diode laser trabeculoplasty for primary open-angle glaucoma and ocular hypertension. Ophthalmology 1989; 100:1614–1618.

149. Traverso CE, Greenidge KC, Spaeth GL. Formation of peripheral anterior synechiae following argon laser trabeculoplasty: A prospective study to determine relationship to position of laser burns. Arch Ophthalmol 1984; 102:861–863.

150. Bellows AR, Grant WM. Cyclocryotherapy in advanced inadequately controlled glaucoma. Am J Ophthalmol 1973; 75:679–684.

151. Lee P-F, Pomerantzeff O. Transpupillary cyclophoto-co-

agulation of rabbit eyes: An experimental approach to glaucoma surgery. Am J Ophthalmol 1971; 71:911–920.

152. Weekers R, Lavergne G, Watillon M, et al. Effects of photocoagulation of ciliary body upon ocular tension. Am J Ophthalmol 1961; 52:156–165.

153. Beckman H, Kinoshita A, Rota AN, et al. Transscleral ruby laser irradiation of the ciliary body in the treatment of intractable glaucoma. Trans Am Acad Ophthalmol Otolaryngol 1972; 76:423–436.

154. Wilensky JT, Welch D, Mirolovich M. Transscleral cyclocoagulation using a neodymium:YAG laser. Ophthalmic Surg 1985; 16:95–98.

155. Schubert HD, Federman JL. A comparison of CW Nd: YAG contact transscleral cyclophotocoagulation with cyclocryopexy. Invest Ophthalmol Vis Sci 1989; 30:536–542.

156. Vogel A, Dlugos CH, Nuffer R, et al. Optical properties of human sclera, and their consequences of transscleral laser applications. Lasers Surg Med 1991; 11:331–340.

157. Barraquer RI, Kargacin M. Nd:YAG laser diascleral cyclophotocoagulation: survival analysis after four years. Dev Ophthalmol 1991; 22:132–137.

158. Suzuki Y, Araie M, Yumita A, et al. Transscleral Nd: YAG cyclophotocoagulation versus cyclocryotherapy. Graefe's Arch Clin Exp Ophthalmol 1991; 229:33–36.

159. Schuman JS, Jacobson JJ, Puliafito CA, et al. Experimental use of semiconductor diode laser in contact transscleral cyclophotocoagulation in rabbits. Arch Ophthalmol 1990; 108:1152–1157.

160. Schuman JS, Noecker JR, Puliafito CA, et al. Energy levels and probe placement in contact transscleral semiconductor diode laser cyclophotocoagulation in human cadaver eyes. Arch Ophthalmol 1991; 109:1534–1538.

161. Simmons RB, Prum BE, Shields SR, et al. Videographic and histologic comparison of Nd:YAG and diode laser contact transscleral cyclophotocoagulation. Am J Ophthalmol 1994; 117:337–341.

162. Gaasterland DE, Abrams DA, Belcher CD, et al. A multicenter study of contact diode laser transscleral cyclophotocoagulation in glaucoma patients. Invest Ophthalmol Vis Sci 1992; 33(Suppl):1019.

163. Berry J. Recurrent trichiasis: Treatment with laser photocoagulation. Ophthalmic Surg 1979; 10(7):36.

164. Campbell DC. Thermoablation treatment for trichiasis using the argon laser. Austr N Z J Ophthalmol 1990; 18:427–430.

165. Hornblass A, Coden DJ. Lasers in oculoplastic and orbital surgery. Int Ophthalmol Clin 1989; 29:265–274.

166. Noe JM, Barsky SH, Geer DE, et al. Port wine stains and the response to argon laser therapy: successful treatment and the predictive role of color, age, and biopsy. Plastic Reconstr Surg 1980; 65:130–136.

167. Apfelberg DB, Maser MR, White DN, et al. Benefits of contact and noncontact YAG laser for periorbital hemangiomas. Ann Plastic Surg 1990; 24:397–408.

168. Bosniak SL, Ginsberg G. Laser eyelid surgery: Evaluating the therapeutic options. Ophthalmol Clin North Am 1993; 6:479–489.

169. Shields JA, Parsons H, Shields CL, et al. The role of photocoagulation in the management of retinoblastoma. Arch Ophthalmol 1990; 108:205–208.

170. Shields JA, Glazer LC, Mieler WF, et al. Comparison of xenon arc and argon laser photocoagulation in the treatment of choroidal melanomas. Am J Ophthalmol 1990; 109:647–655.

171. Vogel M, Schäfer FP, Theuring S, et al. Results of dyelaser photocoagulation of the rabbit fundus. In Gitter KA, Schatz H, Yannuzzi LA, eds. "Laser Photocoagulation of Retinal Disease." San Francisco: Pacific Medical Press, 1988, pp 37–40.

172. Brancato R, Menchini U, Pece A, et al. Dye laser photocoagulation of macular subretinal neovascularization in pathological myopia. Int Ophthalmol 1988; 11:235–238.

173. Anderson RR, Parrish JA: Selective photothermolysis: Precise microsurgery by selective absorption of pulsed radiation. Science 1983; 220:524–527.

174. Krauss JM, Puliafito CA, Lin WZ, et al. Interferometric technique for investigation of laser thermal retinal damage. Invest Ophthalmol Vis Sci 1987; 28:1290–1297.

175. Roider J, Michaud NA, Flotte TJ, et al. Response of the retinal pigment epithelium to selective photocoagulation. Arch Ophthalmol 1992; 110:1786–1792.

176. Tse DT, Dutton JJ, Weingeist TA, et al. Hematoporphyrin photoradiation therapy for intraocular and orbital malignant melanoma. Arch Ophthalmol 1984; 102:833–838.

177. Diamond I, Granelli SG, McDonagh AF, et al. Photodynamic therapy of malignant tumours. Lancet 1972; 2:1175–1177.

178. Kramer M, Miller JW, Michaud N, et al. Photodynamic therapy (PDT) of experimental choroidal neovascularization (CNV) using liposomal benzoporphyrin derivative monoacid (BPD-MA): Refinement of dosimetry. Invest Ophthalmol Vis Sci 1994; 35(Suppl):1503.

179. Howard MA, Hu LK, Gonzalez VH, et al. Photodynamic therapy (PDT) of pigmented choroidal melanoma using a liposomal preparation of benzoporphyrin derivative (BPD). Invest Ophthalmol Vis Sci 1994; 35(Suppl):1722.

180. Destro M, Puliafito CA. Indocyanine green videoangiography of choroidal neovascularization. Ophthalmology 1989; 96:846–853.

181. Guyer DR, Puliafito CA, Monés JM, et al. Digital indocyanine-green angiography in chorioretinal disorders. Ophthalmology 1992; 99:287–291.

182. Slakter JS, Yannuzzi LA, Sorenson JA, et al. A pilot study of indocyanine green angiography-guided laser photocoagulation of occult choroidal neovascularization in age-related macular degeneration. Arch Ophthalmol 1994; 112:465–472.

183. Reichel E, Puliafito CA, Duker JS, et al. Indocyanine green dye-enhanced diode laser photocoagulation of poorly defined subfoveal choroidal neovascularization. Ophthalmic Surg 1994; 25:195–201.

184. Spikes JD. Phthalocyanines as photosensitizers in biological systems and for the photodynamic therapy of tumors. Photochem Photobiol 1986; 43:691–699.

185. Evensen JF, Moan J. A test of different photosensitizers for photodynamic treatment of cancer in a murine tumor model. Photochem Photobiol 1987; 46:859–865.

186. Bauman WC, Monés JM, Tritten J-J, et al. Transpupillary phthalocyanine photodynamic therapy of experimental posterior malignant melanoma. Invest Ophthalmol Vis Sci 1991; 32(Suppl):713.

187. Ozler SA, Nelson JS, Liggett PE, et al. Photodynamic therapy of experimental subchoroidal melanoma using

chloroaluminum sulfonated phthalocyanine. Arch Ophthalmol 1992; 110:555–561.

188. Kliman GH, Puliafito CA, Stern D, et al. Phthalocyanine photodynamic therapy: New strategy for closure of choroidal neovascularization. Lasers Surg Med 1994; 15:2–10.

189. Kliman GH, Puliafito CA, Grossman GA, et al. Retinal and choroidal vessel closure using phthalocyanine photodynamic therapy. Lasers Surg Med 1994; 15:11–18.

190. Miller JW, Stinson WP, Gregory WA, et al. Phthalocyanine photodynamic therapy of experimental iris neovascularization. Ophthalmology 1991; 98:1711–1719.

191. Naoumidis LP, Tsilimbaris MK, Georgiades A, et al. A diode laser mounted on a slit lamp for ophthalmic photodynamic applications of phthalocyanine. Am J Ophthalmol 1993; 115:111–112.

192. Tsilimbaris MK, Pallikaris IG, Naoumidi II, et al. Phthalocyanine mediated photodynamic thrombosis of experimental corneal neovascularization: Effect of phthalocyanine dose and irradiation onset time on vascular occlusion rate. Lasers Surg Med 1994; 15:19–31.

193. Firey PA, Rodgers MAJ. Photoproperties of a silicon naphthalocyanine: A potential photosensitizer for photodynamic therapy. Photochem Photobiol 1987; 45:535–538.

194. Garrett J, Reddy S, Ryan S, et al. Photodynamic therapy (PDT) of experimental ocular melanoma with silicon naphthalocyanine (SlNc) in rabbits. Invest Ophthalmol Vis Sci 1994; 35(Suppl):2120.

195. Zeimer RC, Khoobehi B, Niesman MR, et al. A potential method for local drug and dye delivery in the ocular vasculature. Invest Ophthalmol Vis Sci 1988; 29:1179–1183.

196. Khoobehi B, Peyman GA, Niesman MR, et al. Measurement of retinal blood velocity and flow rate in primates using a liposome-dye system. Ophthalmology 1989; 96:905–912.

197. Khoobehi B, Char CA, Peyman GA. Assessment of laser-induced release of drugs from liposomes: an in vitro study. Lasers Surg Med 1990; 10:60–65.

198. Khoobehi B, Peyman GA, Vo K. Laser-triggered repetitive fluorescein angiography. Ophthalmology 1992; 99:72–79.

199. Ren Q, Simon G, Parel J-M, et al. Laser scleral buckling for retinal reattachment. Am J Ophthalmol 1993; 115:758–762.

200. Burstein NL, Williams JM, Nowicki MJ, et al. Corneal welding using hydrogen fluoride lasers. Arch Ophthalmol 1992; 110:12–13.

201. Khadem JJ, Truong TV, Ernest JT. Laser activated tissue glue. Invest Ophthalmol Vis Sci 1993; 34(Suppl):1247.

202. Wolf MD, Arrindell L, Han DP. Retinectomies treated by diode laser activated indocyanine green dye-enhanced fibrinogen glue. Invest Ophthalmol Vis Sci 1992; 33(Suppl):1316.

203. McClung FJ, Hellwarth RW. Giant optical pulsating from ruby. J Appl Phys 1967; 33:828–831.

204. Krasnov M. Laser-puncture of the anterior chamber angle in glaucoma. Vestn Oftalmol 1972; 3:27–31.

205. Aron-Rosa D, Aron JJ, Greisemann J, et al. Use of the neodymium-YAG laser to open the posterior capsule after lens implant surgery: A preliminary report. J Am Intraocul Implant Soc 1980; 6:352–354.

206. Fankhauser F, Roussel P, Steffen J, et al. Clinical studies on the efficiency of a high power laser radiation upon some structures of the anterior segment of the eye. Int Ophthalmol 1984; 3:129–139.

207. Steinert RF, Puliafito CA, Trokel S. Plasma formation and shielding by three ophthalmic Nd-YAG lasers. Am J Ophthalmol 1983; 96:427–434.

208. Fradin DW, Bloembergen N, Letellier JP: Dependence of laser-induced breakdown field strength on pulse duration. Appl Phys Lett 1973; 22:635–637.

209. Ready JF. "Effects of High-Power Laser Radiation." New York: Academic Press, 1971, pp 133–143, 215–217.

210. Hu C-L, Barnes FS. The thermal-chemical damage in biological material under laser irradiation. IEEE Trans Biomed Eng 1970; 17:220–229.

211. Felix MP, Ellis AT. Laser-induced liquid breakdown—a step-by-step account. Appl Phys Lett 1971; 19:484–486.

212. Lauterborn W. High-speed photography of laser-induced breakdown in liquids. Appl Phys Lett 1972; 21:27–29.

213. Brewer RJ, Rieckhoff KE. Stimulated Brillouin scattering in liquids. Phys Rev Lett 1964; 13:334–336.

214. Cleary SF, Hamrich PE. Laser-induced acoustic transients in the mammalian eye. J Acoust Soc Am 1969; 46:1037–1044.

215. Van der Zypen E, Fankhauser F, Bebie H, et al. Changes in the ultrastructure of the iris after irradiation with intense light. Adv Ophthalmol 1979; 39:59–180.

216. Fujimoto JG, Lin WZ, Ippen IP, et al. Time-resolved studies of Nd:YAG laser induced breakdown: Plasma formation, acoustic wave generation, and caviation. Invest Ophthalmol Vis Sci 1985; 26:1771–1777.

217. Carome EF, Carreira EM, Prochaska CJ. Photographic studies of laser-induced pressure impulses in liquids. Appl Phys Lett 1967; 11:64–66.

218. Mainster MA, Sliney DH, Belcher CD, et al. Laser photodisruptors: Damage mechanisms, instrument design, and safety. Ophthalmology 1983; 90:973–991.

219. Taboada J. Interaction of short laser pulses with ocular tissues. In Trokel S, ed. "YAG Laser Ophthalmic Microsurgery." Norwalk, CT: Appleton-Century-Crofts, 1983, pp 15–38.

220. Smith WL, Liu P, Bloembergen N. Superbroadening in water and deuterium by self-focused picosecond pulses from a neodymium doped YAlG laser. Phys Rev [A] 1977; 15:2396–2403.

221. Anthes JP, Bass M. Direct observation of the dynamics of picosecond-pulse optical breakdown. Appl Phys Lett 1977; 31:412–414.

222. Ashkinadze BM, Vladimirov VI, Likhachev VA, et al. Breakdown in dielectrics caused by intense laser radiation. Sov Phys JETP 1966; 23:788–797.

223. Loertscher H. Laser-induced breakdown for ophthalmic applications. In Trokel S, ed. "YAG Laser Ophthalmic Microsurgery." Norwalk, CT: Appleton-Century-Crofts, 1983, p 39.

224. Sinskey RM, Cain W. The posterior capsule and phacoemulsification. J Am Intraocul Implant Soc 1978; 4:206–207.

225. Steinert RF, Puliafito CA, Kumar SR, et al. Cystoid macular edema, retinal detachment and glaucoma after Nd:YAG laser posterior capsulotomy. Am J Ophthalmol 1991; 112:373–380.

226. Parker WT, Clorfeine GS, Stocklin RD. Marked intraocular pressure rise following Nd-YAG laser capsulotomy. Ophthalmic Surg 1984; 15:103–104.

227. Epstein DL, Jedziniak JA, Grant WM. Obstruction of aqueous outflow by lens particles and by heavy molecular-weight soluble lens proteins. Invest Ophthalmol Vis Sci 1978; 17:272–277.

228. Richter CU, Arzeno G, Pappas HR, et al. Prevention of intraocular pressure elevation following neodymium-YAG posterior capsulotomy. Arch Ophthalmol 1985; 103:912–915.

229. Silverstone DE, Novack GD, Kelley EP, et al. Prophylactic treatment of intraocular pressure elevations after neodymium-YAG laser capsulotomies and extracapsular cataract extraction with levobunolol. Ophthalmology 1988; 95:713–718.

230. Del Priore LV, Robin AL, Pollack IP. Neodymium-YAG and argon laser iridotomy. Long-term follow-up in a prospective, randomized clinical trial. Ophthalmology 1988; 95:1207–1211.

231. Schwartz L: Laser iridectomy. In: Schwartz L, Spaeth G, Brown G, eds. "Laser Therapy of the Anterior Segment: A Practical Approach." Thorofare, NJ: Charles B. Slack, 1984, pp 29–58.

232. Panek WC, Lee DA, Christensen RE. The effects of Nd:YAG laser iridectomy on the corneal endothelium. Am J Ophthalmol 1991; 111:505–507.

233. Robin AL, Pollack IP. Q-switched neodymium-YAG laser iridotomy in patients in whom the argon laser fails. Arch Ophthalmol 1986; 104:531–535.

234. Zborwski-Gutman L, Rosner M, Blumenthal M, et al. Sequential use of argon and Nd:YAG lasers to produce an iridotomy—a pilot study. Metab Pediatr Syst Ophthalmol 1988; 11:58–60.

235. Puliafito CA, Wasson PJ, Steinert RF, et al. Nd-YAG laser surgery on experimental vitreous membranes. Arch Ophthalmol 1984; 102:843–847.

236. Krauss JM, Puliafito CA, Miglior S, et al. Vitreous changes after neodymium-YAG laser photodisruption. Arch Ophthalmol 1986; 104:592–597.

237. Pepose JS, Ubels JL. The cornea. In: Hart WM, ed. "Adler's Physiology of the Eye," 9th ed. St. Louis: Mosby-Year Book, 1992, pp 29–70.

238. Krauss JM, Puliafito CA, Steinert RF. Laser interactions with the cornea. Surv Ophthalmol 1986; 31:37–53.

239. Patel CKN. Interpretation of CO_2 optical laser experiments. Phys Rev Letters 1964; 12:588–590.

240. Beckman H, Fuller TA. Carbon dioxide laser scleral dissection and filtering procedure for glaucoma. Am J Ophthalmol 1979; 88:73–77.

241. Schachat A, Iliff WJ, Kashima HK. Carbon dioxide laser therapy of recurrent squamous papilloma of the conjunctiva. Ophthalmic Surg 1982; 13:916–918.

242. Meyers SM, Bonner RF, Rodrigues MM, et al. Phototransection of vitreal membranes with the carbon dioxide laser in rabbits. Ophthalmology 1983; 90:563–568.

243. Beckman H, Rota A, Barraco R. Limbectomies, keratectomies, and keratostomies performed with a rapid-pulsed carbon dioxide laser. Am J Ophthalmol 1971; 71:1277–1283.

244. Keates RH, Pedrotti LS, Weichel H, et al. Carbon dioxide laser beam control for corneal surgery. Ophthalmic Surg 1981; 12:117–122.

245. Peyman GA, Larson B, Raichand M, et al. Modification of rabbit corneal curvature with use of carbon dioxide laser burns. Ophthalmic Surg 1980; 11:325–329.

246. Keates RH, Levy SN, Fried S, et al. Carbon dioxide laser use in wound sealing and epikeratophakia. J Cataract Refract Surg 1987; 13:290–295.

247. Bachem A. Ophthalmic ultraviolet action spectra. Am J Ophthalmol 1956; 41:969–975.

248. Slavin W. Stray light in ultraviolet, visible, and near-infrared spectral photometry. Anal Chem 1963; 35:561–566.

249. Beaven GH, Holiday ER. Ultraviolet absorption spectra of proteins and amino acids. Adv Prot Chem 1952; 7:319–386.

250. Wetlaufer DB. Ultraviolet spectra of proteins and amino acids. Adv Prot Chem 1962; 17:303–390.

251. Loofbourow JR, Gould BS, Sizer IW. Studies on the ultraviolet absorption spectra of collagen. Arch Biochem 1949; 22:406–411.

252. Smith KC. Ultraviolet radiation effects on molecules and cells. In: Smith KC, ed. "The Science of Photobiology." New York: Plenum, 1985, pp 113–141.

253. O'Brien WJ. Measurement of corneal DNA content. Invest Ophthalmol Vis Sci 1979; 18:538–543.

254. Dougherty AM, Causley GC, Johnson WC. Flow dichroism evidence for tilting of the bases when DNA is in solution. Proc Natl Acad Sci USA 1983; 80:2194.

255. Stone AL. Optical rotary dispersion of mucopolysaccharides III: Ultraviolet circular dichroism and conformational specificity in amide groups. Biopolymers 1971; 10:739–751.

256. Kurzel RB. On the nature of the action spectrum for ultraviolet photokeratitis. Ophthalmic Res 1978; 10:312–315.

257. Buschke W, Friedenwald JS, Moses SG. Effects of ultraviolet irradiation on corneal epithelium: mitosis, nuclear fragmentation, post-traumatic cell movements, loss of tissue cohesion. J Cell Comp Physiol 1945; 26:147–164.

258. Friedenwald JS, Buschke W, Crowell J, et al. Effects of ultraviolet irradiation on the corneal epithelium. J Cell Comp Physiol 1948; 32:161–173.

259. McCann J, Ames BN. Detection of carcinogens as mutagens in the salmonella/microsome test: assay of 300 chemicals: discussion. Proc Natl Acad Sci USA 1976; 73:950–954.

260. Norren DV, Vos JJ. Spectral transmission of the human ocular media. Vision Res 1974; 14:1237–1244.

261. Ringvold A. Damage of the cornea epithelium caused by ultraviolet radiation: A scanning electron microscopic study in rabbit. Arch Ophthalmol 1983; 61:898–907.

262. Taboada J, Mikesell GW, Reed RD. Response of the corneal epithelium to KrF excimer laser pulses. Health Phys 1981; 40:677–683.

263. Zuclich JA. Ultraviolet induced damage in the primate cornea and retina. Curr Eye Res 1984; 3:27–34.

264. Tapaszto I, Vass Z. Alteration in mucopolysaccharide-compounds of tear and that of corneal epithelium caused by ultraviolet radiation. Ophthalmologica 1969; 58(Suppl):343.

265. Koliopoulos JX, Margaritis LH. Response of the cornea to far-ultraviolet light: an ultrastructural study. Ann Ophthalmol 1979; 11:765–769.

266. Regan JD, Trosko JE, Carrier WL. Evidence for excision

of ultraviolet-induced pyrimidine dimers from the DNA of human cells in vitro. Biophys J 1968; 8:319–325.

267. Burlamacchi P. Laser sources. In: Hillenkamp F, Pratesi R, Sacchi CA, eds. "Lasers in Biology and Medicine." New York: Plenum, 1980, pp 1–16.

268. Searles KS, Hart GA. Stimulated emission at 281.8 nm from XeBr. Appl Phys Lett 1975; 27:243–245.

269. McKee T, Nilson JA. Excimer applications. Laser Focus 1982; 18:51–55.

270. Deutsch TF, Geis MW. Self-developing UV photoresist using excimer laser exposure. J Appl Phys 1983; 54: 7201–7204.

271. Koren G, Yeh JT. Emission spectra, surface quality, and mechanism of excimer laser etching of polyimide films. Appl Phys Lett 1984; 44:1112–1114.

272. Srinivasan R, Leigh WJ. Ablative photodecomposition on poly(ethylene terephthalate) films. J Am Chem Soc 1982; 104:6784–6785.

273. Garrison BJ, Srinivasan R. Microscopic model for the ablative photodecomposition of polymers by far-ultraviolet radiation (193 nm). Appl Phys Lett 1984; 44:849–851.

274. Jellinek HH, Srinivasan R. Theory of etching of polymers by far-ultraviolet, high-intensity pulsed laser and long-term irradiation. J Phys Chem 1984; 88:3048–3051.

275. Melcher RL. Thermal and acoustic techniques for monitoring pulsed laser processing. Springer Series in Chemical Physics 1984; 39:418–424.

276. Srinivasan R. Kinetics of the ablative photodecomposition of organic polymers in the far-ultraviolet (193 nm). J Vacuum Sci Tech 1983; B11:923–926.

277. Srinivasan R, Braren B. Ablative photodecomposition of polymer films by pulsed far-ultraviolet (193 nm) laser radiation: Dependence of etch depth on experimental conditions. J Polym Sci Polym Chem Ed 1984; 22:2601–2609.

278. Gorodetsky G, Kazyaka TG, Melcher RL, et al. Calorimetric and acoustic study of ultraviolet laser ablation of polymers. Appl Phys Lett 1985; 46:828–830.

279. Parrish JA. Ultraviolet-laser ablation. Arch Dermatol 1985; 121:599–600.

280. Srinivasan R. Ultraviolet laser ablation of organic polymer films. Springer Series in Chemical Physics 1984; 39:343–354.

281. Srinivasan R, Wynne JJ, Blum SE. Far-UV photoetching of organic material. Laser Focus 1983; 19:62–66.

282. Linsker R, Srinivasan R, Wynne JJ, et al. Far-ultraviolet laser ablation of atherosclerotic lesions. Lasers Surg Med 1984; 4:201–206.

283. Lane RJ, Linsker R, Wynne JJ, et al. Ultraviolet-laser ablation of the skin. Arch Dermatol 1985; 121:609–617.

284. Mohr FW, Grundfest WS, Litvack F, et al. Excimer laser angioplasty. In: Ginsburg R, White JC, eds. Primer on Laser Angioplasty. Mount Kisco, NY: Futura, 1989, pp 181–211.

285. Rowsey JJ, Balyeat HD, Rabinovitch B, et al. Predicting the results of radial keratotomy. Ophthalmology 1983; 90:642–654.

286. Villasenor RA, Salz J, Steel D, et al. Changes in corneal thickness during radial keratotomy. Ophthalmic Surg 1981; 12:341–342.

287. Hoffer KJ, Darrin JJ, Pettit TH, et al. The UCLA clinical trial of radial keratotomy: Preliminary report. Ophthalmology 1981; 88:729–736.

288. Fyodorov SN, Durnev VV. Operation of dosaged dissection of corneal circular ligament in cases of myopia of mild degree. Ann Ophthalmol 1979; 11:1885–1890.

289. Gelender H, Flynn HW, Mandelbaum SH. Bacterial endophthalmitis resulting from radial keratotomy. Am J Ophthalmol 1982; 93:323–326.

290. Swinger CA, Barraquer JI. Keratophakia and keratomileusis—clinical results. Ophthalmology 1981; 88: 709–715.

291. Trokel SL, Srinivasan R, Braren B. Excimer laser surgery of the cornea. Am J Ophthalmol 1983; 96:710–715.

292. Puliafito CA, Steinert RF, Deutsch TF, et al. Excimer laser ablation of the cornea and lens: Experimental studies. Ophthalmology 1985; 92:741–748.

293. Walsh JY, Deutsch TF, Flotte T, et al. Comparison of tissue ablation by pulsed CO_2 and excimer lasers. Paper TuL2. Technical Digest. Conference on Lasers and Electro-Optics, San Francisco, June 9–13, 1986.

294. Kerr-Muir MG, Trokel SL, Marshall J, et al. Ultrastructural comparison of conventional surgical and argon fluoride excimer laser keratectomy. Am J Ophthalmol 1987; 103:448–453.

295. Feld JR, Lin CP, Puliafito CA. Study of the mechanism of excimer laser corneal ablation using calorimetric measurements. Invest Ophthalmol Vis Sci 1993; 34(Suppl):802.

296. Krueger RR, Trokel SL. Quantitation of corneal ablation by ultraviolet laser light. Arch Ophthalmol 1985; 103:1741–1742.

297. Krueger RR, Trokel SL, Schubert HD. Interaction of ultraviolet laser light with the cornea. Invest Ophthalmol Vis Sci 1985; 26:1455–1464.

298. Boettner EA, Wolter JR. Transmission of the ocular media. Invest Ophthalmol 1962; 1:776–783.

299. Peyman GA, Kuszak JR, Weckstrom K, et al. Effects of Xe-Cl excimer laser on the eyelid and anterior segment structures. Arch Ophthalmol 1986; 104:118–122.

300. Puliafito CA, Wong K, Steinert RF. Quantitative and ultrastructural studies of excimer laser ablation of the cornea at 193 and 248 nanometers. Lasers Surg Med 1987; 7:155–159.

301. Fantes FE, Waring GO. Effect of excimer laser radiant exposure on uniformity of ablated corneal surface. Lasers Surg Med 1989; 9:533–542.

302. Berns MW, Liaw L-H, Oliva A, et al. An acute light and electron microscopic study of ultraviolet 193-nm excimer laser corneal incisions. Ophthalmology 1988; 95: 1422–1433.

303. Campos M, Wang XW, Hertzog L, et al. Ablation rates and surface ultrastructure of 193 nm excimer laser keratectomies. Invest Ophthalmol Vis Sci 1993; 34: 2493–2500.

304. Baron WS, Munnerlyn C. Predicting visual performance following excimer photorefractive keratectomy. Refract Corneal Surg 1992; 8:355–362.

305. Dehm EJ, Puliafito CA, Adler CM, et al. Corneal endothelial injury in rabbits following excimer laser ablation at 193 and 248 nm. Arch Ophthalmol 1986; 104:1364–1368.

306. Zabel R, Tuft S, Marshall J. Excimer laser photorefractive keratectomy: Endothelial morphology following

area ablation of the cornea. Invest Ophthalmol Vis Sci 1988; 29(Suppl):390.

307. Nuss RC, Puliafito CA, Dehm EJ. Unscheduled DNA synthesis following excimer laser ablation of the cornea in vivo. Invest Ophthalmol Vis Sci 1987; 28:287–294.

308. Kochevar IE. Cytotoxicity and mutagenicity of excimer laser radiation. Lasers Surg Med 1989; 9:440–445.

309. Müller-Stolzenburg NW, Müller GJ, Buchwald HJ, et al. UV exposure of the lens during 193-nm excimer laser corneal surgery. Arch Ophthalmol 1990; 108:915–916.

310. Cotliar AM, Schubert HD, Mandel ER, et al. Excimer laser radial keratotomy. Ophthalmology 1985; 92:206–208.

311. Steinert RF, Puliafito CA. Corneal incisions with the excimer laser. In: Sanders DR, Hofmann RF, Salz JJ, eds. "Refractive Corneal Surgery." Thorofare, NJ: Charles Slack, 1986, pp 401–410.

312. Marshall J, Trokel S, Rothery S, et al. Photoablative reprofiling of the cornea using an excimer laser: Photorefractive keratectomy. Lasers in Ophthalmology 1986; 1:21–48.

313. Puliafito CA, Stern D, Krueger RR, et al. High-speed photography of excimer laser ablation of the cornea. Arch Ophthalmol 1987; 105:1255–1259.

314. Missotten L, Boving R, François G, et al. Experimental excimer laser keratomileusis. Bull Soc Belge Ophthalmol 1987; 220:103–120.

315. Aron Rosa DS, Boerner CF, Gross M, et al. Wound healing following excimer laser radial keratotomy. J Cataract Refract Surg 1988; 14:173–179.

316. L'Esperance FA, Taylor DM, Del Pero RA, et al. Human excimer laser corneal surgery. Trans Am Ophthalmol Soc 1988; 86:208–275.

317. Hanna KD, Chastang JC, Pouliquen Y, et al. Excimer laser keratectomy for myopia with rotating-slit delivery system. Arch Ophthalmol 1988; 106:245–250.

318. Marshall J, Trokel SL, Rothery S, et al. Long-term healing of the central cornea after photorefractive keratectomy using an excimer laser. Ophthalmology 1988; 95:1411–1421.

319. Munnerlyn CR, Koons JS, Marshall J. Photorefractive keratectomy: A technique for laser refractive keratectomy. J Cataract Refract Surg 1988; 14:46–52.

320. Keates RH, Bloom RT, Ren Q, et al. Fibronectin on excimer laser and diamond knife incisions. J Cataract Refract Surg 1989; 15:404–408.

321. Hanna KD, Chastang JC, Asfar L, et al. Scanning slit delivery system. J Cataract Refract Surg 1989; 15:390–396.

322. Hanna KD, Pouliquen Y, Waring GO, et al. Corneal stromal wound healing in rabbits after 193-nm excimer laser surface ablation. Arch Ophthalmol 1989; 107:895–901.

323. Tuft SJ, Zabel RW, Marshall J. Corneal repair following keratectomy: A comparison between conventional surgery and laser photoablation. Invest Ophthalmol Vis Sci 1989; 30:1769–1777.

324. Goodman GL, Trokel SL, Stark WJ, et al. Corneal healing following laser refractive keratectomy. Arch Ophthalmol 1989; 107:1799–1803.

325. McDonald MB, Frantz JM, Klyce SD, et al. One-year refractive results of central photorefractive keratectomy for myopia in the nonhuman primate cornea. Arch Ophthalmol 1990; 108:40–47.

326. Del Pero RA, Gigstad JE, Roberts AD, et al. A refractive and histopathologic study of excimer laser keratectomy in primates. Am J Ophthalmol 1990; 109:419–429.

327. Fantes FE, Hanna KD, Waring GO, et al. Wound healing after excimer laser keratomileusis (photorefractive keratectomy) in monkeys. Arch Ophthalmol 1990; 108:665–675.

328. Hanna KD, Pouliquen YM, Savoldelli M, et al. Corneal wound healing in monkeys 18 months after excimer laser photorefractive keratectomy. Refract Corneal Surg 1990; 6:340–345.

329. Sher NA, Barak M, Daya S, et al. Excimer laser photorefractive keratectomy in high myopia. A multicenter study. Arch Ophthalmol 1992; 110:935–943.

330. Taylor DM, L'Esperance FA, Warner JW, et al. Experimental corneal studies with the excimer laser. J Cataract Refract Surg 1989; 15:384–389.

331. L'Esperance FA, Taylor DM, Warner JW. Human excimer laser keratectomy: short-term histopathology. J Refract Surg 1988; 4:118–124.

332. McDonald MB, Frantz JM, Klyce SD, et al. Central photorefractive keratectomy for myopia. The blind eye study. Arch Ophthalmol 1990; 108:799–808.

333. Seiler T, Kahle G, Kriegerowski M. Excimer laser (193 nm) myopic keratomileusis in sighted and blind human eyes. Refract Corneal Surg 1990; 6:165–173.

334. Zabel RW, Sher NA, Ostrov CS, et al. Myopic excimer laser keratectomy: a preliminary report. Refract Corneal Surg 1990; 6:329–334.

335. Brancato R, Tavola A, Carones F, et al. Excimer laser photorefractive keratectomy for myopia: results in 1165 eyes. Refract Corneal Surg 1993; 9:95–104.

336. Holschbach A, Derse M, Seiler T, et al. Preliminary two year results of photorefractive keratectomy. Invest Ophthalmol Vis Sci 1993; 34(Suppl):798.

337. Epstein D, Hamberg-Nyström H, Fagerholm P, et al. Three-year follow-up of excimer laser photorefractive keratectomy for myopia. Invest Ophthalmol Vis Sci 1994; 35(Suppl):1650.

338. Tengroth B, Epstein D, Fagerholm P, et al. Excimer laser photorefractive keratectomy for myopia. Clinical results in sighted eyes. Ophthalmology 1993; 100:739–745.

339. Gartry DS, Kerr Muir MG, Lohmann CP, et al. The effect of topical corticosteroids on refractive outcome and corneal haze after photorefractive keratectomy. Arch Ophthalmol 1992; 110:944–952.

340. Stevens JD, Steele AD, Ficker LA, et al. Prospective randomized study of two topical steroid regimes after excimer laser PRK. Invest Ophthalmol Vis Sci 1994; 35(Suppl):1651.

341. Liu JC, McDonald MB, Varnell R, et al. Myopic excimer laser photorefractive keratectomy: An analysis of clinical correlations. Refractive and Corneal Surgery 1990; 6:321–328.

342. Campos M, Hertzog L, Garbus JJ, et al. Corneal sensitivity after photorefractive keratectomy. Am J Ophthalmol 1992; 114:51–54.

343. Ficker LA, Bates AK, Steele AD. Excimer laser photorefractive keratectomy for myopia: 12 month follow-up. Eye 1993; 7:617–624.

344. Piebenga LW, Matta CS, Deitz MR, et al. Excimer photorefractive keratectomy for myopia. Ophthalmology 1993; 100:1335–1345.

345. Seiler T, Holschbach A, Derse M, et al. Complications of myopic photorefractive keratectomy with the excimer laser. Ophthalmology 1994; 101:153–160.

346. Heitzmann J, Binder PS, Kassar BS, et al. The correction of high myopia using the excimer laser. Arch Ophthalmol 1993; 111:1627–1634.

347. Förster W. Time-delayed, two-step excimer laser photorefractive keratectomy to correct high myopia. Refract Corneal Surg 1993; 9:465–467.

348. Binder PS, Anderson JA, Lambert RW, et al. Endothelial cell loss associated with excimer laser. Ophthalmology 1993; 100(9A):107.

349. Carones F, Brancato R, Venturi E, et al. The corneal endothelium after myopic excimer laser photorefractive keratectomy. Arch Ophthalmol 1994; 112:920–924.

350. Krueger RR, Saedy NF, McDonnell PJ. Clinical analysis of topographic steep central islands following excimer laser photorefractive keratectomy (PRK). Invest Ophthalmol Vis Sci 1994; 35(Suppl):1740.

351. Kawesch GM, Maloney RK, Derse M, et al. Contour of the ablation zone after photorefractive keratectomy. Invest Ophthalmol Vis Sci 1992; 33(Suppl):1105.

352. Moreira H, Garbus JJ, Fasano A, et al. Multifocal corneal topographic changes with excimer laser photorefractive keratectomy. Arch Ophthalmol 1992; 110:994–999.

353. Seiler T, Bende T, Wollensak J, et al. Excimer laser keratectomy for correction of astigmatism. Am J Ophthalmol 1988; 105:117–124.

354. McDonnell PJ, Moreira H, Garbus J, et al. Photorefractive keratectomy to create toric ablations for correction of astigmatism. Arch Ophthalmol 1991; 109:710–713.

355. Campos M, Hertzog L, Garbus J, et al. Photorefractive keratectomy for severe postkeratoplasty astigmatism. Am J Ophthalmol 1992; 114:429–436.

356. Taylor HR, Guest CS, Kelly P, et al. Comparison of excimer laser treatment of astigmatism and myopia. Arch Ophthalmol 1993; 111:1621–1626.

357. Gibralter R, Trokel SL. Correction of irregular astigmatism with the excimer laser. Ophthalmology 1994; 101:1310–1314.

358. Lieurance RC, Patel AC, Wan WL, et al. Excimer laser cut lenticules for epikeratophakia. Am J Ophthalmol 1987; 103:475–476.

359. Serdarevic ON, Hanna K, Gribomont A-C, et al. Excimer laser trephination in penetrating keratoplasty: morphologic features and wound healing. Ophthalmology 1988; 95:493–505.

360. Lang GK, Schroeder E, Koch JW, et al. Excimer laser keratoplasty part 2: Elliptical keratoplasty. Ophthalmic Surg 1989; 20:342–346.

361. Gabay S, Slomovic A, Jares T. Excimer laser-processed donor corneal lenticules for lamellar keratoplasty. Am J Ophthalmol 1989; 107:47–51.

362. Serdarevic O, Darrell RW, Krueger RR, et al. Excimer laser therapy for experimental Candida keratitis. Am J Ophthalmol 1985; 99:534–538.

363. Dausch D, Schröder E. Die behandlung von hornhaut- und skleraerkrankungen mit dem excimerlaser: ein vorläufiger erfahrungsbericht. Fortschr Ophthalmol 1990; 87:115–120.

364. Steinert RF, Puliafito CA. Excimer laser phototherapeutic keratectomy for a corneal nodule. Refract Corneal Surg 1990; 6:352.

365. Sher NA, Bowers RA, Zabel RW, et al. Clinical use of the 193-nm excimer laser in the treatment of corneal scars. Arch Ophthalmol 1991; 109:491–498.

366. Chamon W, Azar DT, Stark WJ, et al. Phototherapeutic keratectomy. Ophthalmol Clin North Am 1993; 6:399–413.

367. Bowers RA, Sher NA, Gothard TW, et al. The clinical use of 193 nm excimer laser in the treatment of corneal scars. Invest Ophthalmol Vis Sci 1991; 32(Suppl):720.

368. Kornmehl EW, Steinert RF, Puliafito CA. A comparative study of masking fluids for excimer laser phototherapeutic keratectomy. Arch Ophthalmol 1991; 109:860–863.

369. Klyce SD, Wilson SE, McDonald MB, et al. Corneal topography after excimer laser keratectomy. Invest Ophthalmol Vis Sci 1991; 32(Suppl):721.

370. Loertscher H, Mandelbaum S, Parrish RK, et al. Preliminary report on corneal incisions created by a hydrogen fluoride laser. Am J Ophthalmol 1986; 102:217–221.

371. Thompson KP, Barraquer E, Parel J-M, et al. Potential use of lasers for penetrating keratoplasty. J Cataract Refract Surg 1989; 15:397–403.

372. Peyman GA, Badaro RM, Khoobehi B. Corneal ablation in rabbits using an infrared (2.9-μm) erbium:YAG laser. Ophthalmology 1989; 96:1160–1170.

373. Tsubota K. Application of erbium:YAG laser in ocular ablation. Ophthalmologica 1990; 200:117–122.

374. Seiler T, Berlin M, Genth U. Fundamental mode photoablation (FMP) using an electro-optically Q-switched Er:YAG laser. Invest Ophthalmol Vis Sci 1994; 35(Suppl):2017.

375. Stern D, Puliafito CA, Dobi ET, et al. Infrared laser surgery of the cornea: Studies with a Raman-shifted neodymium:YAG laser at 2.80 and 2.92 μm. Ophthalmology 1988; 95:1434–1441.

376. Stern D, Schoenlein RW, Puliafito CA, et al. Corneal ablation by nanosecond, picosecond, and femtosecond lasers at 532 and 625 nm. Arch Ophthalmol 1989; 107:587–592.

377. Gasset AR, Kaufman H. Thermokeratoplasty in the treatment of keratoconus. Am J Ophthalmol 1975; 79:226–232.

378. Seiler T, Matallana M, Bende T. Laser thermokeratoplasty by means of a pulsed holmium:YAG laser for hyperopic correction. Refract Corneal Surg 1990; 6:335–339.

379. Seiler T. Ho:YAG laser thermokeratoplasty for hyperopia. Ophthalmol Clin North Amer 1992; 5:773–780.

380. Moreira H, Campos M, Sawusch MR, et al. Holmium laser thermokeratoplasty. Ophthalmology 1993; 100:752–761.

381. Chow DR, Chen JC, Saheb NA, et al. Holmium laser scleroplasty—a new idea in refractive surgery. Invest Ophthalmol Vis Sci 1994; 35(Suppl):2021.

382. Simon G, Ren Q. Laser refractive scleroplasty (LRS) for astigmatic correction. Invest Ophthalmol Vis Sci 1994; 35(Suppl):2021.

383. Wapner F, Eaton A, Schubert H, et al. Micropulsed diode laser dye-enhanced thermokeratoplasty. Invest Ophthalmol Vis Sci 1992; 33(Suppl):769.

384. Korn EL. Use of the carbon dioxide laser for removal of lesions adjacent to the punctum. Ann Ophthalmol 1990; 22:230–234.

385. Korn E. Tarsorrhaphy: A laser-assisted approach. Ann Ophthalmol 1990; 22:154–157.

386. Kennerdell JS, Maroon JC. Use of the carbon dioxide laser in the management of orbital plexiform neurofibromas. Ophthalmic Surg 1990; 21:138–140.

387. Bosniak SL, Novick NL, Sachs ME. Treatment of recurrent squamous papillomata of the conjunctiva by carbon dioxide laser vaporization. Ophthalmology 1986; 93:1078–1082.

388. Kennerdell JS, Maroon JC, Garrity JA, et al. Surgical management of orbital lymphangioma with the carbon dioxide laser. Am J Ophthalmol 1986; 102:308–314.

389. Korn EL, Glotzbach RK. Carbon dioxide laser repair of medial ectropion. Ophthalmic Surg 1988; 19:653–657.

390. Gonnering RS, Lyon DB, Fisher JC. Endoscopic laser-assisted lacrimal surgery. Am J Ophthalmol 1991; 111:152–157.

391. Mittelman H, Apfelberg DB. Carbon dioxide laser blepharoplasty—advantages and disadvantages. Ann Plast Surg 1990; 24:1–6.

392. Woog JJ, Metson R, Puliafito CA. Holmium:YAG endonasal laser dacryocystorhinostomy Am J Ophthalmol 1993; 116:1–10.

393. Troutman RC, Véronneau-Troutman S, Jakobiec FA, et al. A new laser for collagen wounding in corneal and strabismus surgery: A preliminary report. Trans Am Ophthalmol Soc 1986; 84:117–130.

394. Nanevicz TM, Prince MR, Gawande AA, et al. Excimer laser ablation of the lens. Arch Ophthalmol 1986; 104:1825–1829.

395. Bath PE, Mueller G, Apple DJ, et al. Excimer laser lens ablation. Arch Ophthalmol 1987; 105:1164–1165.

396. Keates RH, Bloom RT, Schneider RT, et al. Absorption of 308-nm excimer laser radiation by balanced salt solution, sodium hyaluronate, and human cadaver eyes. Arch Ophthalmol 1990; 108:1611–1613.

397. Ross BS, Puliafito CA. Erbium-YAG and holmium-YAG laser ablation of the lens. Lasers Surg Med 1994; 15:74–82.

398. Gailitis RP, Patterson SW, Samuels MA, et al. Comparison of laser phacovaporization using the Er-YAG and the Er-YSGG laser. Arch Ophthalmol 1993; 111:697–700.

399. L'Esperance FA, Mittl RN, James WA. Carbon dioxide laser trabeculostomy for the treatment of neovascular glaucoma. Ophthalmology 1983; 90:821–829.

400. Jaffe GJ, Williams GA, Mieler WF, et al. Ab interno sclerostomy with a high-powered argon endolaser. Am J Ophthalmol 1988; 106:391–396.

401. Berlin MS, Rajacich G, Duffy M, et al. Excimer laser photoablation in glaucoma filtering surgery. Am J Ophthalmol 1987; 103:713–714.

402. Seiler T, Kriegerowski M, Bende T, et al. Partial trabeculectomy with the excimer laser (193 nm). Invest Ophthalmol Vis Sci 1988; 29(Suppl):239.

403. Allan BDS, van Saarloos PP, Russo AV, et al. Excimer laser sclerostomy: The in vitro development of a modified open mask delivery system. Eye 1993; 7:47–52.

404. Margolis TI, Farnath DA, Puliafito CA. Mid infrared laser sclerostomy. Invest Ophthalmol Vis Sci 1988; 29(Suppl):366.

405. Eaton AM, Odrich SA, Schubert HD, et al. Holmium and thulium laser sclerostomy: A comparative study. Invest Ophthalmol Vis Sci 1991; 32(Suppl):860.

406. Iwach AG, Hoskins HD, Drake MV, et al. Update of the subconjunctival THC:YAG (holmium) laser sclerostomy ab externo clinical trial: 30-month report. Ophthalmic Surg 1994; 25:13–21.

407. McAllister JA, Watts PO. Holmium laser sclerostomy: A clinical study. Eye 1993; 7:656–660.

408. Namazi N, Schuman JS, Wang N, et al. Acute and long term effects of THC:YAG sclerostomy with adjunctive antimetabolite therapy in rabbits. Invest Ophthalmol Vis Sci 1992; 33(Suppl):1266.

409. Engel JM, Blair NP, Harris D, et al. Use of the carbon dioxide laser in the drainage of subretinal fluid. Arch Ophthalmol 1989; 107:731–734.

410. Pellin MJ, Williams GA, Young CE, et al. Endoexcimer laser intraocular ablative photodecomposition. Am J Ophthalmol 1985; 99:483–484.

411. Margolis TI, Farnath DA, Destro M. Erbium-YAG laser surgery on experimental vitreous membranes. Arch Ophthalmol 1989; 107:424–428.

412. Lin CP, Stern D, Puliafito CA. High-speed photography of Er:YAG laser ablation in fluid. Invest Ophthalmol Vis Sci 1990; 31:2546–2550.

413. Lin CP, Weaver YK, Birngruber R, et al. Intraocular microsurgery with a picosecond Nd:YAG laser. Lasers Surg Med 1994; 15:44–53.

414. Borirakchanyavat S, Puliafito CA, Kliman GH, et al. Holmium-YAG laser surgery on experimental vitreous membranes. Arch Ophthalmol 1991; 109:1605–1609.

415. Huie TY, Chang CJ, Tso MOM. Localized surgical debridement of RPE by Q-switched neodymium:YAG laser. Invest Ophthalmol Vis Sci 1993; 34(Suppl):959.

416. Chong LP, Kohen L. A retinal laser which damages only the RPE: Ultrastructural study. Invest Ophthalmol Vis Sci 1993; 34(Suppl):960.

417. Roider J, Michaud N, Flotte T, et al. Selective RPE photocoagulation by 1 µsec laser pulses. Invest Ophthalmol Vis Sci 1993; 34(Suppl):960.

418. Lewis A, Palanker D, Hemo I, et al. Microsurgery of the retina with a needle-guided 193-nm excimer laser. Invest Ophthalmol Vis Sci 1992; 33:2377–2381.

419. Webb RH, Hughes GW, Pomerantzeff O. Flying spot TV ophthalmoscope. Applied Optics 1980; 19:2991–2997.

420. Mainster MA, Timberlake GT, Webb RH, et al. Scanning laser ophthalmoscopy: clinical applications. Ophthalmology 1982; 89:852–857.

421. Dreher AW, Weinreb RN. Accuracy of topographic measurements in a model eye with the laser tomographic scanner. Invest Ophthalmol Vis Sci 1991; 32:2992–2996.

422. Weinreb RN, Dreher AW, Bille JP. Quantitative assessment of the optic nerve head with the laser tomographic scanner. Int Ophthalmol 1989; 13:25–29.

423. Bartsch D-U, Intaglietta M, Bille JF, et al. Confocal laser tomographic analysis of the retina in eyes with macular hole formation and other focal macular diseases. Am J Ophthalmol 1989; 108:277–287.

424. Sjaarda RN, Frank DA, Glaser BM, et al. Assessment of vision in idiopathic macular holes with macular microperimetry using the scanning laser ophthalmoscope. Ophthalmology 1993; 100:1513–1518.

425. Woon WH, Fitzke FW, Bird AC, et al. Confocal imaging of the fundus using a scanning laser ophthalmoscope. Br J Ophthalmol 1992; 76:470–474.

426. Weinreb RN, Dreher AW, Coleman A, et al. Histopatho-

logic validation of Fourier-ellipsometry measurements of retinal nerve fiber layer thickness. Arch Ophthalmol 1990; 108:557–560.

427. Dreher AW, Bille JF, Weinreb RN. Active optical depth resolution improvement of the laser tomographic scanner. Applied Optics 1989; 28:804–808.

428. Cioffi GA, Robin AL, Eastman RD, et al. Confocal laser scanning ophthalmoscope: Reproducibility of optic nerve head topographic measurements with the confocal laser scanning ophthalmoscope. Ophthalmology 1993; 100:57–62.

429. Katsumi O, Timberlake GT, Hirose T, et al. Recording pattern reversal visual evoked response with the scanning laser ophthalmoscope. Acta Ophthalmol 1989; 67: 243–248.

430. Timberlake GT, Van de Velde FJ, Jalkh AE. Clinical use of scanning laser ophthalmoscope retinal function maps in macular disease. Lasers Light Ophthalmol 1989; 2:211–222.

431. Wolf S, Arend O, Sponsel WE, et al. Retinal hemodynamics using scanning laser ophthalmoscopy and hemorheology in chronic open-angle glaucoma. Ophthalmology 1993; 100:1561–1566.

432. Frambach DA, Dacey MP, Sadun A. Stereoscopic photography with a scanning laser ophthalmoscope. Am J Ophthalmol 1993; 116:484–488.

433. Scheider A, Kaboth A, Neuhauser L. Detection of subretinal neovascular membranes with indocyanine green and an infrared scanning laser ophthalmoscope. Am J Ophthalmol 1992; 113:45–51.

434. Kuck H, Inhoffen W, Schneider U, et al. Diagnosis of occult subretinal neovascularization in age-related macular degeneration by infrared scanning laser videoangiography. Retina 1993; 13:36–39.

435. Kiryu J, Ogura Y, Shahidi M, et al. Enhanced visualization of vitreoretinal interface by laser biomicroscopy. Ophthalmology 1993; 100:1040–1043.

436. Sawa M, Sakanishi Y, Shimizu H. Fluorophotometric study of anterior segment barrier functions after extracapsular cataract extraction and posterior intraocular lens implantation. Am J Ophthalmol 1984; 97:197–204.

437. Shah SM, Spalton DJ, Allen RJ, et al. A comparison of the laser flare cell meter and fluorophotometry in assessment of the blood-aqueous barrier. Invest Ophthalmol Vis Sci 1993; 34:3124–3130.

438. Sawa M, Tsurimaki Y, Tsuru T, et al. New quantitative method to determine protein concentration and cell number in aqueous in vivo. Jpn J Ophthalmol 1988; 32:132–142.

439. Shah SM, Spalton DJ, Smith SE. Measurement of aqueous cells and flare in normal eyes. Br J Ophthalmol 1991; 75:348–352.

440. Sawa M. Clinical application of laser flare-cell meter. Jpn J Ophthalmol 1990; 34:346–363.

441. Oshika T, Araie M, Masuda K. Diurnal variation of aqueous flare in normal human eyes measured with laser flare-cell meter. Jpn J Ophthalmol 1988; 32:143–150.

442. Oshika T, Kato S, Sawa M, et al. Aqueous flare intensity and age. Jpn J Ophthalmol 1989; 33:237–242.

443. Guex-Crosier Y, Pittet N, Herbort CP. Evaluation of laser flare-cell photometry in the appraisal and management of intraocular inflammation in uveitis. Ophthalmology 1994; 101:728–735.

444. Oshika T. Aqueous protein concentration in rhegmatogenous retinal detachment. Jpn J Ophthalmol 1990; 34: 63–71.

445. Oshika T, Yoshimura K, Miyata N. Postsurgical inflammation after phacoemulsification and extracapsular extraction with soft or conventional intraocular lens implantation. J Cataract Refract Surg 1992; 18:356–361.

446. Altamirano D, Mermoud A, Pittet N, et al. Aqueous humor analysis after Nd:YAG laser capsulotomy with the laser flare-cell meter. J Cataract Refract Surg 1992; 18:554–558.

447. Mermoud A, Pittet N, Herbort CP. Inflammation patterns after laser trabeculoplasty measured with the laser flare meter. Arch Ophthalmol 1992; 110:368–370.

448. Nussenblatt RB, de Smet M, Podgor M, et al. The use of flarephotometry in the detection of cytomegalic virus retinitis in AIDS patients. AIDS 1994; 8:135–136.

449. Yoshitomi T, Wong AS, Daher E, et al. Aqueous flare measurement with laser flare-cell meter. Jpn J Ophthalmol 1990; 34:57–62.

450. Green DG. Testing the vision of cataract patients by means of laser-generated interference fringes. Science 1970; 168:1240–1242.

451. Faulkner W. Laser interferometric prediction of postoperative visual acuity in patients with cataracts. Am J Ophthalmol 1983; 95:626–636.

452. Selenow A, Ciuffreda KJ, Mozlin R, et al. Prognostic value of laser interferometric visual acuity in amblyopia therapy. Invest Ophthalmol Vis Sci 1986; 27:273–277.

453. Palestine AG, Alter GJ, Chan CC, et al. Laser interferometry and visual prognosis in uveitis. Ophthalmology 1985; 92:1567–1569.

454. Spurny RC, Zaldivar R, Belcher CD, et al. Instruments for predicting visual acuity: A clinical comparison. Arch Ophthalmol 1986; 104:196–200.

455. Fish GE, Birch DG, Fuller DG, et al. A comparison of visual function tests in eyes with maculopathy. Ophthalmology 1986; 93:1177–1182.

456. Klett Z, Morris M, Gieser SC, et al. Assessment of contrast sensitivity. Part II: The relationship between objective lens opacity and laser interferometric contrast sensitivity in the cataract patient. J Cataract Refract Surg 1991; 17:45–57.

457. Hitzenberger CK. Optical measurement of the axial eye length by laser Doppler interferometry. Invest Ophthalmol Vis Sci 1991; 32:616–624.

458. Hitzenberger CK, Drexler W, Fercher AF. Measurement of corneal thickness by laser Doppler interferometry. Invest Ophthalmol Vis Sci 1992; 33:98–103.

459. Huang D, Wang J, Lin CP, et al. Micron-resolution ranging of cornea anterior chamber by optical reflectometry. Lasers Surg Med 1991; 11:419–425.

460. Huang D, Swanson EA, Lin CP, et al. Optical coherence tomography. Science 1991; 254:1178–1181.

461. Swanson EA, Huang D, Hee MR, et al. High-speed optical coherence domain reflectometry. Optics Lett 1992; 17:151–153.

462. Swanson EA, Izatt JA, Hee MR, et al. In vivo retinal imaging by optical coherence tomography. Optics Lett 1993; 18:1864–1866.

463. Izatt JA, Hee MR, Huang D, et al. Micron-resolution biomedical imaging with optical coherence tomography. Optics & Photonics News Oct 1993; 14–18.

464. Izatt JA, Hee MR, Huang D, et al. Ophthalmic diagnostics using optical coherence tomography. SPIE Ophthalmic Technologies III 1993; 1877:136–144.

465. Izatt JA, Hee MR, Huang D, et al. High speed in vivo retinal imaging with optical coherence tomography. Invest Ophthalmol Vis Sci 1994; 35(Suppl):1729.

466. Hee MR, Izatt JA, Swanson EA, et al. Optical coherence tomography of the human retina. Arch Ophthalmol 1995; 113:325–332.

467. Puliafito CA, Hee MR, Lin CP, et al. Imaging of macular diseases with optical coherence tomography (OCT). Ophthalmology 1995; 102:217–229.

468. Schuman JS, Hee MR, Puliafito CA, et al. Quantification of nerve fiber layer thickness in normal and glaucomatous eyes using optical coherence tomography: A pilot study. Arch Ophthalmol 1995; 113:586–596.

469. Hee MR, Puliafito CA, Wong C, et al. Optical coherence tomography (OCT) of macular holes. Ophthalmology 1995; 102:748–756.

470. Hee MR, Puliafito CA, Wong C, et al. Optical coherence tomography (OCT) of central serous chorioretinopathy. Am J Ophthalmol 1995; 120:65–74.

471. Izatt JA, Hee MR, Swanson EA, et al. Micrometer-scale resolution imaging of the anterior eye in vivo with optical coherence tomography. Arch Ophthalmol 1994; 112:1584–1589.

472. Prydal JI, Campbell FW. Study of precorneal tear film thickness and structure by interferometry and confocal microscopy. Invest Ophthalmol Vis Sci 1992; 33:1996–2005.

473. Hitzenberger CK, Drexler W, Dolezal C, et al. Measurement of the axial length of cataract eyes by laser Doppler interferometry. Invest Ophthalmol Vis Sci 1993; 34:1886–1893.

474. Riva CE, Ross B, Benedek GB. Laser Doppler measurements of blood flow in capillary tubes and retinal arteries. Invest Ophthalmol 1972; 11:936–944.

475. Riva CE, Feke GT, Eberli B, et al. Bidirectional LDV system for absolute measurement of retinal blood speed. Applied Optics 1979; 18:2302–2306.

476. Milbocker MT, Feke GT. Intensified charge-coupled-device-based eyetracker and image stabilizer. Applied Optics 1992; 31:3719–3729.

477. Grunwald JE. Effect of topical timolol on the human retinal circulation. Invest Ophthalmol Vis Sci 1986; 27:1713–1719.

478. Sullivan PM, Davies GE, Caldwell G, et al. Retinal blood flow during hyperglycemia. A laser Doppler velocimetry study. Invest Ophthalmol Vis Sci 1990; 31:2041–2045.

479. Riva CE, Petrig BL, Grunwald JE. Near infrared retinal laser Doppler velocimetry. Lasers Ophthlamol 1987; 1:211–215.

480. Grunwald JE, Riva CE, Martin DB, et al. Effect of an insulin induced decrease in blood glucose on the human diabetic retinal circulation. Ophthalmology 1987; 94:1614–1620.

481. Sebag J, Delori FC, Feke GT, et al. Effects of optic atrophy on retinal blood flow and oxygen saturation in humans. Arch Ophthalmol 1989; 107:222–226.

482. Grunwald JE, Brucker AJ, Grunwald SE, et al. Retinal hemodynamics in proliferative diabetic retinopathy: A laser Doppler velocimetry study. Invest Ophthalmol Vis Sci 1993; 34:66–71.

483. Pratesi R, Brancato R, Trabucchi G: Miniature laser for retinal photocoagulation: The self-doubling 532 nm neodymium-yttrium aluminum borate (NYAB) microlaser. Invest Ophthalmol Vis Sci 1992; 33(Suppl):1317.

484. Inderfurth JHC, Ferguson RD, Puliafito CA, et al. Reflectance monitoring during retinal photocoagulation in humans—steps toward the development of an automated feedback-controlled photocoagulator. Invest Ophthalmol Vis Sci 1994; 35(Suppl):1374.

485. Inderfurth JHC, Ferguson RD, Frish MB, et al. Dynamic reflectometer for control of laser photocoagulation on the retina. Lasers Surg Med 1994; 15:54–61.

486. Seiler T, Genth U, Holschbach A, et al. Aspheric photorefractive keratectomy with excimer laser. Refract Corneal Surg 1993; 9:166–172.

487. Solomon KD, Chamon W, Green WR, et al. Superficial concentric excimer laser keratectomy in monkey eyes: a histopathologic analysis. Invest Ophthalmol Vis Sci 1993; 34(Suppl):797.

488. Maloney RK, Friedman M, Harmon T, et al. A prototype erodible mask delivery system for the excimer laser. Ophthalmology 1993; 100:542–549.

489. Talamo JH, Gollamudi S, Green WR, et al. Modulation of corneal wound healing after excimer laser keratomileusis using topical mitomycin C and steroids. Arch Ophthalmol 1991; 109:1141–1146.

490. Liu JC, Steinemann TL, McDonald MB, et al. Effects of corticosteroids and mitomycin C on corneal remodeling after excimer laser photorefractive keratectomy. Invest Ophthalmol Vis Sci 1991; 32(Suppl):1248.

491. Lohmann CP, O'Brart D, Patmore A, et al. Plasmin in the tear fluid: A new therapeutic concept to reduce postoperative myopic regression and corneal haze after excimer laser photorefractive keratectomy. Lasers Light Ophthalmol 1993; 5:205–210.

492. Morlet N, Gillies MC, Crouch R, et al. Effect of topical interferon-alpha 2b on corneal haze after excimer laser photorefractive keratectomy in rabbits. Refract Corneal Surg 1993; 9:443–451.

493. Jain S, Hahn TW, Chen W, et al. Modulation of corneal wound healing following 193-nm excimer laser keratectomy using free radical scavengers. Invest Ophthalmol Vis Sci 1994; 35(Suppl):2015.

494. Lohmann CP, MacRobert I, Patmore A, et al. A histopathological study of surgical human specimen of tissue responsible for haze and regression after excimer laser photorefractive keratectomy. Invest Ophthalmol Vis Sci 1994; 35(Suppl):1723.

495. Sher NA, Frantz JM, Talley A, et al. Topical diclofenac in the treatment of ocular pain after excimer photorefractive keratectomy. Refract Corneal Surg 1993; 9:425–436.

496. Derse M, Seiler T. Repeated excimer laser treatment after photorefractive keratectomy. Invest Ophthalmol Vis Sci 1992; 33(Suppl):761.

497. Tengroth B, Fagerholm P, Epstein D, et al. Retreatment of regression after photorefractive keratectomy for myopia. Invest Ophthalmol Vis Sci 1994; 35(Suppl):1724.

498. Seiler T, Jean B. Photorefractive keratectomy as a second attempt to correct myopia after radial keratotomy. Refract Corneal Surg 1992; 8:211–214.

499. Thompson KP, Hanna K, Waring GO. Emerging technologies for refractive surgery: Laser adjustable syn-

thetic epikeratoplasty. Refract Corneal Surg 1989; 5:46–48.

500. Pallikaris IG, Papatzanaki ME, Stathi EZ, et al. Laser in situ keratomileusis. Lasers Surg Med 1990; 10:463–468.

501. Shimmick JK, Koons JS, Telfair WB, et al. Analysis of an offset slit excimer laser delivery system for the treatment of hyperopia. Invest Ophthalmol Vis Sci 1994; 35(Suppl):1487.

502. McDonald M, Telfair WB, Nesburn AB, et al. Excimer laser hyperopia PRK phase I: The blind eye study. Invest Ophthalmol Vis Sci 1994; 35(Suppl):1488.

503. Hogan C, McDonald M, Byrd T, et al. Effect of excimer laser photorefractive keratectomy on contrast sensitivity. Invest Ophthalmol Vis Sci 1991; 32(Suppl):721.

504. Gobbi PG, Carena M, Fortini A, et al. Automatic eye tracker for excimer laser photorefractive keratectomy. Invest Ophthalmol Vis Sci 1994; 35(Suppl):2017.

505. Stern D, Lin W-Z, Puliafito CA, et al. Femtosecond optical ranging of corneal incision depth. Invest Ophthalmol Vis Sci 1989; 30:99–104.

506. Ren Q, Gailitis RP, Thompson K, et al. Corneal refractive surgery using an ultra-violet (213 nm) solid state laser. Proceedings of Ophthalmic Technologies, SPIE 1991; 1423:129–139.

507. Gailitis RP, Ren Q, Thompson KP, et al. Solid state UV laser ablation (213 nm) of the cornea and synthetic epikeratoplasty material. Invest Ophthalmol Vis Sci 1991; 32(Suppl):996.

508. Manns F, Ren Q, Parel J-M, et al. Investigation of an algorithm for photo-refractive keratectomy (PRK) using a scanning beam delivery system. Invest Ophthalmol Vis Sci 1993; 34(Suppl):800.

509. Ren Q, Simon G, Parel J-M, et al. Ultraviolet solid-state laser (213-nm) photorefractive keratectomy. In vitro study. Ophthalmology 1993; 100:1828–1834.

510. Ren Q, Simon G, Legeais J-M, et al. Ultraviolet solid-state laser (213-nm) photorefractive keratectomy. In vivo study. Ophthalmology 1994; 101:883–889.

511. Lin JT. A multiwavelength solid state laser for ophthalmic applications. Proceedings of Ophthalmic Technologies II, SPIE 1992; 1644:266–275.

512. Feld JR, Lin CP, Woods WJ, et al. Cornea ablation studies at wavelengths between 205 and 225 nm using a tunable solid state laser. Invest Ophthalmol Vis Sci 1992; 33(Suppl):1105.

513. Bende T, Jean B, Matallana M, et al. Photoablation with the free electron laser between 2.8 and 6.2 microns wavelength. Invest Ophthalmol Vis Sci 1993; 34(Suppl):1246.

514. Logan RA, O'Day DM, Haglund RF, et al. Preliminary observations on the effects of the free electron laser on corneal tissue. Invest Ophthalmol Vis Sci 1993; 34(Suppl):1246.

515. Fowler WC, Wehrly SR, Imami NR, et al. Keratorefractive change induced by circumferential infrared wavelength ablations utilizing the free electron laser in porcine corneas. Invest Ophthalmol Vis Sci 1994; 35(Suppl):2027.

516. Zysset B, Fujimoto JG, Puliafito CA, et al. Picosecond optical breakdown: tissue effects and reduction of collateral damage. Lasers Surg Med 1989; 9:193–204.

517. Rowsey JJ, Bowyer BL, Margo CE, et al. Intrastromal ablation of corneal tissue using a frequency doubled Nd:YAG laser. Invest Ophthalmol Vis Sci 1993; 34(Suppl):1247.

518. Rowsey JJ, Bowyer BL, Johnson DE, et al. Phoenix laser: Refractive changes in the cat corneal model. Invest Ophthalmol Vis Sci 1994; 35(Suppl):2027.

519. Bado P, Bouvier M, Coe JS: Nd-YLF mode-locked oscillator and regenerative amplifier. Optics Lett 1987; 12:319–321.

520. Frueh BE, Bille JF, Brown SI. Intrastromal relaxing incisions with a picosecond infrared laser. Lasers Light Ophthalmol 1992; 4:165–168.

521. Remmel RM, Dardenne CM, Bille JF. Intrastromal tissue removal using an infrared picosecond Nd:YLF ophthalmic laser operating at 1053 nm. Lasers Light Ophthalmol 1992; 4:169–173.

522. Niemz MH, Hoppeler TP, Juhasz T, et al. Intrastromal ablation for refractive corneal surgery using picosecond infrared laser pulses. Lasers Light Ophthalmol 1993; 5:149–155.

523. Nissen M, Speaker MG, Davidian ME, et al. Acute effects of intrastromal ablation with the Nd:YLF picosecond laser on the endothelium of rabbit eyes. Invest Ophthalmol Vis Sci 1993; 34(Suppl):1246.

524. Brown DB, O'Brien WJ, Schultz RO. Nd:YLF picosecond laser capabilities and ultrastructure effects in corneal ablations. Invest Ophthalmol Vis Sci 1993; 34(Suppl):1246.

525. Cooper HM, Schuman JS, Puliafito CA, et al. Picosecond neodymium:yttrium lithium fluoride laser sclerectomy. Am J Ophthalmol 1993; 115:221–224.

526. Park SB, Kim JC, Aquavella JV. Nd:YLF laser sclerostomy. Ophthalmic Surg 1993; 24:118–120.

527. Frangie JP, Park SB, Aquavella JV. Peripheral iridotomy using Nd:YLF laser. Ophthalmic Surg 1992; 23:220–221.

528. Taboada J, Poirier RH, Yee RW, et al. Intrastromal photorefractive keratectomy with a new optically coupled laser probe. Refract Corneal Surg 1992; 8:399–402.

529. Zelman J: Photophaco fragmentation. J Cataract Refract Surg 1987; 13:287–289.

530. Chambless WS. Neodymium:YAG laser phacofracture: An aid to phacoemulsification. J Cataract Refract Surg 1988; 14:180–181.

531. Maguen E, Martinez M, Grundfest W, et al. Excimer laser ablation of the human lens at 308 nm with a fiber delivery system. J Cataract Refract Surg 1989; 15:414.

532. Haefliger E, Parel J-M, Fantes F, et al. Accommodation of an endocapsular silicone lens (phaco-ersatz) in the nonhuman primate. Ophthalmology 1987; 94:477.

533. Netter FH. "Atlas of Human Anatomy." Summit, NJ: Ciba-Geigy, 1989.

534. Warwick R. "Eugene Wolff's Anatomy of the Eye and Orbit," 7th ed. Philadelphia, PA: W.B. Saunders, 1976.

535. Margolis TI, Duker JS. Laser treatment of retinal vein occlusion. Ophthalmic Practice 1994; 12(1):8–12, 42.

536. Reichel E, Puliafito CA. Indocyanine green (ICG) angiography in the diagnosis and treatment of choroidal neovascularization. New England Eye Center Clinical Modules 1994 1(3):9–10.

Chapter 9

Clinical Applications of Lasers in Otolaryngology—Head and Neck Surgery

Robert H. Ossoff, DMD, MD, Jack A. Coleman, MD, Mark S. Courey, MD, James A. Duncavage, MD, Jay A. Werkhaven, MD, and Lou Reinisch, PhD

Department of Otolaryngology, Vanderbilt University Medical Center, Nashville, Tennessee

INTRODUCTION
History of Lasers in Otolaryngology

To understand the use of lasers today in otolaryngology–head and neck surgery, one must consider the history of lasers and their rapid incorporation into medicine. The history notably begins when Theodore Maiman first achieved lasing in ruby on May 16, 1960, [1]. Following this achievement, only 18 months later, in December 1961, a prototype ruby laser was used to destroy a retinal tumor in a patient [2]. Subsequent nonophthalmologic developments of the medical laser were then influenced by Leon Goldman [3,4], who established a medical laser laboratory at the University of Cincinnati in 1962. Laser surgery equipment was in the marketplace in 1965, less than 5 years after the first working laser was developed in a physics laboratory.

Otolaryngologists—head and neck surgeons—realized the potential of the laser very early. In fact, in the early 1960s they considered different methods to use pulsed laser systems in the middle ear and labyrinth [5,6]. At approximately the same time, Geza Jako began studying the effects of laser energy on human vocal folds [7]. His first attempts at tissue ablation were made with the neodymium-glass laser, with a wavelength of 1.06 μm. The absorption characteristics of the tissue were not suitable for precise excision with this wavelength of light. In 1965, Strully and Yahr [8] tried to enhance the absorption of the tissue by painting the tissue with a copper sulfate solution. The results were still unsatisfactory. They needed higher intensity levels, could produce only small lesions, and were left with significant destruction of the tissue next to the lesion.

It is worthy to note that these initial experiments on human laryngeal tissue were conducted on cadaver specimens with handheld lasers. The use of handheld lasers returns to medical lasers approximately 25 years later.

The desire for a laser that produces discrete wounds in a reproducible manner led to the investigation of the carbon dioxide (CO_2) laser. The

10.6 μm wavelength of the CO_2 laser is highly absorbed by water. Biologic tissue, high in water content, absorbs the laser energy well. The energy is concentrated at the point of laser impact and comparatively minimal spread through surrounding tissue occurs. In addition, the longer wavelength at 10.6 μm shows minimal scattering of the laser light in tissue.

In 1967, Polanyi tested the CO_2 laser in human cadaver larynxes and was encouraged by the ability to produce discrete wounds. These results spurred the development of an endoscopic delivery system so the laser could be tested in vivo [9–11]. Additional refinements lead to the development of an endoscopic delivery system designed to be coupled with the binocular microscope for binocular microlaryngoscopy. In 1972, Jako reported the initial use of this new equipment in a canine model [7,12].

In otolaryngology the most common use of the medical laser is for tissue ablation. The CO_2 laser energy can create intense localized heating sufficient to vaporize both extra- and intracellular water, producing a coagulative necrosis [13–15]. Advantages of the laser include: (1) it can interact remotely with the tissue; it is only necessary to have a line of sight (or optical conduit) between the laser and the tissue, and (2) the laser is gentle in its interaction with tissue when compared to the hammer, mallet, saw, or drill. Due to the minimal damage to tissue adjacent to the ablation site, the CO_2 laser is often the laser of choice. The CO_2 laser offers many advantages to the surgeon, but the hemostatic effects are sometimes suboptimal [16,17]. Other lasers, such as the KTP and the argon (wavelengths of 532 nm and 514–488 nm, respectively), are more effective at hemostasis since their wavelengths are near the absorption maxima of hemoglobin. The balance between precise ablation with minimal adjacent tissue damage and the need for hemostasis prompted much of the subsequent research.

In 1984, Beamis and Shapshay [18] reported on the use of the Nd:YAG laser at 1.06 μm for malignant and vascular lesions in the tracheobronchial tree. Applications of the argon laser and, later, yellow pulsed dye lasers to vascular cutaneus lesion have permitted the successful treatment of port wine stains [19–21]. Finally, the argon dye laser for use in photodynamic therapy offers exciting possibilities in the treatment of early or superficially spreading cancers.

Not only has the choice of lasers and the best wavelength for a given application been carefully considered, but the optimal delivery system for each laser and application has also been investigated. The drive for new and better laser delivery systems comes, in part, from the fact that all medical systems have their limitations. The potential for increased morbidity and mortality is due, to some extent, to these limitations. For instance, in otolaryngology—head and neck surgery, the CO_2 laser is commonly used in microlaryngeal surgery. Vocal cord fibrosis results from prolonged or high intensity exposure to the laser. The excess heat in the larynx can leave a scarred cord when vaporizing normal vocalis muscle [22].

Research continues toward finer control of the laser. This would lead to increased precision in ablation when compared to handheld probes and micro manipulators. This finer control can be achieved with the aid of computers. A computer-directed laser beam would offer greater precision and flexibility in the shape and size of the incision. The currently available Hexascan™ has shown this to be true; however, the Hexascan™ is limited in that only hexagonal excisions can be made [23–25].

Essential Laser Physics for Otolaryngology

What are the characteristics that distinguish a laser from a lamp? There are four basic characteristics. The first is that the light is monochromatic. Although the narrow spectral characteristics of the laser are extremely important in physics and chemistry, the monochromatic nature of the laser is only moderately important in surgery. The promise for selective ablation has never been fully realized. It is still not possible to irradiate a large volume of tissue and have the laser only ablate the diseased tissue and leave the healthy tissue undamaged.

The second property that makes a laser light a laser is that the light is coherent. In medicine, the coherence of laser light is not often exploited. Yet, there are new measurements of the tympanic membrane motion or motion of the vocal folds using interferometric techniques [27] (G. Gardner, personal communication). These novel applications do utilize the coherence of the laser.

Third, the light from a laser is collimated. Of all the laser properties, the collimation is probably the most important. A collimated beam of light focuses to the smallest possible spot, which is diffraction limited. This high concentration of energy is what allows the surgeon to perform laser ablation, the most common application of lasers in medicine.

And fourth, a laser also has high power that can be delivered to a small area. The cross-sectional area of the laser beam can be varied in two ways. First, as the focal length of the lens becomes smaller, there is a decrease in the spot size of the laser in the focal plane. The smaller the focal point, the greater the corresponding power density becomes for any given power output. Second, the surgeon can vary the cross-sectional area of the beam by working either in-focus or out-of-focus. The cross-sectional area of the laser beam is smallest in the focal plane. As the beam becomes defocused, the cross-sectional area of the spot grows larger and thus lowers or decreases the power density for a given output. Therefore, the cross-sectional area of the spot depends on both the focal length of the lens and the working distance from the target tissue the surgeon chooses to use.

Use of the laser with the surgical microscope in otolaryngology-head and neck surgery is normally with a 400 mm focal length lens. This very long focal length lens results in relatively large spot sizes, even in the focal plane. The ablation of tissue by a handheld probe with a 100 mm focal length lens can be dramatically different from the spot used with the microscope. The handheld probe can have a factor of 16 higher fluence due to the smaller spot size.

Tissue Effects

The actual tissue effects produced by the radiant energy of a laser vary with the specific wavelength and pulse structure of the laser used. The interaction of laser energy with living tissue can produce at least three distinct reactions. First, the laser energy can be absorbed by chromophores within the tissue. The absorption of energy by the tissue is then converted to heat. This is the thermal effect seen in most conventional surgical laser systems today.

Second, the radiant energy of a laser can stimulate or react with specific molecules within a cell. This molecule-specific reaction causes a chemical change to occur within the cell. This effect is termed photochemical. An example of a photochemical process is the reaction that occurs with injection of a photosensitizing drug into tissue and the subsequent biochemical effect that is produced when the drug is activated by the laser energy.

Third, the use of short pulses of high intensity laser light can disrupt cellular architecture because of the production of stress transient waves or photo acoustic shock waves. This mechanical disruption of tissue is an example of a nonthermal tissue effect [27].

The radiant energy of a laser produces a thermal effect when it is absorbed by the tissue and converted to heat. If the radiant energy is poorly absorbed by the target tissue, excess thermal damage to adjacent tissues occurs. Reflection of the energy at the tissue surface or transmission of poorly absorbed light through the target tissue makes it necessary to prolong the time of exposure of the target tissue to the laser energy to achieve the desired ablation. This prolonged exposure of the target tissue causes an increased thermal effect with resultant damage to the surrounding non target tissue. When the target absorbs a specific amount of radiant energy to raise its temperature to $\sim 60-65°C$, protein denaturation starts to occur. Blanching of the tissue surface is readily visible, and the deep structural integrity of the tissue is disturbed. When the absorbed laser light heats the tissue to $\sim 100°C$, vaporization of the intracellular water occurs. This causes vacuole formation, cratering, and tissue shrinkage. Carbonization, disintegration, smoke, and gas generation with destruction of the laser radiated tissue occurs at several hundred degrees centigrade.

In the center of the wound created by a CO_2 laser a volume of tissue is vaporized. Here, just a few flakes of carbon debris are noted. Immediately next to this volume is a zone of thermal necrosis measuring ~ 100 µm wide. Next is a volume of thermal conductivity and repair, usually $300-500$ µm wide. Small vessels, nerves, and lymphatics are sealed in the zone of thermal necrosis; the minimal operative trauma combined with the vascular seal probably account for the notable absence of postoperative edema characteristic of laser wounds [28].

Studies comparing the histologic properties of healing and the tensile strength of the healing wound after laser and scalpel-produced incisions on experimental animals have been performed. In 1971, Hall [13] demonstrated that the tensile strength in a CO_2 laser-induced incision was less up to the twentieth day of healing and became the same by the fortieth day. In 1981, Norris [29] studied the healing properties of CO_2 laser incisions on the hog histologically. He showed that scalpel-induced incisions exhibited better tissue reconstruction than laser-induced incisions up to the thirtieth day, after which time both incisions exhibited similar results.

In 1982, Finsterbush et al. [30] measured the tensile strength of CO_2 laser incisions in rabbits and compared them to scalpel wounds. They gently removed the charring and debris on the wound edges before closure. The laser beam-induced wounds were significantly stronger than those done by scalpel for the first 19 days. In 1983, Buell and Schuller [31] created CO_2 laser incisions in pigs and compared them to scalpel incisions. They found the laser wound to be weaker in tensile strength than the scalpel wounds for the first 3 weeks. It is clear that more research is needed to clarify the effects of CO_2 laser energy on wound healing.

TYPE OF LASERS USED IN OTOLARYNGOLOGY

Argon Ion Laser

Various types of lasers are currently used in otolaryngology. These include the argon ion laser (frequently called the argon laser) with wavelengths of 514 and 488 nm. The argon laser is operated in the continuous wave (CW) mode, can be delivered through optical fibers, and is used in cutaneous applications as well as stapedectomies. This laser normally has special electrical power requirements and needs tap water for cooling the laser.

The visible color of the argon laser beam is blue-green. The argon laser energy is poorly absorbed by clear liquids. Hemoglobin and melanin strongly absorb the laser light. The argon laser is presently used to treat vascular cutaneous lesions because of its absorption by melanin and hemoglobin [31].

Absorption of the argon laser energy by the hemoglobin and melanin causes a heating of the surrounding tissue. The heat produced causes destruction of the epidermis and upper dermis. Therefore, the surgeon must minimize the amount of laser energy delivered to the vascular cutaneous lesion to decrease the tendency of scarring in the overlying skin. The technique described by Keller et al. [33,34], called minimal treatment/retreatment, seems ideally suited to limit the scarring in the overlying skin. The method uses the lowest power setting and exposure time necessary to cause a blanching of the vascular cutaneous lesion. The argon laser energy is delivered with a 1-mm spot size in an overlapping beading pattern.

Focusing the argon laser beam to a small spot size results in high power densities sufficient to vaporize tissue. Otologists have used the argon laser to perform stapedectomy procedures because of its ability to be focused to the small spot size [35,36]. Other otologic applications of this laser include lysis of middle ear adhesions [37] and spot welding of grafts in tympanoplasty surgery [38, 39].

The argon laser beam will readily penetrate the eye and be absorbed by the retina. Therefore, special safety glasses must be worn by the patient, surgeon, and all operating room personnel.

KTP Laser

Similar to the argon laser, the potassium titanyl phosphate (KTP or KTP/532) laser lases at 532 nm in a quasi-CW mode and can be delivered through optical fibers. The single wavelength of this KTP laser is centered on a hemoglobin absorption band. The laser normally does not have any special power requirements and does not require external water to cool the laser. The lasing source is a Nd:YAG laser. The Nd:YAG laser rod is continuously pumped with a krypton arc lamp and Q-switched. The 1.06 μm light traverses a frequency doubling potassium titanyl phosphate crystal yielding the 532 nm green light.

Like the argon laser, the radiant energy from the KTP laser is readily transmitted through clear aqueous tissues because it has a low water absorption coefficient. Certain tissue pigments, such as melanin and hemoglobin, absorb the KTP laser light effectively. When low levels of green laser light interact with highly pigmented tissues, a localized coagulation takes place within these tissues. The KTP laser can be selected for procedures requiring precise surgical excision with minimal damage to surrounding tissue, vaporization, or photocoagulation. The power density chosen for a given application determines the tissue interaction achieved at the operative site.

The KTP laser is transmitted through a flexible fiber optic delivery system, which can be used in association with a micromanipulator attached to an operating microscope or free-hand in association with various handheld delivery probes having several different tip angles. These handheld probes facilitate use of the KTP laser for functional endoscopic sinus surgery and other intranasal applications [40], otologic applications [41], and microlaryngeal applications [42]. The optical fiber delivery of the 532 nm laser light can be manipulated through a rigid pediatric bronchoscope as small as 3.0 mm, facilitating lower tracheal and endobronchial lesion treatment in infants and neonates [43]. Examples of handheld KTP laser applications include tonsillectomy [44–48], stapedectomy [49,50], excision of acoustic neuroma [51], and excision of benign and malignant laryngeal lesions [52]. Use of the micromanipulator facilitates middle ear and microlaryngeal laser surgery because it is more conventionally performed using a CO_2 laser. The KTP laser can also be used with an automatic scanning device to treat areas of pigmented dermal lesions, such as port wine stains [23].

Because the visible green light from the KTP laser can penetrate into the eye and cause retinal damage, special wavelength specific safety glasses must be worn by the surgeon and all personnel in the operating room.

Nd:YAG Laser

The neodymium-yttrium aluminum garnet (Nd:YAG) laser at 1.06 μm has the longest penetration depth of any of the surgical lasers. This laser produces a homogenous zone of thermal coagulation and necrosis that may extend 4 mm from the impact site. The CW light can also be delivered through optical fibers. The laser normally does not have any special power requirements and does not need external cooling water.

The primary applications for the Nd:YAG laser in otolaryngology include palliation of obstructing tracheobronchial lesions [53–57], palliation of obstructing esophageal lesions [58], photocoagulation of vascular lesions of the head and neck [59,60], and photocoagulation of lymphatic malformations [61]. The Nd:YAG laser has several distinct advantages in the management of obstructing lesions of the tracheobronchial tree. Hemorrhage is the most frequent and dangerous complication associated with laser bronchoscopy, and its control is extremely important. Control of hemorrhage is more secure with this laser because of its deep penetration in tissue. Nd:YAG laser application through an open, rigid bronchoscope allows for multiple distal suction capabilities simultaneous with laser application and rapid removal of tumor fragments and debris to prevent hypoxemia. Other advantages of the use of this laser with a rigid bronchoscope include ventilatory control of the compromised airway, palpation of the tumor/cartilage interface, use of the bronchoscope tip as a "cookie cutter," and use of the bronchoscope tip to compress a bleeding tumor bed for temporary hemostasis. The flexible fiberoptic bronchoscope is often used through the open, rigid scope to provide pulmonary toilet and more distal laser application after the major airway is secure.

The major disadvantage of the Nd:YAG laser is its less predictable depth of tissue penetration. This laser is used primarily to photocoagulate tumor masses rapidly at power settings in the upper and lower aerodigestive tract of 40–50 W, 0.5–1.0 s exposures. The laser beam is always applied parallel to the wall of the tracheobronchial tree, whenever possible. The rigid tip of the bronchoscope is used mechanically to separate the devascularized tumor mass from the wall of the tracheobronchial tree.

The selection of patients for Nd:YAG laser bronchoscopy should include a flexible fiberoptic bronchoscopic examination of the tracheobronchial tree in addition to tracheal polytomography or computerized tomography. Patients in whom extrinsic compression of the airway can be demonstrated should be excluded from bronchoscopic laser surgery.

Ho:YAG Laser

At slightly longer wavelengths, holmium:YAG (Ho:YAG) lases at 2.1 μm. This is a pulsed laser in the near infrared region of the spectrum and is a relatively new laser that interacts with tissue in a precise manner, like the CO_2 laser. Yet, the 2.1 μm wavelength can propagate through optical fibers. The technology for these lasers is still evolving. The current lasers normally require 220 V and are air cooled.

The short penetration depth of the laser and the pulse structure has shown great promise in orthopedic surgery. In otolaryngology, the Ho:YAG has been considered for facial nerve decompression [62]. Yet, large temperature transients still preclude this procedure. The future applications of this laser will probably involve endoscopic sinus surgery. The optical fiber transmission, short penetration depth, and ability to ablate bone all show promise in endoscopic sinus surgery.

Other Lasers

Other lasers include the flash lamp pumped dye laser (FLDL). This laser operates at 585 nm with pulses of light ~ 0.4 ms long. The parameters have been optimized for the selective treatment of vascular lesions with minimal damage to the dermis. The light is delivered through an optical fiber. The laser normally requires 220 V and cooling water. Another laser developed for cutaneous applications is the argon pumped dye laser [63,64]. Here, the wavelength can be varied from 488 nm through the red region of the spectrum (800 nm). The CW light is delivered through an optical fiber. This laser has special electrical requirements and requires a significant flow of tap water for cooling.

Recent investigations have considered the diode laser. These lasers operate in the red to near infrared region of the spectrum. They are small and require no water for cooling. The lasers operate CW and the light is delivered through an optical fiber. The intensities are relatively low. They have been investigated for photodynamic therapy and tissue welding [65,66].

CO₂ Laser

The workhorse of surgery, the CO_2 laser operates at 10.6 μm. The invisible CO_2 laser beam has a coaxial helium-neon laser beam to act as an indicator of where the CO_2 laser beam will fall. The wavelength of the CO_2 laser has a high coefficient of absorption for water. Therefore, its energy is well absorbed by all soft tissues that are high in water content. The midinfrared light at 10.6 μm cannot propagate through glass optical fibers and is normally delivered through an articulated arm. Silver halide optical fibers for the CO_2 laser as well as waveguides have recently been introduced to the market [67,68]. The applications of these waveguides and fibers are still, for the most part, experimental. The laser energy can be delivered to tissue either through a handpiece for macroscopic surgery or adapted to an operating microscope for microscopic surgery. The universal endoscopic coupler allows for delivery of the laser energy through a rigid bronchoscope [69,70]. Transmission through rigid nonfiberoptic endoscopes facilitates use of the CO_2 laser for bronchoscopy, laparoscopy, and arthroscopy. This laser does not have special electrical requirements and is air cooled.

MICROSCOPIC APPLICATIONS

Laser technology has expanded greatly over the past few years. This translates directly into newer instrumentation available to the laser surgeon. Often hospitals will update their equipment on a regular basis. It is mandatory for the surgeon to be completely familiar with the laser unit before any patient application. Power output, spot size, and therefore power density vary and cannot be extrapolated from one unit to another.

All the laser wavelengths previously discussed may be adapted for use with the binocular operating microscope. The argon, KTP, and Nd:YAG lasers may be used with fiberoptic delivery probes that are fed through a suction catheter and used in either a contact or noncontact mode. The CO_2 and KTP laser have the ability of being delivered by an optical system with a micromanipulator. This allows precise, noncontact delivery at a predetermined focal length.

Microscopic delivery systems for the CO_2 have evolved since the initial endoscopic coupler developed by Polanyi in the late 1960s. In 1968, Jako spearheaded the production of a binocular endoscopic delivery system for use with the binocular microlaryngoscope and operating binocular microscope. These early micromanipulators were large, transmitted light poorly, and often had treatment paths that were not coincident with the optical path. This problem, referred to as the parallax error, has been overcome in later generation micromanipulators by the development of a partially reflective dichroic mirror. This mirror allows reflection of the CO_2 laser while permitting transmission of almost 75% of visible light [71]. The optical path and treatment path are, therefore, coincident. The other advance in micromanipulators has dealt with the reduction of the spot size from 800 μm, in the earliest commercially available manipulators, to 250–300 μm, in the later generation micromanipulators [72]. As the thermal effects of laser applications have become better understood, the desirability of using a smaller spot size for tissue interaction has become evident.

Since the CO_2 laser has its major tissue interaction with intracellular water, the surgical site must be kept free of moisture. It is mandatory for the pathology to be visualized, and for certain areas, mirrors have been designed to assist in this regard, particularly for the under surfaces of the vocal cords. During surgery, the plume created as tissue is irradiated, must be constantly evacuated so as not to deposit carbon debris, raising tissue temperatures and absorption of energy as well as obscuring the field [73].

The helium–neon laser acting as an aiming beam may occasionally be difficult to visualize or not be coaxial with the CO_2 laser. This shortcoming has been rectified in the KTP laser, which uses the same aiming and treatment beam, with the aiming beam attenuated by several orders of magnitude.

LARYNGEAL SURGERY

Over the last 5 or so years, the role of lasers in microlaryngoscopic applications has become better understood. The CO_2 laser has become the laser of first choice for most microlaryngoscopic applications. The advantages of microscopic control and decreased postoperative edema have made this the instrument of choice for many benign laryngeal diseases, such as for removal of recurrent respiratory papillomatosis. Initial disappointment with its inability to cure the disease has been overcome by its ability to precisely remove papilloma and spare normal laryngeal tissue. Other applications include subglottic stenosis, webs, granuloma, and capillary hemangiomas. Surgery for other benign laryngeal disease processes such as polyps, nodules, leukoplakia, and cysts, may also be performed with the CO_2 laser; however, cold knife excision has been shown to produce equal, if not improved, postoperative results. Surgery in the pediatric group for webs, subglottic stenosis, and capillary meningiomas, have all been significantly improved by the precision, preservation of normal tissue, and decreased postoperative edema associated with the CO_2 laser.

A second laser, with potential laryngeal application is the Nd:YAG. The Nd:YAG laser has much more limited application with regard to intralaryngeal use. Specifically, the increased tissue absorption with an increased depth of penetration make this laser ideal for the treatment of vascular lesions, such as cavernous hemangiomas, where hemostasis and vessel coagulation are the treatment goals.

Stenosis

The management of laryngotracheal stenosis is a difficult problem for the otolaryngologist-head and neck surgeon. The first decision, whether open management is necessary or if endoscopic techniques alone are adequate, is probably the most demanding. All patients with laryngotracheal stenosis need staging direct laryngoscopy and bronchoscopy to determine the extent and degree of stenosis. Having the laser readily available during this staging laryngoscopy is advantageous as scaring can be easily removed or incised with the CO_2 laser. Supplemental dilation with the bronchoscope or stent placement may then be beneficial in further management of the stenotic area [74].

Retrospective analysis has determined that stenotic lesions appropriate for endoscopic management have certain features in common [75]. First, all lesions treated with endoscopic techniques must have intact external cartilaginous support. Attempted endoscopic incision or excision of areas of tracheomalacia can have disastrous results if surrounding structures are perforated. Second, lesions appropriate for endoscopic management are usually < 1 cm in vertical length. Favorable results, however, have been reported for lesions up to 3 cm in length when endoscopic incision is combined with prolonged stenting [74,76]. Finally, total cervical tracheal or subglottic stenosis does not usually respond well to endoscopic management. Again, however, successful case reports exist for endoscopic management when it is combined with prolonged stenting of the stenotic area [74].

Endoscopic management of laryngotracheal stenosis relies on mucosal preservation. The two techniques advocated for this task are radial incision with bronchoscopic dilation [74] and the microtrapdoor flap [77–80]. In the first technique, the laser is used to make radial incision, like the spokes of a wheel, in the stenotic area (Fig. 1). Bronchoscopes are then sequentially passed through the stenosis to dilate it (Fig. 2). The incision is carried on until mucoperichondrium is exposed with care exercised to not expose cartilage. The microtrapdoor flap technique utilizes the CO_2 laser to make a horizontal incision in the mucosa overlying the stenosis (Fig. 3). The laser is then used to vaporize the underlying scar tissue (Fig. 4). Either microscissors or the laser can then be used to incise the lateral portions of the inferiorly based flap to permit redraping of the preserved mucosa. Care must be taken to make the mucosal flap thin without destroying the microcirculation. During creation of the lateral incisions, the flap usually contracts so that a U-shape, uncovered area is created. This, however, is smaller than the area that would be created if the entire flap was excised and usually remucosalizes rapidly. The microtrapdoor flap has been used in a sequential, staged manner on circumferential stenosis with fair to good results [77,81].

The development of the microsubglottiscope has facilitated the use of the CO_2 laser in the subglottis and cervical trachea. This specially designed endoscope fits through the vocal folds and permits binocular vision of the entire subglottis and upper cervical trachea. The CO_2 laser can then be attached to the operating microscope via a

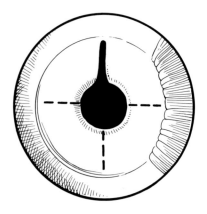

Fig. 1. Radial incisions of stenosis.

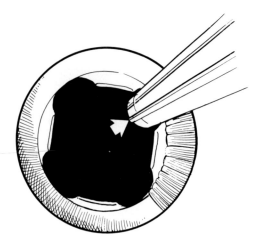

Fig. 2. Endoscope used to dilate stenosis.

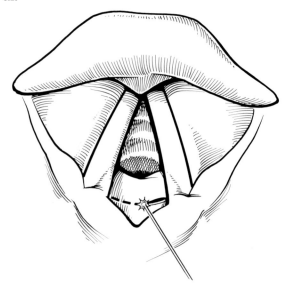

Fig. 3. Horizontal incision in mucosa over stenosis.

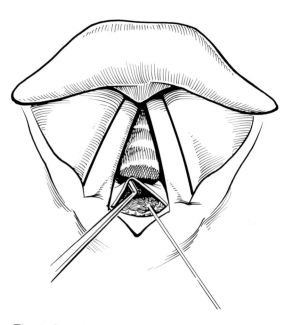

Fig. 4. Scar tissue vaporized in area of stenosis.

micromanipulator and lesions can be approached through a microlaryngoscopic technique as opposed to a bronchoscopic technique. Both adult [82] and pediatric sizes are available [83]. The use of the CO_2 laser is further facilitated by the addition of a smoke evacuation channel and a port for jet Venturi ventilation.

Although the CO_2 laser appears to be the most useful laser for the management of laryngotracheal stenosis, several surgeons are reporting favorable results in lesions treated with the Nd:YAG laser [74,84]. The Nd:YAG laser has the advantage of a fiberoptic delivery system that facilitates its use in otherwise difficult to expose subglottic or cervical tracheal lesions. Secondary to the somewhat unpredictable depth of penetration, however, care must be taken not to produce thermal injury to the underlying cartilage. This is best avoided by using low power settings with a short pulse duration.

Finally, the Ho:YAG laser with a wavelength of 2.1 μm has been used to incise cricoid cartilage in animal models. The endoscopic technique is being explored as an alternative to traditional open cricoid splitting in neonatal and pediatric subglottic stenosis [85].

Bilateral True Vocal Fold Immobility

When true vocal fold immobility is bilateral, treatment is aimed at widening the glottis. Multiple procedures, both open and endoscopic, have been employed, and all have met with variable success. Currently accepted techniques, both open and endoscopic, are aimed at widening the posterior glottis and preserving the integrity of the membranous glottis for voice. Microlaryngoscopic techniques and the CO_2 laser are well suited for this task [86]. Total arytenoidectomy remains the gold standard technique. Success, however, has been reported with other procedures, including posterior cordotomy [87,88] and medial arytenoidectomy [89].

The technique of lasery arytenoidectomy is as follows. Use of the posterior commissure laryngoscope aids in exposing the arytenoid cartilage. After exposure of the posterior commissure, the mucoperichondrium overlying the corniculate cartilage is vaporized, exposing the underlying cartilage. With the laser in the repeat mode (0.1 s) at 2,000 W/cm^2, the corniculate cartilage is vaporized. Next, the mucoperichondrium overlying the apex and upper body of the arytenoid cartilage is vaporized, followed by the vaporization of the apex and upper body. Thereafter, the mucoperichondrium overlying the lower body of the arytenoid is ablated, followed by the vaporization of the lower body of the arytenoid itself (Fig. 5). The lateral ligament is transected, and the cricoid cartilage is exposed. Next, the mucoperichondrium over the vocal process and most of the remaining muscular process are vaporized. Then, the vocal process with an adjacent portion of vocalis muscle and the muscular process up to, but not including, the attachment of the arytenoideus muscle is vaporized. Care must be taken to prevent injury to the mucosa of the interarytenoid cleft. Following this step, a small area lateral to the vocalis muscle is vaporized to help in lateralization of the vocal cord during the healing by secondary intention (Fig. 6).

With regard to the techniques of posterior cordotomy and medial arytenoidectomy, the CO_2 or KTP laser can be used to incise the vocal fold at the junction of the vocal process or shave the medical surface of the arytenoid body, respectively. These techniques can be employed either unilaterally or bilaterally to gain an adequate airway. Their use does not preclude eventual arytenoidectomy if later required to further improve the glottic airway. The reader should be cautioned that any procedure designed to statically open the glottis to improve air flow will, by necessity, decrease voicing. In this respect, rehabilitation of the glottis for air passage is a compromise ac-

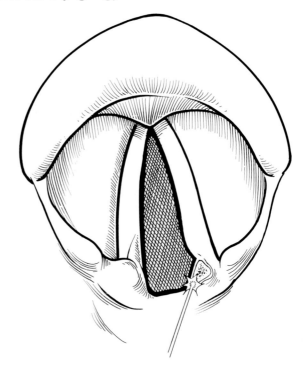

Fig. 5. Cartilage of arytenoid is vaporized after mucosa is ablated.

cepted to eliminate the need for tracheostomy in these patients.

Recurrent Respiratory Papillomatosis

The CO_2 laser has become the standard treatment modality for patients with recurrent respiratory papillomatosis. Some surgeons have reported successful treatment results with the KTP laser for this disorder; however, the less predictable depth of penetration and, therefore, increased potential for thermal injury in surrounding normal tissue make it less than ideal [90]. Although the CO_2 laser cannot cure the disease, its greater absorption and decreased scatter potential in laryngeal tissue account for its greater effectiveness in preserving normal laryngeal structures and maintaining a laryngeal airway.

The first CO_2 laser treatment should be directed at removing as much papilloma from one vocal cord as possible and then as much as possible from the other. Care should be taken to preserve a 2–3 mm strut of covering over the anterior part of one vocal cord. The papilloma overlying the true vocal cord should be vaporized to the vocal ligament. Following the initial CO_2 laser removal of papilloma, a planned repeat operation should be performed in ~ 6 weeks. In a series

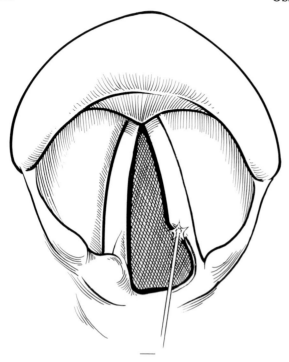

Fig. 6. Lateral vocalis muscle is vaporized to further enlarge the airway.

reported by Ossoff et al. [91], 22 patients underwent 105 CO_2 laser excisions. The intraoperative soft tissue complication rate was zero. The delayed soft tissue complication rate, consisting of two patients with slight true vocal fold scarring and one patient with a small posterior web, was 13.6%. This compares favorably with other published complication rates of 28.7% and 45% [92,93]. The development of the microsubglottiscope allows binocular inspection and has facilitated the treatment of subglottic and cervical extension of respiratory papillomatosis [82].

Two further considerations regarding the treatment of recurrent respiratory papillomatosis are worthy of mention. First, considerable attention has been given to the possible detection of papilloma virus in the laser plume. Conflicting reports exist on both sides of the issue [94,95]. We have treated both surgeons and anesthesiologists for the disease that was manifest only after clinical exposure. Current recommendations to lessen the potential risk of exposure include the use of adequate smoke evacuation and high filtration face masks. The second issue is the management of patients who require multiple laser laryngoscopies for excision on a frequent basis. Treatment intervals then can be based on the rate of reexpression. There are a number of adult and

pediatric patients, however, who cannot be placed into clinical remission with this regimen. Therapeutic trials with interferon alpha N-3 have shown no long-term benefit of administration. A more recent investigation with interferon alpha N-1, however, seems to show more promise in producing remission after a 3–6-month drug trial [96].

Polypoid Degeneration

The treatment of patients with polypoid degeneration includes preoperative and postoperative voice therapy. The patient also should be advised to stop using any laryngeal irritants such as smoking products and alcoholic beverages. For extensive polypoid degeneration that does not resolve with these conservative measures, surgical excision is indicated. The preferred technique involves the elevation of a laryngeal microflap. Gentle medial traction is placed on the polypoid tissue. An incision is made using the CO_2 laser or a microsickle knife on the superior surface of the true vocal fold just medial to the laryngeal ventricle. A flap of epithelium is elevated from lateral to medial with specialized microsurgical instrumentation, and the mucoid material is suctioned. The redundant epithelium is removed using microscissors. The remaining epithelium is placed over the true vocal fold. The patient needs to be advised that a weak, breathy voice will be present for 6–8 weeks postoperatively. Both true vocal folds can be treated with this technique at the same operation if care is taken to preserve a 2–3-mm cuff of epithelium over one true vocal cord at the anterior commissure.

Granulomas

The initial treatment of granulomas of the larynx is directed at treating gastric reflux and teaching vocal relaxation techniques. If the granuloma persists and dysphonia or airway compromise is present, surgical excision is indicated. The posterior commissure should be exposed using a posterior commissure laryngoscope [97]. The granuloma is grasped, and a large portion is excised using the CO_2 laser in the repeat mode (0.1 s) at 2,000 W/cm². The small remnant of granuloma that remains should be vaporized carefully until the granuloma matrix is encountered. This represents the deep level of the dissection and prevents exposure of the underlying vocal process. Care should be taken to remove as much as possible of the charred, carbonaceous debris [98]. Benjamin and Croxson [99] have noted no difference in recurrence rates when granulomas are excised by conventional microlaryngeal or laser techniques.

Nodules

Voice therapy is the treatment of choice for patients with vocal fold nodules. Excision of the nodule may become necessary for fibrotic nodules and those patients who do not improve with voice therapy and have been compliant. Microsurgical, cold knife, excision techniques are the time tested treatment of choice for this disease. The CO_2 laser can be used; however, the potential risk of increased scaring from thermal injury to surrounding tissue exists. If the CO_2 laser is used, it should be set at the lowest power density necessary to vaporize the nodule. No specimen is obtained when the CO_2 laser is used. The preferred technique involves shaving the nodule with half of the laser beam and allowing the other half to fall on the suction platform. The newer generation microspot micromanipulator also helps to facilitate this technique. An excisional biopsy should be performed when there is a question of the pathology.

Malignant Laryngeal Disease

Patients with T1 glottic carcinoma have been treated with external-beam radiation, laryngofissure and cordectomy (hemilaryngectomy), and endoscopic excision. Hemilaryngectomy has been more commonly reserved for patients with large or bulky cancers involving a mobile true vocal cord. It offers equivalent local control rates to radiation therapy, but it alters the voice to some degree. External-beam radiation is the most commonly prescribed treatment modality for patients with early glottic cancer. Local control rates with this form of therapy are in the range of 90% [70]. Before radiation treatment can be started, a direct laryngoscopy and biopsy are necessary to confirm the diagnosis.

Stutsman and McGavran [100] reported a review of serial sections of specimens from patients who had laryngofissure and cordectomy for T1 glottic carcinoma. They found 11 specimens in which there was no tumor and concluded that the biopsy alone had successfully treated these patients. Lillie and DeSanto [101,102] reported on 57 patients with early squamous cell carcinoma of the true vocal cord managed by endoscopic excision and surgical diathermy. Five of these patients did develop recurrent or second primary tumors, four were successfully retreated by endo-

scopic excision, and the fifth patient had a laryngectomy 8 years after the initial endoscopic excision.

In 1975, Strong [103] reported on 11 patients with T1 glottic carcinoma managed by endoscopic excision with the CO_2 laser. He noted no recurrences in this series of patients. Three of the patients had prior radiation therapy. Blakeslee et al. [104] reported on use of the CO_2 laser in the management of patients with T1 glottic carcinoma. Of the 98 patients presented, 68 were able to be treated by CO_2 laser excision only. Five of these patients required a second endoscopic excision for metachronous tumors. In this group of 68 patients (73 cases), the 3-year absolute survival rate was 88%. The CO_2 laser excision was used alone in 35 patients with successful management in 31 (89%); two patients were salvaged with radiation therapy. Two patients died, one from local disease after laryngectomy and one from carcinoma of the lung 1 year after laryngectomy. Thirty-four patients had endoscopic excision followed by radiation; 29 of these were successfully managed (85%), and five developed recurrent disease that required laryngectomy for attempted salvage. There were two deaths from local disease in this group. Four patients had endoscopic excision followed by partial laryngectomy and all were alive at 3 years without disease (100%).

In 1978, Ossoff et al. [70] began using the CO_2 laser to manage patients with early midcordal T1 glottic cancers. Twenty-five previously untreated patients were selected, and 24 were alive and free of disease at three-year follow-up (96%). One patient died of both local and regional recurrence. Seventeen patients were managed with endoscopic excision alone, and all were free of disease at 3 years (100%). Six patients had excision followed by radiation and all were free of disease at 3 years (100%). Two patients had endoscopic excision followed by partial laryngectomy, and one was free of disease at 3 years (50%).

Use of the CO_2 laser in the endoscopic management of patients with early vocal cord carcinoma offers the advantages of precision, hemostasis, and decreased perioperative edema. The endoscopic CO_2 laser excision of midcordal micro- and mini-cancers can be curative, with rates equal to both radiation therapy and laryngofissure with cordectomy. The major advantage of CO_2 laser excision is the ability to differentiate deeply invasive "early midcordal" T1 glottic cancers from those that are truly superficial in nature. Currently, worrisome lesions are biopsied with a cold knife technique. If a frozen section shows severe dysplasia, carcinoma in situ or carcinoma with microinvasion, a cold knife microflap technique is used to excise the involved mucosa with a 2 mm margin. The deep and lateral margins are inspected. If they are free of disease, the laser can be used on low power settings (1,500 W/cm^2) to vaporize the deeper layers of Reinke's space. If the deep margins are involved with disease, the laser can be used in a focused power setting of 2,000 W/cm^2 to excise a portion of the vocal ligament and underlying vocalis muscle for a deep margin. This technique can be used for lesions involving the membranous vocal folds. However, when invasive lesions are present near the anterior commissure or encroaching in the vocal process, partial laryngectomy or radiation therapy is recommended secondary to enhanced lymphatic drainage from these areas and anatomic difficulty in obtaining adequate margins. The need for further treatment will be apparent in cases with deep cancer invasion. The CO_2 laser excisional biopsy can be used repeatedly and does not interfere with further treatment.

Complications of Laser Laryngoscopy

Most laser surgery of the larynx can be highly efficacious and safe as demonstrated by Healy et al. [105]. A complication rate of 0.2% (9 complications in a total of 4,416 patients) can be expected when the appropriate precautions are taken. A similar low complication rate has been reported by Ossoff et al. [106], who noted 12 complications in 204 patients involving all types of CO_2 laser surgery. None of the untoward events were life-threatening; they consisted of six laser-related problems and two minor injuries to OR staff and the remaining complications related to the laryngeal suspension system. Of the six laser-related patient injuries, one was secondary to retained metallic tape in the oropharynx, one was secondary to perichondritis with posterior laryngeal web formation, there was one laser burn of a tooth, and there were two instances of postoperative airway obstruction (one due to edema and one due to a retained pharyngeal pack).

Unfortunately, this experience is not universal, and a survey of one of the senior otolaryngology societies was reported by Fried [73]. Out of 229 questionnaires mailed, a response of 92% was obtained. Of the physicians who responded, 49% had used the laser without complications. An additional 27% did not use the laser at all at the time of the survey. The remaining 49 physicians

had a total of 81 complications. The most frequent was endotracheal explosion, with facial burns being the next most common occurrence. Five cases of pneumothorax and two of subcutaneous emphysema also were reported. Facial burns occurred nine times, and laryngeal subglottic or tracheal stenoses were reported in eight patients. Moreover, it was noted that increased experience with the laser did not necessarily guarantee fewer complications. The greater number of cases performed, the more likely a complication is to occur.

Laser complications directly related to impact from the laser include the most serious of all complications, which is the ignition of the endotracheal tube [73,107–113]. This can occur when the laser acts on the external surface of an unprotected tube or in the dehiscence of a poorly wrapped tube. Combustible items such as a dry cottonoid can be ignited as well. Perforation of the airway with a pneumothorax and subcutaneous emphysema also has been experienced [114].

Secondary laser effect results from tissue alteration as a consequence of the laser or laser instrumentation. Ignition of an endotracheal tube from insufflated tissue entering into the lumen of the tube and causing internal combustion is such an event. An endotracheal tube also may be obstructed by the lasered tissue [115]. Mucosal charring with subsequent airway obstruction as well as hemorrhage, edema, and perichondritis can occur as well [116,117]. The laser beam itself may be reflected off the wall of the laryngoscope either externally or internally, producing subsequent mucosal burns.

Delayed effects that occur because of the surgical procedure include webs of the vocal cord, laryngeal or tracheal stenosis, and glottic incompetence due to excessive tissue removal. This latter situation occurs particularly after removal of a vocal cord carcinoma or arytenoidectomy [118].

Prevention of Complications

The best method of prevention is adequate preparation. It is imperative that all members of the surgical team, including nurses and the anesthesiologist, be familiar with the laser and contingency plans if complications should occur (e.g., endotracheal tube ignition). Equipment should be checked, and the aiming and CO_2 laser beams should be aligned at the outset of each case. The endotracheal tube and its wrapping should be tested. Steroids should be administered to prevent laryngeal edema. All members of the OR staff as well as the patient should have adequate eye protection. The all metal endotracheal tube with saline placed in the distal cuff has been very safe for both CO_2 and KTP laser procedures.

Certain precuations must be taken when performing CO_2 laser surgery. First, to reduce the risk of ocular damage, the patient's eyes should be protected by a double layer of moistened eye pads, and all operating personnel should wear protective glasses. Second, all the patient's exposed skin in the immediate area of the surgical field should be protected by a double layer of moistened surgical towels. Intraoperative cardiac monitoring is necessary, since the procedure may be prolonged and cardiac arrhythmias may be stimulated [119].

The surgeon should use binocular vision whenever possible and keep the laser in the center of the operative field. This avoids reflection off the side of the laryngoscope and allows for increased surgical precision. If, however, the surgical field must encompass more than visualized with the laryngoscope, both the laser and endoscope should be repositioned before lasering is continued. All lasered tissues should be removed so that no char forms. This will prevent excessive tissue damage. Hemorrhage should be controlled. Protection should be afforded to the vocal cord not being operated on. This can be done with cord protectors that are commercially available. This prevents the complication of anterior commissure webbing. Circumferential lasering should be avoided at all costs, since this will lead to laryngeal stenosis. A surgeon must be mindful of the characteristics of the tissue lasered. Vocal cord, tumor, and cartilage have different appearances during lasering. This can be used to the surgeon's advantage to assess the depth of penetration as well as the location within the larynx. Naturally, evacuation of vapor and plume is mandatory for visualization [120]. It should be remembered, however, that difficulties with use of the laser can be avoided if the age-old dictum of adequate preparation, knowledge of the capabilities of the instrumentation, and meticulous techniques are adhered to.

Limitations of Laser Laryngoscopy

Prior to any surgical procedure, the surgeon must consider whether the laser is the best method to treat a particular laryngeal disorder. As noted earlier, such entities as vocal nodules may require no therapy whatsoever. Although the laser is a highly precise instrument, when used in conjunction with the operating microscope, thermal injury, and carbonaceous debris may stimulate submucosal fibrosis that may be unacceptable in certain types of patients, as in the professional voice user. Numerous methods such as the use of forceps or microscissors have withstood the test of time and yield similar results. Moreover, the surgeon must be aware that the laser may not be functional on the particular day of surgery, and alternative plans should be available.

If indeed the laser is felt to be the optimal method of treatment, limitations may be imposed by the patient's particular anatomic configuration. Mandible size and position as well as spinal column flexibility may limit the type of laryngoscope that can be utilized and thereby affect visualization of the larynx. Patients with cervical arthritis, retrognathia, prominent teeth, or hypertrophy of the base of the tongue may be difficult candidates for endoscopy. Patients with ischemic cardiovascular disease may not withstand the prolonged laryngoscopic suspension that stimulates the vagus nerve and may produce subsequent cardiac arrhythmias as well as silent myocardial infarctions. Even in ideal circumstances, laser laryngoscopy may require more time to complete than other surgical techniques. For example, the patient with unstable cardiac disease suspected of having a laryngeal tumor may well best be treated with operative visualization and biopsy by conventional techniques rather than with use of the laser [117].

Patients with chronic obstructive or restrictive pulmonary disease may be difficult to ventilate. In such situations, an endotracheal tube may be mandatory and by its presence may limit laryngeal visualization and access.

BRONCHOSCOPY
Indications

Currently, CO_2 laser bronchoscopy is indicated in the evaluation, treatment, and palliation of multiple disease processes. These include recurrent respiratory papillomatosis, tracheal and bronchial stenosis, acute tracheal and bronchial granulation tissue formation, tracheal membranous webs, and palliation of selected tracheal or bronchial tumors. The surgical techniques used in the treatment of these processes usually involve insertion of the endoscope to the most distal portion of the lesion and an excision or vaporization in a retrograde fashion. Technique, however, may vary and is discussed individually for each lesion as well as the relative indications and contraindications for each disease process.

Recurrent Respiratory Papillomatosis

Recurrent respiratory papillomatosis is a virally mediated disease that affects the upper aerodigestive tract. The virus induces the formation of papillarylike projections that interfere with vocal and respiratory function. It is a mucosal process without deep invasion. Treatment therefore is aimed at removal of the mucosal lesion with minimal injury to the surrounding tissue. The CO_2 laser with its tissue interaction characteristics is well suited to the treatment of this disease. Difficulty, however, arises secondary to the recurrent nature of the disease process. Studies by Pignatari et al. [121] showed that the viral particle is frequently identified in asymptomatic tissue surrounding the symptomatic lesions. This makes ablation of all viral particles impossible and leads to the recurrent nature of the disease.

Tracheal and bronchial disease require treatment with the CO_2 endoscopic coupler for the bronchoscope. Technically the endoscope is inserted in the tracheal bronchial tree. Lesions are visualized with the aid of a bronchoscopic telescope with a 0° and/or 30° angled lens. Starting at the most distal portion of the most distal lesion, lesions are biopsied or vaporized as necessary. Care must be taken not to circumferentially denude tracheal or bronchial mucosa. This will result in cicatricial scarring and airway stenosis. Fortunately, the majority of symptomatic lesions are not confluent and areas of mucosa can be spared between lesions to lessen scar formation. Unnecessarily deep removal will also encourage scarring.

Multiple-stage endoscopies are required for surveillance and palliation. Initially we find it beneficial to perform these endoscopies on a 6-week interval basis. This is continued until good disease control has been achieved. Interval endoscopic evaluations can then be lengthened to 3–6 months depending on the rate of viral expression. Multiple trials with acyclovir and alpha interferon have been undertaken to determine if chemotherapy may provide an alternative or improved form of therapy. Studies with acyclovir indicate no substantial benefit for use in treatment of recurrent respiratory papillomatosis [122]. Interferon therapy has met with limited success. Recommendations are made that only patients with life threatening recurrent respiratory papillomatosis or those requiring surgery more frequently than every 4–6 weeks, may benefit from administration from beta interferon [96].

Tracheal Stenosis

The addition of the CO_2 laser to the endoscopic treatment of tracheal stenosis is a logical application of laser technology. Tissue interaction principles of the laser can be used to facilitate hemostasis in excision or vaporization of endoluminal scar.

The etiology of tracheal stenosis is varied. An exhaustive discussion of the topic is beyond the scope of this review. However, a review of multiple small series of patients indicates that acquired tracheal stenosis from prior endotracheal intubation is probably the most common etiology [74,123–127]. The second most common etiology is prior tracheal surgery. This includes both tracheostomy and tracheal resection [74,124–126], followed by congenital lesions.

Treatment of tracheal stenosis by endoscopic CO_2 laser bronchoscopy has resulted in a success rate of 34% [75] to 77% [124]. This has led surgeons to try to identify factors that are associated with a good endoscopic treatment prognosis. Simpson et al. [75] found that scarring with cicatricial contraction, scarring wider than 1 cm in the vertical dimension, previous history of severe bacterial infection and tracheomalacia with loss of cartilaginous support were associated with poor outcome after attempted endoscopic management. Ossoff et al. [69] confirmed these observations and added carinal involvement to the list of poor prognostic indicators.

Preoperative assessments consisting of history, physical examination, flexible office endoscopy, and radiographic evaluation are imperative before initiation of treatment. Radiographic evaluation with computerized tomography or magnetic resonance imaging will help to identify the condition or involvement of the tracheal cartilage. The endoscopic approach is only appropriate for lesions consisting of endoluminal scar tissue. Endoscopic treatment begins with staging endoscopy to characterize the width, length, and circumferential involvement of the stenosis. In addition, evaluation under negative pressure ventilation is essential to determine the presence or absence of tracheomalacia. This can be performed with either flexible or rigid endoscopy. Once the stenosis has been characterized and the stenotic lesion determined appropriate for laser endoscopic treatment, therapy can begin. Again, as in papilloma, the endoscope is advanced to the most distal aspect of the stenosis. The area is dilated to allow manipulation and the CO_2 laser is used to excise scar tissue. Care must be taken to avoid circumferential mucosal excision as this will lead to worsening contracture. No more than 180° of the lumen is treated at one time. Staged endoscopies can be performed at 4-week intervals. This allows adequate time for remucosalization of the previously excised segment.

In the small series reported by Simpson et al. [75], an average of six endoscopic procedures were required prior to successful relief of obstruction. Long-term follow-up is not available. Ossoff et al. [69] reported on a multiinstitutional assessment of CO_2 laser bronchoscopic therapy of tracheal stenosis. This review covered a 9-month period from September 1982 to June 1983. Twenty-three patients underwent 48 procedures for the treatment of tracheal stenosis. Seventeen of the 23 patients improved with therapy. Eleven of these 17 had in-dwelling tracheostomies at the time of treatment and five of these 11 were eventually decanulated. The other six showed improvement. Six patients were minimally amenable to laser treatment as the initial endoscopy either revealed cicatricial scar or loss of tracheal cartilage with tracheomalacia. In 1989, Shapshay et al. [74] reported on five patients with tracheal and/or subglottic stenosis. Four of these five patients were successfully improved with CO_2 laser bronchoscopy. The fifth patient underwent Nd:YAG bronchoscopy with only minimal improvement. This patient was not treated with the CO_2 laser at the time of reporting.

Granulation Tissue

Tracheal obstruction caused by granulation tissue is amenable to CO_2 laser bronchoscopic resection. Granulation tissue, a reaction to inflammation, is a mass of chronic inflammatory cells with a fibrous matrix. The inciting process can be induced by the tip of the endotracheal tube, tracheotomy tube, from over vigorous suctioning through an endotracheal tube with a traumatic catheter or from over inflation of a respiratory tube cuff. Overinflation produces a shearing force on the tracheal mucosa during movement and can lead to mucosal membrane necrosis or disruption [128].

The chronic inflammation induced by membrane disruption and localized bacterial overgrowth often progresses to perichondritis. This results in perichondrial inflammation with disruption of the blood supply to the cartilage, cartilage resorption, and tracheal collapse. Tracheal granulation tissue should therefore be treated promptly with antibiotics. Failure to achieve a response with antibiotic therapy or progression of the granulation tissue to respiratory compromise may necessitate endoscopy for the removal of the obstructing lesion. Endoscopy is aimed at excision of the lesion with relief of tracheal obstruction and decrease in the tracheal bacterial wound count. Work by Healy [129] suggests improved results in the treatment of tracheal or subglottic stenosis can be achieved when antibiotics are used prophylactically. The importance of the surgical excision of granulation tissue is, therefore, to decrease the bacterial colonization, improve the responsiveness of the infection to systemic antibiotics, and thereby decrease the risk of perichondritis and endotracheal collapse.

As in papilloma, during the excision of granulation tissue by CO_2 laser bronchoscopy, the endoscope is inserted to the most distal portion of the most distal lesion. Excision and/or vaporization is undertaken in a retrograde fashion. Again, care must be taken to avoid circumferential mucosal excision as this will result in cicatricial scar formation and permanent stenosis. Often, staged excisions are necessary to prevent cicatricial scarring. These can be performed at 2–4 week intervals with intervening dilations as necessary to maintain an airway. If possible, tracheostomy should be avoided as this will increase the likelihood of bacterial colonization, and may increase the rate of perichondritis and eventual tracheomalacia [130]. Tracheostomy, however, was not found to be a significant limiting factor to the successful treatment of tracheal stenosis by Ossoff et al. [69]. They found the laser to be particularly useful in the treatment of tracheal granulation tissue and were successful in the treatment of four of four lesions by endoscopic methods. The patients each underwent an average of 1.5 procedures. Beamis, et al. [131] also found the CO_2 laser particularly useful for the excision of tracheal granulation tissue because it is an excellent cutting tool and vaporizes tissue adequately.

Weblike Stenoses

The treatment of tracheal weblike stenoses with the CO_2 laser has been well documented [69,74]. This has been described for use in both the subglottis and trachea. Weblike stenoses are thin, < 1 cm in width, and circumferential. The most common etiology remains previous intubation, and good results can be achieved with laser radial incision and dilation.

Technically, the endoscope is inserted to the lesion. Incisions are made at the 12, 3, 6, and 9 o'clock positions. The bronchoscope is then passed through the incised area of stenosis and rotated 90° from maximal dilation. Often, multiple procedures are required for maintenance of the airway lumen. Using this technique, Shapshay et al. [74] were successful in treating five patients with moderate to severe subglottic and tracheal stenosis. Three of these patients required more than one endoscopic procedure. Ossoff et al. [69] were also successful in treating four of four patients with weblike tracheal stenosis. They required, however, an average of two procedures per patient.

Obstructing Tracheal Malignancy

The treatment of obstructing endobronchial malignant lesions poses a challenge to the bronchologist. Their disease is often recurrent and the pulmonary and medical condition poor. Yet, the symptoms of tracheal bronchial obstruction are severe and palliation to prevent death from suffocation is necessary. Bronchoscopic therapy provides an excellent option for relief of obstruction with relatively minimal morbidity.

As the CO_2 laser was the first laser available to bronchologists, it was the first laser used for the palliation of these lesions. Surgeons, however, quickly found that the vascularity of these tumors made the CO_2 laser less than ideal. Resections were difficult and tedious. Because of the previously mentioned absorptive spectrum of the CO_2 laser, hemostasis is achieved only in blood vessels < 0.5 mm in diameter. The Nd:YAG laser, however, is preferentially absorbed by pigmented tissue, and therefore deeper penetration produces better hemostasis. The majority of surgeons now prefer the Nd:YAG laser for treatment of malignant endobronchial lesions.

Shapshay et al. [132] compared their experience in the endoscopic treatment of tracheal and bronchial malignancies with the CO_2 and Nd:YAG lasers. Of 506 operations performed on 273 patients, they found the Nd:YAG laser to be preferable over the CO_2 laser secondary to improved hemorrhage control. In addition, they were able to use telescopic visualization with the Nd:YAG laser through a rigid bronchoscope, whereas this was not possible with the closed CO_2 laser system.

It is worth noting that they often used the flexible fiberoptic bronchoscope through the open rigid bronchoscope. The open scope served as a conduit for both the laser and the telescope. It also served as a port for the removal of necrotic and excised tumor. Nd:YAG laser bronchoscopy is currently the treatment of choice for the palliation of malignant lesions.

Contraindications

Because of precise tissue interaction and the relatively minimal morbidity of endoscopic CO_2 laser surgery, there are only three contraindications to its use. (1) Patients with circumferential stenosis of the trachea wider than 1 cm in length will probably have unfavorable results [69,74]. Therefore, endoscopic management of these patients should be limited to the initial diagnostic procedure. (2) The second contraindication to CO_2 laser bronchoscopy is tracheomalacia. In patients suffering from tracheal stenosis caused by tracheomalacia or loss of tracheal cartilaginous support, use of the laser bronchoscope can be dangerous. It may result in perforation of the trachea wall with subsequent mediastinitis or rupture of a great vessel. This complication obviously can be devastating. (3) In patients with airway obstruction caused by extrinsic compression of the tracheobronchial tree, there is no amenable form of endoscopic treatment.

LASER-ASSISTED UVULO-PALATOPLASTY

The laser-assisted uvulo-palatoplasty (LAUP) is a technique developed by Dr. Yves-Victor Kamami in Paris, France, in the late 1980s [133] and introduced to the United States in 1992 (JAC), where it has continued to grow in popularity. The procedure is designed to correct snoring caused by airway obstruction and soft tissue vibration at the level of the soft palate by reducing the amount of tissue in the velum and uvula. The procedure is performed over several stages and is performed in an ambulatory setting under local anesthesia.

At the present time the procedure is being looked at very closely by several institutions to determine its place in the treatment of patients with obstructive sleep apnea. The author has preliminary results that show that the place of this procedure in the treatment of sleep apnea patients is very similar to that of the uvulo-palatopharyngoplasty. This procedure does have the advantage that most of the morbidity associated with the uvulo-palatopharyngoplasty is not encountered.

Description Of Procedure

The patient is evaluated completely to determine the degree of severity of airway obstruction during sleep. If one is to consider surgical correction of snoring, a complete evaluation of the patient for sleep apnea should be made and this should include some kind of testing. Apnea cannot be ruled out on the basis of history and physical appearance alone [134,135]. If the patient is found to have apnea, treatment of this condition is mandatory.

One can consider this the equivalent to a dental procedure; so if the patient needs subacute bacterial endocarditis (SBE) prophylaxis, it will need to be administered in conjunction with this procedure. The procedure is performed with the patient sitting in an exam chair in the upright position. A local anesthetic is administered.

The procedure is performed using a CO_2 laser. The CO_2 laser was selected because of its familiarity to most practicing otolaryngologists-head and neck surgeons, as well as its availability to otolaryngologists in the outpatient clinic and office settings. It is a very precise tool insofar as its ability to give very fine incisions, and its tissue interaction is favorable for this type of procedure. Although it is not the best coagulating laser available, it has adequate coagulation for the diameter of most vessels encountered with this procedure. The CO_2 laser is used at a power setting of between 15 and 20 watts in a continuous mode. The beam is used focused for cutting and defocused for ablation and vaporization. A handpiece with a backstop to protect the posterior pharyngeal wall from stray laser energy should be used.

Once the adequate level of anesthesia has been achieved in the soft palate, the CO_2 laser is then used to make bilateral vertical incisions through and through the palate at the base of the uvula (Fig. 7). The length of the backstop on the laser handpiece is the gauge for incision length. The uvula is then reduced by ~ 50% of its length and is reshaped in a curved fashion, as a normal uvula would be shaped (Fig. 8). One can retract the tip of the uvula anteriorly and vaporize the central portion of the uvula muscle while leaving the mucosa intact (Fig. 9). This may result in less postoperative pain. Once this has been accomplished, the procedure is finished.

Vaporization may also be accomplished by an instrument called a "Swiftlase" (Sharplan Lasers,

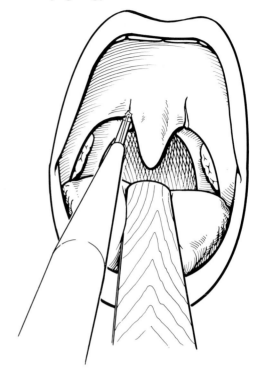

Fig. 7. A through and through incision is made in the palate on each side of the uvula.

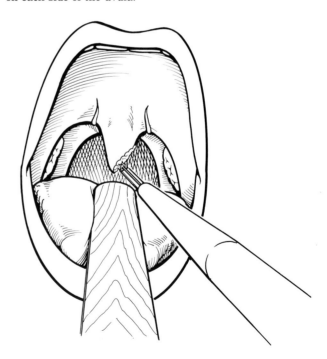

Fig. 8. The uvula is reduced by vaporization.

Allendale, NJ), used in a focused mode and at the same power setting. This instrument rapidly rotates the beam in a 3 mm arch, thus producing less char while ablating the tissue more rapidly.

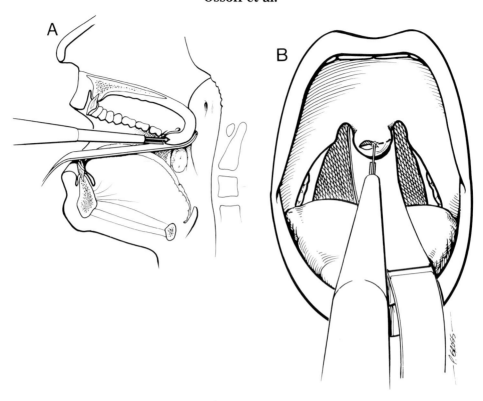

Fig. 9. The center of the uvula is ablated to reduce the tissue bulk.

Postoperative Period

When the patient returns to the clinic, he or she is requested to report on amount of pain, any changes in voice or swallowing, and bleeding and infection. Subjective improvements in sleep are also elicited, as well as any objective changes in snoring. In general, the patients are seen at the time of their next procedure, which is generally within 4 weeks.

Subsequent Procedures

The palate is allowed to heal over the next 3–4 weeks. Subsequent procedures are basically the same as the initial procedure. Nearing the completion of the treatment course, the palate must be examined to determine if attention is needed in other areas. As the retraction occurs, the palate will come anteriorly and superiorly, and this may tether the posterior tonsillar pillars, causing them to medialize. Should this occur and the pillars themselves begin to obstruct the airway, they can be released by making a horizontal incision at the superior aspect of the pillar, through and through the pillar, thus releasing it (Fig. 10). If the tonsils are still present, they can

be superficially vaporized after first anesthetizing this surface.

One may also find that vaporizing lateral to the incision in a crescent-shape manner prevents some of the side-to-side healing that would tend to take place in the palate with just simple through and through incisions (Fig. 11). By reducing side to side healing, more retracting of the palate occurs and this, over the course of the treatment sessions, will reduce the number of sessions necessary to achieve the end result.

Determination of Endpoint

The endpoint for this procedure is determined by any one or combination of the following factors. (1) The patient is satisfied. This occurs when the obstruction is relieved to the extent that the patient's snoring is decreased and the patient does not wish to proceed with any further procedures. As this is an elective procedure, this is a legitimate point at which to stop. (2) The snoring is gone. (3) The patient is unable to make any snorting sound. If the patient still has noisy breathing but is unable to make a snorting sound, this should alert the surgeon that the patient is

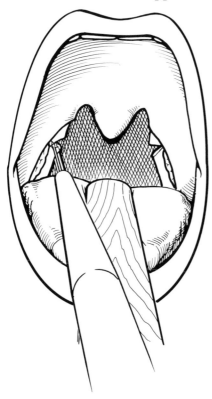

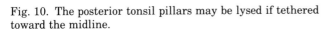

Fig. 10. The posterior tonsil pillars may be lysed if tethered toward the midline.

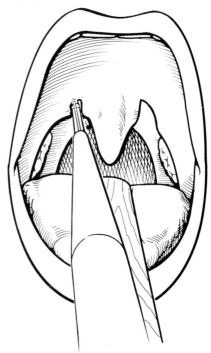

Fig. 11. Crescent-shape ablations are used to further open the airway in a lateral direction.

having noisy breathing from other tissue vibrating, such as in the region of the base of the tongue, and not necessarily at the soft palate. Any further resection of the soft palate after the patient is no longer able to snort will run the risk of excising too much tissue and creating velo-pharyngeal incompetence.

Complications

The complication rate for this procedure has been extremely low. There has been some postoperative bleeding in the immediate post-op period, but it has responded to silver nitrate cauterization.

Permanent voice changes, velopharngeal insufficiency, temporary or permanent nasal reflux, and dehydration from the inability to take food or liquid orally have not been seen with this procedure.

Although there is pain associated with the procedure, it has not been of an incapacitating nature, and all patients have been able to attend classes or work in their normal routine. Most patients have reported some degree of weight loss, the maximum being between 10–15 pounds over

the course of the treatment. In most of our patients, this has been a desirable side effect.

Progression of Relief

The progression of relief is such that one often sees a decrease in the subjective symptoms before seeing a change in the objective symptoms. Usually after the first or second procedures, patients begin to feel that they are sleeping better and they are better rested when they awaken in the morning; their spouses will very often notice an improvement in mood. On the subsequent procedures, one will start to see a decrease in the amount of snoring sounds, to the point that by the third or fourth procedure the snoring has been almost virtually eliminated. Couples who have been sleeping apart are usually back in the same bedroom by the end of the third procedure.

PEDIATRIC OTOLARYNGOLOGY

The use of lasers in the field of pediatric otolaryngology has expanded due to engineering and technical refinements in the lasers and delivery systems. Most applications of lasers within adult otolaryngology are now found within the subspecialty of pediatric otolaryngology. Children, however, cannot be visualized as just "tiny adults."

They possess unique anatomic and pathological differences. Smaller anatomy necessitates smaller and consequently more precise instrumentation and greater precision of thermal effect. Unique differences in the way pediatric tissue heals have also necessitated modifications of those techniques used in adults.

The use of lasers in the field of pediatric otolaryngology may be subdivided into four anatomic regions or applications: (1) glottic/airway, (2) oral/oropharynx, (3) cutaneous, and (4) nasal applications. Developments in each of these anatomic regions have generally followed closely on the discovery of new applications in adults. A different healing process present in children has dictated the development of different techniques for cutaneous laser applications when compared to adults.

The lasers finding general and specific applications within pediatric otolaryngology are the CO_2, Nd:YAG, dye, KTP, and argon lasers. The desired thermal effect for each potential application dictates the selection of laser. As a general rule, many oral and oropharyngeal applications would use a laser with a deeper thermocoagulation to allow sealing of the vessels in this region. Applications in the glottis and airway would generally require a more precise thermal control and, therefore, are usually accomplished with the CO_2 laser. These are general guidelines; the appropriate selection of laser is dependent upon the pathological process to be treated.

Laser units with pulse durations as short as 0.01 s are highly desirable, especially for glottic applications where thermal spread to the underlying vocalis ligament in the true vocal folds is to be minimized. In addition, CO_2 laser units that employ a yellow aiming beam have facilitated visualization down long target path length, such as the rigid ventilating bronchoscope. Many laser units employ a red aiming beam, which may be seen at a distance of 250 mm in a 4 mm ventilating bronchoscope, but from an operating standpoint, a yellow aiming beam is more advantageous.

The microspot micro-manipulator developed for the CO_2 laser has been one of the most important developments in extending the applications of the CO_2 laser in pediatric otolaryngology. The microspot micro-manipulator allows a 250-μm focal spotsize at 400 mm. This is less than 1/3 the size of the first-generation micromanipulator spotsizes. In addition, the newer microspot micromanipulators utilize a "hot mirror" technology, which allows the surgeon to direct the CO_2 beam coincident with the optical path from the microscope [72]. With the use of the microspot micromanipulator, the beam may now be directed down as small a laryngoscope as a 3 mm subglottoscope while providing the surgeon with binocular vision.

CO_2 laser bronchoscopes are now available with internal diameters of as small as 3 mm and external diameters as small as 7.2 mm. This has extended the application of CO_2 laser bronchoscopy to younger individuals with the caveat that a subglottic opening of greater than 7.2 mm is required. For children with a subglottic diameter smaller than this, the neonatal subglottoscope may offer exposure to the cervical trachea with diameters down to $\sim$ 5 mm. Bronchoscopic application in children with tracheas smaller than this is limited to those situations where a laser fiber from an argon or KTP laser may be placed down the side channel of a ventilating bronchoscope.

The small spotsize on the microspot micromanipulator has allowed development of the technique of micro trapdoor flap procedures. With this technique, the mucosa is preserved while scar or lesions that are deep are removed.

The Nd:YAG laser functions at a wavelength that provides deep thermal coagulation. This has allowed its use for vascular lesions and selected hemangiomas. The development of contact fibers for the Nd:YAG laser has been particularly useful for oral cavity work, such as tongue resection. The use of the laser provides adequate coagulation while allowing very precise cutting. These contact fibers are now available for the KTP and argon lasers and have found similar applications in the oral cavity.

The KTP laser has been used with a bare fiber in both the contact mode and a noncontact mode for laser tonsillectomy. It has been found to be very effective in the noncontact mode for those patients with documented bleeding disorders. The KTP laser now also has a dye module, which may be attached to the laser to allow its use for cutaneous photocoagulation of pigmented lesions, such as port wine stains. The flashlamp excited dye laser operating at 582 nm has been especially effective treating port wine stains in children. The older technique of photocoagulation of port-wine stains with shorter wavelengths (below 540 nm) often resulted in excessive scarring for children under 12 years of age. The use of the dye laser has not been associated with as high an incidence of untoward scarring. Both the KTP and the argon laser have been used in limited applications for airway lesions, such as obstructing tumors or granulation tissue in the trachea and bronchi, where the CO_2 laser could not be used. The argon laser also has found application within the field of otology but is not in general use for this within pediatric otolaryngology.

Glottic/Airway Applications

Lasers in pediatrics have found their most widespread applications within the glottis and the airway. Paralleling the use of the CO_2 laser in adults, this laser was also used for children. Laryngoscopes were developed to fit the smaller pediatric anatomy, and the laser is now considered the standard of care for treatment of such lesions as recurrent respiratory papillomatosis. The laser is used for the removal or marsupialization of cysts, coagulation of hemangiomas, and removal of other obstructive lesions such as granulation tissue [136–142]. In addition, with development of the micro trapdoor flaps and the microspot micromanipulator, the CO_2 laser is now used for the treatment of tracheal and glottic stenosis, as well as anterior and posterior glottic webs [78,80,81].

The CO_2 ventilating bronchoscope allows the use of the laser in the distal trachea and bronchi in patients in whom their size is large enough to admit insertion of the bronchoscope. In patients smaller than this, the lasers that are capable of being delivered by fiberoptics may be used down the side channel of a smaller ventilating bronchoscope [143,144].

Oral Cavity/Oropharynx

Although the CO_2 laser is very good at vaporization of tissue, many of the lesions occurring in the oral cavity and oropharynx are very vascular with blood vessels somewhat larger than that capable of being sealed by the CO_2 laser. Therefore, those lasers that allow deeper thermal coagulation have found more applications in the oral cavity.

Tongue resections are especially amenable to the use of the laser. Both contact and noncontact fiberoptic delivery of the argon, KTP, and Nd:YAG lasers may be used in various pathologic conditions of the tongue. One advantage of the use of the laser over that of the electrocautery system is the lack of musculature artefact and motion. We have found the contact fibers to be especially useful for removal of ranula because the lack of motion artefact with the electrocautery allows a more precise dissection while maintaining the cyst wall in many cases. Base of tongue lesions often are very vascular, and although the CO_2 has been used with success, the contact and noncontact modes of the argon, KTP, and Nd:YAG lasers have proven very clinically effective.

Tonsillectomy has been performed using all the major medical lasers, including the CO_2 laser. However, because of the vascularity involved, lasers providing slightly deeper thermo-coagulation are more accepted. A counterpoint is that whereas the procedure may in fact be done using the laser, except in those cases of documented bleeding tendencies such as hemophilia or von Willebrand's disease, the laser is not economically justified.

Cutaneous Applications

As noted earlier, the healing following cutaneus photocoagulations of lesions in children proceeds differently than that in adults. This has led to the development of the newer dye lasers. Their use for the treatment of portwine stains and vascular hemangiomas has been very effective.

Nasal Applications

The use of lasers in endoscopic sinus surgery and in turbinate reduction has not generally expanded into the pediatric realm. The more difficult anatomy and the proximity to vital structures have justified a very cautious exploration of the use of lasers in this region.

There have been many reports of the use of the CO_2 laser in the treatment of choanal stenosis. Technically, it is difficult to use the CO_2 laser in a very small child in whom one would be repairing a choanal stenosis. The overall surgical results have not been significantly better than traditional approaches. Therefore, laser repair of choanal stenosis has not been popularized within pediatric otolaryngology.

OTOLOGY

The first application of lasers in otology was reported in 1967. Sataloff [5] attempted to use a neodymium glass laser for stapedotomy. In vitro work was initially promising but was not extended to clinical applications. Since that time, investigations into the use of the argon, KTP, and CO_2 lasers have led to their practical use within otology and in specific circumstances. Experimental investigations in the use of the erbium YAG (Er:YAG) and Ho:YAG are currently in progress.

Considerable controversy still exists in the field as to which laser is the most appropriate for use in otology, with each having its proponents [145,146]. The controversy can generally be summed up as a concern for thermal effect propagation near the facial nerve or through the stapes footplate into the saccule. Despite experimental evidence of saccular damage with the use of the argon laser in cats, clinically the argon, KTP, and CO_2 lasers have all found applications in stapedotomy [50,147–149]. Case reports of large series of patients have not demonstrated any damage to the vestibulare system.

In theory, the CO_2 laser is highly absorbed by water and should not propagate very deeply into the vestibule after penetrating the stapes. This, indeed, has been found to be the case, but the converse of propagation of the argon and KTP lasers into the vestibule has not been borne out on clinical experience. One explanation is that the use of the optical fibers with the argon and KTP laser has a significantly high divergence after the beam has exited the fiber and, therefore, is not concentrated in any one region. As the fibers are used in close apposition to the footplate and the divergence rapidly falls off as the distance from the fiber is increased, the thermal effect is not seen clinically.

The engineering requirements in the use of the CO_2, argon, and KTP lasers have also generated some controversy. The CO_2 laser must be attached to the micromanipulator by an articulated arm assembly. The micromanipulator must be of a microspot type without parallax error aiming. Despite this, the exact point of focus between the helium neon aiming light and the CO_2 beam is often not coincident. In addition, the use of the microspot micromanipulator on the operating microscope necessitates use of a longer focal length lens (300 mm) and modification of the draping technique on the microscope. The argon and KTP lasers by contrast use a 100-μm fiber on a hand-held probe, which can be placed in close position on the stapes. This technique is more natural to the otologic surgeon.

The laser has shown itself to be possibly the best instrument to use for revision stapes procedures. Any of the lasers allows a noncontact vaporization of scar and adhesions around the prosthesis and footplate, and according to case reports of large series, has significantly decreased postoperative complications in this very difficult procedure. In addition, lasers have found application in primary stapedotomies as an effective alternative to drilling out a thick footplate with minimal trauma [50]. Lasers have also been used with significant clinical success in chronic ear surgery [150]. The ability of the laser to vaporize granulation tissue precisely with minimal bleeding has been very advantageous in this type of procedure as well.

ENDOSCOPIC SINUS SURGERY

To discuss the use of lasers for endoscopic sinus surgery, an understanding of the anatomy and the surgical techniques used today is necessary.

The introduction of sinus endoscopes for the diagnosis and surgical treatment of nasal/sinus disorders occurred in the mid 1980s [151]. Prior to the introduction of the endoscopes, the otolaryngologist-head and neck surgeon relied on the use of a nasal speculum. A reflective head mirror or fiber optic head light was used as the source for illumination of the nasal cavity. The nasal speculum provides excellent anterior rhinoscopy with a clear view of the midline of the nose. The sinus ostia, except for the sphenoid, are all located laterally. The ability to see internally with a nasal speculum is severely limited by the illumination and the examiner's inability to visualize around corners. The sinus endoscopes have a fiber optic light source providing distal illumination. The rigid optic lens system has 0°, 25°, 30°, and 70° angled optics that provide the ability to see laterally.

Circa 1987, advances in computerized tomography allowed for imaging of the paranasal sinuses in the coronal projection. The coronal projection of the sinuses provides the otolaryngologist with anatomical and surgical views of the sinuses. The use of an electronic window technique allows the radiologist to select a specific section of the Hounsfield densities to highlight the bone/soft tissue differences. This electronic window technique is referred to as a bone window when ordering sinus CT scans [152].

The combination of excellent endoscopic visualization of the nasal cavity and sinus ostea along with coronal CT scans resulted in an explosion of case reports on sinus disease [153–156]. Otolaryngologists learned that many patient symptoms of sinus disorders could be correlated with anatomic abnormalities. In addition, the coronal CT scan was able to show these anatomic abnormalities and provide early evidence of sinus inflammation and or infection [157–159].

The CO_2, the KTP, the argon, and Nd:YAG have been used in otolaryngology in many otolaryngology-head and neck surgical procedures. These lasers are also used in the nose and sinuses. The CO_2 laser has been described by Mittleman [160] for use in the treatment of obstruction of the nasal cavity from hypertrophic inferior turbinates and for synechiae of the nasal cavity. The CO_2 laser produces a surface effect by heating and vaporization of intracellular water. This produces a visible tissue effect giving the surgeon visual feedback on tissue destruction. The CO_2 laser energy has been delivered through microscope couplers, hand pieces, and more recently through hollow wave guides. The positive for CO_2 laser use in the nasal cavity is the predictable tissue effect and lack of scattering or transmission within the tissue. The negative is that the CO_2 laser energy can only be delivered in a straight path. In the case of the hollow wave guide, some slight flexion of the wave guide is possible. The transmission of the thermal energy to adjacent structures is of concern. No studies have been done to measure the temperature at the base of skull or on the orbital side of the lamina papyracea.

The Nd:YAG laser is used in otolaryngology for removal of obstructing tracheal bronchial neoplasms and coagulation of large vessels. The Nd:YAG laser energy can be transmitted through fiber optic carriers. The main tissue effect of the Nd:YAG is volume heating. The Nd:YAG laser energy can travel through tissue because of the large scattering coefficient. It also can be transmitted through tissue and is intensely absorbed by dark tissue. The ability to coagulate large vessels has been used to treat hereditary hemorrhagic telangiectasia of the nasal cavity [59]. The dilated vessels seen in the nose in association with this disease are mainly limited to the inferior turbinate and nasal septum.

The advantages of the Nd:YAG laser are its ability to coagulate large vessels and the flexibility of the fiber to bend within the nasal cavity. The disadvantages include the Nd:YAG laser's ability to penetrate deeply within tissue and the ability to be absorbed by dark tissue. The medial rectus muscle is adjacent to the lamina papyracea and is dark in color. The optic nerve is adjacent to the ethmoid sinuses posteriorly, and it courses through the lateral wall of the sphenoid sinus. The anterior cranial fossa is at risk to both thermal effect and direct laser injury. The Nd:YAG laser is not suited for use in the OMC. It can be safely used on the inferior turbinate and nasal septum where risk of injury to vital adjacent structures is not of concern.

The KTP laser is a visible wavelength laser at 532 nm. It will cut tissue and coagulate blood vessels and can be delivered through a fiber optic fiber. The visible light lasers are highly sensitive to color. The darker the color, the more the laser energy is intensely absorbed. The visible lasers also transmit through tissue. The KTP laser has been described for use on the inferior turbinate to coagulate the mucosa and vessels within resulting in a smaller inferior turbinate (Fig. 12) [40]. Colleagues in ophthalmology have used the KTP for Dacrocysto rhinostomy. In this procedure, they use the KTP to remove lacrimal bone over the lacrimal sac. Recent communication with ophthalmologists performing this procedure finds that the KTP use for bone removal is cumbersome and time-consuming. The bone removal is now being done with a bone rongeur.

The advantages of the KTP laser are its ability to pass through a fiber optic carrier. There are many disadvantages to the KTP laser in the nose. The KTP cannot cut tissue easily, and multiple pulses of the laser energy are necessary. As the tissue becomes charred, the KTP laser energy is absorbed, resulting in tissue destruction. The KTP energy does transit through tissue, causing concern for vital structures such as the eye and brain when used in the nose and sinuses. The KTP is similar to the Nd:YAG in that its use in the nose should be limited to the inferior turbinate and septum.

The argon laser has wavelengths between 488 and 514 nm. These wavelengths make the argon very similar to the KTP laser with a wavelength of 532 nm. The tissue effects are also very similar. The only difference is that the argon is a continuous laser and the KTP has been described as a quasicontinuous wave laser. The argon laser energy can be passed through a fiber optic carrier. The argon laser energy is absorbed intensely by darkly colored tissue. The laser energy also transmits through clear tissue for a distance. The argon is suitable for use on the inferior turbinate and nasal septum.

The Ho:YAG laser has a wavelength of 2.1 μm and is a pulsed laser. The extinction length in water is ~ 0.4 mm, which suggests that this laser should react with tissue similarly to the CO_2 laser. The Ho:YAG laser has been studied by Shapshay [161] for its suitability for sinus surgery. This laser will cut through bone and its energy is primarily absorbed by intracellular water simi-

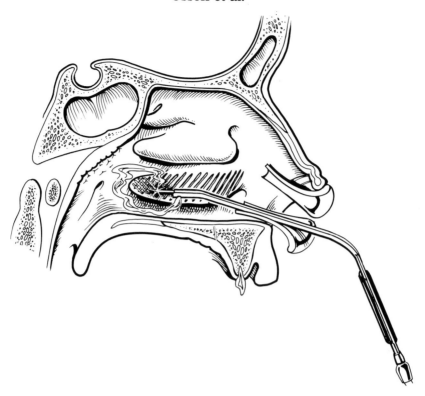

Fig. 12. The inferior turbinate is reduced using a cross hatch pattern.

larly to the CO_2 laser. Two limitations noted by Shapshay [161] are the loss of tissue contact resulting in tactile feedback to the surgeon and the lack of adequate hematosis if bleeding should occur. The Ho:YAG laser energy does not travel beyond the delivery point at the tissue surface. For laser sinus surgery, this would seem to be the best suited of the lasers discussed in this report. The transmission of the heat from the laser impacts has not been studied, but clinical and cadaver studies have not found this to be a problem. The main disadvantage to the use of this laser is that the pulsed delivery of the energy causes a splatter effect on the tissue, making the view through the sinus endoscope difficult. In addition, the inability to palpate the tissue along with the inability to control bleeding have made this laser not well suited for sinus surgery.

There is also work with other materials that lase in the near infrared region of the spectrum, such as the cobalt:magnesium fluoride laser (tunable from 1.8 to 2.14 μm). Alexandrite lasers (750 nm) and titanium sapphire lasers (tunable from 0.6 to 1.0 μm) have also been considered for sinus surgery. In addition, there is a free electron laser operating from 2 to 10 μm. The average output

intensity is normally from 1 to 10 watts [162]. The ability to use this laser in the midinfrared range makes this an exciting research tool for exploration of the ideal wavelength for sinus surgery.

OTHER CONSIDERATIONS IN LASER SURGERY OF THE HEAD AND NECK
Anesthetic Considerations

The surgeon and anesthesiologist are the two principal members of the surgical team and as such should be completely familiar with the equipment being used, the patient being treated, and the anticipated outcome and potential complications. A discussion of the various possible techniques should occur before the operation [22]. The final decision for the particular technique must be compatible with the anesthesiologist's need to ventilate the patient as well as the surgeon's goals so that both can be accomplished readily. If intubation is the anesthetic method chosen, it is incumbent on the surgeon to inspect the endotracheal tube as well as the wrapping used. Both the tube and the wrapping should be tested with the laser. Changes in manufacturing

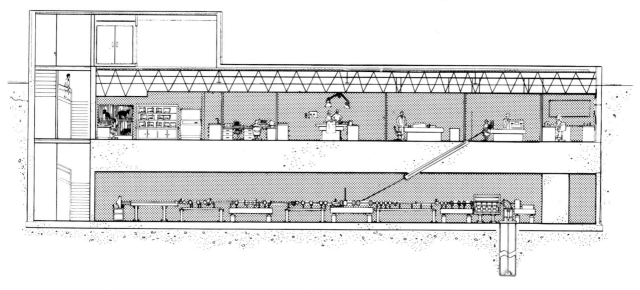

Fig. 13. Interior elevation of the free electron laser facility at Vanderbilt University.

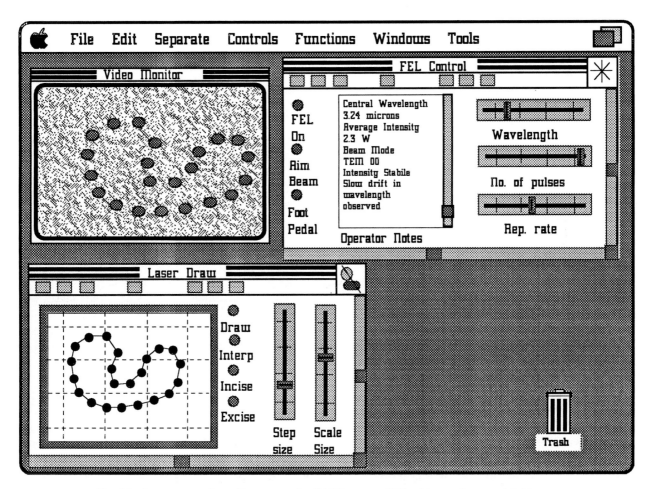

Fig. 14. Appearance of monitor screen for CAST system. Video image of surgical field is in the upper left corner. Lower left corner contains control panel for ablation pattern. Upper right corner shows control panel for the free electron laser.

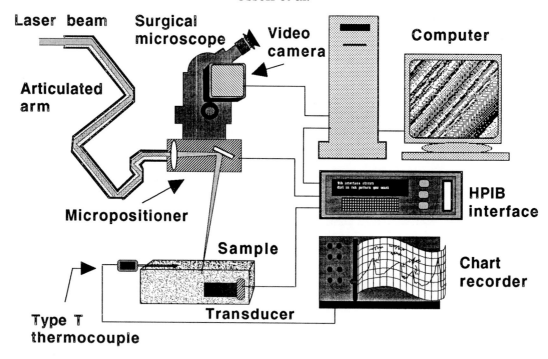

Fig. 15. Diagram of CAST system components.

techniques of the wrapping have altered the content of the reflecting tape used to cover the endotracheal tube. Mylar has been used and will burn upon exposure to the laser beam. Because of this, it should be remembered that not all reflecting tape is alike and necessarily safe. Newer endotracheal tubes are being made available. Some are made of metal but still require an inflatable cuff [163].

The use of a helium-oxygen mixture may ensure further safety during a laser procedure. The helium acts as a heat sink, reducing the combustion point of the endotracheal tube [22]. At high power output, however, even this added benefit may be insufficient to prevent ignition.

The Venturi anesthetic system removes the possibility of endotracheal tube combustion. The injector system may be placed either proximally or distally in the laryngoscope or through a Norton metal endotracheal tube [164–166]. When the insufflation device is placed distally, it may impair the surgeon's visibility. Since this is a cuff-less system, patients with restrictive pulmonary disease may be difficult to ventilate. Moreover, if a tear is produced in the mucosa and a high pressure system is used, particularly when placed distally, the anesthetic agent may dissect outside the airway causing subcutaneous emphysema, pneumomediastinum, or pneumothorax [114].

Usually when esophagoscopy and bronchoscopy are to be performed at the time of laryngoscopy, such as in the staging of new pharyngeal cancers, the Venturi technique cannot be utilized throughout the procedure. Some surgeons prefer to have an endotracheal tube placed at the outset and then switch to Venturi insufflation for the laser portion of the procedure. If an endotracheal tube is to be used during laser surgery, the cuff should be protected by moist cottonoids and filled with saline, which acts as a heat sink should the laser impact on the cuff and cause disruption [167].

A continuous dialogue should occur throughout the operation between the surgeon and anesthesiologist concerning the status of ventilation, the amount of bleeding encountered, the motion of vocal cords, and the timing of laser use in conjunction with respiration. This latter is particularly important when the Venturi system is used.

FUTURE FOR LASER SURGERY

Recently, researchers have begun using infrared spectroscopy to examine tissue. The absorption bands of the molecules can be identified. The water molecule is not the only potential absorber of infrared laser energy. The use of infrared spectroscopy to identify the main tissue molecular components that absorb the laser energy can be used in otolaryngology. A laser that would

TABLE 1. Summary of Laser Use in Otolaryngology

Anatomic site	Lesion	CO_2	KTP	Nd:YAG	Reason
Glottis	Bilateral vocal cord paralysis	1st	2nd		laser arytenoidectomy, coagulation
	Nodules	1st			microspot, precision
	Polyps	1st			microspot, precision
	Reinke's edema	1st			microspot, precision, microflap technique
	T1 mid cordal SCC with no anterior commissure involvement	1st			excisional biopsy
Larynx	Laryngoceles, cysts, granulomas	1st			coagulation, hands-off technique
	Laryngomalacia	1st			aryepiglottic fold division, precision, coagulation
	Obstructing SCC	2nd	1st		debulking airway, staging, coagulation
	Recurrent respiratory papilloma	1st	2nd		hands-off technique, less scarring precision, although KTP may be faster
	Stenoses (glottic, posterior and subglottic)	1st			microtrapdoor techniques
	Suprahyoid supraglottic T1 SSC	1st	2nd		excision with frozen section control
Lingual tonsils	Recurrent tonsillitis, hypertrophy	1st			minimal edema with complete vaporization
Nose	Epistaxis		1st or	1st	fiber delivery, coagulation, hands-off technique
	Osler-Weber-Rendu (HHT)		2nd	1st	coagulation, hands-off technique
	Polyps, concha bullosa		1st		debulking for visualization, coagulation
	Turbinate hypertrophy	1st or		1st	coagulation, less scabbing & scarring
Oral cavity	Carcinoma (verrucous, superficial T1)	1st			less pain & edema, cover a large area
	Lymphangioma	1st	2nd	2nd	minimal edema, coagulation
	Premalignant (leukoplakia, erythroplakia)	1st			vaporization, excision, can cover a large area
	Tongue T1 & limited T2	1st	2nd		less pain & edema, precise cutting, coagulation
Oropharynx	Sleep apnea (UPPP)	1st or	1st		coagulation
	T1 & T2 squamous cell carcinoma	1st	2nd	2nd	precision, coagulation, less edema, or contact tip with Nd:YAG
Palatine tonsils	Recurrent tonsillitis, obstructive apnea	2nd	1st		coagulation (?), less post-op pain
Subglottis	Hemangioma	1st		2nd	defocused beam, shrinkage, coagulation
Trachea	Obstructing malignant lesions	2nd	2nd	1st	debulking, coagulation fiber delivery

vaporize tissue with little heat transmission to the surrounding structure and would not transmit through the tissue would be a significant step in the use of lasers for nearly all types of surgery.

This technique might also be used to differentiate tumor tissue from normal tissue to allow for in vivo microscopic diagnosis and the development of a "smart laser" to treat only tumor-bearing tissue.

Computer-Assisted Surgery Techniques

Using the Vanderbilt free electron laser (FEL) (Fig. 13), we are working on a Computer Assisted Surgical Techniques (CAST) program that will help to control a surgical laser and monitor the types of tissue being ablated [168,169]. We have chosen to couple this CAST program with the FEL because one can select and control many of the laser parameters. In fact, there is a wider range of control with the FEL than with any other laser system. Thus there is the versatility to ablate many different tissues and to control the rate of ablation and the damage to the surrounding tissue. However, it has become clear that techniques developed for the FEL have applications with many surgical laser systems. Therefore, we are attempting to relate our studies to conventional lasers.

The CAST system replaces the joy stick of the micro manipulator on a surgical microscope with servos and computer direction. The image through the surgical microscope is inserted on the computer screen. On the same screen, the surgeon then draws the line or pattern that he or she wishes to incise (Fig. 14). Using the computer together with the laser, the surgeon is capable of making an incision with minimal lateral damage and extreme precision.

The computer is programmed to draw a pattern, stepping the position of the beam with every macropulse from the laser. The stepsize (distance the beam moves between pulses) is controlled by the user. The computer also can move randomly inside an arbitrarily defined boundary.

The image of the surgical field is also on the computer screen. An Ikegami video camera is attached on the side port of the surgical microscope. The image is interfaced to the computer with a Videospigot video input card (Fig. 15).

To operate the FEL at its maximum repetition rate, but avoid the extensive lateral thermal damage from the buildup of heat, we use a microscan micro positioner to move the beam between every pulse. The maximum repetition rate allows for the fastest cutting. The mechanized control of the laser beam also allows us to retrace a given pattern many times along a defined path. Therefore, the ablated line is kept as narrow as possible. Clearly, the added precision of the computer scanning can minimize unwanted lateral damage from a laser incision. The benefits of the CAST system applied to the FEL should also be applicable to conventional lasers.

Computer-assisted surgery does not have to stop with aiming the laser beam. The computer can also monitor the ablation process through the acoustic signals. When tissue is ablated with a pulsed laser, each laser pulse creates a popping sound due to photo acoustic emission. The frequency of the pop depends upon the physical characteristics of the tissue being ablated [170]. A hard tissue produces a higher frequency sound wave. Therefore, one could monitor bone ablation by monitoring the acoustic signal. Once the frequency dropped, the bone would be penetrated and the computer could turn off the laser.

The video image on the computer screen also need not be restricted to a visible light image. The image could be a false color image of temperature gradients from the infrared emission. The image could also be a false color image of ultraviolet fluorescence from tissue. In this system, a particular tissue or tissue type could be enhanced with dyes or a special autofluorescence pattern. The surgeon will be able to "see" the tissue in a new light.

Our computer-assisted surgical techniques system attempts to take full advantage of the FEL. A computer-controlled microscanner has been developed to prevent the accumulation of heat during tissue ablation. This microscanner also permits precise control and the ability to ablate lines or patterns with minimal loss of material. The CAST system can be transported to any of the current surgical laser systems. It will assist the surgeon in making a precise minimum size incision or excision with any laser. It will also reduce lateral thermal damage, especially with those lasers that have a small depth of penetration.

The FEL promises to be an important tool in surgery [171]. In medicine, the importance of the FEL probably will be the flexibility of the laser. We will be able to understand and test ablation models across the spectrum and using a constant laser pulse structure. The FEL will also lead to modifications of surgical lasers and laser delivery systems. The modifications will make the lasers more effective and initiate innovative surgical procedures.

As otolaryngologists have become more comfortable with predicting and controlling the thermal effect of various laser wavelengths, medical lasers have seen rapid acceptance within the field of otolaryngology. The development of new instrumentation and the use of these lasers in residency programs will see a significant growth of their use in the general field of otolaryngology.

REFERENCES

1. Maiman TH. Stimulated optical radiation in ruby. Nature 1960; 187:493.
2. Koester CJ, Snitzer E, Campbell CJ, Rittler MC. Experimental laser retina photocoagulation. J Opt Soc Am 1962; 52:607.
3. Goldman L, Blaney D, Kindel D, Franke EK. Effect of the laser beam on the skin. J Invest Dermatol 1963; 40:121–122.
4. Goldman L, Blaney D, Kindel DJ Jr, Richfield D, Franke EK. Pathology of the effect of the laser beam on the skin. Nature 1963; 197:912–914.
5. Sataloff J. Experimental use of laser in otosclerotic stapes. Arch Otolaryngol 1967; 85:614–616.
6. Hogberg L, Stahle J, Vogel K. The transmission of high-powered ruby laser beam through bone. Acta Societa Medicorum Upsaliensis 1967; 72:223–228.
7. Jako GJ. Laser surgery of the vocal cords: An experimental study with carbon dioxide laser on dogs. Laryngoscope 1972; 82:2204–2216.

8. Strully KJ, Yahr W. Biological effects of laser radiation enhancements by selective stains. Fed Prod 1965; 24:S–81.

9. Bredemeier HC. 1969, Laser accessory for surgical applications, U. S. Patent no. 3,659,613, issued 1972.

10. Polanyi TG, Bredemeier HC, Davis TW Jr. Lasers for surgical research. Med Biol Eng 1970; 8:541–548.

11. Bredemeier HC. 1973, Stereo laser endoscope, U.S. Patent no. 3,796,220, issued 1974.

12. Strong MS, Jako GJ. Laser surgery in the larynx: Early clinical experience with continuous CO_2 laser. Ann Otol Rhinol Laryngol 1972; 81:791–798.

13. Hall RR. The healing of tissues incised by carbon-dioxide laser. Br J Surg 1971; 58:222–225.

14. Fleischer D. Lasers and gastroenterology, a review. Am J Gastroenterol 1984; 79:406–415.

15. Cochrane JPS, Beacon JP, Creasey GH, Russel CG. Wound healing after laser surgery: An experimental study. Br J Surg 1980; 67:740–743.

16. Bellina JJ, Hemmins R, Voroz JI, Ross LF. Carbon-dioxide laser and electrostatic wound study with an animal model: A comparison of tissue damage and healing patterns in peritoneal tissue. Am J Obstet Gynecol 1984; 148:327–334.

17. Fox JL. The use of laser radiation as a surgical "light knife." J Sur Res 1969; 9:199–205.

18. Beamis JF Jr, Shapshay SM. Nd-YAG laser therapy for tracheobronchial disorders. Postgrad Med 1984; 75:173–180.

19. Cosman B. Experience in the argon laser therapy for port-wine stains. Plast Reconstr Surg 1980; 65:119–129.

20. Pickering JW, Butler PH, Ring BJ, Walker EP. Computed temperature distributions around ectatic capillaries exposed to yellow (578 nm) laser light. Phys Med Biol 1989; 34:1247–1258.

21. Tan OT, Carney JM, Margolis R, Seki Y, Boll J, Anderson RR, Parrish JA. Histologic responses of port-wine stains treated by argon, carbon dioxide, and tunable dye lasers: A preliminary report. Arch Dermatol 1986; 122:1016–1022.

22. Ossoff RH, Reinisch L. Complications of Laser Surgery. In: Eisele DW, ed. "Complications in Head and Neck Surgery." Philadelphia: Decker, 1993, pp 306–316.

23. McDaniel DH, Mordon S. Hexascan: A new robotized scanning laser handpiece. Cutis 1990; 45:300–305.

24. McDaniel DH. Clinical usefulness of the Hexascan: Treatment of cutaneous vascular and melanocytic disorders. J Dermatol Surg Oncol 1993; 312–319.

25. Apfelberg DB, Smoller B. Preliminary analysis of histological results of Hexascan device with continuous tunable dye laser at 514 (argon) and 577 nm (yellow). Lasers Surg Med 1993; 13:106–112.

26. Decraemer WF, Dirckx JJ, Funnell WR. Shape and derived geometrical parameters of the adult, human tympanic membrane measured with a phase-shift moiré interferometer. Hear Res 1991; 51:107–121.

27. Doukas AG, McAuliffe DJ, Flotte TJ. Biological effects of laser-induced shock waves: structural and functional cell damage in vitro. Ultrasound Med Biol 1993; 19:137–146.

28. Mihashi S, Jako GJ, Incze J, Strong MS. Laser surgery in otolaryngology: Interaction of the CO_2 laser in soft tissue. Ann NY Acad Sci 1976; 267:263–294.

29. Norris CW, Mullarky MB. Experimental skin incision made with the carbon dioxide laser. Laryngoscope 1982; 92:416–419.

30. Finsterbush A, Rousso M, Ashur H. Healing and tensile strength of CO_2 laser incisions and scalpel wounds in rabbits. Plast Reconstr Surg 1982; 70:360–362.

31. Buell BR, Schuller DE. Comparison of tensile strength in CO_2 laser and scalpel skin incisions. Arch Otolaryngol 1983; 109:465–467.

32. Apfelberg DB, Maser MR, Lash H, Rivers J. The argon laser for cutaneus lesions. JAMA 1981; 245:2073–2075.

33. Keller GS, Doiron D, Weingarten C. Advances in laser skin surgery for vascular lesions. Otolaryngology 1985; 111:437–440.

34. Parkin JL, Dixon JA. Argon laser treatment of head and neck vascular lesions, Otolaryngol Head Neck Surg 1985; 93:211–216.

35. Perkins RC. Laser stapedotomy for otosclerosis. Laryngoscope 1980; 90:228–240.

36. Strunk CL Jr, Quinn FB Jr. Stapedectomy surgery in residency: KTP-532 laser verus argon laser. Am J Otol 1993; 14:113–117.

37. DiBartolomeo JR, Ellis M. The argon laser in otology. Laryngoscope 1980; 90:1786–1796.

38. Escudero LH, Castro AO, Drumond M, Porto SP, Boziniz DG, Penna AF, Gallego-Lluesma E. Argon laser in human tympanoplasty. Arch Otolaryngol 1979; 105:252–253.

39. Hanna E, Eliachar I, Cothren R, Ivanc T, Hughes G. Laser welding of fascial grafts and its potential application in tympanoplasty: An animal model. Otolaryngol Head Neck Surg 1993; 108:356–366.

40. Levine HL. Endoscopy and the KTP/532 laser for nasal sinus disease. Ann Otol Rhinol Laryngol 1989; 98:46–51.

41. Thedinger BS. Applications of the KTP laser in chronic ear surgery. Am J Otol 1990; 11:79–84.

42. Atiyah RA, Friedman CD, Sisson GA. The KTP/532 laser in glossal surgery: KTP/532 clinical update. Laserscope 1988; no 22.

43. Ward RF. Treatment of tracheal and endobronchial lesions with the potassium titanyl phosphate laser. Ann Otol Rhinol Laryngol 1992; 101:205–208.

44. Joseph M, Reardon E, Goodman M. Lingual tonsillectomy: A treatment for inflammatory lesions of the lingual tonsil. Laryngoscope 1984; 94:179–184.

45. Krespi YP, Har-El G, Levine TM, Ossoff RH, Wurster CF, Paulsen JW. Laser laryngeal tonsillectomy. Laryngoscope 1989; 99:131–135.

46. Kuhn F. The KTP/532 laser in tonsillectomy: KTP/532 clinical update. Laserscope 1988; no. 06.

47. Strunk CL, Nichols ML. A comparison of the KTP/532-laser tonsillectomy vs. traditional dissection/snare tonsillectomy. Otolaryngol Head Neck Surg 1990; 103:966–971.

48. Linden BE, Gross CW, Long TE, Lazar RH. Morbidity in pediatric tonsillectomy. Laryngoscope 1990; 100:120–124.

49. Bartels LJ. KTP laser stapedotomy: Is it safe? Otolaryngol Head Neck Surg 1990; 103:685–692.

50. Strunk CL, Quinn FB Jr, Bailey BJ. Stapedectomy techniques in residency training. Laryngoscope 1992; 102:121–124.

51. McGee TM. The KTP/532 laser in otology. KTP/532 clinical update. Laserscope 1988; no. 08.

52. Atiyah RA. The KTP/532 laser in laryngeal surgery KTP/532 clinical update. Laserscope 1988; no. 21.

53. McDougall JC, Cortese DA. Neodymium-YAG laser therapy of malignant airway obstruction. Mayo Clin Proc 1983; 58:35–39.

54. Shapshay SM, Simpson GT. Lasers in bronchology. Otolaryngol Clin North Am 1983; 16:879–886.

55. Toty A, Personne C, Colchen A, Vourc'h G. Bronchoscopic management of tracheal lesions using the Nd:YAG laser. Thorax 1981; 36:175–178.

56. Dumon JF, Reboud E, Garbe L, Aucomte F, Meric B. Treatment of tracheobronchial lesions by laser photoresection. Chest 1982; 81:278–284.

57. Bemis JF Jr, Vergos K, Rebeiz EE, Shapshay SM. Endoscopic laser therapy for obstructing tracheobronchial lesions. Am Otol Rhinol Laryngol 1991; 100:413–419.

58. Flesicher D. Endoscopic laser therapy for gastrointestinal neoplasms. Otolaryngol Clin North Am 1984; 64: 947–953.

59. Shapshay SM, Oliver P. Treatment of hereditary hemorrhagic telangiectasia by Nd-YAG laser photocoagulation. Laryngoscope 1984; 94:1554–1556.

60. Rebeiz E, April MM, Bohigian RK, Shapshay SM. Nd-YAG laser treatment of venous malformations of the head and neck: An update. Otolaryngol Head Neck Surg 1991; 105:655–661.

61. April MM, Rebeiz EE, Friedman EM, Healy GB, Shapshay SM. Laser therapy for lymphatic malformations of the upper aerodigestive tract: An evolving experience. Arch Otolaryngol Head Neck Surg 1992; 118:205–208.

62. Qadir R, Kennedy D. Use of the holmium:yttrium aluminum garnet (Ho:YAG) laser for cranial nerve decompression: An in vivo study using the rabbit model. Laryngoscope 1993; 103:631–636.

63. Cosman B. Experience in the argon laser therapy for port-wine stains. Plast Reconstr Surg 1980; 65:119–129.

64. Parkin JL, Dixon JA. Argon laser treatment of head and neck vascular lesions. Otolaryngol Head Neck Surg 1985; 93:211–216.

65. Spitzer M, Krumholz BA. Photodynamic therapy in gynecology. Obstet Gynecol Clin North Am 1991; 18:649–659.

66. Merguerian PA, Seremetis G, Becher MW. Hypospadias repair using laser welding of ventral skin flap in rabbits: Comparison with sutured repair. J Urol 1992; 148: 667–70; discussion, 671.

67. Kao MC. Video endoscopic sympathectomy using a fiberoptic CO_2 laser to treat plamar hyperhidrosis. Neurosurgery 1992; 30:131–135.

68. Absten GT. Physics of light and lasers. Obstet Gynecol Clin North Am 1991; 18:407–427.

69. Ossoff RH, Duncavage JA, Gluckman JL, Adkins JP, Karlan MS, Toohill RJ, Keane WM, Norris CW, Tucker JA. The universal endoscopic coupler bronchoscopic carbon dioxide laser surgery: A multi-institutional clinical trial. Otolaryngol Head Neck Surg 1985; 93:824–830.

70. Ossoff RH, Sisson GA, Shapshay SM. Endoscopic management of selected early vocal cord carcinoma. Ann Otol Rhinol Laryngol 1985; 94:560–564.

71. Ossoff RH, Werkhaven JA, Raif J, Abraham M. Advanced microspot microslad for the CO_2 laser. Otolaryngol Head Neck Surg 1991; 105:411–414.

72. Shapshay SM, Wallace RA, Kveton JF, Hybels RL, Setzer SE. New microspot micromanipulator for CO_2 la-

ser application in otolaryngology—head and neck surgery. Otolaryn Head Neck Surg 1988; 98:179–181.

73. Fried MP. Limitations of laser laryngoscopy. Otolaryngol Clin North Am 1984; 17:199–207.

74. Shapshay SM, Beamis JF Jr, Drumon JF. Total cervical tracheal stenosis: treatment by laser, dilation, and stenting. Ann Otol Rhinol Laryngol 1989; 98:890–895.

75. Simpson GT, Polanyi TG. History of the carbon dioxide laser in otolaryngologic surgery. Otolaryngol Clin N Am 1983; 16:739–752.

76. Whitehead E, Salam MA. Use of the carbon dioxide laser with the Montgomery T-tube in the management of extensive subglottic stenosis. J Laryngol Otol 1992; 106: 829–831.

77. Beste DJ, Toohill RJ. Microtrapdoor flap repair of laryngeal and tracheal stenosis. Ann Otol Rhinol Laryngol 1991; 100:420–423.

78. Dedo HH, Sooy CD. Endoscopic laser repair of posterior glottic, subglottic and tracheal stenosis by division or micro-trapdoor flap. Laryngoscope 1984; 94:445–450.

79. Duncavage JA, Ossoff RH, Toohill RJ. Laryngotracheal reconstruction with composite nasal septal cartilage grafts. Ann Otol Rhinol Laryngol 1989; 98:565–585.

80. Duncavage JA, Piazza LS, Ossoff RH, Toohill RJ. Microtrapdoor technique for the management of laryngeal stenosis. Laryngoscope 1987; 97:825–828.

81. Werkhaven JA, Weed DT, Ossoff RH. Carbon dioxide laser serial microtrapdoor flap excision of subglottic stenosis. Arch Otolaryngol Head Neck Surg 1993; 119: 676–679.

82. Ossoff RH, Duncavage JA, Dere H. Microsubglottoscopy: An expansion of operative microlaryngoscopy. Otolaryngol Head Neck Surg 1991; 104:842–848.

83. Ward RF, Arnold JE, Healy GB. Flexible minibronchoscopy in children. Ann Otol Rhinol Laryngol 1987; 96: 645–649.

84. Mehta AC, Lee FY, Cordasco EM, Kirby T, Eliachar I, De Boer G. Concentric tracheal and subglottic stenosis: Management using the Nd-YAG laser for mucosal sparing followed by gentle dilatation. Chest 1993; 104:673–677.

85. April MM, Rebeiz EE, Aretz HT, Shapshay SM. Endoscopic holmium laser laryngotracheoplasty in animal models. Ann Otol Rhinol Laryngol 1991; 100:503–507.

86. Ossoff RH, Sisson GA, Duncavage JA, Moselle HI, Andrews PE, McMillan WI. Endoscopic laser arytenoidectomy for the treatment of bilateral vocal cord paralysis, Laryngoscope 1984; 94:1293–1297.

87. Dennis DP, Kashima H. Carbon dioxide laser posterior cordectomy for treatment of bilateral vocal cord paralysis. Ann Otol Rhinol Laryngol 1989; 98:930–934.

88. Kashima HK. Bilateral vocal fold motion impairment: Pathophysiology and management by transverse cordotomy. Ann Otol Rhinol Laryngol 1991; 100:717–721.

89. Crumley RL. Endoscopic laser medial arytenoidectomy for airway management in bilateral laryngeal paralysis. Ann Otol Rhinol Laryngol 1993; 102:81–84.

90. Strong MS, Vaughan CW, Cooperband SR, Healy GB, Clemente MA. Recurrent respiratory papillomatosis management with the CO_2 laser. Ann Otol Rhinol Laryngol 1976; 85:508–516.

91. Ossoff RH, Werkhaven JA, Dere H. Soft-tissue complications of laser surgery for recurrent respiratory papillomatosis. Laryngoscope 1991; 101:1162–1166.

92. Crockett DM, McCabe BF, Shive CJ. Complications of laser surgery for recurrent respiratory papillomatosis. Ann Otol Rhinol Laryngol 1987; 96:639–644.

93. Wetmore SJ, Key JM, Suen JY. Complications of laser surgery for laryngeal papillomatosis. Laryngoscope 1985; 95:798–801.

94. Abramson AL, DiLorenzo TP, Steinberg BM. Is papillomavirus detectable in the plume of laser-treated laryngeal papilloma? Arch Otolaryngol Head Neck Surg 1990; 116:604–607.

95. Garden JM, O'Banion MK, Shelnitz LS, Pinski KS, Bakus AD, Reichmann ME, Sundberg JP. Papillomavirus in the vapor of carbon dioxide laser-treated verrucae. JAMA 1988; 259:1199–1202.

96. Leventhal BG, Kashima HK, Mounts P, Thurmond L, Chapman S, Buckley S, Wold D. Long-term response of recurrent respiratory papillomatosis to treatment with lymphoblastoid interferon alfa-N1: Papilloma Study Group. N Engl J Med 1991; 325:613–617.

97. Ossoff RH, Karlan MS, Sisson GA. Posterior commissure laryngoscope for carbon dioxide laser surgery. Ann Otol Rhinol Laryngol 1983; 92:361.

98. Durkin GE, Duncavage JA, Toohill RJ, Tieu TM, Caya JG. Wound healing of true vocal cord squamous epithelium following CO_2 laser ablation and cup forcep stripping. Otolaryngol Head Neck Surg 1986; 95:273–277.

99. Benjamin B, Croxson G. Vocal cord granulomas. Ann Otol Rhinol Laryngol 1985; 94:538–541.

100. Stutsman AC, McGavran MH. Ultraconservative management of superficially invasive epidermoid carcinoma of the true vocal cord. Ann Otol Rhinol Laryngol 1971; 80:507–512.

101. DeSanto LW. The options in early laryngeal carcinoma. N Engl J Med 1982; 306:910–912.

102. Lillie JC, DeSanto LW. Transoral surgery of early cordal carcinoma. Trans Am Acad Opthalmol Otolaryngol 1977; 77:ORL92–96.

103. Strong MS. Laser excision of carcinoma of the larynx. Laryngoscope 1975; 85:1286‘–1289.

104. Blakeslee, D, Vaughan, CW, Shapshay, SM, Simpson GT, Strong MS. Excisional biopsy in the selective management of T1 glottic cancer: A three-year follow-up study. Laryngoscope 1984; 94:488–494.

105. Healy GB, Strong MS, Shapshay S, Vaughan C, Jako G. Complication of CO_2 laser surgery of the aerodigestive tract: Experience of 4416 cases. Otolaryngol Head Neck Surg 1984; 92:13–18.

106. Ossoff RH, Hotaling AJ, Karlan MS, Sisson GA. CO_2 laser in otolaryngology head and neck surgery: A retrospective analysis of complications. Laryngoscope 1983; 93:1287–1289.

107. Cozine K, Rosenbaum LM, Askanazi J, Rosenbaum JH. Laser-induced endotracheal tube fire. Anesthesiology 1981; 55:583–585.

108. Hirshman CA, Leon D. Ignition of an endotracheal tube during laser microsurgery. Anesthesiology 1980; 53:177.

109. Hirshman CA, Smith J, Indirect ignition of the endotracheal tube during carbon dioxide laser surgery. Arch Otolaryngol 1980; 106:639–641.

110. Meyers A. Complication of CO_2 laser surgery of the larynx. Ann Otol Rhinol Laryngol 1981; 90:132–134.

111. Schramm VL Jr, Mattox DE, Stool SE. Acute management of laser-ignited intracheal explosion. Laryngoscope 1981; 91:1417.

112. Snow JC, Norton ML, Saluja TS, Estanislao AF. Fire hazard during CO_2 laser microsurgery on the larynx and trachea. Anesth Anagl 1976; 55:146–147.

113. Vourc'h G, Tannieres M, Freche G. Ignition of a tracheal tube during laryngeal laser surgery. Anaesthesia 1979; 34:685.

114. Ganfield RA, Chapin JW. Pneumothorax with upper airway laser surgery. Anesthesiology 1982; 56:398–399.

115. Torres LE, Reynolds RC. A complication of use of a microlaryngeal surgery endotracheal tube. Anesthesiology 1980; 53:355.

116. Feder RJ. Laryngeal granuloma as a complication of the CO_2 laser. Laryngoscope 1983; 93:944–945.

117. Fried MP, Kelly JH, Strome M. "Complications of Laser Surgery of the Head and Neck." Chicago: Yearbook Medical Publishers, 1986.

118. Fried MP. Complications of CO_2 laser surgery of the larynx. Laryngoscope 1983; 93:275–278.

119. Strong MS, Vaughan CW, Mahler DL, Jaffe DR, Sullivan RC. Cardiac complications of microsurgery of the larynx: Etiology, incidence and prevention. Laryngoscope 1974; 84:908–920.

120. Alberti PW. The complications of CO_2 laser surgery of otolaryngology. Acta Otolaryngol 1981; 91:375–381.

121. Pignatari S, Smith EM, Gray SD, Shive C, Turek LP. Detection of human papillomavirus infection in diseased and nondiseased sites of the respiratory tract in recurrent respiratory papillomatosis patients by DNA hybridization. Ann Otol Rhinol Laryngol 1992; 101:408–412.

122. Morrison GA, Evans JN. Juvenile respiratory papillomatosis: Acyclovir reassessed. Int J Pediatr Otorhinolaryngol 1993; 26:193–197.

123. Bagwell CE, Marchildon MB, Pratt LL. Anterior cricoid split for subglottic stenosis. J Pediatr Surg 1987; 22:740–742.

124. Koufman JA, Thompson JN, Kohut RI. Endoscopic management of subglottic stenosis with the CO_2 surgical laser. Otolaryngol Head Neck Surg 1981; 89:215–220.

125. Strong MS, Healy GB, Vaughan CW, Fried MP, Shapshay S. Endoscopic management of laryngeal stenosis. Otolaryngol Clin North Am 1979; 12:797–805.

126. Shapshay SM, Beamis JF Jr, Hybels RL, Bohigian RK. Endoscopic treatment of subglottic and tracheal stenosis by radial laser incision and dilation. Ann Otol Rhinol Laryngol 1987; 96:661–664.

127. Johnson DG, Stewart DR. Management of acquired tracheal obstructions in infancy. J Pediatr Surg 1975; 10:709–717.

128. Nagaraj HS, Shott R, Fellows R, Yacoub U. Recurrent lobar atelectasis due to acquired bronchial stenosis in neonates. J Pediatr Surg 1980; 15:411–415.

129. Healy GB. An experimental model for the endoscopic correction of subglottic stenosis with clinical applications. Laryngoscope 1982; 92:1103–1115.

130. Sasaki CT, Horiuchi M, Koss N. Tracheostomy-related subglottic stenosis: bacteriologic pathogenesis. Laryngoscope 1979; 89:857–865.

131. Beamis JF Jr, Vergos K, Rebeiz EE, Shapshay SM. Endoscopic laser therapy for obstructing tracheobronchial lesions. Ann Otol Rhinol Laryngol 1991; 100:413–419.

338   **Ossoff et al.**

132. Shapshay SM, Dumon JF, Beamis JF Jr. Endoscopic treatment of tracheobronchial malignancy: Experience with Nd-YAG and CO_2 lasers in 506 operations. Otolaryngol Head Neck Surg 1985; 93:205–210.

133. Kamami Y-V. Laser CO_2 for snoring: Preliminary results. Acta Oto-rhino-laryngologic Beg 1990; 44:451–456.

134. Croaker BD, Allison GL, Saunders NA, Henley MJ, McKeon JL, Allen KM, Gyulay SG. Estimation of the probability of disturbed breathing during sleep before a sleep study. Am Rev Respir Dis 1990; 142:14–18.

135. Young T, Palta M, Dempsey J, Skatrud J, Weber S, Badr S. The occurrence of sleep disordered breathing among adults. N Engl J Med 1993; 328:1230–1235.

136. Mizono G, Dedo HH. Subglottic hemangiomas in infants: Treatment with CO_2 laser. Laryngoscope 1984; 94:638–641.

137. Bagwell CE. CO_2 laser excision of pediatric airway lesions. J Pediatr Surg 1990; 25:1152–1156.

138. Werkhaven J, Maddern BR, Stool SE. Post-tracheotomy granulation tissue managed by carbon dioxide laser excision. Ann Otol Rhinol Laryngol 1989; 98:828–830.

139. Healy GB, McGill T, Strong MS. Surgical advances in the treatment of lesions of the pediatric airway: The role of the carbon dioxide laser. Pediatrics 1978; 61:380–383.

140. Seid AB, Park SM, Kearns MJ, Gugenheim S. Laser division of the aryepiglottic folds for severe laryngomalacia. Int J Pediatr Otorhinolaryngol 1985; 10:153–158.

141. Werkhaven J, Ossoff RH. Surgery for benign lesions of the glottis. Otolaryngol Clin North Am 1991; 24:1179–1199.

142. Karlan MS, Ossoff RH. Laser surgery for benign laryngeal disease. Surg Clin North Am 1984; 64:981–994.

143. Shapshay SM. Laser applications in the trachea and bronchi: A comparative study of the soft tissue effects using contact and noncontact delivery systems. Laryngoscope 1987; 97:Part 2, suppl 41.

144. Werkhaven JA, Lee-Polis S. Bronchoscopy methods make pediatric cases practical. Clinical Laser Monthly 1991; 119–121.

145. Lesinski SG. Lasers for otosclerosis. Laryngoscope 1989; 99:Part 2, suppl 46.

146. Clark WC, Robertson JH, Gardner G. Selective absorption and control of thermal effects: A comparison of the laser systems used in otology and neurotology. Otolaryngol Head Neck Surg 1984; 92:73–79.

147. Vollrath M, Schreiner C. Influence of argon laser stapedotomy on inner ear function and temperature. Otolaryngol Head Neck Surg 1983; 91:521–526.

148. Coker NJ, Ator GA, Jenkins HA, Neblett CR, Morris JR. Carbon dioxide laser stapedotomy. Arch Otolaryngol 1985; 111:601–605.

149. Coker NJ, Ator GA, Jenkins HA, Neblett CR. Carbon dioxide laser stapedotomy: A histopathologic study. Am J Otolaryngol 1986; 7:253–257.

150. McGee TM. The argon laser in surgery for chronic ear disease and otosclerosis. Laryngoscope 1983; 93:1177–1182.

151. Kennedy DW, Zinreich SJ, Rosenbaum AE, Johns ME. Functional endoscopic sinus surgery: Theory and diagnostic evaluation. Arch Otolaryngol Head Neck Surg 1985; 111:576–582.

152. Zinreich SJ, Mattox DE, Kennedy DW, Chisholm HL, Diffley DM, Rosenbaum AE. Concha bullosa: CT evaluation. J Comput Assist Tomogr 1988; 12:778–784.

153. Schaefer SD, Manning SD, Close LG. Endoscopic paranasal sinus surgery: indications and considerations. Laryngoscope 1989; 99:1–5.

154. Kennedy DW, Zinreich SJ, Shaalan H, Kuhn F, Naclerio R, Loch E. Endoscopic middle meatal antrostomy: Theory, technique, and patency. Laryngoscope 1987; 97:1–9.

155. Rice DH. Basic surgical techniques and variations of endoscopy sinus surgery. Otolaryngol Clin North Am 1989; 22:713–726.

156. Ragheb S, Duncavage J. Maxillary sinusitis: Value of endoscopic middle meatus antrostomy versus Caldwell-Luc procedure. Operative Techniques in Otolaryngol Head Neck Surg 1992; 3:129–133.

157. Sonkens JW, Harnsberger R, Blanch GM, Babbel RW, Hunt S. The impact of screening sinus CT on the planning of functional endoscopic sinus surgery. Otolaryngol Head Neck Surg 1991; 105:802–813.

158. Nass RL, Holliday RA, Reede DL. Diagnosis of surgical sinusitis using nasal endoscopy and computerized tomography. Laryngoscope 1989; 99:1158–1160.

159. Teatini G, Simonetti G, Savolini U, Masala W, Meloni F, Rovasio S, Dedola GL. Computed tomography of the ethmoid labyrinth and adjacent structures. Ann Otolog Rhinol Laryngol 1987; 96:239–250.

160. Mittleman H. CO_2 laser turbinectomy for chronic, obstructive rhinitis. Lasers Surg Med 1982; 2:29–36.

161. Shapshay SM, Rebeiz EE, Bohigian RK, Hybels RL, Aretz HT, Pankratov MM. Holmium:yttrium aluminum garnet laser-assisted endoscopic sinus surgery: Laboratory experience. Laryngoscope 1991; 101:142–149.

162. Brau C. Free-electron lasers. Science 1988; 239:115–1121.

163. Norton ML. Anesthesia problems in laser surgery, of the head and neck. Chicago: Yearbook Medical, 1986.

164. Gofarth AJ, Cooke JE, Putney FJ. An anesthesia technique for laser surgery of the larynx. Laryngoscope 1983; 93:822–823.

165. Ruder CB, Rapheal NL, Abramson AL. Oliverio RM Jr. Anesthesia for carbon dioxide laser microsurgery of the larynx. Otolaryngol Head Neck Surg 1981; 89:732–737.

166. Woo P, Strong MS. Venturi jet ventilation through the metal endotracheal tube: A nonflammable system. Ann Otol Rhinol Laryngol 1983; 92:405–407.

167. LeJeune FE Jr, Guice C, LeTard F, Marice H. Heat sink protection against lasering endotracheal cuffs. Ann Otol Rhinol Laryngol 1982; 91:606–607.

168. Ossoff RH, Reinisch L. Computer assisted surgical techniques: A vision for the future of laryngeal and otolaryngology-head and neck surgery. J Otolaryngol (in press).

169. Reinisch L, Mendenhall M, Charous S, Ossoff RH. Computer assisted surgical techniques utilizing the Vanderbilt free electron laser. Laryngoscope (in press).

170. Reinisch L, Ossoff RH. Acoustic effects during ablation, Proc. Laser-Tissue Interaction III. Jacques SL, Katzir A, eds. SPIE 1993; 1882:112–121.

171. Reinisch L, Mendenhall MH, Ossoff RH. Medical delivery systems for the Vanderbilt free electron laser. SPIE 1994; 2131:266–277.

Chapter 10

Clinical and Preclinical Photodynamic Therapy

Anita M.R. Fisher, PhD, A. Linn Murphree, MD, and Charles J. Gomer, PhD

Clayton Ocular Oncology Center, Childrens Hospital Los Angeles, and Departments of Pediatrics, Ophthalmology, and Radiation Oncology, University of Southern California School of Medicine, Los Angeles, California

INTRODUCTION

Medical interest in the cytotoxic responses of photosensitizers has been recorded as early as 1900 [1–4]. However, the synthesis of hematoporphyrin derivative (HPD), a complex porphyrin mixture with reported tumor-localizing properties, by Schwartz in the 1950s [5], can be regarded as the beginning of modern photodynamic therapy (PDT). In the following years, experimental and pilot clinical studies evaluated hematoporphyrin and HPD for both diagnosis and therapy of malignant tumors [6–11]. Pioneering efforts in clinical HPD photosensitization were made by Dougherty [12,13], whose reports of a series of cancer patients treated by this technique appeared from 1978 onward. In 1980, Hayata and coworkers [14] were the first to apply fiberoptic endoscopic laser irradiation to treat early endobronchial lung cancer with PDT. Early studies, being anecdotal, tended to vary treatment conditions, but by the late 1980s, investigators using PDT for malignancies of the lung [15], esophagus [16], and bladder [17] were documenting staging, dosing, and tumor response with a goal of achieving standardization of this relatively new therapy.

In the past 15 years, several thousand cancer patients have undergone HPD- or DHE-mediated PDT, although the majority have not been part of prospective clinical trials. At the same time, second-generation photosensitizers and improved clinical laser delivery systems have been developed. After the completion of Phase III randomized trials, many ongoing at present, the status of PDT in comparison with conventional oncology treatment modalities will be known. PDT is being integrated into multimodality regimens, with the distinct advantage that photosensitizer injection and laser irradiation can be repeated multiple times.

There are also a number of nononcologic applications in which PDT is being evaluated. It is undergoing preclinical and clinical testing for its ability to inactivate viruses, to treat atherosclerotic lesions, and also to treat skin disorders such as psoriasis and portwine stains.

PHOTOSENSITIZER DEVELOPMENT

Classes of Photosensitizers

Most clinical PDT experience comes from using the porphyrin variants, HPD and DHE. The active components of HPD were identified by Dougherty et al. [18] to be dihematoporphyrin ethers and esters (DHE). The commercial preparation of DHE, known as porfimer sodium, or Photofrin, contains <20% of inactive monomers and >80% of the active porphyrin dimers and oligomers. However, Photofrin remains a complex mixture with inherent variability, and it has the further limitation of weak light absorption at wavelengths above 600 nm. In addition, Photofrin has the side effect of causing prolonged cutaneous photosensitivity. These properties provided incentives for developing new photosensitizers. The next generation of clinical photosensitizers ideally will provide rapid plasma and tissue clearance, enhanced tumor to normal tissue selectivity, comparable photoactivation efficiency, and superior light absorption of visible red and near infrared light. Theoretically, these developments will lead to more selective treatment of large malignant lesions than is currently possible with Photofrin-mediated PDT.

A growing number of second-generation photosensitizers are being synthesized, which can be activated at wavelengths of light >650 nm. A nonexhaustive list of classes of compounds includes porphyrin and chlorin derivatives, purpurins, benzoporphyrins, phthalocyanines, and naphthalocyanines. The chlorins include many categories and are reviewed in detail elsewhere [19,20]. Chlorins are derived either by modifying a porphyrin (reducing one of the pyrrolic rings of the porphyrin macrocycle) or from chlorophyll as the starting material for synthesis. Purpurins are formally chlorins, since they have one reduced pyrrole group, as well as a fused five-membered isocyclic ring [21]. Benzoporphyrin derivatives are also formally chlorins, since they have a reduced pyrrole ring, as well as a fused six-membered isocyclic ring [22]. Phthalocyanines have been synthesized specifically for PDT [23]. They commonly incorporate a diamagnetic metal ion, usually zinc or aluminium, to enhance triplet photosensitizer yields and lifetimes in order to increase photodynamic activity [24,25]. Naphthalocyanines (absorption maxima 770 nm) have red shifted absorption spectra compared with phthalocyanines (maxima 670 nm). However, the properties of zinc and aluminium naphthalocyanines differ from their phthalocyanine counterparts in having high aggregation and photochemical instability, resulting in the naphthalocyanines being relatively photoinactive in vitro [24].

Second-generation photosensitizers undergoing clinical investigation include benzoporphyrin derivative mono-acid ring A (BPD-MA), mono-aspartyl chlorin e6 (NPe6), meso-tetra(hydroxyphenyl)chlorin (mTHPC), tin etiopurpurin (SnET2), and 5-amino-levulinic acid (ALA). The structures of these compounds and DHE are shown in Figure 1. Light at 650 nm is used to activate mTHPC, 660–665 nm is used to activate the chlorin and purpurin derivatives NPe6 and SnET2, and 690 nm light to activate BPD-MA. ALA is a precursor of protoporphyrin IX (PpIX) in heme biosynthesis, and endogenous PpIX produces effective photosensitization when activated by 630 nm light.

Tissue Distribution Studies

Considerable information on porphyrin tissue distribution has been obtained from preclinical animal studies [26–29], in addition to pharmacokinetic studies in humans [30–32]. Following intravenous injection, DHE has a biphasic plasma clearance in humans; an initial elimination half-life of 12–22 hours and a second half-life of 5–6 days have been reported [31,32]. The maximal therapeutic ratio for DHE between tumor and normal tissue varies between 24 and 96 hours. Many second-generation photosensitizers, such as NPe6 and BPD-MA, have a more rapid rate of clearance [33,34]. Consequently, photosensitizer injection and laser irradiation can be performed on the same day. DHE and NPe6 are primarily excreted unchanged through the feces, whereas BPD-MA is metabolized to an inactive form prior to excretion through the feces [27,33, 34]. Animal studies show that organ retention of these drugs is most persistent in reticuloendothelial tissues, such as liver, spleen, and kidney [26,33]. Levels in these tissues exceeded tumor levels at all time intervals after drug administration. Adrenal glands, pancreas, and bladder also retain high amounts of DHE. Skin and muscle take up relatively low levels of porphyrin and normal brain tissue has minimal uptake [27,28].

Transport in the blood of hydrophilic photosensitizers (hematoporphyrin monomers, tetrasulphonated porphyrins, and phthalocyanines) is mostly via albumen and globulins. These sensitizers localize in the stroma of tumor, vascular, and normal tissue. More hydrophobic photosensitizers (hematoporphyrin oligomers, mono and un-

A

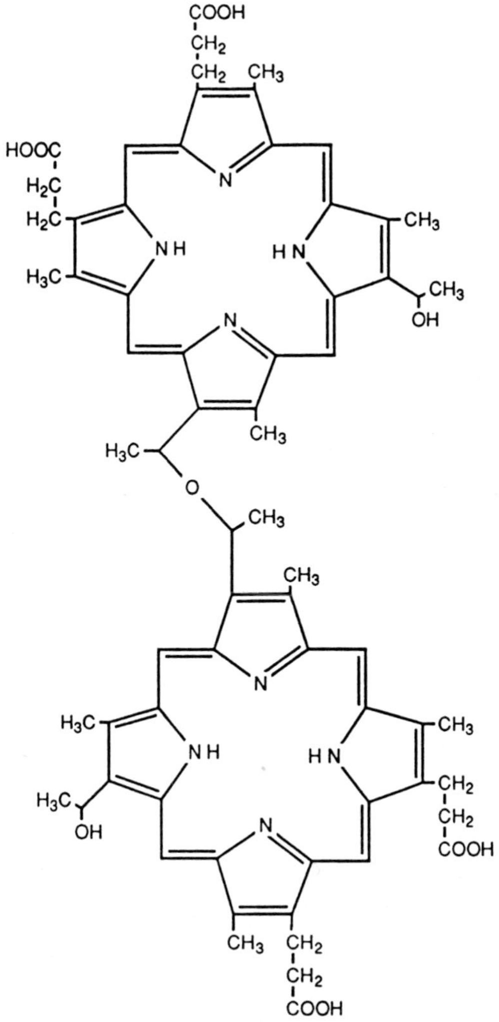

B

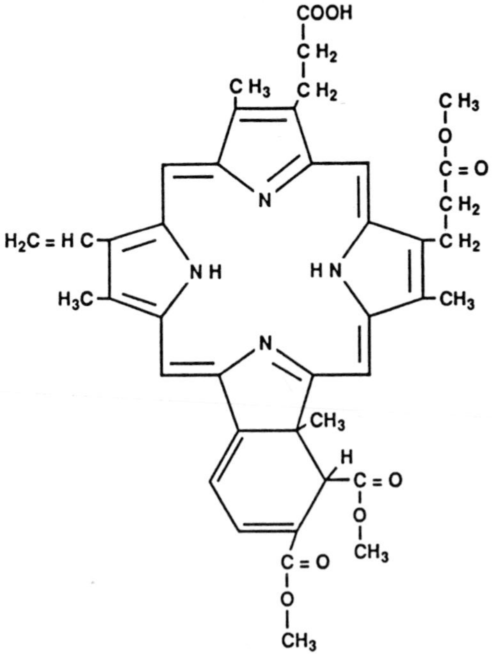

C

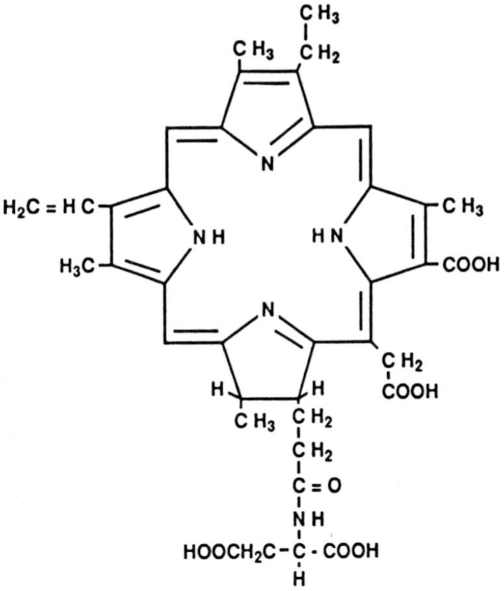

D

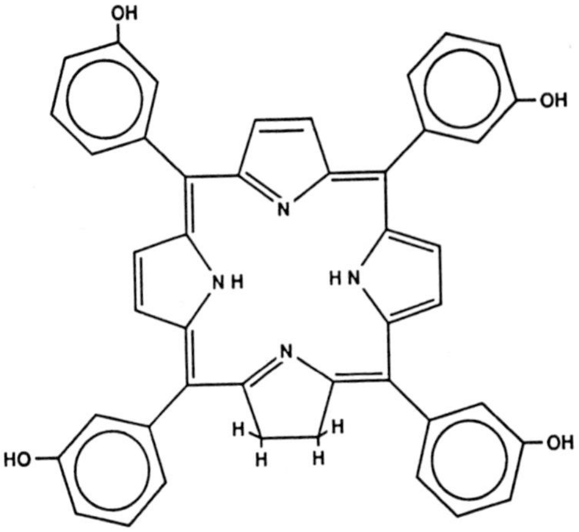

E

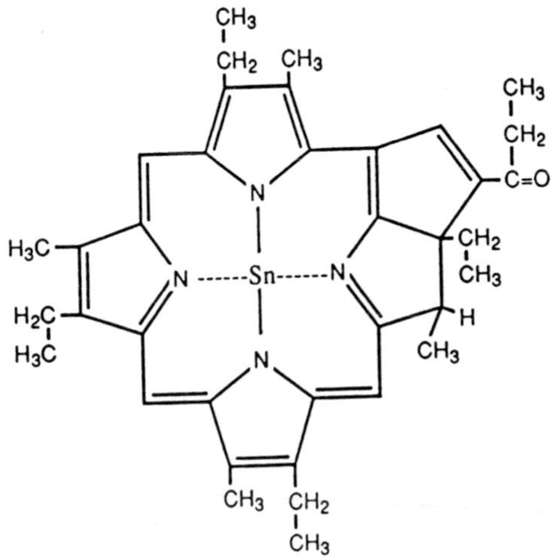

F

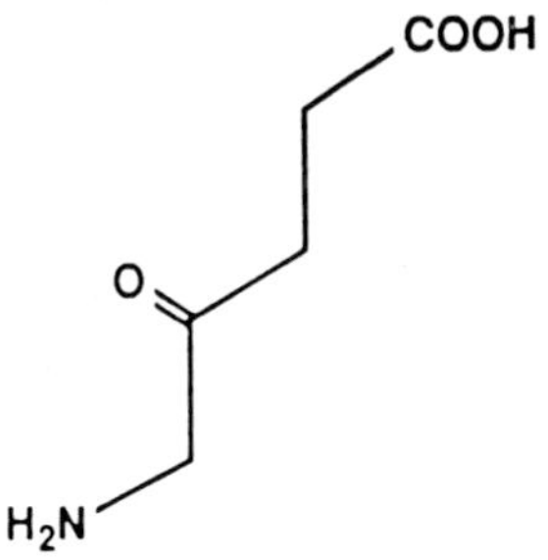

Fig. 1. Chemical structures for (**A**) dihematoporphyrin ether, DHE; (**B**) benzoporphyrin derivative monoacid ring A, BPD-MA; (**C**) mono-aspartyl chlorin e6, NPe6; (**D**) meta-tetra (hydroxyphenyl) chlorin, mTHPC; (**E**) tin etiopurpurin, SnET2; and (**F**) 5-amino-levulinic acid, ALA.

substituted phthalocyanines) are preferentially incorporated in the lipid portion of plasma lipoproteins [35]. Dyes with affinity for low density lipoproteins (LDL) are taken up by cells, at least in part, by receptor-mediated endocytosis. Lipoprotein-carried dyes are mostly deposited in endocellular loci, including mitochondria, lysosomes, and plasma membrane [35]. Otherwise, tightly aggregated dyes partly circulate as unbound pseudomicellar structures, which can enter cells by pinocytosis and localize in macrophages [35].

Photosensitizer Targeting

Approaches to improve the selective localization of photosensitizers in tumors involve binding the dye to targeting molecules such as antibodies, liposomes, and lectins [36,37]. The various conjugation strategies are described elsewhere [38,39]. The methods rely on the targeting molecule having high affinity for a tumor-associated antigen or receptor.

Plasma lipoproteins were found to play a major role in the in vivo transport of all classes of photosensitizers that are moderately or highly hydrophobic [40]. The low density lipoproteins (LDL) are of particular interest because they are recognized by specific receptors (e.g., the apo B/E receptor), which would result in LDL-bound photosensitizers being efficiently released to cells via apo B/E receptor-mediated endocytosis [41]. The process would favor cells that have a high content of LDL receptors, such as highly mitotic cells, including tumor cells, and endothelial cells [42]. In agreement with this, a correlation was seen between the extent of a photosensitizer's association with LDL and the efficiency of tumor targeting [40]. Therefore, various methods to enhance the LDL-mediated mechanism have been investigated, including formulation of photosensitizer in liposomes, lipid emulsions, inclusion complexes such as cyclodextrin, as well as preincorporation of the drug with LDL. Hematoporphyrin and zinc phthalocyanine incorporated into various liposomes show highly increased delivery to lipoproteins and high tumor uptake, compared with when administered in saline [40]. Photofrin prepared in LDL shows the same findings [40]. Benzoporphyrin derivative analogs, which naturally bind to the lipoprotein fractions when mixed with human plasma, have enhanced tumor uptake and tumor eradication when prebound to low density or high density lipoproteins [43]. BPD-MA is formulated in liposomes to achieve efficient tumor

photosensitization [44]. ALA encapsulated in liposomes and injected into tumor-bearing mice induced higher endogenous porphyrin accumulation in the tumors and maximal tumor/skin ratios, compared with injection of free drug [45]. However, selectivity indexes cannot be extrapolated directly to humans, since interspecies LDL plasma concentration and receptor activity varies widely. Rabbits and dogs show more similar patterns of plasma lipoproteins to humans than do commonly used mice and rat models [42].

Photoimmunotherapy, also termed "antibody-targeted photolysis," is another targeting technique in which antitumor monoclonal antibodies (MAb) are used as carriers for photosensitizers [36,46,47]. In preparing the conjugates, the goal is to preserve activity of the MAb conjugate and maximize the number of photosensitizer molecules bound to the MAb. For example, a conjugate of MAb-dextran-chlorin achieves a higher ratio of photosensitizer to antibody than is obtainable with direct attachment. This conjugate was used to show that binding at high concentration to the plasma membrane was photodynamically effective and that the chlorin did not need to enter the cells [36]. In contrast, MAb delivery of most drugs and toxins requires internalization. The mechanism of photolysis appears to involve release of singlet oxygen by the conjugate, although the actual target sites of MAb-photosensitizer conjugates are unknown [36,47]. The cell membrane is probably a principal target of MAb-targeted singlet oxygen damage, and cytoplasmic constituents close to the membrane may also be affected. The technique can use a variety of photosensitizers (it is not necessary for the sensitizer to have tumor-localizing properties) and offers theoretical advantages, including sensitizer dose reduction and minimal or no skin photosensitivity, compared with systemic injection of free drug. The clinical role of MAb delivered photosensitizer is not yet defined, although animal models show in vivo effectiveness [47]. The biodistribution of the photosensitizer BPD, conjugated to a MAb specific for A549 human squamous cell carcinoma, was altered compared to injection of free BPD [48]. The results demonstrated that the sensitizer and antibody did not dissociate in vivo. In addition, the MAb-BPD conjugate showed specificity for the A549 tumor, in terms of its kinetics of tumor tissue accumulation of BPD compared with normal tissues.

A preliminary report of MAb-targeted photodynamic cancer treatment was documented in three patients with advanced ovarian carcinoma, by Schmidt et al. [49]. A disulfonated zinc phthalocyanine was coupled by ester linkage to an anti-CA-125 antibody, since the patients all had elevated serum levels of the CA-125 tumor-associated antigen. The MAb-ZnPc conjugate was instilled in the peritoneum 72 hours before surgical tumor reduction and laser irradiation. After treatment, tumor cells were sampled for ultrastructural studies to detect signs of PDT damage.

For clinical application, there are several issues to address, in particular: (1) whether a large-size MAb-photosensitizer conjugate can reach cells in a solid tumor, (2) whether significant tumor cell antigen heterogeneity will arise, and (3) whether the host immune response will limit the technique. Methods to overcome each of these problems exist, such as use of small Fab or $(Fab')_2$ antibody fragments linked to the sensitizer and use of multiple MAbs to recognize different antigens. MAbs can be recognized as foreign proteins and become ineffective when neutralized. To decrease immunogenicity, it is desirable to use human antibodies and perhaps also to apply tolerance induction methods for reducing the immune response [50].

PHOTOCHEMISTRY AND PHOTOBIOLOGY
Type I and Type II Photochemistry

Upon absorption of a photon of light, a photosensitizer will be excited to a high energy singlet state. Singlet photosensitizer can decay back to its ground state, resulting in fluorescence emission. Alternatively, it can form triplet sensitizer, a slightly lower energy state, and longer lived excited species, by electron spin conversion in the process called intersystem crossover [51]. The fluorescent properties of photosensitizers have been useful for visualizing tumor localization and delineation of the malignant lesion. However, photodynamic action is dependent on intersystem crossover being the predominant process. The most efficient photosensitizers for PDT have a high triplet quantum yield and long triplet half-life. Triplet photosensitizer can undergo either Type I (electron or hydrogen atom transfer) or Type II (energy transfer) photochemical reactions. Transfer of energy to molecular oxygen is thought to be the primary photochemical reaction in porphyrin-mediated PDT. This results in the in situ generation of singlet oxygen $(^1O_2)$ [52]. The scheme for type II photochemical reactions is shown in Figure 2.

Type I reactions probably occur also, porphyrins being most likely to undergo electron transfer processes with production of superoxide anions (O_2^-) [51]. Hydroxyl radicals and O_2^- have been detected during PDT reactions [53].

The highly reactive oxygen products of Type I and II reactions produce damage initially at the site of photosensitizer localization, due to their very short lifetimes in a biological environment. Unfortunately, it has been difficult to identify the initial target sites, because photochemical reactions can produce radical chain auto-oxidation and further oxidative reactions, leading to varying types of intracellular damage [51].

Cellular Targets of PDT

Subcellular sites of photodynamic damage include the plasma membrane and many organelle membranes, in particular the mitochondria [54]. Following DHE-mediated PDT, fluorescence and electron microscopy show immediate changes in mitochondria, with progressive swelling and structural disruption. Biochemical analysis has shown that PDT inactivates membrane-bound mitochondrial enzymes such as cytochrome C oxidase and succinate dehydrogenase, and inhibits respiration [55–57]. Damage to endoplasmic reticulum membranes is similarly observed, ultrastructurally and biochemically, with inactivation of acyl coenzyme A [58]. Plasma membrane depolarization and inactivation of transmembrane pumps, such as the Ca^{2+}/ATPase and the Na^+/K^+ ATPase, is observed following porphyrin PDT [59,60]. Chlorin, benzoporphyrin, and phthalocyanine photosensitizers cause damage to lysosomes, resulting in hydrolytic enzyme leakage [61]. It is probable that multiple sites and types of cellular photooxidation result from photodynamic treatment using the current photosensitizers, as none of the drugs are site-specific [54].

Damage to DNA has been demonstrated by measurement of single-strand breaks and sister chromatid exchanges, but this does not appear to be a critical determinant of cytotoxicity [62,63]. Cell sensitivity to DHE photosensitization was comparable in human fibroblast cells whether proficient or deficient in DNA damage repair [64]. The quantity of DNA–protein crosslinks (rather than DNA–DNA crosslinks) was thought to be a factor in the differential sensitivity to PDT in mouse lymphoma cell lines [65]. It was noted that one of the most sensitive lymphoma cell strains had a mutated thymidine kinase gene locus after PDT treatment [66]. However, mutation and car-

Type II Porphyrin Photochemistry

$$
\begin{array}{lll}
\text{porphyrin} + h\upsilon & \longrightarrow & {}^{1}\text{porphyrin} \qquad\qquad \text{(absorption \& excitation)}\\
{}^{1}\text{porphyrin} & \longrightarrow & \text{porphyrin} + h\upsilon \qquad \text{(fluorescence)}\\
{}^{1}\text{porphyrin} & \longrightarrow & \text{porphyrin} \qquad\qquad \text{(nonradiative decay)}\\
{}^{1}\text{porphyrin} & \longrightarrow & {}^{3}\text{porphyrin} \qquad\qquad \text{(intersystem crossover)}\\
{}^{3}\text{porphyrin} & \longrightarrow & \text{porphyrin} + h\upsilon \qquad \text{(phosphorescence)}\\
{}^{3}\text{porphyrin} + {}^{3}O_2 & \longrightarrow & \text{porphyrin} + {}^{1}O_2 \qquad \text{(energy transfer)}\\
{}^{1}O_2 + \text{substrate} & \longrightarrow & \text{oxidized substrate} \quad \text{(photooxidation)}
\end{array}
$$

$h\upsilon$ = light quantum

^{1}porphyrin = singlet excited state porphyrin

^{3}porphyrin = triplet excited state porphyrin

${}^{3}O_2$ = ground state oxygen (triplet state)

${}^{1}O_2$ = singlet oxygen

Fig. 2. Type II photochemical reactions involved in the cytotoxic action of porphyrin PDT.

cinogenic transformation levels were measured as unchanged after a wide range of porphrin-mediated photosensitization doses [67].

Interestingly, PDT induces the expression of several types of stress proteins in cells, including heat shock proteins (HSP) and glucose-regulated proteins (GRP), although the specific response varies as a function of the photosensitizer and sensitizer incubation conditions [68–70]. Cells exposed to DHE and light, after a long incubation protocol to allow intracellular localization of drug, show induction of GRP78, GRP94, and hemeoxygenase (HO). NPe6 PDT and SnET2 PDT induce GRPs and HO, as well as HSP70 and HSP25. The induction of stress genes by PDT appears to be at the transcriptional level, but the complex problem of what target damage is responsible for induction of each stress gene is yet to be determined.

Apoptosis is also induced by PDT and appears to involve a signal transduction pathway originating at the cell membrane. Oleinick et al. [71,72] demonstrated characteristic DNA fragmentation, chromatin condensation, and activation of a constitutive endonuclease in phthalocy-anine and porphyrin photosensitized cells. Inositol triphosphate (IP$_3$) release was measured as a result of phospholipase C activation by PDT. The pathway is thought to follow IP$_3$ release, rise in free intracellular Ca^{2+}, activation of phospholipase A$_2$, and subsequent release of arachidonic acid. One of the metabolic products of arachidonic acid presumably activates an apoptotic endonuclease. Importantly, apoptosis has also been identified in vivo as an early event in tumor shrinkage following DHE or phthalocyanine-mediated PDT [73]. The significance of apoptosis in the clinical PDT response compared with necrotic cell death is unknown.

Vascular Destruction Versus Direct Tumor Cell Kill

Experimental studies indicate that vascular injury plays a major role in tumor destruction following PDT. The in vivo response of porphyrin-mediated PDT is characterized by rapid onset of vascular stasis, vascular hemorrhage, and both direct and anoxia-induced tumor cell death. In a study examining perfusion of mouse tumors after

Photofrin PDT, tumor regrowth delay correlated with treatment protocols that cause the most severe reduction in tumor blood flow [74]. Vasculature destruction also appears to be the major effect following chlorin and phthalocyanine photosensitization, with tumor cell death occurring secondary to vascular shutdown [75]. Henderson et al. [76] used an in vivo/in vitro technique to demonstrate the time course of PDT events. In tumors removed soon after HPD PDT treatment, the cells were clonogenically viable, but viability decreased with longer intervals of sampling. Tumor cell death was occurring later from oxygen and nutrient deprivation, following early vascular injury.

Endothelial cells and macrophages are known to be particularly sensitive to photosensitization. Irradiation of sensitized mast cells and macrophages causes release of vasoactive inflammatory agents and cytokines, including prostaglandins, lymphokines, and thromboxanes [77, 78]. These inflammatory mediators seem to play an important role in the microvascular response to PDT, since administration of cyclooxygenase inhibitors not only inhibits their release, but also inhibits PDT-induced vascular damage and tumor destruction [79,80]. However, there does not seem to be any significant difference in photosensitivity between tumor and normal vascular endothelium [81].

It is likely that the mechanism of PDT tumor destruction in human tumors is not always the same as found using transplanted animal tumors. One reason is that spontaneous tumors have marked differences in vascular and stromal structures. It has been suggested that in the clinical situation, the vascular effects may be less responsible for tumor destruction than direct killing of tumor cells. An initial increase in blood flow can sometimes occur, seen in preliminary human tumor blood flow studies [82]. Also, direct cell kill effects might be underestimated from the mechanistic studies in animals. Histological evaluation of tumors following PDT shows clear demarcation of tissue necrosis, corresponding to depth of light penetration and not consistent with vascular occlusion causing cell kill [82]. Ultimately, the relative contributions from tumor cell and vascular photosensitization will depend to some extent on the time interval employed between drug injection and light irradiation and drug dose. The photosensitizer type is a particularly important factor due to their variation in clearance kinetics and tissue compartment localization [77].

Tumor Selectivity of PDT

PDT offers a degree of tumor selectivity with minimal systemic side effects. Factors contributing to selectivity include: (1) preferential photosensitizer localization in neoplastic tissues, and (2) precise laser light irradiation of the tumor region. The first factor cannot be relied upon using current photosensitizers to produce selective photodynamic treatment of the malignant lesion, since the amount of differential localization between tumor and normal tissue is highly variable. There are several theories regarding the mechanisms whereby photosensitizers can accumulate or be retained in neoplastic tissue more than in the adjacent normal tissue. It is probable that more than one mechanism is operating.

The majority of data on in vitro cell studies indicate that normal cells and cells of varying oncogenic potential take up similar levels of photosensitizer [83]. Cationic intramitochondrial dyes are an exception, capable of producing selective in vitro photolysis, due to increased dye incorporation by carcinoma cells [84]. Tissue physiology is clearly important, since Chan et al. [85] transplanted the same tumor (colorectal carcinoma) to different organs in mice and found significant variation in in vivo ClAlPc uptake. Henderson and Dougherty [82] suggest that simple pooling and retention of photosensitizer could occur as a result of the typically large interstitial space and poor lymphatic network characteristic of tumor tissue, in comparison with normal tissues having lower interstitial, higher vascular spaces [86]. The tumor localization properties of anionic dyes, such as hematoporphyrin derivatives and phthalocyanines, are thought to involve tissue factors such as low pH, and increased amounts of macrophage infiltration and newly synthesized collagen [83]. The density of lipoprotein receptors was proposed as a more specific mechanism for increased uptake, whereby LDL-bound photosensitizer rapidly enter neoplastic cells by receptor-mediated endocytosis [87]. However, uptake assisted by LDL binding is not the only explanation since protoporphyrin associates well with lipoproteins but is a poor tumor localizer. Several other dyes, such as TPPS and uroporphyrin, are reported to be good tumor localizers, although they associate poorly with lipoproteins.

The drug concentration ratio depends on the tissue. The highest tumor to normal tissue ratios of Photofrin have been reported in the brain, which might be due to a breakdown in the blood-brain barrier at the tumor site [88]. In skin, the tumor to normal tissue ratio of Photofrin in rodent models is <2:1. However, human malignant skin lesions have shown more selectivity in treatment response than rodent models [82]. In reticuloendothelial tissues where uptake of current photosensitizers is high, there is no time interval that produces a useful ratio. Understanding the mechanisms for preferential uptake is mainly important for attempting to improve tumor targeting of sensitizers. Methods of targeting photosensitizers using carrier molecules or delivery systems may prove worthwhile as a means to increase tumor selectivity.

Combined Use of PDT and Hyperthermia

In general, the reason for using nonthermal power densities for photodynamic treatment is to exploit the potential selectivity of PDT by irradiating tumors at a time when the photosensitizer is retained in higher concentrations than the surrounding normal tissue. This allows undefined tumor margins to be lasered more safely. Clinically, combined hyperthermia and PDT tend not to be employed, although simultaneous treatment could be achieved simply by using higher dose rates of light during PDT.

From experimental studies, hyperthermia (HT) has been proposed to be a useful adjunct to photodynamic therapy for some applications, since the two treatments can be synergistic. In vitro and in vivo experiments indicate that the therapeutic response is synergistic or superadditive only within a short window, when HT is applied before, during or immediately after PDT [89,90]. The following mechanisms have been suggested for the synergistic response that follows the specific treatment sequence of PDT followed by HT. The rapid vascular destruction caused by PDT can hinder heat dissipation by blood circulation and increases the temperature differential between tumor and normal surrounding tissue [91]. At the cellular level, PDT and HT may have targets in common, particularly membranes. The proteins of the plasma membrane and mitochondrial membranes undergo structural transitions at hyperthermic temperatures [91]. Despite PDT and HT having similarities in their subcellular targets and denaturing effects on proteins, there is no evidence that the two modalities share mechanisms of cytotoxicity. Cross resistance to PDT is not observed in temperature resistant murine fibrosarcoma cell lines [92].

Heat applied before PDT may be a less effective combination in vivo, since the vascular modifications due to HT, such as hemorrhage, could drastically decrease light penetration in the tumor [91]. Heat-induced capillary collapse could significantly decrease oxygenation in the tumor microenvironment, which would theoretically impair the efficiency of photodynamic action [91].

Advocating against combined PDT and HT to obtain improved tumor control, injury to normal tissue can also be increased as a result of vascular effects common to both treatments. An experimental model showed that combined treatment of PDT followed by HT required an interval of more than 21 days between modalities to minimize normal skin necrosis [93].

LIGHT IRRADIATION
Laser and Nonlaser Sources

Incandescent filament (tungsten) and arc (xenon, mercury) lamps were used in early clinical PDT studies. It seems likely that nonlaser sources of light will continue to have a useful role, even though they supply relatively broad spectrum light. Lasers have become the standard light source for most clinical PDT applications largely because the laser beam can be efficiently coupled into single optical fibers, ideal for inserting in flexible endoscopes and for interstitial use.

Laser light is monochromatic, and the wavelength chosen depends on the specific photosensitizer and application. The absorption spectrum of DHE includes a high Soret band absorption (370–410 nm) with progressively smaller Q bands (505, 540, 580, and 630 nm) [94]. The 514 nm output of the argon laser is suitable for PDT applications where tissue penetration requirements are minimal, such as in certain cancers of the peritoneal cavity or bladder. Although Photofrin absorption is minimal for 630 nm light, this wavelength is routinely used for Photofrin-mediated PDT because light penetration in tissue is greater than at the shorter wavelength Q bands [95]. The argon ion laser-pumped dye laser has been the most widely used laser system to produce 630 nm light. In the visible red spectrum, the choices of gas and solid state laser with sufficient power for PDT treatment are limited. The gold vapor laser (GVL) emitting at 628 nm can generate over 1W of power. Optically pumped dye lasers remain a popular light source for PDT, since single dyes can cover a significant range of wavelengths. The tunability is an obvious advantage of dye lasers over the GVL, since the output wavelength can be altered accordingly to suit new drugs with varying absorption properties.

Argon ion laser-pumped dye laser (ADL). This has been the most widely used light source for clinical PDT and emits continuous wave (CW) light. Medical ADL systems have minimized the requirement for precise optical alignment of the dye laser. Argon lasers are termed small frame (7–10 W) or large frame (20–25 W) and generate 1–2 W or 3–4 W of red light, respectively, out of the dye laser. This light can be coupled with 80–90% efficiency into single 200–400 μm fibers. Rhodamine B is a relatively stable dye with long-lasting lifetimes, most commonly employed in the ADL to obtain 630 nm light; DCM (4 dicyanomethylene-2-methyl-6-dimethylaminostyryl-4H-pyran) and Kiton red are other dyes of choice for obtaining light of this wavelength.

Gold vapor laser (GVL). The GVL produces a pulsed output at 628 nm. Compared to dye lasers, GVL are tolerant to misalignment and easy to operate. The laser pulse duration is typically 50–100 nsec and pulse repetition frequencies tend to be in the range 4–20 kHz for commercial systems. Average output powers range from 1.5 W to 9 W. The fixed wavelength output of 628 nm matches Photofrin absorption, although it would be possible to use this laser for new photosensitizers, by converting the plasma tube to a copper vapor laser for pumping a tunable dye laser.

Copper vapor laser-pumped dye laser (CVDL). The copper vapor laser is also a pulsed system with pulse structures similar to the GVL. The output from the copper laser at 510 and 578 nm would be useful only in surface PDT treatments. Its high pulse repetition frequency and high average pulse power make it suitable as a pump laser for dyes with emission in the red and near infrared. A negative feature of this pulsed laser output is a large beam divergence, requiring a larger diameter fiber (1,000 μm) for light delivery. Like the ADL, its most important characteristic is its tunability, particularly useful when new drugs are approved.

Excimer laser-pumped dye laser (EDL). This laser system is widely used by Japanese clinicians in their Phase III registration studies using Photofrin. XeCl or XeF gas is excited to produce UV line output, which is then used for pumping rhodamine or DCM dye to produce 630 nm light. The excimer laser is a high power pulsed laser, capable of megawatt peak output of 10–100 ns pulse duration. The EDL has a low repetition rate (maximum 80 Hz).

Solid state lasers. The neodymium:YAG (Nd:YAG) laser emitting at 1,064 nm or frequency doubled to emit at 532 nm has applications in surgical specialties, the wavelength of choice depending on 1,064 nm light having excellent penetration properties through hemoglobin, whereas 532 nm light does not. With regard to suitability for PDT, frequency doubled operation can be used to pump a dye laser resulting in tunable pulsed laser output. A combination system has been assembled intended specifically for this application, in which a KTP doubled Nd:YAG laser (line output at 532 nm) is used to pump a dye laser to emit light at 630 nm. The average power is 3–4 W from the KTP-dye laser system. The repetition rate is 25 kHz and the pulse width is 470 nsec. Alternatively, Nd:YAG has several minor lines, such as 1,318 nm, which can be frequency doubled to provide 659 nm light.

Tunable solid state lasers have advanced considerably in the past 5 years and are being tested experimentally for PDT use. They can only generate far-red/near infrared light, so they are potential laser sources for matching to second- and third-generation photosensitizers. The titanium:sapphire (Ti:Al$_2$O$_3$) laser has three sets of optics to cover the wavelength range 690–1,100 nm; the alexandrite lasers have a working range 720–800 nm.

Diode lasers. Major progress in the use of semiconductor laser diodes for PDT has been gained by making phased arrays of the output beams from multiple low power diodes to make a sufficiently high power coherent beam. Diode lasers are a portable size and represent convenient light sources. Most development is on the GaAlAs diodes, usually operating in the wavelength range of 780–850 nm with 1–5 W output. Diode laser systems emitting at 660–700 nm have been developed, but the power output is lower. Diode arrays have considerable potential for PDT involving current sensitizers (NPe6, BPD) and new sensitizers with absorption in the far-red region. The quality of the output beam is relatively divergent compared to the other laser systems described, making it more difficult to couple to fiber optics.

Comparison of CW and Pulsed Lasers for PDT

There are few prospective studies comparing CW and pulsed laser systems for PDT. In general, it has been demonstrated that both types of laser light can be used for therapy. There is insufficient information for the new laser systems being introduced and, therefore, further evaluation will be required in this regard. Controlled studies are required to determine biological equivalence for the EDL and solid-state lasers with the ADL, in terms of PDT efficacy and safety. Pulsed lasers operating at very high repetition rate represent a quasi-CW mode. Differences in effects may be expected with pulsed lasers that have a high peak power per pulse.

Several studies have been conducted to directly compare the ADL (630 nm light) and GVL (628 nm) [96–98]. One experimental study used a cell culture and a murine tumor response assay [96]. Both laser systems were tested using 400 mW output (average pulse power of 400 mW), coupled to a 400 μm fiber to create a 1 cm diameter spot. The GVL had a 50 ns pulse width and repetition frequency of 10–14 kHz. The lasers were equivalent in in vitro cytotoxicity and in tumoricidal efficiency. For clinical usage, which generally required ~1 W of power, the GVL was easier to operate [97]. Output needed to be coupled to a 600μm diameter fiber (compared to 200 μM with the dye laser), which can be a disadvantage if the large, less flexible fiber reduces the maneuvreability of endoscopes. Otherwise, light applied continuously or in a pulsed mode appeared to make no difference to the results of patient PDT treatments. A recent study compared the ADL and GVL for treatment of virally induced papillomas in rabbits [98]. The GVL produced a faster rate of initial response following PDT, but ultimately there were no differences in overall cure rate, histology assessment, or viral DNA analysis from involved tissues using either laser system.

Barr et al. [99] compared three lasers for photodynamic effectiveness using normal rat colon as an in vivo model and aluminium sulphonated phthalocyanine as the photosensitizer. An ADL system (DCM dye), a 10 kHz repetition CVDL (Oxazine72/Rhodamine G dye), and a 5 Hz repetition flashlamp-pumped dye laser (cresol violet dye) were evaluated. Each laser was tuned to emit 100 mW at 675 nm, coupled to a 200-μm fiber. The ADL and CVDL were comparable at producing damage, measured as the radius of necrosis in histology sections. The CVDL pulses were 40 ns width and 10 mJ energy. The flashlamp-pumped dye laser produced 2 μs, 20 mJ pulses, and failed to produce a photodynamic effect. The most likely explanation for the ineffectiveness of this laser was that the higher energy, microsecond pulses produced saturation of the phthalocyanine. Specifically, the pulse energy was

able to pump most of the ground state photosensitizer to an excited state and deplete the ground state population, so that subsequent pulse energy is not used efficiently. Saturation pumping is a common process for phthalocyanines because they have a high absorption coefficient. However, the flashlamp-pumped dye laser was also found to be ineffective for PDT mediated by HPD in a murine tumor model, despite HPD having a lower absorption coefficient and lower potential for saturation [100].

A direct comparison has also been made between the ADL and the pulsed KTP-pumped dye laser [101]. Both dye lasers were tuned to emit 630 nm light and the output coupled to a 200 μM fiber. The lasers were tested over the range 0–400 J/cm^2 using a power density of 75 mW/cm^2. They were shown to be biologically equivalent in several types of experimental systems, including in vivo tumor response, murine skin photosensitization, and in vitro cytotoxicity. Furthermore, tumor temperature levels during laser exposure, amount of DHE photobleaching, and induction of cellular stress protein synthesis were observed to be identical using either laser system.

Laser Dosimetry and Delivery

The clinical effectiveness of PDT for solid tumors depends in large part on the transmission of adequate light throughout the tumor tissue. The aim is to disperse low power light uniformly, either over the surface area or into the volume of tissue, to initiate the photochemical process without inducing side-effects, such as thermal damage of adnexal structures. This is in contrast to surgical laser treatments, in which light is focused for cutting, coagulating, or photoacoustical effects. In PDT, further requirements of the delivery systems are to make them: (1) compatible with other clinical instrumentation, such as endoscopes and stereotactic devices, (2) to incorporate light output monitoring and dosimetry devices, and (3) to tailor the light spatial distribution to match the tumor shape and size in each patient [102].

The light dose chosen for PDT depends on the size, location, and type of tumor. Using Photofrin and 630 nm light, typical radiant exposures are 25–300 J/cm^2 for surface treatment and 100–400 J/cm for interstitial applications, with maximum irradiances of 200 mW/cm^2 or 400 mW/cm, respectively [103]. This has generally been attained using laser sources having an output power of 1–2 W. However, higher power lasers (at least 5 W) may be required during intracavitary PDT, involving treatment of large surface areas in pleural and peritoneal cavities.

Power requirements are not likely to be much less with second-generation photosensitizers either, since the rationale for these is to allow treatment of larger tumors by exploiting their higher extinction coefficient and longer wavelength activation. Another situation in which a higher light dose is required than normal is during differential photobleaching of photosensitizer in tumor and adjacent normal tissues [104]. The technique can potentially improve the therapeutic ratio of PDT and it involves significant photosensitizer dose reduction. The light dose needs to be increased more than proportionally to achieve equivalent photodynamic tumor destruction.

Laser delivery systems differ depending on the application. Rather than simply using an expanded laser beam from a bare fiber, more uniform irradiation is obtained by fitting a microlens to the fiber for forward surface illumination [105,106]. For treating thicker lesions and tumors within the body, the use of interstitial laser irradiation is required. The fiber can be directly inserted into the tumor mass, either by point insertion or inside a needle using a flat cut fiber tip, or by insertion of spherical and cylindrical diffusing tips. If several sites are to be irradiated, translucent nylon catheters can be surgically implanted for subsequent laser treatments.

The concept of "photodynamic dose" and contributing factors have been described by Wilson [107]. During patient follow-up, a wide range in tumor response is seen. Factors responsible for heterogeneity are speculated to include differences in photosensitizer uptake and light transmission within the tumor, and variation in tumor tissue sensitivity depending on cell composition, vascularity, and oxygenation. Techniques to measure light fluence within tissue, photosensitizer concentration, and tumor tissue oxygenation are being developed to assist patient PDT treatments.

Several workers [105,107] have identified the requirement for incorporation of light monitoring and dosimetry instruments into clinical delivery systems as the next essential step to gain information from each patient treated with PDT. Invasive and noninvasive devices will be able to provide real-time information during the laser procedure. Direct noninvasive measurement of drug concentration in a tissue can be based on quantitative fluorometry or reflectance spectro-

photometry, although these only provide average values. Transcutaneous DHE levels in an animal model were measured using a hand-held fluorometer and showed a good correlation with fluorescence measurements of DHE in skin biopsy specimens [108]. Similarly, noninvasive measurement of local oxygen concentration can be made during treatment. Tromberg et al. [109] used transcutaneous oxygen electrodes in rabbits transplanted with VX-2 skin carcinomas. PDT using low light doses caused a reversible decrease in oxygen tension, whereas large fluences caused long-term irreversible hypoxia.

There are ongoing attempts to make in vivo measurements of singlet oxygen ($^1O_2$) production, by monitoring its luminescence emission at 1,270 nm, since $^1O_2$ is generally accepted as a key intermediate in the photodynamic effect [110]. It is thought that a minimum threshold level of $^1O_2$ (or photoactivated species) is required to produce tumor necrosis. So far, it seems in a cell or tissue environment, the extremely short lifetime of singlet oxygen (<0.5 μs) prevents reliable detection with present infrared detectors [111,112].

PHOTODYNAMIC THERAPY APPLICATIONS IN CANCER TREATMENT
Current Status of Clinical Photofrin PDT

PDT has been used to treat several thousand cancer patients as an investigational modality. Recently, Canada received Board of Health approval for the use of Photofrin-mediated PDT for treating superficial bladder cancer. In addition, The Netherlands has permitted licenses for treating lung and esophageal cancers with Photofrin PDT. Further regulatory submissions for a variety of applications have been made in Japan, Belgium, Germany, Denmark, and Greece. A product license for PDT specifies not only the photosensitizing drug, but also the laser type and the fiberoptic devices for producing and delivering the light [113].

The following Phase I and II trials are underway or near completion in the United States: for breast metastases, gynecological tumors, cutaneous cancers, Carcinoma In Situ (CIS), Kaposi's sarcoma, and papillomatosis, plus Phase I/II trials for intraperitoneal and intrapleural (intracavitary) PDT. Phase III trials in the United States, Canada, and Europe are evaluating Photofrin PDT for treatment of endobronchial lung cancer, esophagus, superficial bladder cancer, and prophylaxis of bladder cancer following transurethral resection (TUR) of tumors. Japan has Phase III clinical trials in progress for early stage lung, esophagus, gastric, bladder, and cervical cancers.

Clinical Studies of PDT Using HPD/Photofrin

This section reviews the current status of clinical PDT treatment using Photofrin (DHE) or its predecessor, HPD. Details are given for specific laser delivery systems designed for the specific cancer type. Clinical outcomes are mostly described as complete response (CR; no tumor present grossly and microscopically), partial response (PR; >50% decrease in all tumors treated), with the remainder of lesions representing progressive disease. Follow-up times vary in each study.

Endobronchial lung cancer. The lung cancer mortality rate remains high, despite increased screening and early detection. This disease is thought to be multicentric; patients have a high risk of developing another primary lung tumor even after complete resection of the original lesion [114,115]. This means that surgical treatment of initial early stage lung cancer has become as conservative as possible to preserve lung tissue. Surgical resection can be totally successful at removing the original lesion, but patients frequently have coexisting pulmonary or cardiovascular disease, making them a high surgical risk [114,115].

PDT represents a local therapeutic modality that can produce complete responses and cure of centrally located early stage endobronchial lung cancer [116,117]. Results from ~500 patients with this disease have been reported to produce complete and partial response rates ranging from 70–100% [118]. Superficial disease at the time of treatment is an essential factor for long-term effectiveness. PDT is useful for patients who cannot undergo surgery, as well as for palliation of advanced endobronchial malignancy. Patients with endobronchial tumor obstruction recruited in Phase III studies are randomized to receive either palliative Nd:YAG treatment or Photofrin PDT. Clean-up bronchoscopy is routinely scheduled 24–48 h after PDT to prevent complications of pulmonary obstruction, due to mucosal plugs and necrotic tissue.

McCaughan et al. [119] reported treatment of 31 patients (49 tumor sites) with endobronchial cancer using HPD and Photofrin PDT. All patients had been pretreated with or were unsuitable for conventional surgery, radiation therapy, and chemotherapy. An ADL system was used to supply the 630 nm light using a flexible bronchoscope, incorporating a biopsy channel. The results were promising in that 37% had a complete response and only 4% had progressive disease at 1 month after treatment.

By 1989, Kato et al. [120] had treated 165 patients with lung cancer by PDT, using an argon-dye laser and an excimer-dye laser as light sources. Forty patients did not have disease evident on chest X-ray, but endoscopically were classified as having early stage lung cancer. The majority of the 165 patients received additional surgery, radiotherapy, or chemotherapy, but a total of 26 patients (with 30 lesions) received PDT as the sole treatment. All lesions in the PDT-only group showed complete remission initially, with 16 patients remaining disease-free and three patients classified as 5-year "cures." Ono et al. [121] treated 36 patients with biopsy specimens positive for malignancies of the trachea and bronchus; again not all identifiable on chest X-ray. HPD was administered 72 hours before laser treatment under fiberoptic bronchoscope delivery. The range in response was a complete response with no recurrent disease in 16 patients and death of 20 patients related to the disease. Follow-up ranged from 37–109 months. Cortese [114] has treated > 60 lung cancer patients with PDT. Patients were not deemed suitable for this treatment if lymph nodes were known or suspected to be involved. Some of their patients were suitable for conventional surgery but received PDT as a first-line treatment instead. Twelve of 13 such patients demonstrated a complete response after one or two PDT sessions, and these were all superficial tumors. The one tumor treated that showed only a partial response was a bulky, exfoliative lesion.

A study in Japan was recently reported of 39 patients with early lung cancer, treated with Photofrin and light irradiation delivered by EDL through a flexible bronchoscope [122]. Cure rates were high for small (< 1 cm length) lesions, with a complete response in 32 of 40 lesions. Sutedja et al. [123] performed a pilot study of Photofrin PDT on 26 patients. The group with Stage I disease had a CR rate of ten of 11 patients. The patients with Stage III disease had little clinical benefit, showing either partial response or tumor progression. The four patients who died (within 6 months of PDT) had previously failed radiation therapy, Nd:YAG laser, and brachytherapy.

Okunaka et al. [124] had treated 145 lung cancer patients with PDT and reported the effectiveness of Photofrin PDT in 13 patients with multiple primary bronchial carcinoma. Three patients had only early stage lesions and received no surgery additional to PDT, whereas ten patients required surgery for advanced lesions. Patient survival ranged 14 to 87 months, with seven alive at the time of report.

Shimatani et al. [125] treated seven patients, mostly with Stage I early lung cancer, with PDT by administering the Photofrin by bronchial arterial infusion (BAI). For this pilot study, the Photofrin dose was 0.7 mg/kg, about one-third of the usual dose employed. An EDL emitting 630 nm light was used at a dose of 100 J/cm^2, via fiberoptic bronchoscope at 72 h after BAI. Complete remission was achieved in five Stage I cases and a partial response achieved in two patients, which were a recurrence case and an advanced stage case.

Gastrointestinal cancer. This group includes esophageal, gastric, and colorectal cancer. Early stage esophageal lesions are treatable by surgery. Advanced disease involving varying degrees of esophageal obstruction carries a mortality of 10–20% after surgery, and many different palliative techniques have been introduced to relieve dysphagia. These include combinations of dilation, stents, Nd:YAG laser, BICAP thermal probes, and radiation therapy [126]. None of the available treatments offer long-term survival if esophageal cancer is advanced at the time of diagnosis, so early diagnosis is essential.

PDT appears promising for treating early or superficial esophageal tumors and as a palliative treatment for malignant dysphagia [127]. A Phase III trial for esophageal cancer includes patients with partially obstructing esophageal lesions. The patients are randomized to Photofrin PDT or Nd:YAG laser treatment. Patients with completely obstructive disease can receive Photofrin PDT as part of a Phase II single-arm protocol [118]. PDT is also being evaluated for the condition known as Barrett's esophagus, in which columnar epithelium replaces normal malpighian epithelium [128,129]. The incidence of carcinoma is 10% in these patients. Currently, two patients with Barrett's esophagus with early adenocarcinomas have been treated with Photofrin PDT [129]. Variation in response was noted because of insufficient light delivery to esophageal folds.

Overholt and colleagues [130] have developed a cylindrical esophageal balloon device for delivering circumferential light to the center of the lumen for PDT of esophageal cancer. The balloon is specifically intended to distend and flatten

esophageal folds. Inside the balloon is a clear tube for holding a cylinder diffuser-tip fiber. Three isotropic probes on the outside of the balloon measure the delivered light dose to the esophageal mucosa. Uniform light irradiation was achieved, compared to use of the cylindrical diffuser without the balloon device.

In Japan, 80 patients with upper gastrointestinal tumors were treated with HPD and ADL light delivered endoscopically [131]. PDT was most effective for superficial esophageal cancer and poorly defined gastric cancer lesions. Okunaka et al. [132] treated 20 patients by PDT, six with early superficial esophageal carcinoma, and 14 had advanced invasive disease. PDT was performed through a biopsy channel of the gastroscope. Treatment was effective for early esophageal cancer (4/6 had complete remission), whereas advanced cancer patients experienced only improvement in dysphagia. McCaughan (133) reported the results of 40 patients receiving PDT as palliative treatment; 19 had adenocarcinomas, 19 squamous cell carcinomas, and two had melanoma lesions of the esophagus. The treatment goal was to improve swallowing in the patients, which proved to be of short-term benefit. Average survival time was 7.7 months for adenocarcinoma and 5.8 months for squamous cell carcinoma. In China, 142 patients with a variety of advanced gastrointestinal tumors were treated with HPD 48–72 h before ADL (630 nm light) treatment [134]. Fifteen patients showed CR (10.6%) and 53 showed PR (37.3%).

Gastric cancer normally presents in advanced form in most parts of the world and is associated with high mortality. Japan has implemented screening protocols involving endoscopic ultrasound and biopsy, with the result that early diagnoses are being made and the mortality rate has decreased [135]. Early gastric cancer is conventionally treated by surgery, and in Japan, patients have received PDT who refused surgery. Kato et al. [136] treated 19 patients (20 adenocarcinoma lesions) with Stages I–III gastric cancer, using HPD or Photofrin PDT. Red (630 nm) light supplied by an ADL or EDL was delivered through a fiber passed down the instrument channel of a gastrofiberscope. A CR was reported in 11 of the 19 patients (60%). Incomplete responses were thought to be due to inadequate light dosage, either because of the tumor's location or because of extensive or invasive growth into the muscular layer.

Colorectal cancer is treated by surgery as the

treatment of choice, but prognosis for recurrence depends on degree of spread outside the colon or rectum. By the time deep tumor invasion is present, treatment is intended to be palliative using Nd:YAG thermal ablation therapy to control hemorrhage or obstruction [137]. Barr et al. [138] reported the results of ten patients with inoperable colorectal disease treated with HPD PDT as an alternative to Nd:YAG laser therapy. The advantage of PDT over thermal ablation appeared to be preservation of the submucosal collagen layer. As a result, the colon retained mechanical strength, which removed the risk of perforation (the potential complication after Nd:YAG laser), and healing by rapid regeneration occurred. The conclusion of this study [138] was that a combination of Nd:YAG laser for tumor debulking and PDT for small or residual disease might produce optimal results.

Superficial bladder cancer. This cancer can present as papillary tumors or as carcinoma in situ (CIS). Papillary bladder cancer is conventionally treated by transurethral resection (TUR). The recurrence rate is high (ranging 40–70%) following TUR, and prophylactic intravesical chemotherapy has been found to significantly improve the long-term response [139]. PDT Phase III trials are underway for prophylaxis of recurrent papillary bladder cancer. After TUR of tumors, patients receive Photofrin (2 mg/kg) and low dose light (15 J/cm^2) to the whole bladder [118]. CIS is a high grade and aggressive manifestation of transitional cell carcinoma of the bladder, which previously indicated cystectomy [140]. However, intravesical BCG therapy now produces uniformly good responses, so that cystectomy is no longer the appropriate initial treatment [140]. A Phase II study for CIS is being performed in Europe and the United States of America in which PDT is an alternative to cystectomy. Patients receive Photofrin followed by whole bladder PDT, using the parameters described above for the Phase III (papillary bladder cancer) trial [118].

Irradiation of the whole bladder (or sometimes combined focal and whole bladder irradiation) is now the preferred procedure for PDT, because bladder cancer is often multifocal. The superficial tumors are often difficult to detect cytoscopically, so there is a risk of missing tumors with focal irradiation only [102]. Several methods are used for uniform irradiation of the whole bladder. Intralipid is a fat emulsion that acts as a light-scattering medium and makes it possible to use a flat cut fiber for laser treatment. Otherwise,

many investigators use a spherical diffuser-tip fiber, which can emit light isotropically. Specially designed double balloon catheters can be used to position the tip. Unsoeld et al. [141] have reported on a new type of balloon coated with a light-scattering material, exhibiting ~90% reflectivity. It is inserted into the bladder, then filled with water so it unfolds spherically. Marijnissens group [142,143] developed a delivery system using a modified cystoscope to introduce a fiber with diffusing tip into the bladder and three nylon catheters that unfold in different directions along the bladder wall. Each catheter incorporates an isotropic light detector providing a measure of integrated light dose.

Nseyo et al. [144] described the development of an intravesical laser catheter (IVLC) delivery and monitoring system. The IVLC provides several advantages compared to simply positioning the light by cystoscopy and ultrasound. Mainly, it protects against nonuniform photoirradiation. The system automatically results in the tip being positioned within the center of the bladder. Inflation of the catheter's balloon transforms an asymmetrical bladder into a sphere of known diameter. A light sensor is incorporated in the balloon wall to monitor light fluence and dose and is computer controlled to adjust the total dose.

Nseyo reviewed results of PDT for papillary bladder cancer and reported that eradication rates depend on the tumor size [145]. Widespread micropapillary disease and tumors <2 cm diameter can be completely eradicated. When all patients were included in the assessment, single PDT treatment produced CR rates of 70–95%.

Jocham et al. [146] treated 20 patients with recurrent superficial CIS by whole bladder PDT. Cases that were resistant to intravesical BCG therapy and chemotherapy proved to be highly sensitive to this modality. Six of the 20 patients treated with PDT alone remained free of disease during a 5-year follow-up. The remainder of the patients received TUR and Nd:YAG laser therapy additional to PDT in order to achieve remission. Nseyo [145] reports the response rate of CIS treated by whole bladder PDT (total 37 patients) to be CR 88%, with an incidence of 25% recurrence during a 12–60-month follow-up. In patients undergoing PDT prophylactically, the recurrence rate was 31% with a median time of 18 months to recurrence.

Guo [147] reported on the treatment of 40 patients with superficial bladder tumors (104 lesions). Argon green light (514 nm) was chosen for irradiation, even though tissue penetration is only around 1 mm [148]. Light was delivered locally to visible lesions either by surface or interstitial fibers. The whole bladder was subsequently irradiated with 2–3.5 J/cm^2 green light to reach small multifocal tumors. All patients showed CR initially, and seven of 40 patients had recurred during the reported follow-up period of 7–34 months.

Brain tumors. Surgical excision is the primary treatment for most brain tumors, although the success rate is dependent on the tumor type, degree of encapsulation, and location. Typically, the most malignant tumors, such as glioblastomas, are not encapsulated and postoperative radiation therapy is indicated [88]. Local recurrence of the tumor is the main reason for treatment failures. Median survival is <1 year from time of diagnosis [149]. Nd:YAG laser hyperthermia is also currently under evaluation for residual and recurrent tumors [150].

PDT has been used most often as a treatment to prevent recurrence of supratentorial high grade gliomas after surgical resection, but it is possible that PDT may be of value in other intracranial tumors such as low grade gliomas. Pineal gland and pituitary gland tumors may be treated with PDT as an adjuvant therapy, since complete excision is often difficult [88]. The use of photodynamic therapy in combination with stereotactic equipment is an exciting possibility for treating small, deep-seated unresectable gliomas [150]. A direct correlation has been measured between the grade of glioma and porphyrin level in the tumor. The levels were highest in glioblastoma multiforme (mean 5.9 µg HPD/g tumor wet weight) and lower for the intermediate grade anaplastic astrocytoma (2.4 µg/g) and low grade astrocytoma (1.6 µg/g). Uptake into normal brain tissue of HPD sensitized patients was 0.2 µg/g [151]. The blood-brain barrier is thought to play a role in attenuating the delivery of photosensitizer, so that some brain tumor cells will be spared. Intratumoral injection may be advantageous compared to intravenous administration of photosensitizer [152].

Light delivery systems have been developed for treating brain tumors by PDT. It is important to shield the laser tip and prevent local charring. A device for delivery of light to postresection tumor beds was developed by Muller and Wilson [153–155]. Over 50 patients with malignant supratentorial gliomas have received intraoperative PDT by this group. Patients were injected with porphyrin photosensitizer, and 18–24 h later a craniotomy with tumor resection was performed. The resultant cavity was photoirradiated through an inflatable balloon applicator filled with intralipid to scatter light. The device also comprised intrinsic light detection. Muller and Wilson [153] determined light penetration depth to be 2.9 mm depth in tumor and 1.5 mm depth in normal brain. It will be necessary to develop new light delivery devices for treating areas of brain to several cm depth. For 12 of the 50 patients, a complete immediate response to PDT was achieved. The median survival for this group was 17 months. In 33 cases, which were all primary malignancies, a partial response was noted and median survival was 6.5 months.

Perria et al. [156] treated eight recurrent brain tumor patients with intraoperative PDT who had all previously undergone surgical resection and radiation therapy. HPD was given 24 h before surgery and the residual tumor bed exposed to red light. Survival in a few patients appeared to be lengthened, although all patients ultimately had recurrence. Kaye et al. [157] reported a series treating 45 patients, consisting of 37 glioblastomas, seven anaplastic astrocytomas, and one metastasic lung lesion. A laser dose escalation study was performed, using light generated by an ADL for 15 patients and GVL for 30 patients. Results were comparable with both lasers. The need for high light doses in the treatment of brain tumors by PDT has been recognized, as well as the use of combined intracavitary and interstitial photoillumination [149].

Gynecological cancer. Current treatment options for superficial noninvasive gynecological cancer include surgery, cryotherapy, Nd:YAG laser, and CO$_2$ laser vaporization [158]. The majority of gynecology patients treated with PDT have had cervix or vaginal carcinomas. A few patients with local endometrial and ovarian carcinomas have also been treated [118]. Most studies have comprised only a small number of gynecological cancer patients [118]. A series of 21 patients with recurrent tumors was reported by Lele et al. [159]. Endoscopic or surface delivery of light was employed. All patients experienced significant discomfort at the treatment site. CR was achieved in nine patients and PR was obtained in two patients. Optimization of PDT for gynecological lesions is required, particularly in regard to light delivery.

Head and neck cancer. Head and neck malignancies are treated at present by surgery with radiation therapy and/or chemotherapy. Local or regional recurrence of tumor is common, and further surgery is usually carried out [160]. Initially, only patients with advanced disease (Stages III and IV) were treated with PDT [161]. The treatments, intended to be palliative, met with limited success. Results of PDT for superficial and early tumors of the head and neck are considerably more promising, often saving patients from additional surgery [162]. PDT also appears promising as an adjuvant intraoperative treatment of recurrent head and neck carcinomas [163]. Generalization of the laser procedure is difficult because of the varying geometries of these cancers. Forward surface photoirradiation or cylinder-diffusing delivery systems inserted through a laryngoscope are usually used.

A preliminary investigation of PDT efficacy was carried out in 12 patients with squamous cell carcinomas localized in the nasopharynx, palate and uvula, larynx and retromolar trigone [164]. One patient had no response, and the remainder showed a CR (50%) or PR (50%). Feyh et al. [165,166] reported a study of 94 patients with various superficial head and neck tumors (disease status ranged CIS-T2. HPD was injected 48 hours before 630 nm light treatment. A CR of 95% was confirmed histologically 2 months after PDT. Five patients relapsed during follow-up (maximum 4.5 years). Biel [162] reported on the PDT treatment of 49 patients. All 26 patients with CIS and T1 laryngeal or nasopharyngeal carcinomas obtained a complete response. Three patients recurred, whereas 23 patients remained disease-free for up to 32 months. Eight patients with T2 and T3 carcinomas obtained CR or PR, but all cases recurred locally. Treatment of advanced cancer in four patients resulted in regrowth occurring within 1–3 months. Wenig et al. [167] evaluated HPD PDT for squamous cell carcinoma of the head and neck in 26 patients. The CR rate was 76% during the 48-month follow-up.

A small study examined PDT as an aduvant treatment to surgery in comparison with radical surgery alone [163]. Four patients with recurrent infiltrating carcinomas of the head and neck received Photofrin 48 hours before total surgical excision and laser irradiation (50 J/cm^2) of the resection bed. Follow-up was 6–8 months, during which all patients remained free of disease. Therefore, the results of intraoperative PDT appear promising, especially since Stages III and IV infiltrating carcinomas have a high rate of recurrence (>50%) after surgical and radiotherapy treatments.

Ocular cancer. In adults, the commonest ocular malignancy is choroidal melanoma, with prognosis depending on histological type and tumor size at diagnosis. Enucleation is the primary treatment for large lesions, although ocular brachytherapy and local surgical resection can be tried in an attempt to preserve the eye [168,169]. Retinoblastoma is the most common eye tumor in childhood. A variety of treatments are used, particularly in bilateral cases of retinoblastoma in an attempt to salvage the vision in at least one eye. Options apart from enucleation include external beam radiation, episcleral brachytherapy, and chemotherapy with or without laser hyperthermia [170].

The accessibility of ocular tumors and the optical properties of the eye are compatible for PDT. Preclinical and clinical reports evaluated PDT using transpupillary and transscleral delivery of laser light [171,172]. The transpupillary route produces direct photosensitization of the tumor mass, whereas transscleral delivery is intended to destroy the choroidal blood supply to choroidal melanomas.

Several groups have reported their preliminary clinical results for small numbers of patients. The largest series included 24 patients with choroidal, iris, or ciliary body melanomas treated with HPD PDT [171]. Red (630 nm) light was delivered both transpupillary and transsclerally. All small to medium-size tumors (<1,000 mm^3) tumors responded initially, and some complete responses were achieved during a 7 year follow-up. Larger tumors recurred and required enucleation. Murphree et al. [173] treated seven choroidal melanoma patients, one iris melanoma, one ciliary body melanoma, and six retinoblastoma patients with ocular PDT. Complete responses were obtained in two amelanotic melanomas, whereas responses in pigmented choroidal melanomas were minimal due to attenuation of the light. Retinoblastoma tumors without evidence of vitreous seeding initially responded, but were not cured long term. Avascular tumor seeds in the vitreous did not respond to PDT, presumably because they contained insufficient HPD and/or had insufficient oxygen available for the photodynamic process.

Cutaneous and subcutaneous cancer. Conventional treatments for cutaneous and subcutaneous malignancies include surgery, radiation, and chemotherapy. Satisfactory cure rates can be achieved with current modalities, but alternative modalities are necessary for extensive or multiple lesions, such as superficial basal cell carcinomas (BCC) and Bowen's disease [174]. The results of widespread surgical excision and irradiation can be cosmetically unacceptable for a patient.

McCaughan et al. [175] reported on 27 patients with cutaneous and subcutaneous malignancies (a total of 248 lesions) treated by PDT. Diagnoses included BCC, squamous cell carcinoma, metastatic breast cancer, malignant melanoma, liposarcoma, and Bowen's disease. The total CR observed during a 1-year follow-up was 48%. Carruth [161] also found this modality to be effective against Bowen's disease and multiple BCC in a pilot study. The initial clinical response of all patients was excellent, but recurrence developed in BCC lesions. Wilson et al. [176] carried out a prospective study in 37 patients to determine the effectiveness of Photofrin PDT for primary or recurrent basal cell tumors (151 tumors). A CR rate of 88% was achieved with one treatment session. Jones et al. [177] treated six patients with Bowen's disease, with Photofrin and red light, achieving 100% CR after 12 months of follow-up. Lowdell et al. [178] reported their results of treating nine patients with PDT. Fifty cutaneous or subcutaneous tumors, with volumes of up to 60 cm^3, were treated with interstitial irradiation. Another 22 tumors in these patients received surface irradiation. The total CR rate in this study was 81%. Khan et al. [179] treated a series of 37 patients with cutaneous metastatic breast carcinoma. Effective PDT was achieved using a reduced Photofrin dose of 0.75 mg/kg with the light dose increased to 180 J/cm^2. The conclusions from skin malignancy studies are that the size of the lesions is an important determinant of response, as well as the observation that PDT can produce superior healing of normal tissue without scarring.

Kaposi's sarcoma. HIV-positive patients are susceptible to various types of malignancy, but AIDS-related Kaposi's sarcoma (KS) is the most common and is an aggressive form of sarcoma. Chemotherapy or immunotherapy, radiotherapy, and surgical excision have been used with limited success [180]. KS is a multicentric tumor of vascular endothelial cell origin, which suggests PDT will be effective when mediated by photosensitizers that damage endothelium. Light delivery is either by surface irradiation for diffuse superficial lesions or interstitial for nodular lesions. Schweitzer [180] has treated eight KS patients with Photofrin PDT. Treatment was in-

tended primarily to control large lesions in the oral cavity, either alone or after debulking surgery. Short-term palliation was achieved and the lesions could be retreated. Biel [162] treated two patients with extensive KS of the hard and soft palate, with at least two sessions of PDT. Response was variable; the flat lesions responded, but nodular lesions showed no response.

Comparison of Photofrin PDT and Laser Thermal Ablation as Single Treatments

This section compares PDT and laser thermal ablation therapy (using the Nd:YAG laser) for treating malignant lesions. Randomized clinical trials are being carried out that make this comparison.

McCaughan [181] compared PDT and Nd:YAG laser treatments for endobronchial and esophageal malignancies. Laser treatment times during bronchoscopy were comparable, although Nd:YAG laser reduced the size of obstruction more at the end of a treatment. After clean-up bronchoscopy following PDT, the degree of obstruction was similar. A distinct difference in tissue reaction was observed for the two modalities several days posttreatment. PDT created a fibrinous plug that could be lifted off the bronchus in large pieces. The YAG laser typically produced a burn with coagulated and charred tissue, which was more difficult to remove because it fragmented. PDT was technically easier to perform than thermal laser resection and coagulation, since it was associated with lower risks of bronchial or esophageal perforation. In the case of obstructive emergencies, the disadvantage of PDT that the photosensitizer needs to be administered 1 or 2 days prior was overcome by same day injection and laser. Nd:YAG therapy was considered more effective for debulking large or bleeding lesions, whereas PDT was superior for treating small or residual tumor, producing necrosis cleanly to the bronchus wall. Treatment of patients with thermal ablation followed by PDT a few weeks later utilizes the advantages of both techniques.

In Norway, the Nd:YAG laser is used effectively to produce cures in selected cases of bladder cancer (CIS and recurrent transitional cell carcinoma), as an alternative to TUR. Nseyo [182] discussed Nd:YAG therapy and PDT for treatment of superficial bladder cancer. Thermal ablation produced thick tumor necrosis to a depth of 5–6 mm and sealed lymphatic drainage, which may prevent tumor dispersion. However, energy-dependent injury to contigous organs such as the bowel were possible following laser ablation. The YAG laser is also occasionally used for palliation of locally invasive bladder cancer, when curative cystectomy was contraindicated. PDT using whole bladder laser irradiation was less penetrating than YAG and was suitable for CIS and recurrent superficial lesions following TUR, producing 90–98% response rates. It represents a useful alternative modality for superficial disease.

Intracavitary PDT

Laser treatment of malignancies in the peritoneal and pleural cavity via intraoperative PDT is currently being examined. A Phase I study was initiated using intracavitary PDT for peritoneal carcinomatosis [183]. Patients received DHE 48 hours before laparotomy and debulking surgery, then were treated with light to intra-abdominal surfaces using 0.2–0.5% intralipid to enhance light diffusion. Photodiodes were sewn into the peritoneal cavity for in situ dosimetry. DeLaney et al. [184] reported the results of 54 patients treated as part of the Phase I study. Initially, 630 nm light at 2.8–3 J/cm^2 was used, but small bowel edema occurred with perforation in three cases. Light dose escalation was achieved by using green (514 nm) light, up to 3.75 J/cm^2. No small bowel complications occurred.

Intraoperative PDT was extended to treatment of pleural malignancies, such as mesothelioma or isolated pleural metastases [183]. Similarly, laser light was delivered to the thoracic cavity and photodiodes were sewn into the chest area. The postoperative course in patients was unchanged, and the efficacy of PDT as an intraoperative adjuvant therapy awaits results of future prospective clinical trials.

Sindelar et al. [185] also report on the use of intra-abdominal PDT for disseminated malignant disease, in 23 patients. Following resection, 630 nm light was delivered to peritoneal surfaces at escalating doses ranging from 0.2 to 3 J/cm^2. Viscera were anatomically isolated for laser exposure. Six patients were disease-free after 18 months. Five patients had significant treatment complications.

These preliminary studies suggest that intracavitary PDT will be evaluated in Phase II and III studies to determine efficacy for these types of tumors that have a typically high risk of recurrence. The goal is to convert surgical partial responses to complete responses. Regional toxicity may be a potential concern. Several experimental studies have evaluated the thresholds for damage and toxicity to abdominal organs [186]. Dose ranges were defined in each study that would not result in normal tissue necrosis. Pelton et al. [187] exposed large pleural surfaces to PDT and produced a spectrum of tissue specific injury in intrathoracic organs. Therefore, the risk of complications from locoregional toxicity after intracavitary PDT is currently unknown.

Bone Marrow Purging

Autologous and allogeneic bone marrow transplantation are used to treat leukemias and selected solid tumors. Autologous transplantation offers several advantages, notably avoiding the risk of graft rejection, viral infections, and lymphoproliferative disorders from graft manipulation. Unfortunately, relapse rates tend to be higher in autologous marrow grafts [188].

PDT is one of the newer techniques for extracorporeal bone marrow purging, and several photosensitizers have been proposed for photodynamic treatment of remission marrow, including DHE, BPD, ClAlPc, and merocyanine 540 (MC 540). Bone marrow grafts consist of free-flowing single cells in suspension, which are amenable to uniform exposures of photosensitizer and light. A significant advantage of this technique is that the drug can be removed before reinfusion of the treated cells into the patient, thus avoiding systemic photosensitization. MC 540 has been widely tested in preclinical models. The dye preferentially binds to electrically excitable cells, leukemia/lymphoma cells, and some virus transformed cells [188]. Under conditions that preserve 50% of human pluripotent hematopoietic progenitor cells, PDT can reduce the concentration of clonogenic promyelocytic leukemia cells and CML by up to 8 log [189]. Purging of non-Hodgkin's lymphoma (NHL) from autologous marrow grafts has been specifically explored [190]. MC 540 PDT produced 4–5 log eradication in vitro of patient-derived NHL, at doses which preserved ~50% of normal hematopoietic progenitor cells. MC 540 is the first agent to be evaluated in a Phase I clinical trial, for purging of leukemia and lymphoma cells [191]. The clinical application of MC 540 PDT found that several-fold higher doses were tolerated than used in preclinical models.

In addition, T- and B-cell immunity were found to be suppressed by MC 540 sensitized photoirradiation [192]. As a result, treatment may affect immune reconstitution in autologous marrow graft recipients. In allogeneic grafts, these immunomodulatory effects could reduce graft rejection in the situation of partially mismatched marrow transplants.

Clinical and Preclinical Studies of Second-Generation Photosensitizers

Benzoporphyrin derivative. BPD is synthesized from protoporphyrin and has an absorption peak at 690 nm four times greater than Photofrin's absorption at 630 nm. The mono-acid form has more photodynamic potency than di-acids [193], and the mono-acid was used for all studies described in this review. BPD uses lipoproteins for localization in vivo and particularly associates with tumor cell membranes [194]. Like all sensitizers, BPD does not have specific affinity for tumor tissue, reaching higher concentrations in the liver, spleen, and kidney. BPD has the purported advantage, in addition to its 690 nm absorption, of a favorable distribution between tumors and normal skin within a few hours of injection [195]. This property is expected to result in less skin photosensitivity as a side effect: BPD-MA is showing promise in Phase I/II clinical trials for skin tumors. Similar selectivity in BPD uptake by tumor cell lines (5–10-fold increase) occurs in activated T lymphocytes, compared to normal splenic lymphocytes [196]. Since activated T cells are responsible for the symptoms of most autoimmune diseases, preclinical studies are being carried out as a possible treatment for autoimmune conditions such as systemic lupus erythematosus [196]. BPD is undergoing preclinical testing for its ability to photoinactivate retroviruses in cells and blood [197], and also to treat atherosclerosis [196].

Mono-aspartyl chlorin e6. NPe6 is a chlorin photosensitizer with properties of very short term photosensitivity and a high extinction coefficient at 664 nm. Interestingly, preclinical studies found that PDT-mediated tumor cures correlated with the plasma concentrations of NPe6 rather than the tumor tissue levels of photosensitizer [198]. Maximal tumor response was achieved by irradiating tumors at 4–6 hours after sensitizer administration. NPe6 has been examined in a preliminary clinical study to patients with superficial malignancies [199]. Patients had diagnoses of primary or metastatic skin, oro- and nasopharynx cancer. Drug was injected 4–8 hours prior to irradiation with 664 nm light. Overall, CR was achieved in 11 of 20 tumors treated, four were PR, and the remainder were no responses. The maximum tumor necrosis was measured as 8 mm, whereas normal tissue had 1 mm necrosis or less,

indicating relative tumor selectivity by NPe6 PDT at the treatment times used. This was in spite of high NPe6 levels in the circulation and normal skin during treatment. Drug elimination was complete by 4 weeks after drug administration in all patients.

Meta-tetra(hydroxyphenyl)chlorin. mTHPC was synthesized and evaluated in preclinical studies by Berenbaum [200]. In rodent models, mTHPC was found to have both improved tumor tissue selectivity and antitumor activity compared to DHE. It has an absorption peak at 652 nm. Initial clinical results with mTHPC were published by Ris et al. [201] following treatment of patients with chest malignancies. Initially, two patients received an injection of mTHPC and 652 nm laser irradiation. Parameters were 0.3 mg/kg mTHPC, 48 h prior to light exposure of 10 J/cm². Biopsy samples showed tumor infarction 10 mm deep due to tumor vessel thrombosis, and the concentration of chlorin sensitizer was 14 times higher in mesothelioma tumor tissue than normal tissues. A further eight patients with diffuse malignant mesothelioma received intraoperative PDT to the thoracic cavity following unilateral pleurectomy and lobectomy [201,202]. The patients developed recurrences, although mostly in untreated areas. The conclusions drawn from the intraoperative treatments were that the procedure is feasible, but significant morbidity can occur when large areas are treated. Optimization of the therapeutic ratio is essential in order to prevent extensive damage to normal tissues during intracavitary mTHPC PDT.

Tin etiopurpurin. SnET2 is a metallochlorin with potent photosensitizing properties [203, 204]. It is hydrophobic and requires solubilization in a suitable drug delivery system, such as a lipid emulsion, for in vivo use. SnET2 has an absorption peak at 660 nm, which is used for photodynamic treatment. It is purported to produce significantly reduced photosensitization of normal tissue compared with DHE at the therapeutic dose [205]. Tissue distribution properties and clearance kinetics are comparable for both drugs, and similar drug injection to laser intervals can be employed for treatment [205]. Preclinical results are sufficiently encouraging that SnET2 is commencing Phase I/II clinical trials in the United States.

Amino-levulinic acid. Administration of exogenous ALA enhances the biosynthesis of endogenous PpIX for production of heme in certain types of cells and tissues [206]. The subsequent conversion of PpIX to heme is a relatively slow step, resulting in transient accumulation of protoporphyrin to sufficient levels that it can act as a photosensitizer.

Preclinical studies have been carried out to investigate ALA administration by topical application, intradermal injection, subcutaneous injection, intraperitoneal injection, and orally [207]. Systemic routes produce generalized photosensitivity, but are required for tumors that are too thick to be reached by local administration. Loh et al. [208] found comparable kinetics of PpIX in animals after intravenous and oral ALA administration. PpIX predominantly accumulated in mucosa of skin, colon, and bladder, with little in the submucosa and smooth muscle layers. Subsequent light treatment resulted in mucosal ablation only. Three patients were administered oral ALA, and biopsy samples demonstrated preferential PpIX accumulation after 4–6 h [208]. Following topical application of ALA (10% oimtment) to BCC lesions, fluorescence measurements showed PpIX accumulation only in normal skin after 4 hours. A 12-hour interval was required in order for tumor cells situated in lower dermis to become maximally fluorescent [209].

Several clinical studies have been reported evaluating topical ALA mediated PDT for treatment of cutaneous malignancies [207,210–213]. Topical solution (20%) of ALA is applied before same-day laser irradiation with 630 nm light. Bowen's disease lesions and BCC lesions show the highest response. One clinical trial showed a CR rate of 90% and PR rate of 7.5% in the first 80 BCC patients treated [207]. Similarly, Bowen's disease lesions obtained a CR of 89% at 18 months follow-up [211]. Warloe et al. [211] reported on 11 patients with 94 lesions of BCC, treated with ALA PDT. At 3 months post-PDT, 90 lesions (96%) were evaluated to be CR, although 13% had required more than a single PDT treatment. Lesions thicker than 3 mm may achieve a 40–50% CR [216,218]. Metastatic lesions (adenocarcinoma and melanoma) and noduloulcerative BCC lesions have shown consistently poor resposes [210,213a]. Superior cosmetic results appear to be obtained using ALA PDT in the studies.

NONONCOLOGIC APPLICATIONS OF PHOTODYNAMIC THERAPY
PDT of Viral Diseases

The first photodynamic studies on viruses were on bacteriophage, where it was found that penetration of the sensitizing dye was a variable factor [214]. A number of animal viruses, including adenoviruses and vaccinia viruses, were shown to be inactivated by PDT. Resistant viruses could be made sensitive to PDT by incubating with dye under conditions that increased viral coat permeability [215]. The earliest patient treatments were for herpes simplex viral infections of the skin, using neutral red dye and white light [216]. The efficacy of antiviral PDT is still undergoing preclinical investigation, using various photosensitizers and light delivery systems.

Papillomavirus. PDT has been proposed as a possible treatment for papillomas of the larynx. Laryngeal papillomavirus lesions are initially benign but can become serious and potentially life-threatening. The lesions are surgically removed, but typically the disease is marked by multiple recurrences and a prolonged clinical course [217]. Disease occurs with equal incidence in children and adults.

Abramson et al. [218] treated 33 patients with laryngeal papillomatosis using DHE PDT. The severest cases responded without recurrence during follow-up. Feyh et al. [165] treated 21 patients with recurrent laryngeal papillomatosis as part of a pilot study of HPD PDT for malignant superficial cancers of the head and neck. The study showed a CR rate of 95% over 4 years of follow-up. Although these results appear promising, PDT cannot remove latent infection of papillomavirus in normal tissue. The risk/benefit ratio of PDT treatment for the more frequent problem of cutaneous and genital warts remains undetermined.

HIV and blood-borne viruses. There is an accumulating amount of data that PDT can be used to effectively eliminate pathogenic enveloped viruses from infected cells, cell-free suspensions, and whole blood (219–222). Susceptible viruses include human immunodeficiency virus type I (HIV-1), herpes simplex virus type I/II (HSV-1,HSV-2) type I, human cytomegalovirus (CMV), measles, and simian virus (SIV).

The photosensitizers being evaluated for PDT-mediated viral inactivation include DHE, BPD, aluminium phthalocyanine, and merocyanine 540 (MC 540). Photoinactivation is thought to occur by oxidative modification of the lipid and protein components of the viral envelope. The mechanism of MC 540 antiviral activity has been most studied [223,224]. The available data suggest that MC 540 PDT damage to the virus envelope, in the form of extensive cross-linking, interferes with early events in the infectious process, the ability of the virus to adhere and to penetrate the cell. Since these photosensitizers do not target the nucleic acid of the virus, they are ineffective against non-enveloped viruses, such as poliovirus type I and human adenovirus-2 [219]. One advantage of dyes that do not interact with viral DNA is that they do not have inherent mitogenic properties.

PDT is being evaluated as a potential blood transfusion sterilizing system against pathogenic organisms. Obviously, the formed elements and noncellular components of blood must not be functionally damaged by the treatment. Some loss of activity of coagulation proteins such as factor VIII and von Willebrand factor is acceptable. The expense and complexity of implementing PDT as a sterilization system in a blood bank environment are also important factors that have to be considered [219]. Matthews et al. [220] did not detect damage to erythrocytes, complement factors, and immunoglobulins directly after DHE and BPD mediated PDT of blood, cells, and viral suspensions. Sieber et al. [221] demonstrated MC 540 PDT inactivation of a wide variety of viruses at concentrations that caused little photosensitivity of red cells, factor VIII, and von Willebrand factor. Naturally infected blood (with HIV-1) and spiked human blood have been tested after BPD PDT [225]. Free virus and infected (activated) leukocytes were effectively treated, whereas red cells and uninfected leukocytes were spared.

In another study by North et al., the red cells showed potassium leakage and IgG binding, indicating some damage occurred from photodynamic treatment [222]. This observation together with incomplete free HIV kill in their model system suggests that commercial sterilization of blood and blood products might not be feasible. However, the preferential sensitivity of activated cells (like leukocytes) is considered a real advantage since HIV replicates only in activated CD4 positive T cells [222]. Studies that exploit this result are planned to evaluate PDT as a treatment to reduce the HIV burden in patients. Extracorporeal treatment of blood or leukocytes in HIV-infected individuals seems to stabilize or improve immune function, perhaps by a stimulatory effect of the inactivated virus or by modulation of activated leukocytes. PDT would provide a beneficial treatment modality in this respect.

PDT of Atherosclerosis

Atherosclerotic vascular disease is the leading cause of death in the world [226]. The possibility of treating atherosclerosis with PDT is based on the observation that atherosclerotic plaques take up higher concentrations of porphyrin than normal vessel wall. Preclinical studies showed that DHE, NPe6, and TPPS were found mainly in the interstitial space of plaques, not intracellularly [226]. The drugs were absent in the normal vessel wall and the wall underlying the plaques, which suggests these structures will not be damaged. BPD uptake was measured in atherosclerotic human arteries in vitro and in miniswine arteries in vivo, and again showed potential for treating atherosclerosis [227].

Vincent et al. [228] treated atherosclerotic plaques in miniswine with Photofrin PDT and 630 nm light, using a circumferential diffusing fiber tip. At 2 weeks post-PDT, angiography showed an average reduction in stenosis in 6/8 vessels from 71% to 19%. Interestingly, locally applied photosensitizer through a porous balloon catheter showed very high concentrations in the intima region in animals [229]. The advantage of local administration is that PDT would be feasible immediately after angioplasty and without adverse systemic effects.

Arterial intimal hyperplasia (IH) is the specific condition of restenosis in arteries and veins that were earlier treated for stenosis by transluminal angioplasty or bypass graft surgery. At present, no treatment exists for IH [230]. Smooth muscle cell proliferation in the intima, stimulated by platelet adhesion, is involved in the development of IH. It is possible that it might eventually be treatable by PDT [230,231]. Choroaluminium phthalocyanine PDT was evaluated for its ability to obliterate the IH response in a carotid artery model in the rat. The sensitizer was preferentially retained in the artery with induced IH. Circumferential homogeneous light was then applied to the whole artery. In contrast to untreated arteries, PDT-treated arteries showed a marked decrease in smooth muscle cell growth, as well as normal elastic luminae. Studies are required to determine if the positive response is maintained long term [231]. Interestingly, one study found a significant growth suppressive effect from DHE alone (in the absence of light) on smooth muscle cells from atherosclerotic primary stenosing and restenosing lesions, although the mechanism is unknown [232].

PDT of Skin Disorders

Psoriasis. Psoriasis is a common dermatological disorder in which the epidermal cells overproliferate, resulting in a clinical picture ranging from localized scaling plaques to generalized exfoliation of the skin. Treatment by PUVA phototherapy is an effective established method of controlling the increased cell proliferation. PUVA treatment comprises application of psoralen compounds (either topical or systemic 8-methoxypsoralen) to produce a photoadditive effect with UVA light [233].

Tin protoporphyrin (SnPP) photodynamically activated by UVA light has been proposed for treatment of psoriasis [234]. Repeated doses of UVA can be given for several weeks following a single injection. The photosensitivity of SnPP was investigated in 31 patients. Thresholds for UVA and visible light were lower after SnPP administration, but the UVB threshold was unchanged by this sensitizer. Mild erythema and mild conjunctivitis were experienced lasting several weeks to 3 months.

The first reported treatment with hematoporphyrin and light for psoriasis vulgaris was in 1937 [235]. Since then, there have been a few case reports using either systemic or topically applied photosensitizer. Berns et al. [236] treated one patient with HPD PDT, reporting that the psoriatic skin partially cleared. Treatment of 17 patients with palmoplantar psoriasis was evaluated by Pres et al. [237] using topical HPD ointment application and white light irradiation. All lesions responded, either significantly or totally resolving. In a recent pilot study, three patients with chronic psoriasis were treated every other day with PDT using topical 10% ALA [238]. No significant adverse effects occurred, and the lesions cleared with a similar time course as patients treated with dithranol. PDT using topical photosensitizer appears to be a beneficial psoriasis treatment, applicable to treat large surface areas.

Portwine stain. Portwine stain (PWS) is a congenital vascular lesion consisting of an abnormal set of capillaries in the upper dermis with a normal overlying epidermis. It most commonly occurs on the face and neck region. Treatment of PWS in the past included an array of modalities, such as skin grafting, ionizing radiation, and cryosurgery, all of which caused cosmetic scarring [239]. The introduction of the argon laser represented a major advance in PWS treatment. The blue-green lines of the argon laser correspond to hemoglobin absorption. The light is converted to thermal energy in the dilated ectatic capillaries and produces thrombosis in these vessels. Unfortunately, the epidermis receives some irreversible damage, since melanin and collagen absorb light. Use of longer wavelengths, such as 577 nm, has been shown to be preferable and leave less scarring. The extinction coefficient of oxyhemoglobin is higher than at 514 nm, whereas melanin absorption is minimized.

It may be possible to obtain selectivity using a photosensitizer and appropriate wavelength light, as shown in a chicken comb model by Orenstein et al. [240]. They used time intervals of 1–4 hours between Photofrin and blue (405 nm) light in order to confine damage to the vascular compartment. Fluorescence of HPD, indicating localization, was seen in a facial portwine stain by Keller et al. [241] in a patient who was being treated with PDT for bladder cancer. There do not seem to have been any patient series carried out of PDT treatment for benign vascular dermal lesions.

SUMMARY

After decades of basic and clinical research, PDT is on the verge of becoming an established cancer treatment modality. Its role will emerge when current Phase III clinical trials of Photofrin-mediated PDT are completed and treatment is in practice. The first product license approvals have been granted (outside the United States) for treatment of endobronchial, esophageal cancer, and superficial bladder cancers. Meanwhile, intracavitary PDT is still at the preliminary stages, but so far it appears promising. Certainly, some malignant diseases are more suitable than others with regard to whether complete eradication is possible. Very bulky lesions and tumors inaccessible to light irradiation remain untreatable by PDT. The efficacy and safety of PDT determined by clinical trial are not the only factors determining its future success, but also how the existing treatments for a disease compare. Development of resistance to PDT has not been noted in any patient tumors, which is a distinct advantage over some other anticancer modalities. Also, long-term morbidity does not arise to restrict the number of repeat treatments.

PDT is now being evaluated for wider applications, outside malignant solid tumor treatment. At the beginning of the century, photochemotherapy was realized to be potentially useful for a variety of indications, when photosensitization was first being observed in enzymes, viruses, cells, animals, and plants. Nononcologic applications of PDT are mostly at the preclinical stage and include viral inactivation in blood, modulation of immune function in autoimmune diseases, reduction in atherosclerosis lesions, and treatment of benign skin disorders. It is not possible to say at present which of these diseases or conditions will benefit most from PDT.

Development of second-generation photosensitizers is continuing, and dyes have already been designed with improved photodynamic properties. The side effect of skin photosensitivity can be diminished by dyes that absorb only in the far-red spectrum. Nonsystemic administration of drug or targeting techniques may also eliminate photosensitivity side effects. Classes of sensitizers that have been evaluated photochemically and biologically include porphyrins, chlorins, purpurins, and phthalocyanines. The most promising examples are being developed commercially. The technical development of user-friendly light sources, whether laser or nonlaser, is as important to the clinical applications of PDT as the choice of photosensitizer. Diode lasers generating sufficient power in the far-red visible region are only just becoming available for clinical use. In addition, specialized laser delivery systems continue to be developed, with respect to the specific site being treated. The methodology and technology used for photodynamic treatment of patients can be expected to change significantly for many years ahead. PDT is truly a dynamic process.

REFERENCES

1. Raab O. Uber die wirkung fluoreszierenden stoffen. Infusuria Z Biol 1900; 39:524–546.
2. Hausmann W. The sensitising action of hematoporphyrin. Biochem Z 1911; 30:176.
3. Blum HF. "Photodynamic Action and Diseases Caused by Light." New York: Rhineholt 1941 (reprinted, Hafner, 1964).
4. Figge FHJ, Weiland GS, Manganiello LOJ. Cancer detection and therapy. Affinity of neoplastic, embryonic and traumatized tissues for porphyrins and metalloporphyrins. Proc Soc Exp Biol Med 1948; 68:181–188.
5. Dougherty TJ, Henderson BW, Schwartz S, Winkelman JW, Lipson RL. Historical Perspective. In Henderson BW, Dougherty TJ, eds.: "Photodynamic Therapy, Basic Principles and Clinical Applications." New York: Dekker, 1992, pp. 1–18.
6. Lipson RL, Baldes EJ. The photodynamic properties of a particular hematoporphyrin derivative. Arch Dermatol 1960; 82:517–520.
7. Lipson RL, Baldes EJ, Olsen AM. Hematoporphyrin derivative: A new aid for endoscopic detection of malignant disease. J Thorac Cardiovasc Surg 1961; 42:623–629.
8. Gregorie HB, Horger EO, Ward JL. Hematoporphyrin derivative fluorescence in malignant neoplasms. Ann Surg 1968; 167:820–828.
9. Diamond I, Granelli SG, McDonah AF, Nielson S, Wilson CB, Jaenicke R. Photodynamic therapy of malignant tumors. Lancet 1972; 2:1175–1177.
10. Dougherty TJ, Grindey G, Flel R. Photoradiation therapy II: Cure of animal tumors with hematoporphyrin and light. J Natl Cancer Inst 1974; 55:115–121.
11. Kelly JF, Snell ME, Berenbaum MC. Photodynamic destruction of human bladder carcinoma. Br J Cancer 1975; 31:237–244.
12. Dougherty TJ, Kaufman JE, Goldfarb A, Weishaupt KR, Boyle D, Mittleman A. Photoradiation therapy for the treatment of malignant tumors. Cancer Res 1978; 38:2628–2635.
13. Dougherty TJ. Photodynamic therapy (PRT) of malignant tumors. CRC Crit Rev Biochem 1984; 2:83–116.
14. Hayata Y, Kato H, Konaka C, Ono J, Takizawa N. Hematoporphyrin derivative and laser photoradiation in the treatment of lung cancer. Chest 1982; 81:269–277.
15. Kato H, Kawate N, Kinoshita K, Yamamoto H, Furukawa K, Hayata Y. Photodynamic therapy of early stage lung cancer. In: "Photosensitizing Compounds: Their chemistry, biology and clinical use." Ciba Foundation Symposium. Chichester: Wiley, 1989, pp. 183–197.
16. Okunaka T, Kato H, Conaka C, Yamamoto H, Bonaminio A, Eckhauser ML. Photodynamic therapy of esophageal carcinoma. Surg Endoscopy 1990; 4:150–153.
17. Prout GR, Lin CW, Benson R, Nseyo UO, Daly JJ, Griffin PP, Kinsey J. Photodynamic therapy with hematoporphyrin derivative in the treatment of superficial transitional cell carcinoma of the bladder. N Engl J Med 1987; 317:1251–1255.
18. Dougherty TJ, Potter WR, Weishaupt KR. The structure of the active component of hematoporphyrin derivative. In Doiron DR, Gomer CJ, eds.: "Porphyrin Localization and Treatment of Tumors." New York: Alan R Liss, 1984, pp 301–314.
19. Spikes JD. Chlorins as photosensitizers in biology and medicine. J Photochem Photobiol B:Biol. 1990; 6:259–274.
20. Pandey RK, Bellnier DA, Smith KM, Dougherty TJ. Chlorin and porphyrin derivatives as potential photosensitizers in photodynamic therapy. Photochem Photobiol 1991; 53:65–72.
21. Morgan AR. Reduced porphyrins as photosensitizers: synthesis and biological effects. In Henderson BW, Dougherty TJ, eds. "Photodynamic Therapy, Basic Principles and Clinical Applications." New York: Dekker, 1992, pp. 157–172.
22. Richter AM, Waterfield E, Jain AK, Sternberg ED, Dolphin D, Levy JG. In vitro evaluation of phototoxic properties of four structurally related benzoporphyrin derivatives. Photochem Photobiol 1990; 52:495–500.
23. Rosenthal I. Phthalocyanines as photodynamic sensitizers. Photochem Photobiol 1991; 53:859–870.
24. van Lier JE, Spikes JD. The chemistry, photophysics and photosensitizing properties of phthalocyanines. Ciba Foundation Symposium. 1989; 146:17–26.
25. van Lier JE. Phthalocyanines as sensitizers for PDT of cancer. In D. Kessel, ed.: "Photodynamic Therapy of Neoplastic Disease," Vol. 1. Boca Raton, CRC Press, 1990, pp. 279–291.
26. Gomer CJ, Dougherty TJ. Determination of 3H and 14C hematoporphyrin derivative distribution in malignant C and normal tissue. Cancer Res 1979; 39:146–151.

362   Fisher et al.

27. Bellnier DA, Ho YK, Pandey RK, Missert JR, Dougherty TJ. Distribution and elimination of Photofrin II in mice. Photochem Photobiol 1989, 50:221–228.

28. Pantelides ML, Moore JV, Blacklock NJ. A comparison of serum kinetics and tissue distribution of photofrin II following intravenous and intraperitoneal injection in the mouse. Photochem Photobiol 1989; 49:67–70.

29. Quastel MR, Richter AM, Levy JG. Tumor scanning with indium-111 dihaematoporphyrin ether. Br J Cancer 1990; 62:885–890.

30. Gilson P, Ash P, Driver I, Feather JW, Brown SB. Therapeutic ratio of photodynamic therapy in the treatment of superficial tumors of skin and subcutaneous tissues in man. Br J Cancer 1988; 58:665–667.

31. Brown SB, Vernon DI. The quantitative determination of porphyrins in tissues and body fluids: Applications in studies of photodynamic therapy. In D. Kessel, ed.: "Photodynamic Therapy of Neoplastic disease," Vol. 1. Boca Raton: CRC Press, 1990, pp 109–208.

32. Kessel D, Nseyo U, Schulz V, Sykes E. Pharmacokinetics of Photofrin II distribution in man. SPIE Optical Methods for Tumor Treatment and Early Diagnosis 1991; 1426:180–187.

33. Gomer CJ, Ferrario A. Tissue distribution and photosensitizing properties of mono-L-aspartyl chlorin e6 in a mouse tumor model. Cancer Res 1990; 50:3985–3990.

34. Richter AM, Jain AK, Canaan AJ, Waterfield E, Sternberg ED, Levy JG. Photosensitizing efficiency of two regioisomers of the benzoporphyrin derivative monoacid ring A. Biochem Pharmacol 1992; 43:2349–2358.

35. Jori G. In vivo transport and pharmacokinetic behavior of tumor photosensitizers. Ciba Foundation Symposium 1989; 146:78–86.

36. Oseroff AR, Ara G, Ohuoha D, Aprille J, Bommer JC, Yarmush ML, Foley J, Cincotta L. Strategies for selective cancer photochemotherapy: Antibody targeted and selective carcinoma cell photolysis. Photochem Photobiol 1987; 46:83–96.

37. Jiang FN, Allison B, Liu D, Levy JG. Enhanced photodynamic killing of target cells by either monoclonal antibody or low density lipoprotein mediated delivery systems. J Controlled Release 1992; 19:41–58.

38. Jiang FN, Jiang S, Liu D, Richter A, Levy JG. Development of technology for linking photosensitizers to a model monoclonal antibody. J Immunol Methods 1990; 134:139–149.

39. Klyashchitsky BA, Nechaeva IS, Ponomaryov GV. Approaches to targetted photodynamic tumor therapy. J Controlled Release 1994; 29:1–16.

40. Jori G, Reddi E. The role of lipoproteins in the delivery of tumour-targeting photosensitizers. Int J Biochem 1993; 25:1369–1375.

41. Maziere JC, Santus R, Morliere P, Reyftmann JP, Candide C, Mora L, Salmon S, Maziere C, Gatt S, Dubertret L. Cellular uptake and photosensitizing properties of anticancer porphyrins in cell membranes and low and high density lipoproteins. J Photochem Photobiol B 1990; 6:61–68.

42. Jori G. Low density lipoproteins—Liposome delivery systems for tumor photosensitizers in vivo. In Henderson BW, Dougherty TJ, eds.: "Photodynamic Therapy, Basic Principles and Clinical Applications." New York: Dekker, 1992, pp 173–186.

43. Allison BA, Pritchard PH, Richter AM, Levy JG. The plasma distribution of benzoporphyrin derivative and the effects of plasma lipoproteins on its biodistribution. Photochem Photobiol 1990; 52:501–507.

44. Allison BA, Waterfield E, Richter AM, Levy JG. The effects of plasma lipoproteins on in-vitro tumor cell killing and in-vivo tumor photosensitization with benzoporphyrin derivative. Photochem Photobiol 1991; 54:709–715.

45. Fukuda H, Paredes S, Batlle AM. Tumour localizing properties of porphyrins: In vivo studies using free and liposome encapsulated aminolevulinic acid. Comparative Biochem and Physiol 1992; 102:433–436.

46. Mew D, Wat CK, Towers GHN, Levy JG. Photoimmunotherapy: Treatment of animal tumors with tumor-specific monoclonal antibodies-hematoporphyrin conjugates. J Immunol 1983; 130:1473–1477.

47. Yarmush ML, Thorpe WP, Strong L, Rakestraw SL, Toner M, Tompkins RG. Antibody-targeted photolysis. Crit Rev Ther Drug Carrier Systems 1993; 10:197–252.

48. Jiang FN, Richter AM, Jain AK, Levy JG, Smits C. Biodistribution of a benzoporphyrin derivative-monoclonal antibody conjugate in A549-tumor-bearing nude mice. Biotech Therapeutics 1993; 4:43–61.

49. Schmidt S, Wagner U, Popat S, Schultes B, Eilers H, Spaniol S, Biersack J, Krebs D. Photodynamic therapy in gynecological oncology. In Spinelli P, Dal Fante M, Marchesini R, eds.: "Photodynamic Therapy and Biomedical Lasers." Excerpta Medica, International Congress Series 1011. 1992, pp 327–332.

50. Shockley TR, Lin K, Nagy JA, Tompkins RG, Dvorak HF, Yarmush ML. Penetration of tumor tissue by antibodies and other immunoproteins. Ann NY Acad Sci 1991; 618:367–382.

51. Foote CS. Mechanisms of photooxidation. In Doiron DR, Gomer CJ, eds.: Porphyrin Localization and Treatment of Tumors. New York: Alan R Liss. 1984, pp 3–18.

52. Weishaupt K, Gomer CJ, Dougherty T. Identification of singlet oxygen as the cytotoxic agent in photoinactivation of a murine tumor. Cancer Res 1976; 36:2326–2329.

53. Buettner GR, Need MJ. Hydrogen peroxide and hydroxyl free radical production by hematoporphyrin derivative, ascorbate and light. Cancer Lett 1985; 25:297–304.

54. Gomer CJ, Rucker N, Ferrario A, Wong S. Properties and applications of photodynamic therapy. Rad Res 1989; 120:1–18.

55. Kessel D. Photosensitization with derivatives of hematoporphyrin. Int J Rad Biol 1986; 49:901–907.

56. Kessel D. Sites of photosensitization by derivatives of hematoporphyrin. Photochem Photobiol 1986; 44:489–493.

57. Hilf R, Smail DB, Murant RS, Leakey PB, Gibson SL. Hematoporphyrin derivative induced photosensitivity of mitochondrial succinate dehydrogenase and selected cytosolic enzymes of R3230 AC mammary adenocarcinomas of rats. Cancer Res 1984; 44:1483–1488.

58. Candide C, Maziere J, Santus R, Maziere C, Morliere P, Reyftman J, Goldstein S, Dubertret L. Photosensitization of Wi26-VA4 transformed human fibroblasts by low density lipoprotein loaded with Photofrin II: Evidence for endoplasmic reticulum alteration. Cancer Lett 1989; 44:157–161.

59. Specht K, Rodgers M. Depolarization of mouse myeloma

cell membranes during photodynamic action. Photochem Photobiol 1990; 51:319–324.

60. Dubbelman T, vanSteveninck J. Photodynamic effects of hematoporphyrin derivative on transmembrane transport systems of murine L929 fibroblasts. Biochim Biophys Acta 1984; 771:201–207.

61. Spikes JD. Chlorins as photosensitizers in biology and medicine. Photochem Photobiol B: 1990; 6:259–274.

62. Gomer CJ. DNA damage and repair in CHO cells following hematoporphyrin photoradiation. Cancer Lett 1980; 11:161–167.

63. Moan J, Waksvik H, Christensen T. DNA single-strand breaks and sister chromatid exchanges induced by treatment with hematoporphyrin and light or by X-rays in human NHIK 3025 cells. Cancer Res 1980; 40:2915–2918.

64. Gomer CJ, Rucker N, Murphree AL. Differential cell photosensitivity following porphyrin photodynamic therapy. Cancer Res 1988; 48:4539–4542.

65. Ramakrishnan N, Oleinick NL, Clay ME, Horng MF, Antunez AR, Evans HH. DNA lesions and DNA degradation in mouse lymphoma L5178Y cells after photodynamic treatment sensitized by chloroaluminium phthalocyanine. Photochem Photobiol 1989; 50:373–378.

66. Evans HH, Rerko RM, Mencl J, Clay ME, Antunez AR, Oleinick NL. Cytotoxic and mutagenic effects of the photodynamic action of chloroaluminium phthalocyanine and visible light in L5178Y cells. Photochem Photobiol 1989; 49:43–47.

67. Gomer CJ, Rucker N, Murphree AL. Transformation and mutagenic potential of porphyrin photodynamic therapy in mammalian cells. Int J Rad Biol 1988; 53:651–659.

68. Gomer CJ, Ferrario A, Rucker N, Wong S, Lee AS. Glucose regulated protein induction and cellular resistance to oxidative stress mediated by porphyrin photosensitization. Cancer Res 1991; 51:6574–6579.

69. Gomer CJ, Luna M, Ferrario A, Rucker N. Increased transcription and translation of heme oxygenase in chinese hamster fibroblasts following photodynamic stress or Photofrin II incubation. Photochem Photobiol 1991; 53:275–279.

70. Fisher AMR, Ferrario A, Gomer CJ. Adriamycin resistance in chinese hamster fibroblasts following oxidative stress induced by photodynamic therapy. Photochem Photobiol 1993; 58:581–588.

71. Oleinick NL, Agarwal ML, Antunez AR, Larkin HE, He J. Signal transduction in PDT-induced apoptosis. In Spinelli P, Dal Fante M, Marchesini R, eds.: "Photodynamic Therapy and Biomedical Lasers." International Congress Series 1011, Excerpta Medica, 1992, pp 755–759

72. Oleinick NL, Agarwal ML, Berger NA, Berger SJ, Cheng MF, Mukhtar H, Rihter BD, Zaidi SIA. Signal transduction and metabolic changes during tumor cell apoptosis following phthalocyanine sensitized photodynamic therapy. In: SPIE Optical Methods for Tumor Treatment and Detection 1993; 242–247.

73. Zaidi SIA, Oleinick NL, Zaim MT, Mukhtar H. Apoptosis during photodynamic therapy induced ablation of RIF-1 tumors in C3H mice. Photochem Photobiol 1993; 58:771–776.

74. van Geel IP, Oppelaar H, Oussoren YG, Stewart FA. Changes in perfusion of mouse tumours after photodynamic therapy. Int J Cancer 1994; 56:224–228.

75. Nelson JS, Liaw LH, Orenstein A. Mechanism of tumor destruction following photodynamic therapy with hematoporphyrin derivative, chlorin and phthalocyanine. J Natl Cancer Inst 1988; 80:1599–1605.

76. Henderson BW, Waldow SM, Mang TS, Potter WR, Malone PB, Dougherty TJ. Tumor destruction and kinetics of tumor cell death in two experimental mouse tumors following photodynamic therapy. Cancer Res 1985; 45:572–576.

77. Henderson BW, Bellnier DA. Tissue localization of photosensitizers and the mechanism of photodynamic tissue destruction. Ciba Foundation Symposium 1989; 146:112–125.

78. Henderson BW, Donovan JM. Release of prostaglandin E2 from cells by photodynamic treatment. Cancer Res 1989; 49:6896–6900.

79. Reed MWR, Wieman J, Doak KW, Pietsch CG, Schuschke. The microvascular effects of photodynamic therapy: Evidence for a possible role of cyclooxygenase products. Photochem Photobiol 1989; 50:419–423.

80. Fingar VH, Wieman TJ, Doak KW. Role of thromboxane and prostacycline release on photodynamic therapy induced tumor destruction. Cancer Res 1990; 50:2599–2603.

81. Reed MWR, Wieman TJ, Schuske DA, Tseng MT, Miller FN. A comparison of the effects of photodynamic therapy on normal and tumor blood vessels in the rat microcirculation. Rad Res 1989; 119:542–552.

82. Henderson BW, Dougherty TJ. How does photodynamic therapy work? Photochem Photobiol 1992; 55:145–157.

83. Moan J, Berg K. Photochemotherapy of cancer: Experimental research. Photochem Photobiol 1992; 55:931–948.

84. Oseroff AR, Ohuoha D, Ara G, McAuliffe D, Foley J, Cincotta L. Intramitochondrial dyes allow selective in vitro photolysis of carcinoma cells. PNAS (USA) 1986; 83:9729–9733.

85. Chan WS, Marshall JF, Hart IR. Effect of tumor location on selective uptake and retention of phthalocyanines. Cancer Lett 1989; 44:73–77.

86. Jain RK. Transport of molecules in the tumor interstitium: A review. Cancer Res 1987; 47:3039–3051.

87. Kessel D. Porphyrin-lipoprotein association as a factor in porphyrin localization. Cancer Lett 1986; 33:183–188.

88. Kaye AH, Hill JS. Photoradiation therapy of brain tumors: Laboratory and clinical studies. In Morstyn G, Kaye AH, eds.: "Phototherapy of Cancer." Harwood Academic, Chur, Switzerland 1990, pp 101–118.

89. Mang TS, Dougherty TJ. Time and sequence dependent influence of in vivo photodynamic therapy survival by hyperthermia. Photochem Photobiol 1985; 42:533–540.

90. Waldow SM, Henderson BW, Dougherty TJ. Potentiation of photodynamic therapy by heat: Effect of sequence and time interval between treatments in vivo. Lasers Surg Med 1985; 5:83–94.

91. Frietas I, Pontiggia P, Baronzio GF, McLaren JR. Perspectives for the combined use of photodynamic therapy and hyperthermia in cancer patients. Adv Exp Med Biol 1990; 267:511–520.

92. Gomer CJ, Rucker N, Wong S. Porphyrin photosensitivity in cell lines expressing a heat-resistant phenotype. Cancer Res 1990; 50:5365–5368

93. Moore JV, West CM, Haylett AK. Vascular function and tissue injury in murine skin following hyperthermia and photodynamic therapy, alone and in combination. Br J Cancer 1992; 66:1037–1043.

94. Wijesekera TP, Dolphin D. Some preparations and properties of porphyrins. In Kessel, D, ed.: "Methods in Porphyrin Photosensitization." New York: Plenum, 1985, pp 229–266.

95. Wilson BC, Jeeves WP, Lowe DM. In vivo and postmortem measurements of the attenuation spectra of light in mammalian tissues. Photochem Photobiol 1985; 43:2153–2159.

96. Cowled PA, Grace R, Forbes IJ. Comparison of the efficacy of pulsed and continuous wave red laser light in induction of photocytotoxicity by hematoporphyrin derivative. Photochem Photobiol 1984; 39:115–117.

97. McKenzie AL, Carruth JAS. A comparison of gold vapour and dye lasers for photodynamic therapy. Lasers Med Sci 1986; 1:117–120.

98. Shikowitz MJ. Comparison of pulsed and continuous wave light in photodynamic therapy of papillomas: An experimental study. Laryngoscope 1992; 102:300–310.

99. Barr H, Boulos PB, MacRobert AJ, Tralau CJ, Phillips D, Bown SG. Comparison of lasers for photodynamic therapy with a phthalocyanine photosensitizer. Lasers Med Sci 1989; 4:7–12.

100. Bellnier DA, Lin CW, Parrish JA, Mock PC. Hematoporphyrin derivative and pulse laser photoradiation. In Doiron DR, Gomer CJ, eds.: "Porphyrin Localization and Treatment of Tumors." New York: Alan R Liss, 1984, pp 533–540.

101. Ferrario A, Rucker N, Ryter SW, Doiron DR, Gomer CJ. Direct comparison of in-vitro and in-vivo Photofrin-II mediated photosensitization using a pulsed KTP pumped dye laser and a continuous wave argon ion pumped dye laser. Lasers Surg Med 1991; 11:404–410.

102. Star WM, Wilson BC, Patterson MS. Light delivery and optical dosimetry in photodynamic therapy of solid tumors. In Henderson BW, Dougherty TJ, eds.: Photodynamic Therapy: Basic Principles and Clinical Applications. New York: Dekker, 1992, pp 335–368.

103. Ainsworth MD, Piper JA. Laser systems for photodynamic therapy. In Morstyn G, Kaye AH, eds.: "Phototherapy of Cancer." Harwood Academic, Chur, Switzerland 1990, pp 37–72.

104. Potter WR, Mang TS, Dougherty TJ. The theory of photodynamic therapy dosimetry: consequences of photodestruction of sensitizer. Photchem Photobiol 1987; 46:97–101.

105. Doiron DR. Instrumentation for Photodynamic Therapy. In Chester AN, Martellucci S, Scheggi AM, eds.: "Laser systems for Photobiology and Photomedicine." NATO ASI Series. New York: Plenum, 1991, pp 229–230.

106. Doiron DR. Photophysics of and instrumentation for porphyrin detection and activation. In Doiron DR, Gomer CJ, eds.: "Porphyrin Localization and Treatment of Tumors." New York: Alan R Liss, 1984, pp 41–73.

107. Wilson BC. Photodynamic Therapy: Light Delivery And Dosage For Second-Generation Photosensitizers. In: "Photosensitizing Compounds: Their Chemistry, Biology and Clinical Use." Ciba Foundation Symposium 1989, 146:60–73.

108. Bernstein EF, Friauf WS, Smith PD, Cole JW, Solomon RE, Fessler JF, Thomas GF, Black C, Russo A. Transcutaneous determination of tissue dihematoporphyrin ether content: A device to optimize photodynamic therapy. Arch Dermatol 1991; 127:1794–1798.

109. Tromberg BJ, Orenstein A, Kimel S, Barker SJ, Hyatt J, Nelson JS, Berns MW. In vivo tumor oxygen tension measurements for the evaluation of the efficiency of photodynamic therapy. Photochem Photobiol 1990; 52:375–385.

110. Gorman AA, Rodgers MAJ. Current perspectives of singlet oxygen detection in biological environments. J Photochem Photobiol B:Biol 1992; 14:159–176.

111. Truscott TG, McLean AJ, Phillips AMR, Foulds WS. Detection of haematoporphyrin derivative and haematoporphyrin excited states in cell environments. Cancer Lett 1988; 41:31–35.

112. Patterson MS, Madsen SJ, Wilson BC. Experimental tests of the feasibility of singlet oxygen luminescence monitoring in vivo during photodynamic therapy. J Photochem Photobiol. B. 1990; 5:69–84.

113. Marcus SL, Dugan MH. Global status of clinical photodynamic therapy: the registration process for a new therapy. Lasers Surg Med 1992; 12:318–324.

114. Cortese DA, Edell ES, Silverstein MD, Offord K, Trastek VF, Pairolero PC, Allen MS, Deschamps C. An evaluation of the effectiveness of Photodynamic Therapy (PDT) compared to surgical resection in early stage roentgenographically occult lung cancer. In Spinelli P, Dal Fante M, Marchesini R, eds.: "Photodynamic Therapy and Biochemical Lasers." International Congress Series 1011, Excerpta Medica, 1992, pp 15–22.

115. Furuse K, Fukuoka M, Kato H, Horai T, Kubota K, Kodama N, Kusunoki Y, Takifuji N, Okunaka T, Konaka C, Wada H, Hayata Y. A prospective phase II study on photodynamic therapy with Photofrin II for centrally located early-stage lung cancer. J Clin Oncol 1993; 11:1852–1857.

116. Kato H, Konaka C, Kawate H, Shinohara K, Kinoshita M, Naguchi M, Ootomo S, Hayata Y. Five year disease-free survival of lung cancer patients treated only by photodynamic therapy. Chest 1986; 90:768–770.

117. Edell ES, Cortese DA. Detection and Phototherapy of Lung Cancer. In Morstyn G, Kaye AH, eds.: "Phototherapy of Cancer." Harwood Academic, Chur, Switzerland 1990, pp 185–198.

118. Marcus S. Photodynamic Therapy of Human Cancer. Proc IEEE 1992; 80:869–889.

119. McCaughan JS Jr, Hawley PC, Bethel BH, Walker J. Photodynamic therapy of endobronchial malignancies. Cancer 1988; 62:691–701.

120. Kato H, Kawate N, Kinoshita K, Yamamoto H, Furukawa K, Hayata Y. Photodynamic therapy of early stage lung cancer. In: Photosensitizing Compounds: Their Chemistry, Biology and Clinical Use. Ciba Foundation Symposium, 1989; 146:183–197.

121. Ono R, Ikeda S, Suemasu K. Hematoporphyrin derivative photodynamic therapy in roentgenographically occult carcinoma of the tracheobronchial tree. Cancer 1992; 69:1696–1701.

122. Furuse K, Okunaka T, Sakai H, Konaka C, Kato H, Aoki M, Wada H, Nakamura S, Horai T, Kubota K. Photodynamic Therapy (PDT) in roentgenographically occult lung cancer by Photofrin II and excimer dye laser. Jap J Cancer Chemo 1993; 20:1369–1374.

123. Sutedja T, Baas P, Stewart F, Van Zandwijk N. A pilot study of Photodynamic Therapy in Patients with inoperable Non-Small Cell Lung cancer. Eur J Cancer 1992; 28a:1370–1373.

124. Okunaka T, Kato H, Konaka C, Kawate N, Bonaminio A, Yamamoto H, Ikeda N, Tolentino M, Eckhauser ML, Hayata Y. Photodynamic therapy for multiple primary bronchogenic carcinoma. Cancer 1991; 68:253–258.

125. Shimatani H, Kato H, Okunaka T, Konaka C, Sakai H, Yamada K. Bronchial arterial infusion of Photofrin for PDT. In Spinelli P, Dal Fante M, Marchesini R, eds.: "Photodynamic Therapy and Biomedical Lasers." International Congress Series 1011, Excerpta Medica. 1992, pp 426–430.

126. Overholt BF. Photodynamic therapy and thermal treatment of esophageal cancer. Gastrointest Endoscopy Clin N America 1992; 2:433–455.

127. Overholt BF. Laser and photodynamic therapy of esophageal cancer. Sem Surg Oncol 1992; 8:191–203.

128. Spinelli P, Falsitta M. Barrett's esophagus: characteristics and evaluation of risk of malignancy. Annali Italiani Di Chirurgia 1990; 61:531–537.

129. Overholt B, Panjehpour M, Tefftellar E, Rose M. Photodynamic therapy for treatment of early adenocarcinoma in Barrett's esophagus. Gastrointest Endoscopy 1993; 39:73–76.

130. Panjehpour M, Overholt BF, DeNovo RC, Sneed RE, Petersen MG. Centering balloon to improve esophageal photodynamic therapy. Lasers Surg Med 1992; 12:631–638.

131. Tajiri H, Oguro Y. Laser endoscopic treatment for upper gastrointestinal cancers. J Laparoendoscopic Surg 1991; 1:71–78.

132. Okunaka T, Kato H, Conaka C, Yamamoto H, Bonaminio A, Eckhauser ML. Photodynamic Therapy of esophageal carcinoma. Surgical Endoscopy 1990; 4:150–153.

133. McCaughan JS Jr. Photodynamic therapy of skin and esophageal cancers. Cancer Invest 1990; 8:407–416.

134. Jin ML, Yang BQ, Zhang W, Ren P. Review of Photodynamic Therapy for gastrointestinal tumours in the past 6 years in China. J Photochem Photobiol B. 1990; 7:87–92.

135. Pass HI. Photodynamic therapy in oncology: Mechanisms and clinical use. JNCI 1993: 85:443–456.

136. Kato H, Sakai H, Kawaguchi M, Okunaka T, Konaka C. Experiences with Photodynamic Therapy in early gastric cancer. Onkologie 1992; 15:232–237.

137. Eckhauser ML. Laser therapy of colorectal carcinoma. Surg Clin N America 1992; 72:597–607.

138. Barr H, Bown SG, Krasner N, Boulos PB. Photodynamic Therapy for colorectal disease. Int J Colorectal Dis 1989; 4:15–19.

139. Benson RC. Phototherapy of bladder cancer. In Morstyn G, Kaye AH, eds.: "Phototherapy of Cancer." Harwood Academic, Chur, Switzerland 1990, pp. 199–214.

140. Lamm DL. Carcinoma in situ. Urologic Clin N Amer 1992; 19:499–508.

141. Unsoeld E, Baumgartner R, Beyer W, Jocham D, Stepp H. Fluorescence detection and photodynamic treatment of photosensitized tumors in special consideration of urology. Lasers Med Sci 1990; 5:207–212.

142. Marijnissen JPA, Jansen H, Star WM. Treatment system for whole bladder wall photodynamic therapy with in vivo monitoring and control of light dose rate and dose. J Urol 1989; 142:1351–1355.

143. Marijissen JPA, Star WM, Zandt HJA, D'Hallewin MA, Baert L. In situ light dosimetry during whole bladder wall photodynamic therapy: clinical results and experimental verification. Phys Med Biol 1993; 38:567–582.

144. Nseyo UO, Lundahl SL, Merrill DC. Whole bladder photodynamic therapy: critical review of present-day technology and rationale for development of intravesical laser catheter and monitoring system. Urol 1990; 36:398–402.

145. Nseyo UO. Photodynamic therapy. Urol Clin N Amer 1992; 19:591–599.

146. Jocham D, Baumgartner R, Stepp H, Unsoeld E. Clinical experience with the integral photodynamic therapy of bladder carcinoma. J Photochem Photobiol. B: 1990; 6:183–187.

147. Guo YC. Improved argon laser photodynamic therapy for superficial bladder tumor: Experimental research and clinical analysis. Chinese J Oncol 1990; 12:75–77.

148. Bellnier DA, Prout GR, Lin C. Effect of 514nm Argon ion laser radiation on hematoporphyrin derivative treated bladder tumor cells in vivo and vitro. JNCI 1985; 74:617–625.

149. Muller P, Wilson B. Photodynamic therapy of brain tumors. J Photochem Photobiol B. 1991; 9:117–125.

150. Powers SK. Current status of lasers in neurosurgical oncology. Sem Surg Oncol 1992; 8:226–232.

151. Kaye AH, Hill JS. Photodynamic therapy of brain tumors. Ann Acad Med, Singapore 1993; 22:470–481.

152. Noske DP, Wolbers JG, Sterenborg HJCM. Photodynamic therapy of malignant glioma. A review of literature. Clin Neurol Neurosurg 1991; 93:293–307.

153. Muller PJ, Wilson BC. Photodynamic therapy of malignant brain tumors: clinical effects, postoperative ICP and light penetration of the brain. Photochem Photobiol 1987; 46:929–935.

154. Muller PJ, Wilson BC. Photodynamic therapy of malignant brain tumors. Lasers Med Sci 1990; 5:245–251.

155. Muller PJ, Wilson BC. Photodynamic therapy of malignant brain tumors. Can J Neurol Sci 1990; 17:193–198.

156. Perria C, Carai M, Falzoi A, Orunesu G, Rocca A, Massarelli G, Francaviglia N, Jori G. Photodynamic therapy of malignant brain tumors: clinical results of, difficulties with, questions about, and future prospects for the neurosurgical applications. Neurosurg 1988; 23:557–563.

157. Kaye AH, Morstyn G, Apuzzo M. Photoradiation therapy and its potential in the management of neurological tumors: A review. J Neurosurg 1988; 69:1–14.

158. Bhatta N, Isaacson K, Bhatta KM, Anderson RR, Schiff I. Comparative study of different laser systems. Fertility and Sterility 1994; 61:581–591.

159. Lele SB, Piver HS, Mang TS, Dougherty TJ, Tomczak MJ. Photodynamic therapy in gynecologic malignancies. Gynecol Oncol 1989; 34:350–352.

160. Gluckman JL, Zitsch RP. Photodynamic therapy in the management of head and neck cancer. Cancer Treatment and Research 1990; 52:95–113.

161. Carruth JAS. Photodynamic therapy of tumours involving the skin and the head and neck. In Morstyn G, Kaye AH, eds.: "Phototherapy of Cancer." AH. Harwood Academic, Chur, Switzerland 1990, pp 173–184.

162. Biel MA. Photodynamic therapy and the treatment of

neoplastic diseases of the head and neck; an update. In: SPIE Optical Methods for Tumor Treatment and Detection. 1994; 2133:39–52.

163. Biel MA. Photodynamic therapy as an adjuvant intraoperative treatment of recurrent head and neck carcinomas. In: SPIE Optical Methods for Tumor Treatment and Detection. 1994; 2133:53–59.

164. Schweitzer VG. Photodynamic therapy for treatment of head and neck cancer. Otolaryngol—Head And Neck Surg 1990; 102:225–232.

165. Feyh J, Gutmann R, Leunig A. Photodynamic laser therapy in the field of otorhinolaryngology. Laryngo-Rhino-Otologie 1993; 72:273–278.

166. Feyh J, Goetz A, Mueller W, Koenigsberger R, Gastenbauer E. Photodynamic therapy in head and neck surgery. J Photochem Photobiol. B. 1990; 7:353–358.

167. Wenig BL, Kurtzman DM, Grossweiner LI, Mafee MF, Harris DM, Lobraico RV, Prycz RA, Appelbaum EL. Photodynamic therapy in the treatment of squamous cell carcinoma of the head and neck. Arch Otolaryngol—Head And Neck Surg 1990; 116:1267–1270.

168. Foulds WS. Current options in the management of choroidal melanoma. Trans Ophthalmol Soc, U.K. 1983; 103:28–34.

169. Foulds WS. Management of intraocular melanoma. Br J Ophthalmol 1990; 74:559–560.

170. Murphree ALM, Francis FL. Chapter 27: Retinoblastoma. In Ryan SJ, ed.: "Retina. Volume I: Tumors of the Retina." St. Louis: C.V. Mosby, 1994, pp 571–626.

171. Bruce RA, McCaughan JS. Lasers in uveal melanoma. Ophthalmol Clinics of N America 1989; 2:597–604.

172. Gomer CJ, Liu G, Szirth BC, Morinelli E, Murphree AL. Photodynamic therapy of ocular tumors. In Morstyn G, Kaye AH, eds.: "Phototherapy of Cancer." Harwood Academic, Chur, Switzerland 1990, pp 119–132.

173. Murphree AL, Cote M, Gomer CJ. The evolution of photodynamic therapy in the treatment of intraocular tumors. Photochem Photobiol 1987; 46:919–923.

174. Lui H, Anderson RR. Photodynamic therapy in dermatology: recent developments. Dermatol Clin 1993; 11:1–13.

175. McCaughan JS Jr, Guy JT, Hicks W, Laufman L, Nims TA, Walker J. Photodynamic therapy for cutaneous and subcutaneous malignant neoplasms. Arch Surg 1989; 124:211–216.

176. Wilson BD, Mang TS, Stoll H, Jones C, Cooper M, Dougherty TJ. Photodynamic therapy for the treatment of basal cell carcinoma. Arch Dermatol 1992; 128:1597–1601.

177. Jones CM, Mang T, Cooper M, Wilson BD, Stoll HL. Photodynamic therapy in the treatment of Bowen's disease. J Am Acad Dermatol 1992; 27:979–982.

178. Lowdell CP, Ash DV, Driver I, Brown SB. Interstitial photodynamic therapy: Clinical experience with diffusing fibres in the treatment of cutaneous and subcutaneous tumours. Br J Cancer 1993; 67:1398–1403.

179. Khan SA, Dougherty TJ, Mang TS. An evaluation of photodynamic therapy in the management of cutaneous metastases of breast cancer. Eur J Cancer 1993; 29A:1686–1690.

180. Schweitzer VG. Photodynamic therapy for treatment of AIDS-related mucocutaneous Kaposi's sarcoma. In Spinelli P, Dal Fante M, Marchesini R, eds.: "Photodynamic Therapy and Biomedical Lasers." Interna-

tional Congress Series 1011, Excerpta Medica 1992, pp 49–64.

181. McCaughan JS. Photodynamic therapy versus Nd:YAG laser treatment of endobronchial or esophageal malignancies. In Spinelli P, Dal Fante M, Marchesini R, eds.: "Photodynamic Therapy and Biomedical Lasers." International Congress Series 1011, Excerpta Medica 1992, pp 23–36.

182. Nseyo UO. Thermal lasers and PDT in urology. In Spinelli P, Dal Fante M, Marchesini R, eds.: "Photodynamic Therapy and Biomedical Lasers." International Congress Series 1011, Excerpta Medica 1992, pp 43–47.

183. Pass HI, DeLaney TF. Innovative photodynamic therapy at the National Cancer Institute: Intraoperative, intracavitary treatment. In Henderson BW, Dougherty TJ: "Photodynamic Therapy: Basic Principles and Clinical Applications." New York: Dekker, 1992, pp 287–302.

184. Delaney TF, Sindelar WF, Tochner Z, Smith PD, Friauf WS, Thomas G, Dachowski L, Cole JW, Steinberg SM, Glatstein E. Phase I study of debulking surgery and photodynamic therapy for disseminated intraperitoneal tumors. Int J Rad Oncol Biol Phys 1993; 25:445–457.

185. Sindelar WF, Delaney TF, Tochner Z, Thomas GF, Dachoswki LJ, Smith PD, Friauf WS, Cole JW, Glatstein E. Technique of photodynamic therapy for disseminated intraperitoneal malignant neoplasms. Phase I Study. Arch Surg 1991; 126:318–324.

186. Evrard S, Aprahamian, Marescaux J. Intra-abdominal photodynamic therapy: from theory to feasibility. Br J Surg 1993; 80:298–303.

187. Pelton JJ, Kowalyshyn MJ, Keller SM. Intrathoracic organ injury associated with photodynamic therapy. J Thoracic Cardiovascular Surgery 1992; 103:1218–1223.

188. Sieber F, Krueger GJ. Photodynamic therapy and bone marrow transplantation. Sem Hematol 1989; 26:35–39.

189. Atzpodien J, Gulati SC, Clarkson BD. Comparison of the cytotoxic effects of merocyanine 540 on leukemic cells and normal human bone marrow. Cancer Res 1986; 46:4892–4895.

190. Itoh T, Messner HA, Jamal N, Tweedale M, Sieber F. Merocyanine 540 sensitized photoinactivation of high grade non-Hodgkin's lymphoma cells: potential application in autologous BMT. Bone Marrow Transplant 1993; 12:191–196.

191. Sieber F. Marrow purging by merocyanine 540 mediated photolysis. Bone Marrow Transpl 1987; 2:29–33.

192. Lum LG, Yamagami M, Giddings BR, Joshi I, Schober SL, Sensenbrenner LL, Sieber F. The immunoregulatory effects of merocyanine 540 on in vitro human T and B lymphocyte functions. Blood 1991; 77:2701–2706.

193. Richter AM, Waterfield E, Jain AK, Allison B, Sternberg ED, Dolphin D, Levy JG. Photosensitizing potency of structural analogues of benzoporphyrin derivative (BPD) in a mouse tumour model. Br J Cancer 1991; 63:87–93.

194. Jamieson CHM, McDonald WN, Levy JG. Preferential uptake of benzoporphyrin derivative by leukemic versus normal cells. Leuk Res 1990; 14:209–219.

195. Richter AM, Cerruti-Sola S, Sternberg ED, Dolphin D, Levy JG. Biodistribution of tritiated benzoporphyrin derivative (3H-BPD-MA), a new potent photosensitizer, in normal and tumor-bearing mice. J Photochem Photobiol 1990; 5:231–244.

196. Richter AM, Chowdary R, Ratkay L, Jain AK, Canaan AJ, Meadows H, Obochi M, Waterfield D, Levy JG. Non-oncologic potentials for photodynamic therapy. SPIE 1993; 2078:293–304.

197. North J, Coombs R, Levy J. Photoinactivation of HIV by benzoporphyrin derivative. In Spinelli P, Dal Fante M, Marchesini R, eds.: "Photodynamic Therapy and Biomedical Lasers." International Congress Series 1011, Excerpta Medica 1992, pp 103–110.

198. Gomer CJ, Ferrario A. Tissue distribution and photosensitizing properties of mono-L-aspartyl chlorin e6 in a mouse tumor model. Cancer Res 1990; 50:3985–3990.

199. Allen RP, Kessel D, Tharratt RS, Volz W. Photodynamic therapy of superficial malignancies with NPe6 in man. In Spinelli P, Dal Fante M, Marchesini R, eds.: "Photodynamic Therapy and Biomedical Lasers." International Congress Series 1011, Excerpta Medica 1992, pp 441–445.

200. Berenbaum MC. Comparison of hematoporphyrin derivatives and new photosensitizers. In: Photosensitizing Compounds: Their Chemistry, Biology and Clinical Use. New York: John Wiley & Sons. Ciba Foundation Symposium, 1989, pp 33.

201. Ris HB, Altermatt HJ, Inderbitzi R, Hess R, Nachbur B, Stewart JC, Wang Q, Lim CK, Bonnett R, Berenbaum MC. Photodynamic therapy with chlorins for diffuse malignant mesothelioma: Initial clinical results. Br J Cancer 1991; 64:1116–1120.

202. Ris HB, Altermatt HJ, Nachbur B, Stewart JCM, Wang G, Lim CK, Bonnett R, Althaus U. Clinical evaluation of photodynamic therapy with mTHPC for chest malignancies. In: Photodynamic Therapy and Spinelli P, Dal Fante M, Marchesini R, eds. "Photodynamic Therapy and Biomedical Lasers." International Congress Series 1011, Excerpta Medica, 1992, pp 421–425.

203. Morgan AR, Garbo GM, Keck RW, Selman SH. New photosensitizers for photodynamic therapy: Combined effect of metallopurpurin derivatives and light on transplantable bladder tumors. Cancer Res 1988; 48:194–198.

204. Morgan AR, Garbo GM, Keck RW, Eriksen LD, Selman SH. Metallopurpurins and light: Effect on transplantable rat bladder tumors and murine skin. Photochem Photobiol 1990; 51:589–592.

205. Morgan AR, Garbo GM, Krivak T, Mastroianni M, Petousis NH, St Clair T, Weisenberger M, van Lier JE. New sensitizers for PDT. SPIE Optical Methods for Tumor Treatment and Early Diagnosis 1991; 1426:350–355.

206. Kennedy JC, Pottier RH, Pross DC. Photodynamic therapy with endogenous protoporphyrin IX: Basic principles and present clinical experience. J Photochem Photobiol 1990; 6:143–148.

207. Kennedy JC, Pottier RH. Endogenous protoporphyrin IX, a clinically useful photosensitizer for photodynamic therapy. J Photochem Photobiol B: 1992; 14:275–292.

208. Loh CS, Macrobert AJ, Bedwell J, Regula J, Krasner N, Bown SG. Oral versus intravenous administration of 5-aminolaevulinic acid for photodynamic therapy. Br J Cancer 1993; 68:41–51.

209. Szeimies RM, Sassy T, Landthaler M. Penetration potency of topical applied delta-aminolevulinic acid for photodynamic therapy of basal cell carcinoma. Photochem Photobiol 1994; 59:73–76.

210. Cairnduff F, Stringer MR, Hudson EJ, Ash DV, Brown SB. Superficial photodynamic therapy with topical 5-aminolaevulinic acid for superficial primary and secondary skin cancer. Br J Cancer 1994; 69:605–608.

211. Warloe T, Peng Q, Moan J, Qvist HL, Giercksky KE. Photochemotherapy of multiple basal cell carcinoma with endogenous porphyrins induced by topical application of 5-amino levulinic acid. In Spinelli P, Dal Fante M, Marchesini R, eds: "Photodynamic Therapy and Biomedical Lasers." International Congress Series 1011, Excerpta Medica, 1992, pp 449–453.

212. Svanberg K, Andersson T, Killander D. Photodynamic therapy of human skin malignancies and laser induced fluorescence diagnostics utilizing Photofrin and delta-amino levulinic acid. In: Spinelli P, Dal Fante M, Marchesini R, eds. "Photodynamic Therapy and Biomedical Lasers." International Congress Series 1011, Excerpta Medica, 1992, pp 436–440.

213a. Wolf P, Rieger E, Kerl H. Topical photodynamic therapy with endogenous porphyrins after application of 5-aminolevulinic acid: An alternative treatment modality for solar keratoses, superficial squamous cell carcinomas and basal cell carcinomas. J Am Academy Dermatol 1993; 28:17–21.

213b. Shanler SD, Buscaglia DA, van Leengoed H, Wan W, Whitaker JE, Mang TS, Barcos M, Stoll HL, Oseroff AR. PDT with topical amino-levulinic acid (ALA) for the treatment of patch and plaque stage cutaneous T cell lymphoma. J Invest Dermatol 1994; 102:615.

214. Spikes JD. Photosensitization. In Smith KC: "The Science of Photobiology." New York: Plenum, 1977, pp 96.

215. Wallis C, Melnick JL. Photodynamic inactivation of animal viruses: A review. Photochem Photobiol 1965; 4:159–170.

216. Felber TD, Smith EB, Knox JM, Wallis C, Melnick JL. Photodynamic inactivation of Herpes simplex. JAMA 1973; 223:289–292.

217. Abramson AL, Waner M, Brandsma J. The clinical treatment of laryngeal papillomas with hematoporphyrin therapy. Arch Otolaryngol—Head And Neck Surg 1988; 114:795–800.

218. Abramson AL, Shikowitz MJ, Mullooly VM, Steinberg BM, Amella CA, Rothstein HR. Clinical effects of photodynamic therapy on recurrent laryngeal papillomas. Arch Otolaryngol-Head And Neck Surg 1992; 118:25–29.

219. Sieber F, O'Brien JM, Gaffney DK. Antiviral effects of photosensitizing merocyanine dyes: Implications for transfusion and bone marrow transplantation. Sem Hematol 1992; 20:79–87.

220. Matthews JL, Sogandares-Bernal F, Judy M, Gulliya K, Newman J, Chanh T, Marengo-Rowe A. Inactivation of viruses with photoactive compounds. Blood Cells 1992; 18:75–89.

221. Sieber F, O'Brien JM, Gaffney DK. Merocyanine sensitized photoinactivation of enveloped viruses. Blood Cells 1992; 18:117–127

222. North J, Neyndorff H, Levy JG. Photosensitizers as virucidal agents. J Photochem Photobiol B: 1993; 17:99–108.

223. O'Brien JM, Singh RJ, Feix JB, Kalyanaraman B, Sieber F. Action spectra of the antileukemic and antiviral activities of merocyanine 540. Photochem Photobiol 1991; 54:851–854.

224. O'Brien JM, Gaffney DK, Wang TP, Sieber F. Merocyanine 540 sensitized photoinactivation of enveloped viruses in blood products: Site and mechanism of phototoxicity. Blood 1992; 80:277–285.

225. North J, Coombs R, Levy J. Photoinactivation of HIV by benzoporphyrin derivative. In Spinelli P, Dal Fante M, Marchesini R, eds.: "Photodynamic Therapy and Biomedical Lasers." International Congress Series 1011, Excerpta Medica, 1992, pp 103–110.

226. Vincent GM, Fox J, Hill S, Ding H-W. Photodynamic therapy of atherosclerotic vascular disease. In Spinelli P, Dal Fante M, Marchesini R, eds.: "Photodynamic Therapy and Biomedical Lasers." International Congress Series 1011, Excerpta Medica, 1992, pp 209–213

227. Hsiang YN, Crespo MT, Richter AM, Jain AK, Fragoso M, Levy JG. In vitro and in vivo uptake of benzoporphyrin derivative into atherosclerotic plaque. In Spinelli P, Dal Fante M, Marchesini R, eds.: "Photodynamic Therapy and Biomedical Lasers." International Congress Series 1011, Excerpta Medica, 1992, pp 214–218.

228. Vincent GM, Mackie RW, Orme E, Fox J, Johnson M. In vivo photosensitizer enhanced laser angioplasty in atherosclerotic miniswine. J Clin Laser Med Surg 1990; 8:59–61.

229. Gonschior P, Erdemci A, Gerheuser F, Gonschior G-M, Goetz A, Hofling B. Local application of photosensitive dyes in arterial vessels. In Spinelli P, Dal Fante M, Marchesini R, eds.: "Photodynamic Therapy and Biomedical Lasers." International Congress Series 1011, Excerpta Medica, 1992, pp 238–243.

230. Ortu P, LaMuraglia GM, Roberts WG, Schomaker KT, Deutsch TF, Flotte TJ, Hasan T. Treatment of arterial intimal hyperplasia with photodynamic therapy. In Spinelli P, Dal Fante M, Marchesini R, eds.: "Photodynamic Therapy and Biomedical Lasers." International Congress Series 1011, Excerpta Medica, 1992, pp 225–232.

231. Ortu P, LaMuraglia GM, Roberts WG, Flotte TJ, Hasan T. Photodynamic therapy of arteries: A novel approach for the treatment of experimental intimal hyperplasia. Circulation 1992; 85:1189–1196.

232. Dartsch PC, Ischinger T, Betz E. Differential effect of Photofrin II on growth of human smooth muscle cells from nonatherosclerotic arteries and atheromatous plaques in vitro. Arteriosclerosis 1990; 10:616–624.

233. Epstein JH. Chapter 7: Photomedicine. In Smith, KC: The Science of Photobiology. New York: Plenum Press, 1977, pp 201.

234. Emtestam L, Angelin B, Berglund L, Drummond GS, Kappas A. Photodynamic properties of Sn protoporphyrin: Clinical investigations and phototesting in human subjects. Acta Dermato-Venereologica 1993; 73:26–30.

235. Silver H. Psoriasis vulgaris treated with hematoporphyrin. Arch Dermatol Syph 1937; 36:1118–1119.

236. Berns MW, Rettenmaier M, McCullough J. Response of psoriasis to red laser light (630 nm) following systemic injection of hematoporphyrin derivative. Lasers Surg Med 1984; 4:73–77.

237. Pres H, Meffert H, Sonnichsen N. Photodynamic therapy of psoriasis palmaris et plantaris using a topically applied hematoporphyrin derivative and visible light. Dermatol Monats 1989; 175:745–750.

238. Boehncke WH, Sterry W, Kaufmann R. Treatment of psoriasis by topical photodynamic therapy with polychromatic light. Lancet 1994; 343:801.

239. Aronoff BL. Lasers in cutaneous disease. Sem Surg Oncol 1989; 5:57–60.

240. Orenstein A, Nelson JS, Liaw LH, Kaplan R, Kimel S, Berns MW. Photochemotherapy of hypervascular dermal lesions: A possible alternative to photothermal therapy. Lasers Surg Med 1990; 19:334–343.

241. Keller GS, Doiron DR, Weingarten C. Advances in laser skin surgery for vascular lesions. Arch Otolaryngol 1985; 111:437–440.

Chapter 11

Laser Safety

David H. Sliney, PhD

Laser Microwave Division, U.S. Army Environmental Hygiene Agency, Aberdeen Proving Ground, Maryland

INTRODUCTION

With the increasing variety of lasers and the number of wavelengths now available, safe laser use can become a more complex issue [1]. The extent of potentially hazardous reflections, the type of eye protection, and the ancillary hazards can vary considerably with the type of laser and the procedure. However, in all cases, the laser surgeon and hospital staff must be concerned with both the protection of the patient and the protection of the operating room staff (including the surgeon). Patient safety is assured by limiting needless exposure to adjacent tissues (by choice of wavelength and to a large extent by surgical technique), using noncombustible materials adjacent to the beam, and by protecting the patients' eyes. Safety of the operator and assistants requires concern for both system safety design and means to limit potentially hazardous reflections. Environmental hazards from the smoke produced by vaporizing tissue must be minimized by local exhaust ventilation or fume extractors. The pathogenicity and chemical toxicity of vaporized tissue have been the subject of a number of investigations, as discussed later. Safety standards for medical laser applications have been issued that consider all of these potential hazards and their control measures [1–8]. The current consensus standard in the United States, the American National Standard Z136.3-1988, *Safe Use of Lasers in Health Care Facilities* [4], is now under review for a revision due for a vote in 1995. The revision should offer a realistic and balanced approach to medical laser safety, without needless control measures. This can be achieved only if the entire community of laser surgeons, nurses, biomedical engineers, and hospital administrators participate in the development of the consensus standard.

As with other electrical or electronic equipment, surgical lasers in the clinical environment pose safety problems. Potential hazards of electrical shock exist, requiring appropriate grounding, and other electrical safety procedures are essential. However, there are no particularly unique electrical safety problems associated with laser use, and biomedical engineers and medical electronics technicians familiar with safe installation of electrical and electronic equipment in hospital and health care environments should have no difficulty in providing guidance for the safe electrical use of laser equipment [9].

Like electrosurgical techniques, a laser can produce potentially hazardous airborne contaminants from the photovaporization of tissues. Unfortunately, the vaporized tissue ("smoke") from laser surgery has often been referred to as "laser smoke" or the "laser plume," suggesting that it is unique to laser surgery. This emphasis on the laser origin has frequently led to the result that vaporized tissue fragments from bone saws and pyrolysis products of tissue from electrosurgery have been overlooked as having the same degree of hazard. Vaporized tissue in sufficient quantities must receive special attention, and local exhaust ventilation almost always will be required [9–10]. The pyrolysis products are similar to those resulting from the barbecue of meats. They contain toxic by-products and known carcinogens such as nitrosamines. A number of studies have measured the concentration of potentially hazardous airborne contaminants in the laser operating room, with the result that concentrations are shown to be kept below permissible concentrations with appropriate exhaust ventilation [1].

The one hazard that is truly unique to the laser and that requires special attention results from the laser beam itself—the optical radiation hazard. Unlike other light sources, the laser beam may be collimated and directed over some distance; hence the area of potential hazard may not be limited to the immediate surgical site. Unwarranted fears often accompany the introduction of lasers into the surgical theater or the clinical environment. Therefore, proper appreciation of the real laser beam hazard is necessary for each member of the medical staff so that realistic safety precautions are followed [10–18]. In recent years, the Occupational Safety and Health Administration (OSHA) has emphasized the critical importance of informing and educating the worker on workplace risks, and this is clearly important with regard to laser use [19].

Laser hazards depend upon the laser in use, the environment, and the personnel involved with the laser operation (the operator, ancillary personnel, and patient). The laser hazard is roughly defined by the hazard classification (1 through 4), whereas the other factors must be analyzed in each situation. A basic understanding of laser biological effects and hazards is necessary to assess intelligently laser hazards in the operating room. Once the hazards are understood, the safety measures are obvious.

BIOLOGICAL HAZARDS OF LASER BEAMS
Eye Hazards

Because of its special optical properties, the human eye is considered the most vulnerable to laser light. Aside from the oral mucosa, the only living tissue exposed to the environment is the cornea and conjunctiva. Without the comparative protective features of the stratum cornea of the skin, the eye is exposed to the harsh environment of sun, wind, dust, ultraviolet radiation, and intense light. The eye has a natural protective mechanism in its lid reflex, which limits the retinal exposure to very intense visible light or to intense exposure from infrared rays, which raise the temperature of the cornea. However, some laser beam intensities are so great that injury can occur faster than the protective action of the lid reflex, which occurs between 0.2 and 0.25 second [9].

Laser hazards to the eye depend most predominantly upon wavelength as shown in Figure 1. Obviously, laser energy cannot damage tissue unless the light energy is able to penetrate to and be absorbed in that structure. For this reason, rays in the visible and near infrared (visible and IR-A band), which can be transmitted through clear ocular media and be absorbed in the retina, can, in sufficient intensity, damage the retina. The high collimation of a laser beam permits the rays to be focused to an extremely small spot on the retina. The image size of such a point at the retina is of the order of 10–20 μm (smaller than the diameter of a human hair). For this reason, lasers operating between 400 and 1,400 nm are particularly dangerous to the retina. This spectral region is often referred to as the retinal hazard region, since the increased concentration of light after entering the eye and falling on the retina is of the order of 100,000. Hence, a collimated beam of 1 W/cm^2 at the cornea will focus to a small spot with an irradiance of 100 kW/cm^2. Although damage to such a small region of the retina may seem insignificant at first, it is important to realize that certain parts of the retina, as, e.g., the central retina, the macula, and its fovea (cen-

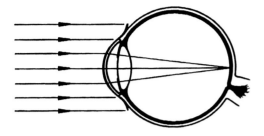

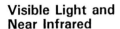

**Visible Light and
Near Infrared**

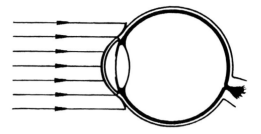

**Far UV and Infrared
[UV-B, C, IR-B & C]**

Fig. 1. The biological effects of optical radiation upon the eye depend upon the absorption properties, which vary with the spectral region.

ter of the macula), are extremely small areas responsible for critically important high acuity vision. If these areas are damaged by laser radiation, substantial loss of vision can result.

The image area alone may not be the only site of damage, but as a result of heat flow and mechanical (acoustic) transients, the tissue surrounding the image site may also be damaged, leading to more severe consequences upon visual function. For example, it was not uncommon for an individual to lose almost total function in an eye exposed to a very small amount of energy (several hundred microjoules) when a laser is accidentally imaged on the fovea. Instead of a normal visual acuity of 20/20, the visual acuity in such accidental situations has often been recorded as 20/200 following the accident. Fortunately, in most accidents, only one eye is exposed to a collimated beam. However, any visual loss is generally permanent since the neural tissue of the retina has very little ability for repair.

At wavelengths outside of the retinal hazard region, in both the ultraviolet and far infrared regions of the spectrum, injury to the anterior segment of the eye is possible. Certain spectral bands may injure the lens (notably at wavelengths between 295 and 320 nm and wavelengths between 1 and 2 µm). Injury to the cornea is possible from a wide range of wavelengths in the ultraviolet and most of the infrared at wavelengths beyond 1,400 nm. Injury to the cornea is normally very superficial, involving only the corneal epithelium, and with the cornea's high metabolic rate, repair occurs within a day or two, and total recovery of vision will occur. If, however, significant injury occurs in deeper corneal layers

in the stroma or endothelium and in the germinative layers of the cornea, corneal scars can result, leading to permanent loss of vision unless a corneal transplant can be effected. In this regard, because of deeper tissue penetration, the use of the 1.44, 1.54 µm, and 2.1 µm infrared wavelengths may actually pose a greater risk for permanent injury than the 10.6 µm CO_2 laser wavelength [9].

Excimer lasers operating in the ultraviolet are now entering the surgical arena. Certain excimer lasers pose a particular hazard to the cornea, and the 308 nm Xe-Cl excimer laser can be considered additionally dangerous as it can produce an immediate cataract of the lens. The argon, krypton, KTP, copper vapor, gold vapor, helium-neon (He-Ne), and neodymium:YAG (Nd:YAG) lasers are all potentially hazardous to the retina. The erbium:YAG, erbium:YLF, holmium:YAG, hydrogen-fluoride, carbon-dioxide, and carbon-monoxide lasers are all potentially hazardous to the cornea because wavelengths that cause corneal damage are not reconcentrated by the eyes as are wavelengths in the retinal hazard region. The thresholds for injury of the cornea are generally much higher than those that may injure the retina. Table 1 lists permissible occupational exposure limits for most of the commonly used surgical lasers [2–8].

Skin Hazards

The skin is less vulnerable to injury than the eye. However, it should be remembered that the probability of accidental exposure to some part of the skin from a reflected laser beam is far greater than to the small area occupied by the eye. Injury

TABLE 1. Selected Occupational Exposure Limits (MPE's) for Some Lasers[a]

Type of laser	Principal wavelength(s)	MPE (eye)
Argon-fluoride laser	193 nm*	3.0 mJ/cm^2 over 8 h
Xenon-chloride laser	308 nm	40 mJ/cm^2 over 8 h
Argon ion laser	488, 514.5 nm	3.2 mW/cm^2 for 0.1 s
Copper vapor laser	510, 578 nm	2.5 mW/cm^2 for 0.25 s
Helium-neon laser	632.8 nm	1.8 mW/cm^2 for 1.0 s
Gold vapor laser	628 nm	1.0 mW/cm^2 for 10 s
Krypton ion laser	568, 647 nm	
Neodymium:YAG laser (primary λ)	1,064 nm	5.0 μJ/cm^2 for 1 ns to 50 μs / No MPE for t < 1 ns 5 mW/cm^2 for 10 s
Neodymium:YAG laser (secondary λ)	1,334 nm	40 μJ/cm^2 for 1 ns to 50 μs / 40 mW/cm^2 for 10 s
Pulsed Nd:YAG (1.44 μm),	1.44 μm	0.1 J/cm^2 for 1 ns to 1 ms
Pulsed holmium laser	2.1 μm	
CW holmium laser	2.1 μm	100 mW/cm^2 for 10 s to 8 h, limited area
CW carbon monoxide laser	~5 μm	10 mW/cm^2 for >10 s for most of body (skin)
Carbon dioxide laser	10.6 μm	

[a]All standards/guidelines have MPE's at other wavelengths and exposure durations.
*Sources: ANSI Standard Z-136.1-1993; ACGIH TLVs (1993) and IRPA.
Note: to convert MPE's in mW/cm^2 to mJ/cm^2, multiply by exposure time t in seconds, e.g., the He-Ne or Argon MPE at 0.1 s is 0.32 mJ/cm^2.

to the skin can occur from either photochemical damage mechanisms (predominant in the ultraviolet end of the spectrum) or by thermal mechanisms (predominant in the infrared end of the spectrum). For example, erythema ("sunburn") results from injury to the epidermis—and to some extent, the dermis as well—and originates from a photochemically initiated event. Skin protection can be much easier for UV excimer lasers if the hazard is understood [20]. First-, second-, and third-degree skin burns can be induced by visible and infrared laser beam exposure, producing thermal injury, and the same irradiances that can produce a severe thermal burn can also ignite fabrics and burn plastics [1].

The severity of the injury depends upon the length of exposure and the penetration depth of the laser radiation. Generally, if the exposure lasts for a second or more, a pain response elicits a jerking movement to move the exposed tissue away from the laser beam, thereby limiting the exposure duration to a second or less. High power laser beam exposure will not result in a deep tissue burn at CO_2 wavelengths if the exposure time is extremely short, since the penetration depth of the CO_2 laser beam is very shallow (of the order 20 μm) and, in fact, does not penetrate the normal thickness of the stratum corneum. Injury to the epidermis from the CO_2 laser is by heat conduction from the stratum corneum to deeper layers.

However, short pulsed exposure to 1,064 nm Nd:YAG laser radiation, which penetrates several millimeters into tissue, can cause a deep, severe burn at a radiant exposure just above burn threshold, albeit at a much higher threshold than for a CO_2 laser burn. A holmium laser (2.1 μm) and a KTP (doubled YAG: 532 nm) or argon (488 and 514.5 nm) laser would produce a burn depth intermediate between CO_2 and Nd:YAG [9].

Clearly, the focal spot of a focused surgical laser or the concentrated beam irradiance at the tip of an optical fiber is designed to ablate or vaporize tissue and will be hazardous to skin if located near the focal spot. Skin injury also can occur as a result of ignition of clothing by a reflected laser beam with tragic consequences. Significant skin injuries from accidental exposure to industrial or medical lasers rarely occur; at least, they are rarely reported. Actual thresholds of injury to the skin are normally of the order of joules-per-square centimeter, and this level of exposure does not occur outside of the focal zone of a surgical laser.

REFLECTIONS AND PROBABILITY OF EXPOSURE

An examination of laser accident records indicates that the source of accidental ocular exposure is most frequently a reflected beam. Figure 2

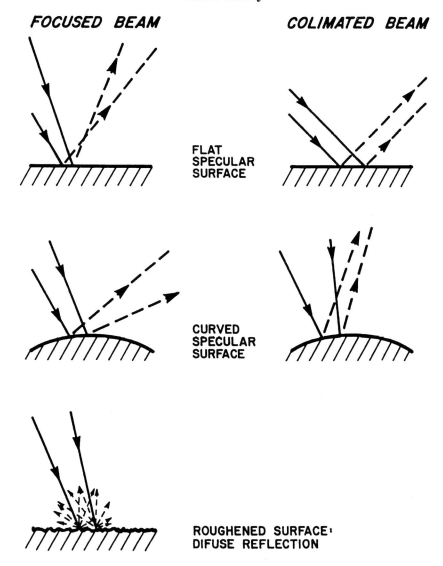

FOCUSED BEAM   COLIMATED BEAM

FLAT
SPECULAR
SURFACE

CURVED
SPECULAR
SURFACE

ROUGHENED SURFACE:
DIFUSE REFLECTION

Fig. 2. Examples of reflections of laser radiation from specular (mirror like) surfaces (e.g., metallic instrument surfaces).

illustrates the types of mirrorlike (specular) laser beam reflections that can occur from the flat or curved surfaces, which are characteristic of metallic instruments used in other surgical procedures. Skin injury of the hand holding an instrument is also possible. Normally, the collimated beam is considered the most hazardous type of reflection, but at very close range, a diverging beam may pose a greater likelihood of striking the eye [1,20,21].

A number of steps can be taken to minimize the potential hazards to both the patient and surgical staff. Preventive measures will depend upon the type of laser. The most common type employed today in most surgical applications is the

CO_2 laser. Since the CO_2 laser wavelength of 10.6 μm is in the far-infrared spectral region—and invisible—the presence of hazardous secondary beams could go unnoticed. This added hazard resulting from an infrared laser beam's lack of visibility is common to other infrared lasers, such as the 2.1 μm holmium or the 1,064 nm Nd:YAG laser. Because there have been a number of serious retinal injuries caused by improper attention to safety with Nd:YAG lasers [1,9], the use of the Nd:YAG laser must be approached with even greater caution than the CO_2 laser. By contrast, the argon laser and the second harmonic Nd:YAG (sometimes referred to as the "KTP") laser emit highly visible, blue-green, (488, 514.5, and 532

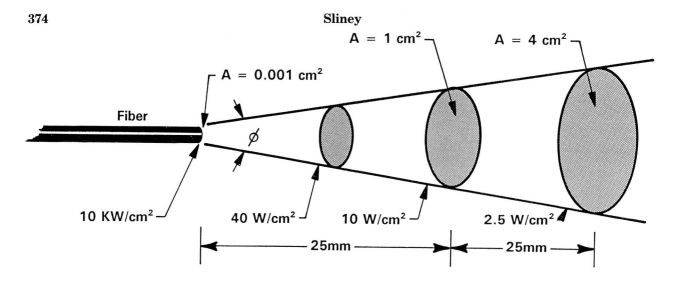

Fig. 3. Beam irradiance of a laser beam as a function of distance from an endoscopic laser fiber. Note the rapid decrease of beam irradiance beyond the focal point.

nm) beams, and in some ways pose a lesser potential hazard.

Most current surgical lasers, such as the CO_2, Nd:YAG, holmium, or argon, are continuous-wave (CW), or nearly so. Even the so-called super-pulse laser is quasi-CW compared to single-pulse ophthalmic laser photodisruptors, dermatological pulsed dye lasers, or some experimental excimer ablative lasers. The biological effects and potential hazards from high-peak power-pulsed lasers are quite different from those of CW lasers. This is particularly true of lasers operating in the *retinal hazard region* of the visible (400–760 nm) and near-infrared spectrum (IR-A: 760–1,400 nm) as shown in Figure 1. The severity of retinal lesions from a visible or near-infrared (IR-A) CW laser is normally considered to be far less than from a q-switched laser. Another major factor that influences the potential hazard is the degree of beam collimation. Almost all surgical lasers are focused, thereby limiting the hazardous area (referred to as the "nominal hazard zone" in ANSI Z-136.1)[2]. An exception is the highly collimated beam from many argon laser photocoagulators, which may remain hazardous at quite some distance from the instrument [20].

Reflections are most serious from flat mirrorlike (specular) surfaces—characteristic of many metallic surgical instruments. Many surgical instruments now have black anodized or sandblasted, roughened surfaces to reduce (but not eliminate) potentially hazardous reflections. The surface roughening is generally more effective than the black (ebonized) surface, since the beam is diffused. However, combining a black surface with roughening provides increased protection, and adding a black polymer finish has been shown to offer the greatest protection [21].

It should be noted that both the surface finish and reflectance seen in the visible spectrum do *not* indicate those qualities in the invisible far-infrared spectrum. In fact, a roughened surface that appears to be quite dull and diffuse at shorter, visible, or IR-A wavelengths, will always be much more specular at far-infrared wavelengths (e.g., at 10.6 μm). This results from the fact that the relative size of the microscopic structure of the surface relative to the incident wavelength determines whether the beam is reflected as a specular or diffuse reflection [1,9,21].

A specularly reflected beam with only 1% of the initial beam's power can still be quite hazardous. Hence the rougher the surface of an instrument likely to intercept the beam, the safer the reflection. For example, even a 1% reflection of a 40-watt (40 W) laser beam is 400 mW! It is somewhat surprising that there have been few cases reported of eye injuries to residents and other persons observing Nd:YAG laser surgery without eye protectors. Hazardous specular reflections from a laser beam emerging from an endoscopic optical fiber are limited in extent because the beam rapidly diverges as shown in Figure 3.

Most invisible beam surgical lasers have a visible alignment beam. Infrared lasers most often make use of a low-power coaxial He-Ne (632.8 nm) red laser. It is desirable where feasible for this alignment beam to be 1 mW (milliwatt) or less, since the maximum CW, visible laser beam power that can safely enter the eye within the aversion response (i.e., within the blink reflex, etc. of 0.25 second) is 1 mW.

Patient Safety

Laser safety regulations do not apply to the exposure of the patient at the target site for surgery. However, accidental exposure to the patient from misdirection of the laser beam should be of concern and can result in injury of eye and skin [1]. Ignition of drapes can be particularly hazardous to the patient who is under anesthesia and unable to warn the OR staff of the sensation of heat. Details of accidents are often not published because of litigation, but anecdotal reports indicate that misfiring of a laser when not in use or undetected breakage of optical fibers has led to drape fires and serious injuries of patients. Procedural methods, such as the use of the standby switch or proper placement of the laser footswitch, can reduce the number of such accidents but never completely eliminate them. Preparations for extinguishing fires and the moistening of drapes must always be part of the OR safety SOP.

Accidental injury of the eye is of particular concern when lasers are used in or near the eyes and where exposure of the eye itself is not intended. Special eye shields are available for patient protection.

Patient safety has been of particular concern to head-and-neck surgeons using the laser near the trachea. As a result of a number of fatal injuries to patients from ignition of airway tubes, the means to reduce ignition have been addressed by anesthesiologists and manufacturers of endotracheal tubes [22–27]. The reduction of ignition depends upon avoiding the use of combustible materials, e.g., by use of metal tubes, but, unfortunately, at least some part of the airway frequently remains as a plastic or rubber element. Training of the surgical staff in prevention of endotracheal tube fires becomes essential in the field of head-and-neck surgery.

Safety of the Surgeon

Normally, the surgeon views the target tissue through the optics of an endoscope, an operating microscope, colposcope, slit-lamp biomicroscope, etc., and the reflections are safely attenuated within the optics. Under such indirect viewing conditions, the surgeon or laser operator is normally not highly susceptible to injury due to proper design of the laser instrument. However, if the laser is accidentally actuated when the surgeon is not looking through the viewing optics, he or she will be as at risk as any other person in the room. Additionally, with hand-held laser delivery systems, one should remember that the surgeon's hand is the closest to the laser target and therefore it is closest to potentially hazardous reflections from adjacent surgical instruments (e.g., metal retractors).

Safety of the Surgical Staff

Nurses, other surgical assistants, and operating room staff are potentially exposed to misdirected laser beams. Lasers have been accidentally initiated when the beam delivery system was directed other than at the patient, a foot switch was accidentally pressed, or similar errors have occurred, and the beam directed at a person. Accidental firing of a laser has also occurred because of confusion created by multiple foot switches positioned below an operating room table. The laser foot switch should be covered and clearly identified. Assistants are potentially exposed to secondary reflections from surgical devices, whereas the surgeon's eyes are protected by viewing through an optical delivery system. For example, a gynecologic surgeon may direct the laser beam while viewing through a colposcope, and the surgeon's eyes are protected by filtration in the viewing optics. Reflections from the cornea or the contact lens used in ophthalmic surgery may be hazardous to assistants or bystanders in line of view of the contact lens to a distance of 1–2 m. The operating microscope used in laser microsurgery by a number of specialties would protect the eyes of the surgeon if properly designed, whereas, assistants, and bystanders may be exposed to potentially hazardous reflections from surgical instruments inserted into the beam path.

Safety of Other Bystanders

Bystanders in the surgical facility or outpatient laser facility who are present to observe or to calm the patient (e.g., a patient's relative) may be susceptible to exposure from reflected laser beams in the same manner as a surgical assistant or nurse. In addition, because of lack of training or knowledge about the laser surgical procedure bystanders may be at greater risk by inadvertently placing themselves in a dangerous position. These individuals should always be provided with laser eye protectors.

Service Personnel Susceptibility

Service personnel are particularly susceptible to laser injury since they often gain access to collimated laser beams from the laser cavity itself or by opening up the beam delivery optics and gaining access to collimated laser beams prior to the beam focusing optics or fiber-optic beam delivery system. Once the laser beam leaves the delivery system and comes rapidly to a focus, it then diverges again, or if emerging from a fiber, it also rapidly diverges. The zone where the beam is concentrated to a level sufficient to pose a severe hazard to the eyes or skin (the Nominal Hazard Zone, or NHZ), is normally a limited zone of 1–2 m near the beam focal point. However, a collimated laser beam, as the raw beam for most laser cavities, or a specular reflection from a turning mirror or Brewster window in the laser console may be emitted from the laser cabinet when the service person gains access. Several serious eye injuries have occurred to service personnel exposed to secondary, collimated, invisible 1064 nm Nd:YAG laser beams when the service personnel gained access to the laser cavity.

OCCUPATIONAL EXPOSURE LIMITS

Relevant ELs for lasers of interest are given in Table 1 and are calculated or measured at the cornea. If the laser beam is <7 mm in diameter, it is assumed that the entire beam could enter the dark-adapted pupil and one can express the maximal safe power or energy in the beam (in the 0.4–1.4 μm retinal hazard region); it is the EL multiplied by the area of a 7-mm pupil, i.e., 0.4 cm^2. For example, for the visible CW lasers, an exposure limited by the natural aversion response of 0.25 s is 2.5 mW/cm^2, and this EL multiplied by 0.4 cm^2 results in the limiting power of 1.0 mW. This 1 mW value has a special significance in laser safety standards, since it is the Accessible Emission Limit (AEL) of Class 2, i.e., the dividing line between two laser safety hazard classifications: Class 2 and Class 3 [2–8]. In the new 1993 standards, a 3.5 mm aperture was introduced for use with CW infrared lasers operating at wavelengths greater than 1,400 nm [3,8].

Laser Hazard Classification

As noted, any CW visible laser (400–700 nm) that has an output power < 1.0 mW is termed a Class 2 (low risk) laser and could be considered more or less equivalent in risk with staring at the sun, at a tungsten-halogen spotlight, or at other bright lights that can cause a photic maculopathy (central retinal injury). Only if one purposely overcomes their natural aversion response to bright light, can a Class 2 laser pose a real ocular hazard. An aiming beam or alignment laser operating at a total power above 1.0 mW would fall into hazard Class 3 and could be hazardous *even if viewed momentarily within the aversion response time.* A subcategory of Class 3, termed Class 3a, consists of lasers from 1–5 mW in power, and these lasers pose a moderate ocular hazard under viewing conditions where most of the beam enters the eye. Class 3b is then the subcategory that comprises, among certain pulsed lasers, CW visible lasers that emit between 5–500 mW output power. Even momentary viewing of Class 3b lasers is potentially hazardous to the eye.

Only lasers that are totally enclosed or that emit extremely low output powers fall into Class 1 and are safe to view. Any CW laser with an output power above 0.5 W (500 mW) falls into Class 4. Class 4 lasers are considered to pose skin or fire hazards as well as eye hazards if not properly used. The purpose of assigning hazard classes to laser products is to simplify the determination of adequate safety measures, i.e., Class 3a measures are more stringent than Class 2 measures and Class 4 measures, more stringent than Class 3b measures. Virtually all surgical lasers fall into Class 4.

Laser Eye Protectors

Laser eye protectors provide the principal means to assure against ocular injury from the direct or reflected laser beams in the operating room [28–42]. Although the eyes of the laser operator may be inherently protected by viewing optics, this should always be ascertained from the manufacturer of the viewing optics. In this regard, ordinary optical glass protects against all wavelengths shorter than ~300 nm and > 2,700 nm [9]. Laser protective filters may be obtained for endoscopes and other viewing optics for the spectral region between these two spectral bands. Eye protectors are available as spectacles, wrap-around lenses, goggles, and related forms of eyewear. It is important that the eyewear be marked with the wavelengths and optical densities provided at those wavelengths. The markings must be clearly understood by all of the operating room staff. The proper use of eyewear and the meaning of the eye-protector markings are key subjects for laser safety training of the staff.

Clear plastic safety glasses with side shields that are known to be made of polycarbonate are suitable for use with the CO_2 laser, but should be marked by the laser safety officer with an indication of the optical density, e.g., "OD = 4 at CO_2 wavelength of 10.6 μm." Although some LSOs may be uneasy about marking eye protectors not sold as "laser" eye protection because of perceived legal concerns, studies of plastic eye protectors show clearly that polycarbonate is far superior in burn-through resistance than other plastics, and such a marking is quite justifiable for CO_2 lasers up to at least 100 W power [28]. Some manufacturers of laser eye protection and some laser safety specialists have made a major issue of burn-through times of plastic eye protectors. However, with the powers generally used in laser surgery of 100 W or less, burn-throughs are probably unrealistic, since the wearer would certainly move their head within a second after detecting a flame shooting from the goggle. Indeed, the skin will incur a serious burn at levels below plastic burn-through irradiances [28,29,41].

Skin protection is seldom a serious concern other than for the hands located near the focal zone of an open-beam laser. If Xe-Cl, 308-nm lasers are employed, scattered UVR would be of concern, and the skin should be covered [43–48]. Most tightly woven fabrics will have an attenuation factor exceeding 10^4, or an optical density exceeding 4 [43].

RESPIRATORY PROTECTION

Probably no issue has caused more concerns in surgical laser safety than the potential hazards from breathing airborne contaminants produced during the vaporization of tissues. Although photocoagulation does not produce a smoke plume, any laser (or electrosurgical) cutting will produce gasses and particulates that must be evaluated as a potential respirable hazard. Studies of the production of both the chemical toxicity of pyrolysis products and the potential viability of infectious particulates (e.g., viral fragments) have shown real cause for concern unless very good local exhaust ventilation and respiratory protection are employed [45–53].

Several medical equipment suppliers offer splash-proof, full-face protection to protect against splash of patients with viral infection [54]. Although normally not designed as laser protection, the shields (particularly if polycarbonate) will offer some protection against exposure

from reflected CO_2 laser radiation. However, thin, lightweight transparent plastic filters may be more susceptible to burn-through. The ultimate protection would, of course, be afforded by wearing a self-contained respirator. As protection against airborne contaminants, several manufacturers provide variously configured self-contained respiratory devices, but these are very cumbersome and have only rarely been seriously suggested (or worn) in a surgical setting. The best protection can never be foolproof, and with appropriate training, most surgical staffs recognize the importance of using good fume extraction. If additional concern exists because of pathogenicity, the wearing of a high-performance face mask provides a still greater level of protection. Hazards from laser gasses are normally controlled by system enclosure, and in some instances, with exhaust ventilation, as with excimer laser systems [55].

Other Ancillary Hazards to the Patient

Besides breathing some airborne contaminants, a patient may experience increased blood levels of methemoglobin even during endoscopy. It has been suggested by Ott [56] that this increase results through peritoneal absorption as well as through the respiratory tract. Clearly, a balanced review of benefits vs. risks will provide the best choice in surgery, and the benefits of laser surgery have generally far outweighed the new risks. However, the review is always required with the introduction of new technologies in any type of surgery.

SAFETY ADMINISTRATION AND TRAINING

The practical implementation of a laser safety program, which includes a laser safety training program, cannot be treated in detail here. Other reviews of the subject treat these aspects in detail [1,4,10–18]. Clearly, the design of a safety program depends largely upon the size of the institution and the variety and number of lasers in use. An office practice might have only a safety SOP and a designated LSO; a large institution frequently benefits from a laser safety committee. In the end, the importance of a well-trained staff cannot be overemphasized. Accidents can be only prevented by a well-trained staff and an administrative policy that encourages a sustained effort toward safe laser use.

CONCLUSIONS

The potential exposure levels to the eye and skin from scattered laser radiation from most surgical laser applications are substantially below a threshold for injury, and only the direct beam or specular reflections are of concern. Only with UV lasers should one be seriously concerned with chronic exposure and delayed effects. The surgical laser user can be assured that today a consensus exists almost worldwide regarding the appropriate laser safety measures to preclude injury from acute or chronic effects. Procedural controls requiring the use appropriate eye protection when needed and control of vaporized tissue byproducts requires both a well-trained surgeon and OR staff. As with many other applications of lasers in industry and research, laser safety training is of crucial importance.

REFERENCES

1. Sliney DH, Trokel SL. "Medical Lasers and Their Safe Use." New York: Springer-Verlag, 1992.
2. ACGIH, TLV's, Threshold Limit Values and Biological Exposure Indices for 1993–1994, American Conference of Governmental Industrial Hygienists, Cincinnati, OH, 1993.
3. ANSI, Safe Use of Lasers, Standard Z-136.1-1993, American National Standards Institute, Laser Institute of America, Orlando, FL, 1993.
4. ANSI, Safe Use of Lasers in Health Care Facilities, Standard Z-136.3-1988, American National Standards Institute, Laser Institute of America, Orlando, FL, 1988 [under revision in 1994].
5. British Standards Organisation, Radiation Safety of Laser Products and Systems, Standard BS4803, London, BSI, 1984.
6. World Health Organization [WHO], Environmental Health Criteria No. 23, Lasers and Optical Radiation, joint publication of the United Nations Environmental Program, the International Radiation Protection Association and the World Health Organization, Geneva, 1982.
7. IRPA, International Non-Ionizing Radiation Committee, Guidelines for Limits of Human Exposure to Laser Radiation, Health Physics 1985; 49(5):341–359.
8. International Electrotechnical Commission, Radiation Safety of Laser Products, Equipment Classification, and User's Guide, Document WS 825-1, IEC, Geneva, 1993.
9. Sliney DH, and Wolbarsht ML. "Safety with Lasers and Other Optical Sources." New York: Plenum, 1980.
10. Ball KA. "Medical Lasers: The Perioperative Challenge." St Louis: Mosby, 1991.
11. Lundergan D, Smith S. Nurses administrative responsibilities for lasers. AORN August 1983; 217–222.
12. Mackety CJ. The laser committee: Its role in quality assurance. Health Care Strategic Management, 1984.
13. Pfister J. A Guide To Lasers in the O.R.: A Manual for OR Personnel. Education Design, 1983.
14. Steffers V. Safety checklist documents responsibilities of the laser nurse. Clin Laser Month 1984; 2:55.
15. Fisher JC. Principles of Safety in Laser Surgery and Therapy. In: Baggish MS, ed. "Basic and Advanced Laser Surgery in Gynecology," Norwalk, CT: Appleton-Century-Crofts, 1985, p 88.
16. Holmes JA. Summary of safety considerations for the medical and surgical practitioner. In: Apfelberg DB, ed. "Surgical Lasers." New York: Springer-Verlag, 1986, pp 69–95.
17. Cayton MM. Nursing responsibilities in laser surgery. Medical Instrumentation 1983; 17:419.
18. Carruth JAS, McKenzie AL, Wainwright AC. Clinical laser safety. In: Atsumi K, ed. "New Frontiers in Lasers in Medicine and Surgery." Amsterdam: Elsevier Science, 1983.
19. US Department of Labor, title 29, Codes of Federal Regulations. Occupational Health and Safety.
20. Sliney DH, Mainster MA. Potentially hazardous reflections to the clinician during photocoagulation. Am J Ophthalmol 1987; 103(6):758–760.
21. Wood RL, Sliney DH, Basye RA. Laser reflections from surgical instruments. Lasers Surg Med 1992, 12:675–678.
22. Fried MP, Mallampati SR, Liu FC, Kaplan S, Caminear DS, Samonte BR. Laser resistant stainless steel tracheal tube: Experimental and clinical evaluation. Lasers Surg Med 1991, 11:301–306.
23. Schramm VL Jr, Mattox DE, and Stool SE. Acute management of laser-ignited intratracheal explosion. Laryngoscope 1991, 91:1417–1426.
24. Birch AA. Anesthetic considerations during laser surgery. Anesth Analg 1974; 52:53–58.
25. Nolt ML, Devos V. New endotracheal tube for laser surgery of larynx. Ann Otol Rhinol Laryngol 1978; 87:554–557.
26. Woo P, Vaughn C. Small metal cuffless venturi ventilation system for use of laser surgery. Otolaryngol Head Neck Surg 1983; 91:497.
27. Wong KC, Oykman PF. Anesthetic considerations in laser surgery. In: Dixon JA, ed. "Surgical Applications of Lasers." Chicago: Yearbook Medical, 1983.
28. Sliney DH, Sparks SD, Wood RL. The protective characteristics of polycarbonate lenses against CO_2 laser radiation. J Laser Appl 1992; 5(1):49–52.
29. Envall KR, Coakley JM, Peterson RW, and Landry RJ. Preliminary evaluation of commercially available laser protective eyewear. U.S. Dept of Health, Education, and Welfare, Bureau of Radiological Health, DHEW Publication (FDA) 1975; 75–8026:32.
30. Eriksen P, Galoff PK. Measurements of laser eye protective filters. Health Physics 1989; 56(3):741–742.
31. Galoff PK, Sliney DH. Evaluation of laser eye protectors in the ultraviolet and infrared. In: Court L, Duchene A, Courant D, eds. "Proceedings of First International Symposium on Laser Biological Effects and Exposure Limits {Lasers et Normes de Protection}, Paris, Nov 24–26, 1986, Paris: Commissariat a l'Energie Atomique, Fontenay-aux-Roses 1988; 356–366.
32. Holst GC. Proper selection and testing of laser protective materials. Am J Opt 1973: 50; 477–483.
33. Lyon TL, and Marshall WJ. Nonlinear properties of optical filters—Implications for laser safety. Health Physics 1986; 51:95–96.
34. Robinson AA, Marshall JJ, Dudevoir SG. Study of saturation in commercial laser goggles. SPIE Proceedings 1990; 1207:202–213.

35. Scherr AE, Tucker RJ, Greenwood RA. New plastics absorb at laser wavelengths. Laser Focus 196; 5:26–48.

36. Sliney DH, Le Bodo H. Laser eye protectors. J Laser Appl 1990; 2:9–13.

37. Spencer DJ, Bixler HA. IR laser radiation eye protector. Rev Sci Instr 1972; 43:1545–1546.

38. Swearengen PM, Vance, WF, Counts DL. A study of burn-through times for laser protective eyewear. Am Ind Hyg Assoc J 1988; 49:608–612.

39. Swope, CH. Design considerations for laser eye protection. Arch Envir Health 1970; 20:184–187.

40. Williams DR, Some comments on the properties of absorptive lenses. J Am Opt Assn 1970; 41:82–91.

41. Yeo R. Laser eye protection I. Optics Laser Tech 1989; 21(4):257.

42. Zwick H, Belkin M, Beatrice ES. Effects of broadbanded eye proection on dark adaptation. In: Court L, Duchene A, Courant D, eds. "Proceedings of First International Symposium on Laser Biological Effects and Exposure Limits {Lasers et Normes de Protection}," Paris, Nov 24–26, 1986, Paris: Commissariat a l'Energie Atomique, Fontenay-aux-Roses, 1988; 356–366.

43. Sliney DH, et al. Transmission of potentially hazardous actinic ultraviolet radiation through fabrics. App Ind Hyg 1987; 2(1):36–44.

44. Parish JA, Pathak MA, Fitzpatrick TB. Protection of skin from germicidal ultraviolet radiation in the operating room by topical chemicals. New Engl J Med 1971; 284; 1257–1258.

45. Baggish MS, Poiesz BJ, Joret D, Williamson P, Refai A. Presence of human immunodeficiency virus DNA in laser smoke. Lasers Surg Med 1991; 11:197–203.

46. Baggish MS, Elbakry M. The effect of laser smoke on the lungs of rats. Am J Obstetr Gyn 1987; 156:1260–1265.

47. Bellina JH, Stjernholm RL, Kurpel JE. Analysis of emissions after irradiation with carbon dioxide laser. Reprod Med 1982; 27:268.

48. Dickes J. Face masks as protection from laser plume. AORN J 1989; 50:520–522.

49. Garden JM, O'Banion KM, Scheinitz LS, Pinski KS, Bakus AD, Reichmann ME, Sundberg JP. Papillomavirus in the vapor of carbon dioxide treated verrucae. JAMA 1988; 259:1199–1202.

50. Sawchuck WS, Weber PH, Lowry DE, Dzubowq LM. Infectious papilomavirus in the vapor of warts treateed with carbon dioxide laser or electrocoagulation: Detection and protection. J Am Acad Derm. 1989; 21:41–49.

51. Voorhies RM, Lavyne MH, Strait TA, et al. Does the CO_2 laser spread viable brain tumor cells outside the surgical field? Neurosurgery 1984; 60:892.

52. Miller GW, Geraci J, Shumrich DA. Smoke evacuation for laser surgery. Otolaryngol Head Neck Surg 1983; 92: 582.

53. Kokasa JM, Eugene J. Chemical composition of laser-tissue interaction smoke plume. J Laser Appl 1989; 1:59–63.

54. American National Standards Institute, Safety Code for Head, Eye, and Respiratory Protection, ANSI Z-2.1, American National Standards Institute, New York, 1978.

55. Sliney DH. Safety of ophthalmic excimer lasers with an emphasis on compressed gases. Refractive Corneal Surg 1991; 7:308–314.

56. Ott D. Smoke production and smoke reduction in endoscopic surgery: Preliminary report. End Surg 1993; 1:230–232.

Chapter 12

Laser Tissue Welding: A Comprehensive Review of Current and Future Clinical Applications

Lawrence S. Bass, MD, **and Michael R. Treat**, MD

*Division of Plastic Surgery (L.S.B.), Division of Laparoendoscopic Surgery (M.R.T.),
Columbia University, College of Physicians & Surgeons, New York, New York*

INTRODUCTION

Laser welding, a developing technique with applications in almost all surgical specialties, is undergoing a transition from laboratory experimentation to accepted clinical practice. The laboratory delineation of the laser welding phenomenon has included exploring the types of tissues that could be welded, the wavelengths that may be of use, and the best laser parameters for each application. Answering these questions has been made more difficult by the fact that each of the major groups investigating these problems has proceeded with different experimental models and conditions. Despite these difficulties, over the past few years a general consensus has emerged regarding the important principles underlying tissue welding. We review these principles and give an overview of welding technique and applications. The second part of this review covers the specific clinical applications in detail.

PRINCIPLES AND THEORY
Why Weld?

Conventional tissue closure methods include sutures, staples, or clips. Laser tissue welding is a technology that, under optimum circumstances, can be faster, less traumatic, and easier to apply than conventional tissue closure methods. Let us first consider the features of conventional tissue closure methods.

Mechanical Closure Methods

Sutures are a superbly flexible technology that can be adapted to almost any tissue conditions encountered. In addition, sutures are inexpensive, reliable, and readily available. However, sutures do create tissue injury during passage of the needle and tying the knot. By their very nature, sutures result in a foreign body being left in the tissue. This tissue injury and foreign body reaction can result in inflammation, granuloma formation, scarring, and stenosis. Sutures in and of themselves do not produce a watertight closure. In addition, the application of sutures involves a complex series of movements [1] that may be difficult or tedious to execute in microsurgical or minimally invasive endoscopic applications. The physical manipulations required to place sutures are the ultimate example of a skill-intensive, literally handcrafted approach. As with any handcrafted technique, the results obtained by an average pair of hands may not be as good as those achieved by more skilled hands, and in any event the results will vary from case to case. In fact, the optimum employment of sutures involves the judicious estimation of and control over many variables, including suture tension and spacing.

Compared to sutures, mechanical methods of tissue closure, such as staples or clips, have the advantage of a more uniform result [2], since tissue tension and staple spacing are determined by the stapling device itself. However, these mechanical methods suffer the major disadvantage of being a "one-size-fits-all" approach. Unlike handcrafted sutures, staples and clips have only a limited range of adaptability in the face of different conditions such as tissue thickness and friability. On the plus side, compared to sutures, staples and clips are well suited to application via endoscopes and laparoscopes. However, as the size of minimally invasive instrumentation is further reduced and as more difficult applications, such as vascular anastomosis, are attempted, mechanical tissue closure methods are encountering fundamental barriers based on the inherent physical limitations of very small mechanical devices. These limitations stem in part from the fact that these stapling/clipping devices require a surprisingly large amount of force in order to form the staple or clip into its closed configuration. Mechanical devices capable of exerting these large forces while maintaining precision of alignment are difficult to build in the small size range.

Other Closure Methods

Besides sutures, staples, and clips, other closure techniques have been tested. These include biological and nonbiological adhesives as well as coupling devices of various types.

For most applications, adhesives have not been able to provide adequate strength and have had problems with tissue reactivity [3,4], toxicity [5], or infection [6]. In addition, conventional tissue adhesives have poor handling properties and permit little control over the bonding process. On the plus side, compared to laser welding, eye safety is not an issue. Large areas such as flaps and grafts can be rapidly treated compared with laser techniques.

The couplers approach has been tried for over 100 years. An archetypal example of this technology is the "Murphy button." Current incarnations of this device include the Biodegradable Anastomotic Ring® ("BAR") [7] for gastrointestinal anastomosis and the 3-M Precise Microanastomotic System® [8]. The use of controlled-rate absorbable materials in the BAR has attracted considerable clinical interest. However, couplers generically suffer from size inflexibility. Also, coupling devices often involve the sacrifice of some length of the structure being anastomosed, and in some applications this can be a serious drawback.

As shown in detail in this section, laser tissue closure methods can transcend the limitations of sutures and mechanical closure devices.

It is generally accepted that welding is a photothermal process. While lasers offer advantages such as precise spatial and temporal confinement of the applied energy, other sources of heat such as radiofrequency energy can be used to produce tissue welds [9,10].

BEGINNINGS OF LASER TISSUE WELDING
Laser Welding: Definition

Laser welding is the process of using laser energy to join or bond tissues. In general, this energy results in some alteration of the molecular structure of the tissues being joined. The altered tissue molecules can form bonds of one sort or another with their neighbors.

Early Concepts

Interest in laser tissue welding is not new. Laboratory and experimental clinical attempts at laser welding have been carried out over more than 15 years [11]. Although these earlier attempts have ultimately not achieved widespread clinical use, it is worthwhile to review them.

Very early experience with the use of electrocautery energy [10], and later laser energy [12], indicated the feasibility of repairing linear venotomies, but arterial anastomosis remained unreliable. The first reproducible experimental use of vascular laser welding was reported by

Jain and Gorisch [11]. In 1979, they studied the use of a Nd:YAG laser for microvascular anastomosis in rat carotid and femoral arteries. This was followed in 1984 by a small series of clinical cases [13] reported in a brief letter in *Lancet*. In this remarkable communication, Jain not only described his clinical approach but also mentioned several technical insights that anticipated experimental and theoretical work of the next 10 years.

CO₂ Laser Welding

Variations on Jain's basic approach were carried out using the CO_2 laser. Most early laser welding experiments employed this wavelength because of its availability and familiarity for most surgeons [14]. Microvascular anastomosis again served as the tissue model. These early attempts were successful in achieving a stable bond some of the time but suffered from an increased rate of aneurysms [15] and dehiscence. The initial strength of the repair was significantly lower than suture anastomoses [16]. Laser repairs did demonstrate the ability to grow [17] and suggested the possibility of reduced intimal hyperplasia [18] and increased vessel wall compliance.

Current theories of the welding process allow us to understand the limitations of these approaches. Consider a simple Beer's law model for the heating of tissue by a given laser wavelength. In the Beer's law model, the amount of laser energy penetrating a given thickness of tissue declines exponentially according to an absorption coefficient α. $F_x = F_0 e^{-\alpha x}$ where F_x is the fraction of incident fluence, F_0, which is present at depth x in the tissue.

The CO_2 wavelength is very strongly absorbed by water (large absorption coefficient relative to water). Since water is a large constituent of most tissues, most of the CO_2 energy is absorbed in the outermost layers of the tissue, and exponentially little of that energy is available for heating of the deeper layers. Another way to express this concept is the *optical penetration depth* ($1/\alpha$), which is the depth at which 50% of the incident energy will be absorbed. The optical penetration depth for CO_2 in water is ~13 μm [19,20]. Thus with a short pulse of light (pulsed welding is discussed below), only a small portion of the apposed surfaces would be heated. Due to the high absorption, the outermost tissue layers are "overcooked," whereas the deeper layers are hardly affected at all (see Fig. 1). The resulting bond is weak, since the full thickness of the tissue is not employed in the bond. If the energy is further in-

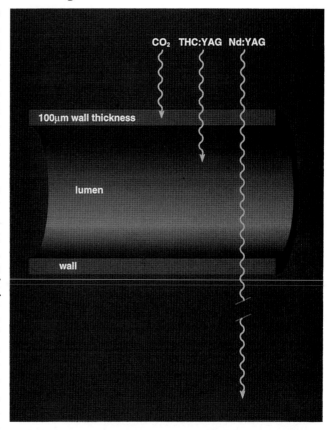

Fig. 1. The CO_2 laser has a very short optical penetration depth relative to the THC:YAG and the Nd:YAG. This diagram is only approximate, since it neglects the absorptive/scattering effects of tissue pigments and intraluminal blood.

creased in a short pulse to try to heat the deeper layers, the ablation threshold at the surface may be exceeded with little additional deep heating. Alternatively, if the duration of exposure is increased (e.g., CW exposure), thermal buildup occurs transmitting heat not only to the deep layers but also laterally producing a large zone of injury. The outer layers are excessively heated, which results in tissue contraction, cell death, and weakening of the bond. Therefore, except for extremely thin tissues, CO_2 is a poor choice of wavelength and unlikely to yield a reliable high strength bond. Even in a microvessel with a wall thickness of ~100 μm, CO_2 light will not provide even heating.

Argon Laser Vascular Welding

In an attempt to produce more uniform tissue heating, and therefore stronger bonds, other wavelengths have been employed, notably argon [21,22] and Nd:YAG [23,24]. Compared to CO_2, these wavelengths produce deeper and more uni-

TABLE 1. Absorption Characteristics of Commonly Available Medical Lasers*

Laser	α (water) (cm^{-1})	α (tissue) (cm^{-1})	OPD[a] (water) (μm)	OPD[a] (tissue) (μm)
CO_2 (10.6μm)	950	600	11	17
Er:YAG (2.94 μm)	4,500	2,700	2	4
Ho:YAG (2.06 μm)	70	35	143	286
Nd:YAG (1.32 μm)	1.2	8	8,333	1,250
Nd:YAG (1.06 μm)	0.1	4	100,000	2,500
Ga:Al:As diode (810 nm)	0.01		1,000,000	
doubled Nd:YAG (532 nm)		12		833
argon (514.5 nm)		14		714
argon (488.0 nm)		20		500

*Modified from EHTL, reprinted with permission.
[a]Optical penetration depth

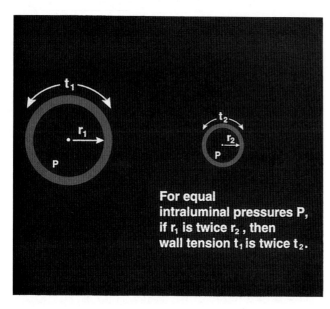

Fig. 2. Diagram of wall tension as a function of vascular radius at a given intraluminal pressure. If the radius of the larger vessel is twice that of the smaller vessel, the wall tension is twice times as great. This effect means that it is more difficult to weld larger vessels successfully.

form tissue heating (Table I) [25]. It was hoped that these deeper penetrating wavelengths would be better suited to weld structures larger and thicker than microvessels. A technique of laser welding was developed using the argon laser for medium-size vessels [26] and intestine [27]. Rodney White [28,29] has performed a small clinical series of arteriovenous anastomoses using the argon laser. Long-term follow-up of these patients has shown satisfactory results. His technique and results are discussed in more detail later under Cardiovascular Surgery.

Despite these encouraging early clinical results, there were serious difficulties with this type of application. The wall stress in larger diameter

vessels is much greater than in smaller vessels as a consequence of LaPlace's law [30]. $P = n \Sigma T/r$ where P is intraluminal pressure, n is the degrees of freedom, ΣT is wall thickness, and r is the radius of the vessel (see Fig. 2).

This medium-size vessel system is therefore a much more difficult test of weld strength than the microvessel models. The relatively high degree of success achieved in these medium-size vessel welding attempts is therefore all the more impressive. However, the anastomoses so created were of variable strength and reliability. This variability was probably due to difficulty in accurately dosing laser energy in the face of confounding factors such as variations in the amount of hemoglobin present, local tissue thickness, and state of hydration. There was a narrow margin between a successful and an unsuccessful weld. Too little laser energy resulted in a weak or nonexistent bond, whereas excessive laser energy resulted in excessive drying and shrinkage of the tissue proteins, which reduced weld flexibility and strength. To prevent overheating, White's group used constant water irrigation of the operative site with an IV cannula. This irrigation technique was intended to ameliorate or "smooth out" the transmural temperature profile. Unfortunately, this method of tissue welding depended on the skill and experience of the operator even more than with sutures, especially considering the relative ease of suture placement in these fairly large vessels. These difficulties prevented the widespread adoption of this technique.

Another noteworthy attempt at using a wavelength with more spatially uniform absorption properties than CO_2 was the use of 1.320 μm Nd:YAG laser [31]. Absorption of this wavelength is mediated both by water and hemoglobin. Dew [31] suggested that this dual absorption characteristic provided a balance to the amount of energy absorbed, regardless of local variations in the amount of tissue hemoglobin. The typical optical penetration depths obtained in tissue were thought to be comparable to most tissue types studied by early laser welders. In addition to the dual absorption characteristics of this wavelength, Dew's strategy relied on dosage-response tables that were used to predetermine the optimum amount of laser energy for a given application based on tissue type and thickness. A computer system controlled pulse duration and laser power to produce predictable tissue heating.

In the microvessel arena, Bass et al. [32] employed the concept of matching laser optical penetration depth to the target thickness. Using a THC:YAG laser (wavelength 2.15 μm, optical penetration depth 285 μm), they repaired microvessels with an average wall thickness of 100 μm. This allowed uniform heating of the vessel wall without excessive total energy deposition on the adventitial surface. The pulsed delivery mode of the THC:YAG was stated to further control the spread of thermal injury (see Fig. 3a). The concept of matching laser optical penetration with wall thickness to achieve uniform and transmural heating was reiterated by LaMuraglia et al. [33], who used a Raman shifted Nd:YAG laser (1.9 μm) to weld small vessels. The concept of pulsed energy delivery is discussed in more detail below.

MECHANISMS OF TISSUE WELDING

Although much time and effort have been expended in bringing tissue welding to clinical practice, there are still major gaps in our understanding of the actual mechanism involved. This lack of basic understanding has been a major obstacle to progress, but several studies have attempted to define the mechanism.

Shober et al. [34] provided the first insight into the underlying process involved in thermal tissue welding. In 1986, they published a study that evaluated electron micrographs of collagen from rat carotid arteries after Nd:YAG welding. They demonstrated loosening of the collagen triple helix and some sort of interaction between collagen strands (see Fig. 4). They concluded that collagen "bonding" was responsible for laser welding. White's group confirmed this finding with argon laser welding of vessels [35]. They correlated this with the surface temperature observed using infrared cameras and their argon laser welding technique. This study suggested that maximum tissue temperature during laser welding with ar-

gon wavelengths was 48.8°C, whereas it was significantly higher (84.0°C) with the CO_2 laser [36]. These differences in surface temperature may be necessary to achieve the same core tissue temperature given the differences in tissue absorption between these two wavelengths. The accuracy of the argon reading is questionable due to the water irrigation used during argon welding but probably gives a realistic trend compared with CO_2.

Anderson's group at the Wellman Laboratory performed detailed studies of the reaction of bovine collagen tendon slices to precisely controlled amounts of heat delivered in a waterbath [37–39]. Electron micrographic morphologic studies suggested that the welding process occurred as a result of the unraveling of collagen bundles at the cut ends of the disks, with subsequent partial interdigitation of these unravelled ends across the cut. They found that optimum weld strength was obtained at 62.2 ± 2°C. In evaluating their results, it is important to realize that the experimental conditions do not relate closely to what is used in most clinical or experimental welding studies. Apposition forces of 9.6×10^5 dynes/cm^2 were used. These would be destructive to many tissue types that we seek to laser weld. As apposition pressure is reduced, optimum weld temperature increases. Optimum tensile strength at this temperature and compression required 30 min of heating. At higher temperatures, less heating time was required to reach peak weld strength.

One of the main controversies in the early stages of laser welding mechanism study was the issue of covalent versus noncovalent bonding. White's group demonstrated the presence of a novel high molecular weight protein band in SDS-PAGE gel electrophoresis of argon laser-welded guinea pig skin and the presence of low molecular weight novel protein bands in argon laser welded canine arteriovenous fistulae [40]. They concluded that covalent protein bonding and degradation take place during laser welding. Helmsworth [41] used a gel preparation of EHS basement membranes containing type IV collagen and demonstrated that exposure to argon ion laser light at 500–3,000 J/cm^2 at 0°C, fluences used for welding, produced formation of disulfide bonds. Whereas this was not laser welding per se, they theorized that disulfide bonding was central to laser welding. Bass and his group [42] addressed this issue in a series of experiments in which rat tail tendons (>90% type I collagen) were welded with diode laser (810 nm) light and

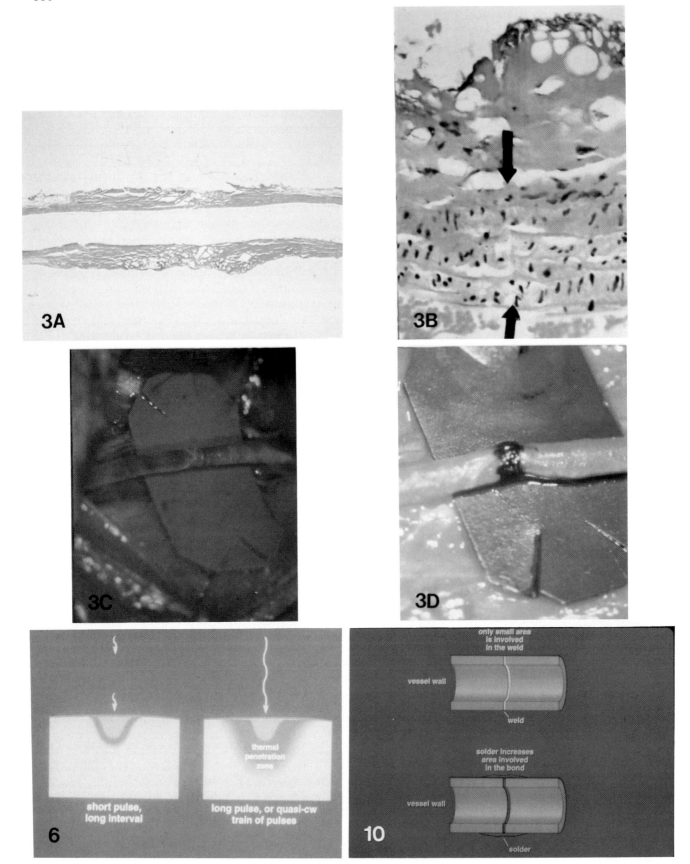

Figs. 3, 6, and 10.

indocyanine green dye (ICG). The laser-exposed collagen was subjected to SDS-polyacrylamide gel electrophoresis following a selection of enzyme degradations as well as circular dichroism studies. Collagen was denatured, uncoiling the native triple helical structure. This correlates with the changes observed in the electron microscopy studies. No helicity was reformed on cooling. No low or high molecular weight fragments indicative of covalent bond cleavage or formation were observed (see Fig. 5). Whereas the interpretation of these experiments is, of course, limited to the laser and tissue system employed, this work strongly suggests that noncovalent bonding is the major mechanism in current laser tissue welding protocols. This means that whereas covalent bond cleavage or formation may take place during laser welding, it is not *necessary* for weld strength. Sufficient heat must be produced to denature the

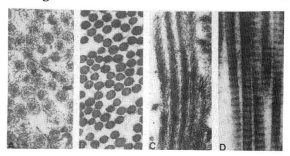

Fig. 4. Shown are a transverse and longitudinal transmission electron micrographs of collagen in laser-welded (**a,c**) and control (**b,d**) rat carotid arteries. The welded specimens demonstrate a loss of some of the well-defined structure of the collagen. This morphologic change is presumed to be a manifestation of the unraveling of the collagen triple helix × 32,000. From Schober R, Ulrich F, Sander T, Durselen H, Hessel S. Laser induced alteration of collagen substructure allow microsurgical tissue welding. Science 1986; 232:1421–1422. Reprinted with permission.

protein present, however. The temperatures required to denature collagen are known. They vary with the type of collagen and with the degree of crosslinking (which increases with aging). Nonetheless, required tissue temperatures are in the range of 60–80°C. The higher temperatures observed in most experiments utilizing clinical techniques compared with those in Anderson's experimental study may relate to welding nontransected collagen surfaces together, to differences in core tissue temperature and sensor measurement, or to differences in compression, length of heating, and evenness of heating with a laser as opposed to a water bath.

Pulsed Laser Welding

The effect of other, discontinuous heating profiles has not been fully assessed, but it is clear from experimental and theoretical considerations that pulsed delivery of laser energy can minimize collateral thermal damage [43]. The relative merits of using laser light versus other forms of heat exposure must be considered. Laser light offers instant on/off exposure with highly accurate spatial control of energy delivery. Unfortunately, the ultimate tissue temperature generated by the laser light is not exactly predictable due to variations in many local factors including tissue absorption and thermal conductivity.

An important concept in understanding the utility of pulsed delivery is the thermal relaxation time (T_r) of the tissue [44]. This tissue-dependent factor is a measure of the rate at which heat can be diffused to surrounding tissue to pre-

Fig. 3. (**a**) Longitudinal section of the THC:YAG laser anastomosis 1 hour after creation. There is uniform transmural heating to weld the entire thickness of the vessel together (hematoxylin, phloxine, saffron stain, × 25). From Bass LS, Treat MR, Dzakonski C, Trokel SL. Sutureless microvascular anastomosis using the THC:YAG laser: A preliminary report. Microsurg 1989; 10:189–193. Reprinted with permission. (**b**) Longitudinal section at 1 hour of rat carotid artery end-to-end anastomosis, which was laser-soldered using the 810 nm gallium-aluminum-arsenide diode laser and indocyanine green-protein solder. Even though the solder shows extensive thermal damage including evidence suggestive of water boiling, the underlying vessel wall is essentially normal. The welded line, indicated by arrows, is barely discernable (hematoxylin, phloxine, and saffron, × 250). (**c**) Immediate postoperative view of an end-to-end rat carotid artery anastomosis produced with the 2.15-μm thulium-holmium-chromium:YAG laser. No charring or distortion is seen. The clinical endpoint of welding is a slight tanning and drying of tissue, as shown in this THC:YAG welded micro-vessel. See (a) for reference. (**d**) Immediate postoperative view of a rat carotid artery end-to-end anastomosis produced with an 810 nm diode laser and indocyanine green-protein solder. The band of solder acts as a "biological band-aid" to hold the vessel ends together without charring or significant thermal injury to the vessel. See insert for color representation.

Fig. 6. When the pulse is shorter than the thermal relaxation time of the tissue and the interval between pulses is long, relative spatial confinement of heat from that pulse occurs. If the pulse is longer than the thermal relaxation time, or if the tissue experiences a quasi-CW train of pulses, then local thermal build-up occurs, resulting in a larger zone of thermal injury. See insert for color representation.

Fig. 10. Solder increases lasered bond strength by increasing the percentage of edge to edge surface contact as well as greatly increasing the overall area involved in the bond (sleeve effect). See insert for color representation.

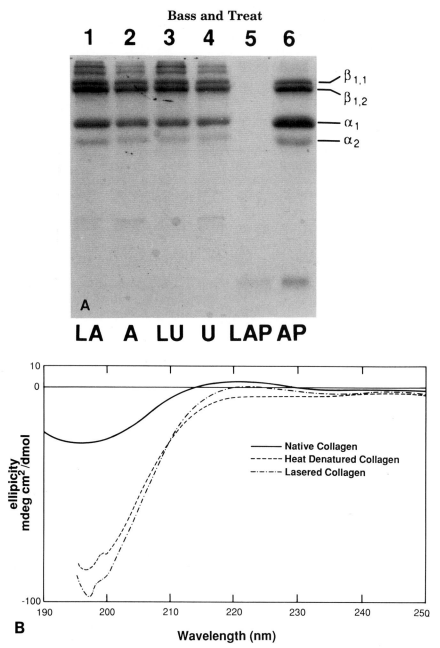

Fig. 5. (**A**) SDS PAGE of lasered (L) and nonlasered rat tail tendon. Lane 1: lasered acetic acid (a) extraction. Lane 2: nonlasered, acetic acid extraction. Lane 3: lasered, urea (U) extraction. Lane 4: nonlasered, urea extraction. Lane 5: lasered, acetic acid extraction, pepsin (P) incubation. Lane 6: nonlasered acetic acid extraction, pepsin incubation. No difference is seen between lasered and nonlasered specimens on urea extraction. Alpha and beta bands are markedly reduced after pepsin incubation in lasered specimens. This suggests that collagen is denatured during laser welding without renaturation on cooling and without formation of novel covalent bonds. From Bass LS, Moazami N, Pocsidio J, Oz MC, LoGerfo P, Treat MR. Changes in type I collagen following laser welding. Lasers Surg Med 1992;12:500–505. (**B**) Ellipticity (mdeg cm²/dmol) of collagen purified from rat tail tendon. Helical structure is demonstrated in native collagen by the area under the curve peaking at 222 nm. Heat-denatured collagen is devoid of helicity. Laser-treated collagen possesses minimal helical structure. See (a) for reference.

vent local thermal buildup. Ideally, in welding as in ablation, the laser pulse width (exposure time) must be shorter than the thermal relaxation time for the input energy to provide maximum effect at the target site with minimal collateral thermal damage due to diffusion of that energy into areas not involved in the weld (see Fig. 6) [45]. However, pulse interval (time between exposures) must be longer than the thermal relaxation time to allow heat to fully dissipate before any more is added, preventing local thermal buildup to levels that would overheat the tissues involved in the weld. The concepts of wavelength-dependent tissue absorption, optical penetration depth, and thermal relaxation time allow the rational selection of laser wavelengths and exposure parameters. Parameters can be selected to provide maximum weld strength with minimal tissue injury. This is an extension of the concept of *selective photothermolysis* enunciated by Anderson and Parrish [46]. Although this concept was presented for tissue ablation, it is equally applicable to the spatial and temporal confinement of the energy required for optimum tissue welding. These principles are useful to obtain a rough idea of the parameters needed as they do not account for scattering, refraction, and blood flow variations, to name just a few additional effects [47].

Actual application of these principles is complicated by the fact that absorption changes during welding as tissue temperature increases [48] and protein is denatured. Thermal diffusion also changes due to changes in circulation and tissue conductivity during welding. Thus simple baseline values of tissue properties may not reliably predict the parameters for optimum outcome. A real-time method of clearly recognizing the required endpoint would be very useful. This method would be based on an understanding of the mechanism of tissue welding and of the physical and optical changes that occur in the tissue during this process. Mathematical models of the welding process can be a useful guide to parameter selection, but given the complex and variable nature of the details of the clinical welding process, we feel that empirical trials of laser parameters must be the ultimate measure of success. This must be done for each wavelength, tissue type, and thickness to be treated.

Insights into the mechanism can help select preferred laser parameters. Both empirical studies and theoretical considerations suggest that laser welding can be produced with almost any laser wavelength that produces a photothermal effect and tissue heating. However, the penetration of the wavelength should approximately match tissue thickness to provide even heating. Controlled heating will be greatly facilitated by pulsing the laser light. The preferred pulse widths and intervals for this are just now being

investigated. The ability to vary pulse width is a significant issue in selecting a laser for welding. The preferred power densities and spot sizes vary with the clinical application selected. Proper control of tissue apposition and laser energy delivery is currently controlled by the surgeon using hand-held laser energy delivery to visually determined endpoints. Various adjunctive techniques such as tissue solders, chromophores to enhance photoabsorption, tissue feedback control systems, and mechanical apposition devices are likely to be useful ensure that the greatest speed and strength are realized. Some of these advances are reviewed in the following section.

IMPROVING LASER TISSUE WELDING

Visually controlled native tissue welding is a finicky process in large part because we cannot always a priori specify the laser parameters needed for an optimum weld, nor can we recognize empirically when that weld has been achieved. Energy levels and exposure times that may work very well with certain tissues may not be the best for other situations. The parameter window for optimum native tissue welding is apparently very small [38]. Furthermore, clinically used end-point is usually a color or surface texture change in the welded tissues; these grossly visible changes (see Fig. 3c) are probably well past the ideal endpoint. Once the tissue has been heated and denatured, the process cannot be reversed. If the tissues are "overcooked" producing a suboptimal weld, revision can be accomplished only by debriding the overcooked tissue to expose fresh tissues edges. In a clinical setting, this is not always possible and is always undesirable.

Laser Soldering

Compared to native tissue welding, laser soldering using biological glues based on proteins and other compounds can provide greater bond strength, lesser collateral damage, and a bigger parameter window for achieving a successful bond. Laser soldering is a bonding technique in which a proteinaceous solder material is applied to the surfaces to be joined followed by application of laser light to seal the solder to the tissue surfaces. Early studies were carried out by Krueger [49], who used argon laser coagulation of blood to assist in small vessel anastomosis, by Poppas [50], who used egg white albumin and a CO_2 laser in a rat urethroplasty model, and by Wang [51,52],

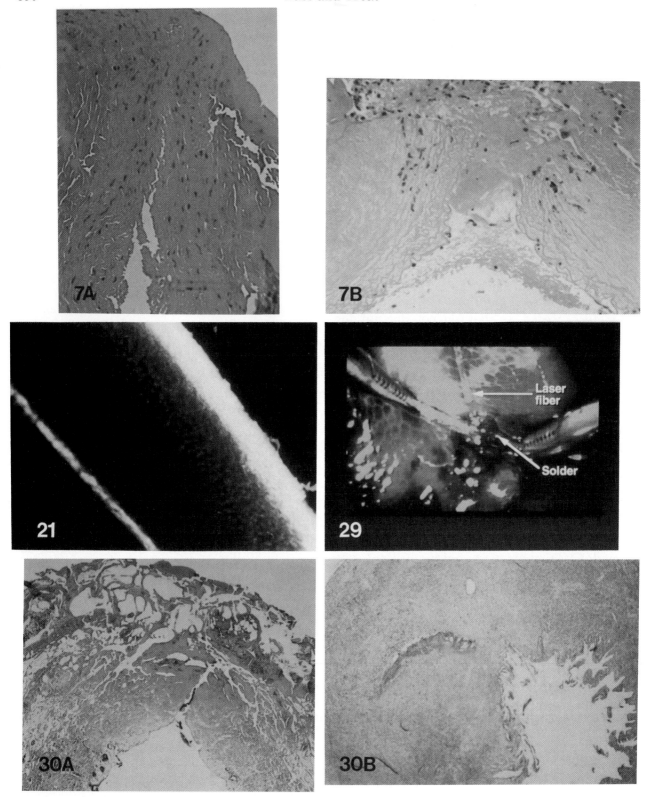

Figs. 7, 21, 29 and 30.

who used blood and also human cryoprecipitate and a CO_2 laser in rat femoral microarterial anastomosis. These studies showed that soldering produced reliable tissue welds with increased strength [49,52] and decreased rate of stricture [50] and of aneurysms [52]. Other studies compared suture closure, fibrin (non-lasered) glue repairs, and laser soldering [53,54]. These studies demonstrated increased weld strength coupled with decreased thermal injury. Coaptation or apposition demands were also greatly reduced (see Figs. 3, 7).

Dye-enhanced Laser Soldering

A newer soldering technique incorporated the added principle of photoenhancement as described in conjunction with Oz [55,56]. An absorbing chromophore is added to the solder to focus light absorption in the solder and not in nontarget tissue. This enhanced absorption in the solder al-

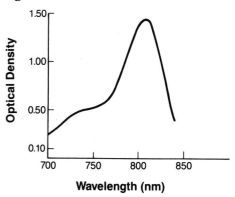

Fig. 8. The absorption curve of indocyanine green dye in an aqueous albumin solution shows a peak at 805 nm. The peak absorption of this dye in a pure aqueous solution is ~770 nm. From Oz MC, Chuck RS, Johnson JP, Parangi S, Bass LS, Nowygrod R, Treat MR. Indocyanine green dye enhanced vascular welding with the near infrared diode laser. Vasc Surg 1990; 24(8):564–570. Reprinted with permission.

Fig. 7. (a) Transverse section at postop day 7 of a longitudinal rabbit aortotomy, which was welded using an argon laser without solder. Note the eosinophilic hyalinization throughout the media, which is representative of extensive thermal damage (hematoxylin, phloxine, and saffron stain, × 20). (b) Transverse section at postop day 7 of a longitudinal rabbit aortotomy which was laser-soldered using an argon laser and fluorescein isothiocyanate-protein solder. Note that the eosinophilic change indicative of thermal damage is essentially limited to the solder and that the vessel media is unaltered. Also, the solder has filled a slight gap caused by imperfect coaptation of the vessel edges (hematoxylin, phloxine, and saffron stain, × 20). See insert for color representation.

Fig. 21. Porcine femoral articular cartilage shows good penetration of the photochemical cross-linking dye following 30 minutes of exposure to a 0.98 mM concentration in 20% Cremophor EL. Courtesy of M.M. Judy. See insert for color representation.

Fig. 29. A longitudinal choledochotomy in the miniswine as viewed through the laparoscope. The cut edges are being apposed in preparation for laser soldering. Welding can be performed endoscopically with relative ease compared with suturing. See insert for color representation.

Fig. 30. Laser-soldered canine common bile duct at postoperative day 2 (a) exhibits significant thermal changes in the solder on the surface of the bile duct. There is little distortion of bile duct contour and only superficial thermal changes in the duct itself. On postoperative day 7 (b), mucosal resurfacing is complete. Solder is nearly resorbed and inflammatory response is minimal. Hematoxylin and eosin stain, × 25. From Bass LS, Libutti SK, Oz MC, Rosen J, Williams MR, Nowygrod R, Treat MR. Canine choledochotomy closure with diode laser-activated fibrinogen solder. Surgery 1994; 115(3): 398–401. Reprinted with permission. See insert for color representation.

lows a lower power density to be used (see Fig. 8). Several advantages accrue, including the ability to use a smaller, lower power laser that is less expensive to purchase and run and less of an eye safety hazard. Also, collateral thermal damage is reduced.

The use of a dye-enhanced laser solder produces an additional advantage. In the effort to produce predictable clinical outcomes, laser parameters have been carefully studied and tightly controlled. Variation in tissue absorption and thermal properties can only partially be accounted for due to variation in tissue hydration, fat content, pigmentation, thickness, and vascularity. Solder with a known concentration of chromophore represents a target with relatively predictable absorption and thermal diffusion characteristics. By combining careful control of laser exposure parameters and known solder absorption characteristics, the likelihood of reproducible welding is maximized.

Use of fibrinogen-based solders like cryoprecipitate in humans raised concerns over infection risks, stability, and handling properties. The need for a solder that was clinically usable led Bass and his group [57,58] to develop an albumin-based solder material made of sterile FDA approved precursors, producing improved strength and handling characteristics (Table 2; see Fig. 9).

The solder serves to increase bond strength in another important way, beyond the stabilizing and broadening of the parameter window. The surface area of a soldered repair is much greater

TABLE 2. Immediate Mean Tensile Strength: Laser Solders Compared with Laser Welding and Fibrin Glue (g/cm^2) (BLET)

Composition	Tensile strength
None (laser welding)	<100
Indocyanine green 1.0%	<100
Fibrinogen & thrombin (no laser-fibrin glue)	<100
Fibrinogen 70% & indocyanine green 0.5%	113
Albumin 25% & indocyanine green 0.5%	250
Albumin 12% & hyaluronate 0.5% & indocyanine green 0.5%	441
Albumin 25% & dextran 15% & indocyanine green 0.5%	386
Collagen 13% & hyaluronate 0.3% & indocyanine green 0.5%	531

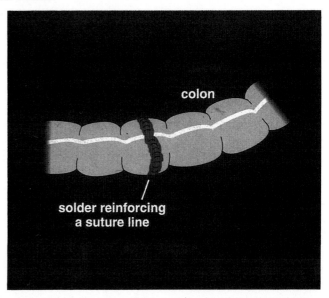

Fig. 11. Solder can be used to reinforce or seal a suture line that might otherwise leak.

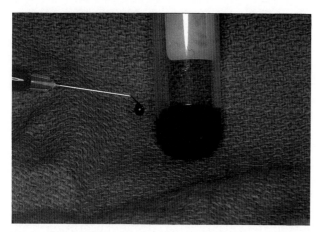

Fig. 9. The handling characteristics of this protein-based solder can be tailored to suit a variety of delivery methods including application by cannula or direct mass application. From Treat MR, Oz MC, Bass LS. New technologies and future applications of lasers: Getting the right tool for the right job. In: "Surgical Clinics of North America." Philadelphia: W.B. Saunders, 1992, pp 705–742. Reprinted with permission.

than that of a welded repair due to the physical presence of the solder not just at the edges of the structures to be joined but also along the sides (see Fig. 10). The presence of solder can increase the available bonding area by a factor of several hundred, with a corresponding increase in overall bond strength.

Solder can be used for several additional applications beyond tissue bonding. Bleeding surfaces like a raw liver bed or the interstices of a vascular graft can be sealed for hemostasis. Leaky anastomoses that surgeons are unable or unwilling to laser weld can be sealed and rendered watertight using solder as a reinforcing

layer over sutures or staples. Such laser-assisted tissue sealing (LATS) could reduce the risk of anastomotic leaks in high risk procedures (see Fig. 11). The solder can be imbued with a variety of pharmacologic agents and thus serve purposes beyond sealing. For example, the solder can be used to perform localized delivery of high doses of anti-inflammatory agents, growth factors, angiogenic agents, antibiotics, anticoagulants, and other factors. Inclusion of cellular elements instead of drugs could allow production of healing patches, substitutes for cartilage, bone or skin grafts or organoids [59,60].

IMPROVEMENTS IN LASER ENERGY DELIVERY
Solid-State Lasers

Completely solid-state diode laser systems offer several advantages compared to flashlamp-pumped crystal lasers or lasers employing gaseous or fluid lasing media. These semiconductor systems can be made much smaller and require much less power than other laser technologies (see Fig. 12). Admittedly, diode laser systems do not compare to other laser technologies in terms of peak power output and therefore are not suitable for certain high power photoablative tasks. However, their power output capabilities are steadily increasing with refinements in diode laser manufacturing and at the present time are well within the requirements for tissue welding,

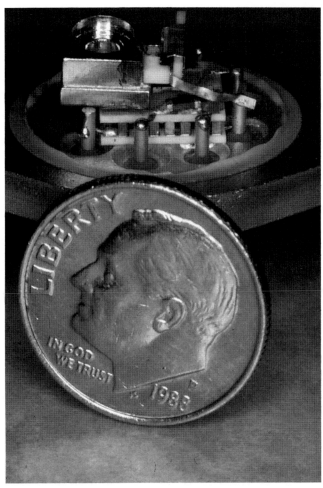

Fig. 12. The actual lasing element of a diode laser is the size of a pinhead and can be contained along with driver electronics on a single semiconductor chip.

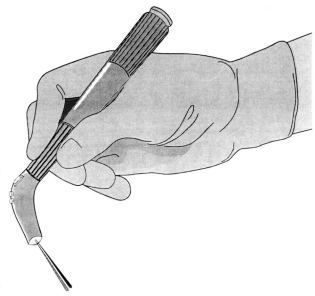

Fig. 13. The ability to laser weld or solder with low powers in conjunction with energy gathering dyes makes it possible to employ diode laser systems that are portable, hand-held, and battery powered. Courtesy of B.A. Soltz, Conversion Energy Enterprises.

sophisticated driver electronic circuitry. This allows the easy implementation of embedded microprocessor control and real-time feedback systems.

One last advantage of diode lasers has yet to materialize completely, namely, the potential for very inexpensive units to be made in large quantities. These semiconductor units could ultimately be made cheaply enough to be disposable or disposable after a certain number of uses.

Automated Dosimetry (afferent control)

The visual end-point in laser welding correlates with tissue desiccation or shrinkage. As noted above, this is probably somewhat beyond the optimal end-point. Afferent control relates to input of tissue parameters as in the Dew system (tissue type, thickness), which allows the computer prospectively to control pulse width and power density. The disadvantages of this approach are enumerated above, relating to an inability to accommodate variations in tissue. Nonetheless, in clinical applications where tissue variation is less common or pronounced, this could provide significant improvement in outcome for laser welding novices. We have been unable to demonstrate a difference in weld strength or thermal injury between afferent control and an experienced operator even in a very reproducible

particularly when energy gathering dyes are employed. It is possible with existing diode laser technology to build welding units that are completely handheld and battery powered (61) (see Fig. 13).

At present, there is a modest variety of diode laser wavelengths to chose from in the visible and infrared. However, for dye-enhanced tissue welding, there is a least one excellent match between a readily available diode wavelength (810 nm) and a biocompatable dye (indocyanine green). All of these wavelengths are readily coupled to fiberoptic delivery systems, which is a very important consideration for some applications such as endoscopic surgery.

Another important feature of these solid-state lasers is that they interface very well with laboratory model where afferent control would be expected to perform ideally.

The clinical utility of this approach is being tested in FDA-monitored clinical trials of 1,320 μm tissue welding for closure of breast biopsy skin incisions [62]. The surgeon presets the tissue type and thickness in the system, which then controls the power density and pulse width of the laser exposure. The surgeon can expose the repair site to as many pulses as seem necessary to obtain a repair. Initial results suggest that even with a fair amount of variability in surgeon technique, tissue closure can be reliably achieved. Long-term results will be needed to evaluate the time savings, complication rates, cost, and cosmetic result compared with conventional suture closure.

Laser in Charge (closed loop feedback)

In theory, feedback control of the welding process would allow attainment of the optimum end-point. Feedback control involves sensors to measure some physical characteristic in the tissue that is related to the degree of completion of the welding process. Measurement of a physical or optical parameter that indicates progression of the welding process is linked with control of laser exposure. These parameters can be measured by sensors that are applied to the weld surface or embedded in the tissue (Fig. 14) [63]. Temperature also can be measured optically [64], at least at the surface of the tissues being joined. Accuracy, response time, and sampling errors (both spatial and temporal) are factors affecting the workability of such systems. For example, because of surface cooling effects due to thermal conductivity of surrounding tissue and due to laser light scattering and reflection, there are significant problems associated with using surface temperature to indicate what is going on in the depth of the weld [65]. An embedded temperature sensor may give falsely low or high readings depending on its location in relation to the temperature distribution profile within the tissue. Also, exactly what the preferred tissue temperature is remains controversial, varying with apposition pressure, tissue type, and chemical composition, and perhaps age of the tissue. In addition, there may not be a single, well-defined temperature at which a total phase transition to denaturation of protein takes place. There is a continuum that relates to temperature and the time at that temperature. Whether this is an Arrhenius type of relationship or otherwise remains to be seen. Despite these limitations, experimental thermal-

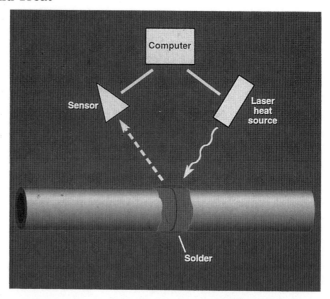

Fig. 14. Ideally, real-time optical monitoring of structural changes in the welded tissue can be used by an embedded microprocessor to regulate the laser parameters being applied to the tissue.

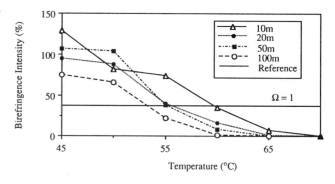

Fig. 15. Temperature dependence of birefringence intensity with exposure times indicated in minutes. From Pearce J, Thomsen S, Vijverberg H, McMurray T. Kinetics for birefringence changes in thermally coagulated rat skin collagen Proc of SPIE 1993; 1876:180–186. Reprinted with permission.

based feedback systems are being developed. Katzir and colleages [66] has tested an optical feedback system in experimental bladder welding. This utilized a CO_2 laser and semiflexible optical fibers for infrared feedback (radiometry), which sensed tissue temperature and controlled laser exposure duration [66]. Stewart and LaMuraglia [67] have done preliminary work in evaluating a 1.9 μm laser coupled to an infrared thermometer system in a closed loop.

Optical methods based on protein structural changes may be a better approach. The orderly triple helical structure of native (unheated) colla-

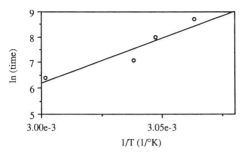

Fig. 16. Arrhenius plot for birefringence loss. From Pearce J, Thomsen S, Vijverberg H, McMurray T. Kinetics for birefringence changes in thermally coagulated rat skin collagen. Proc of SPIE 1993; 1876:180–186. Reprinted with permission.

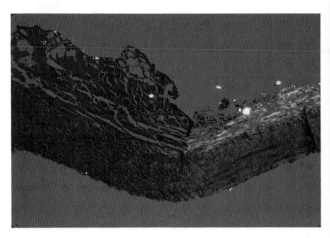

Fig. 17. Rabbit aorta weld viewed through polarizing filters shows normal birefringence in the unexposed tissue on the right half of the specimen, but loss of light on the left (laser exposed) portion. Loss of birefringence occurs when collagen is denatured by heating or otherwise. This phenomenon may form the basis of an optical means for detecting when a weld is complete. Courtesy of S. Thomsen, M.D.

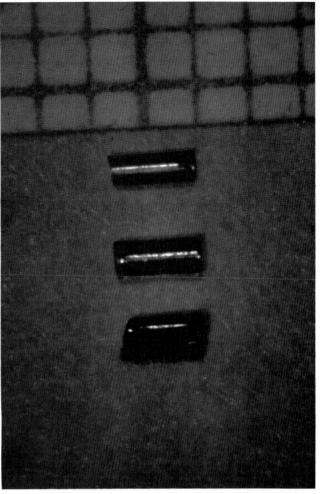

Fig. 18. Stents within the lumen of hollow structures can be used to provide a temporary framework to ensure complete coaptation of the edges during welding or soldering. Currently, there are several biocompatable materials that can be designed to dissolve over whatever time frame is desired. The design of absorbable coaptation devices is an area where much opportunity exists for innovation and possible commercial development.

gen produces birefringence. During heating, collagen denatures, losing some of its orderly structure and its birefringence (Figs. 15–17). Loss of birefringence has been suggested as an end-point for laser welding that is independent of an arbitrary temperature determination (68, 69) This can be expected to correlate with weld strength; feedback systems are being developed and tested experimentally.

Other optical sensing methods exist and have the potential to be applied to tissue welding. These methods are based on protein phase transitions associated with protein denaturation [70].

The capability of producing reliable, strong welds regardless of tissue variation is a likely prospect once appropriate feedback systems are developed and tested. When this state of techno-

logical sophistication is realized, laser welding is likely to replace sutures not only in applications in which a strict advantage is obtained but also in applications where sutures are adequate but welding is faster and easier.

BEYOND THE LASER
Delivery Systems

Accurate coaptation of tissue edges is essential for laser welding. Obviously, if the surfaces are not in contact, no weld will be formed. Even a small gap in the repair can act as a lead point for

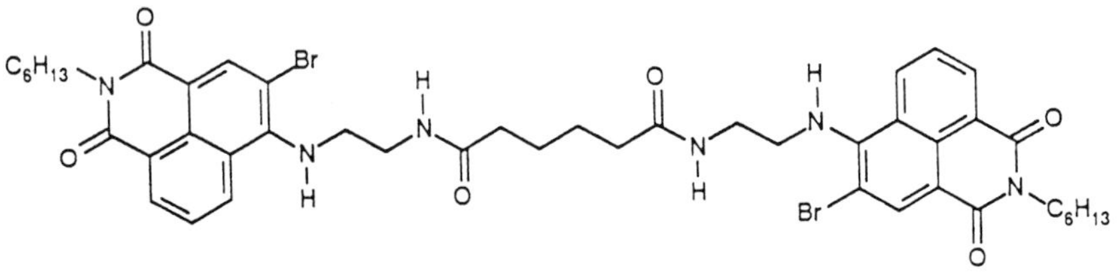

Fig. 19. Chemical structure of a hydrophobic 1,8 napthalimide dye that is used for photochemical crosslinking of tissue when activated with 420 nm light. Courtesy of M.M. Judy.

failure of the entire anastomosis. Solder, which can fill or bridge tissue gaps, can ameliorate but not completely eliminate this problem. This phenomenon has been observed ruefully by many attempting laser vascular anastomosis. Dissolvable stents have been used [24,71–73] to coapt microvessels and intestine (see Fig 18). After the repair is complete, the stent dissolves leaving the repair intact. Mechanical apposition devices have also been developed. These hold the tissue edges together while laser energy is applied. Despite the clearly demonstrated utility of such systems [74], no one has followed through with commercial development of these much needed systems.

Related to the need for precise apposition of the tissue edges is the role of pressure in enhancing weld strength. More experimental work needs to be done to balance the issues of tissue injury and weld strength in selecting the best apposition pressures for particular tissue systems.

PHOTOCHEMICAL WELDING

Efforts are underway to weld using photochemical cross-linking agents. These produce covalent cross links that should be stronger in theory than the noncovalent interactions produced by photothermal welding. Whether this goal is realizable in fact will depend on the density of cross links produced during the welding process. Photochemical welding has the additional advantage of bonding without heat and its associated tissue damage. Judy's group [75] has demonstrated the production of covalent cross links in type I collagen using brominated 1,8 naphthalimide dyes activated by 450 J/cm^2 of light at 420 nm. The materials tested to date have been lipid soluble and are delivered in a Cremophor® base. More hydrophilic compounds are being produced [76] to allow easier delivery and treatment of a wider variety of tissues. Initial studies used frozen dura for in vitro testing (see Figs. 19–21).

Questions that remain to be answered in this area include the toxicity and in vivo response to photochemical welding as well as tensile strength changes during healing. Other tissue models need to be investigated regarding strength, healing, and the ability to cross-link or transilluminate in the required tissue configuration for that type of surgery. The length of exposure required must also be evaluated for practicability during routine surgical application.

HEALING AFTER LASER WELDING

To review the effects of laser welding, one must consider two separate events. First, the tissue injury created at the time of laser welding represents the maximum injury. Second, the body's response to this injury must be studied and compared with suture repairs. Low temperature thermal injury can produce both nonlethal and lethal cellular effects [77]. Enzymes in the cell can be denatured resulting in cell death without any abnormal appearance on light microscopy. By 48–72 hours, signs of cell death will appear.

The whitening changes that are often taken as the end-point of welding represent a range of effects of thermal coagulation, including irreversible alterations of proteins, organelles, and membranes. These include hyperchromasia, cell shrinkage, membrane rupture, hyalinization, and loss of birefringence in collagen. Since elastin is not denatured until 140°C is reached, more controlled forms of laser welding should be able to prevent destruction of the elastic lamellae [77].

Wound healing in laser repairs proceeds by the same basic mechanisms used in suture repairs. There are, however, some temporal differences that have been observed, such as maximum injury shortly after the time of with an early inflammatory response and removal of necrotic tissue if any. Suture repairs have less initial injury but a sustained response to foreign material. Ini-

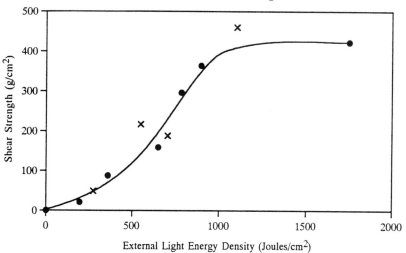

Fig. 20. Variation of shear strength with energy density of a photochemical dura mater weld. X = 457.9 nm argon ion laser light. ● = 420 nm filtered light from a xenon arc lamp. Courtesy of M.M. Judy.

tial resolution of tissue edema and inflammation takes place. Necrotic tissue is then replaced by the formation of scar.

Collagen deposition in Nd:YAG treated compared with thermally burned pig skin demonstrated increased collagen synthesis in the first 7–14 days in both groups. However, after that there was decreased synthesis in the laser group with normal collagenolytic activity but increased synthesis with normal collagenolytic activity in the burned group [78]. Epidermal cell outgrowth from CO_2 laser cut skin explants was delayed approximately 3 days compared with scalpel cut explants, with a similar rate of growth once initiated [79]. A similar 3-day delay in epithelialization was seen in CO_2 laser-ablated wounds compared with dermatome-created wounds [80].

In contrast, in actual laser-welded skin closures, a higher mean collagen concentration (by hydroxyproline assay) and mean tensile strength were seen in argon laser rat skin closures at day 5 compared with diode laser closures and suture closures [81]. By 28 days, diode laser closures were significantly stronger than either argon or suture closures (see Fig. 22). Low power Nd:YAG laser has been shown to have a stimulatory effect on collagen synthesis by fibroblasts, whereas high power Nd:YAG exposures have an inhibitory effect [82].

White et al. [83] compared healing in canine femoral and carotid arteries using argon ion, Nd:YAG, and CO_2 lasers. Suture repairs at 4–5 weeks showed granulomatous reaction around

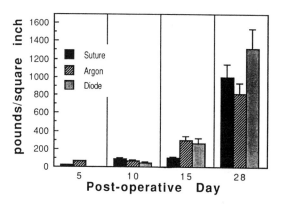

Fig. 22. Mean stress at failure (pounds/in^2) for the three groups studied. Error bars reflect ±S.E.M. Argon is significantly ($P < 0.05$) greater than suture at 5 days. Diode is significantly less than argon and suture at 10 days ($P < 0.05$). Both argon and diode are significantly superior to suture at 15 days ($P < 0.05$). At 28 days, suture is superior to argon ($P < 0.05$) but is similar to diode. From Wider TM, Libutti SK, Greenwald DP, Oz MC, Yager JS, Treat MR, Hugo NE. Skin closure with dye-enhanced laser welding and fibrinogen. Plast Reconstr Surg 1991; 88(6):1018–1025. Reprinted with permission.

the sutures with elevated collagen production and elastin disorientation. Argon laser repairs had minimal inflammatory response, near normal collagen content, but a persistent minimal gap in elastin fibers at the anastomotic site. Laser repairs show earlier resurfacing than suture repairs in blood vessels [84] and bile ducts [85].

The variation in effects on collagen synthesis in onset and rate in these studies demonstrates the impact of laser parameters and end-points on the extent of injury and the degree of biological response and emphasizes the importance of precise parameter control in producing the most desirable outcome. In the next section, we show how application of these principles can effect reliable tissue welding.

CLINICAL AREAS REVIEW

Reviewing clinical applications of laser welding is largely a discussion of potentials. However, the scope of applications is huge. Despite this, laser welding will not replace sutures across the board. There are some applications where laser welding will provide definitive advantages, some where it will be useful sometimes or as a reinforcement ("belt and suspenders"), and some where sutures are likely to remain the preferred technique. This will be influenced by the sophistication of exposure control and coaptation systems that are developed and approved, reducing requirements for operator skill and experience.

Put another way, the advantages of laser welding—reduced inflammation, faster healing, watertightness, greater ease and speed—have more impact on clinical outcome in some applications than others. Clinical attention should be focused in these key areas, such as the following four major categories: (1) microsurgery, (2) watertight applications, (3) endoscopic applications, and (4) cosmetic applications.

Delicate structures such as those treated in microsurgery can suffer failure from even small amounts of tissue injury. Any technique that produces more controlled tissue injury would be advantageous. A great deal of skill and training is required to successfully perform these types of repairs. The surgeon must keep maintaining these skills with laboratory practice or clinical cases. Thus these types of operations can be offered only by a small number of surgeons with recent experience. With welding, the technical demands are reduced along with reduced operating time. These include microvascular, nerve, vas deferens, and fallopian tube repairs as well as eye surgery.

Suture repairs are never completely watertight. The gaps between sutures and the needle holes leak in 100% of repairs. Most of the time this is subclinical, i.e., it does not produce an adverse outcome. However, in some applications the tolerance for leakage is very small. Laser welding/soldering is useful for producing a completely watertight bond or for sealing a sutured or stapled repair to render it watertight. These include

vascular applications to limit blood leakage or to seal vascular grafts, gastrointestinal and urologic applications such as esophagus, stomach, small and large intestine, bile ducts, ureters, urethra, bladder, and pulmonary structures like bronchus and lung resections.

Suturing is slow and difficult endoscopically. There are limitations to the extent of stapler miniaturization. Laser welding is readily performed endoscopically. This may extend the range of procedures that can be converted from the open to endoscopic approach.

A major limitation to the clinical application of tissue welding techniques is strength. Because of the disordered nature of collagen interactions in current welding schemes, there is a limit to peak weld strength. This can be enhanced by chemical cross-linking agents and solders to a certain extent. Most studies report strengths at time zero of 0.5 kg/cm^2 or less. Much higher weld strengths (1.5–4 kg/cm^2) can be obtained in vitro in the laboratory setting [38], but the conditions used are not suitable for living tissue. This means that whereas laser welding is useful for all the types of applications described above, it is not currently feasible for high tensile strength applications.

Let us take a look at the status of tissue welding in the individual clinical areas. We note any pertinent experimental results, any clinical trials of which we are aware, and also any likely potential applications in this specialty.

Cardiovascular Surgery

There has been extensive effort expended to perform primary vascular anastomosis in small and medium-size vessels. This has included CO_2 [86], argon [87], as well as diode [88,89] lasers. Vascular anastomosis has been effective in laboratory studies using the following models: canine femoral arteries and veins, rabbit aorta, and canine femoral arteriovenous fistulae (see Figs. 23, 24).

Clinical experimentation with CO_2 laser welding was initiated in 1985 by Okada [90,91]. His first patient was a 44-year-old woman in chronic renal failure for whom an arteriovenous (radial artery-cephalic vein) fistula was created using low power (20–40 milliwatts) CO_2 laser and a few (typically four) stay sutures. A follow-up report by Okada in 1987 stated that 35 patients had undergone CO_2 laser arteriovenous and arterio-arterial anastomosis without complications due to the laser. This series included four patients

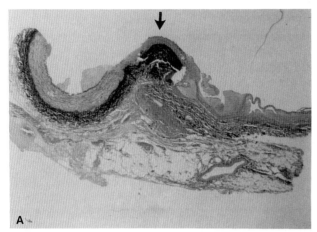

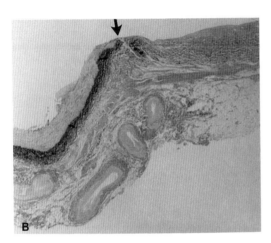

Fig. 23. Comparison of conventional arteriovenous fistula with nonabsorbable suture anastomosis (a) and argon laser welded fistula with absorbable stay sutures (b) at 24 weeks. Not the absence of thickening and inflammatory response in the laser repair compared with the suture repair. From White RA. Applications of laser technology to vascular disease. In Vieth, Hobson, Williams, and Wilson, eds. "Vascular Surgery: Principles and Practice," 2nd ed. New York: McGraw-Hill, 1993, pp 316–331. Reprinted with permission.

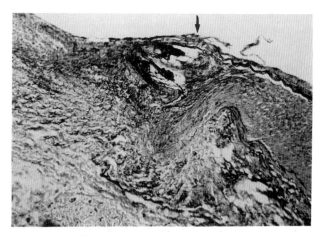

Fig. 24. Histologic section of laser-welded human arteriovenous fistula at a postoperative interval of 5 months. The arrow indicated the transition zone from artery to vein. Toluidine blue stain, × 29. From White RA. "Applications of Laser Technology to Vascular Disease," In: Vieth, Hobson, Williams, and Wilson, eds. "Vascular Surgery: Principles and Practice," 2nd ed. New York: McGraw-Hill, 1993; pp 316–331. Reprinted with permission.

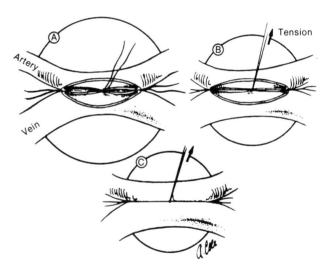

Fig. 25. Technique of laser welding of vein-artery anastomoses. Sutures are placed at the apexes of the incisions and at the middle of the posterior wall (A); tension on the suture at the middle of the posterior wall opposes the edges of the repair for welding (B); suture is placed in the middle of the anterior wall and apposes the edges for welding (C). From White RA, Kopchok G, Donayre C, White G, Lyons R, Fujitani R, Klein ST, Uitto J. Argon laser-welded arteriovenous anastomoses. J Vasc Surg 1987; 6:447–53. Reprinted with permission.

who underwent femoro-popliteal or proximal popliteal-distal popliteal bypass using a saphenous vein graft.

Clinical studies have been performed more recently using radial artery arteriovenous fistulae with argon laser [28] and laser soldering using KTP and diode lasers [92].

White and colleagues performed a clinical series of arteriovenous anastomoses using the argon laser at a power of approximately 0.5 watts [28,29]. The technique involved four-stay sutures that divided the anastomosis into quadrants (Fig. 25). A visual end-point was used to determine weld completion. Patients have been followed by physical exam and duplex scanning. After 4 1/2

years of follow-up, seven of the 10 patients continue to have functioning fistulae without evidence of hematomas, false aneurysms, or stenosis. Three patients have required delayed fistula revision, which was felt to be due to inadequate de-

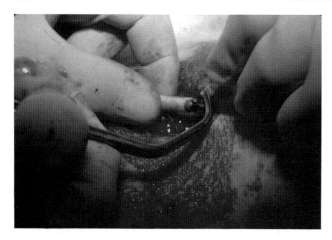

Fig. 26. An 810 nm diode laser is being used to seal an indocyanine green-protein solder to the sutured interface between polytetrafluoroethylene and artery. This will eliminate leakage from suture holes, gaps between sutures and graft interstices.

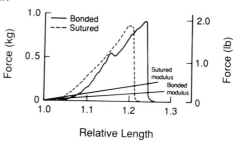

Fig. 27. A typical set of readings for laser-assisted fibrinogen bonded and sutured aorta from the stress-strain apparatus. As the tissue is strained, the rate of development of force (modulus) and the maximum force (tensile break), represented by the apex of the curve, are demonstrated graphically. From Ashton RC, Oz MC, Lontz JF, Matsumae M, Taylor R, Lemole GM, Shapira N, Lemole GM. Laser-assisted fibrinogen bonding of vascular tissue. J Surg Res 1991; 51: 324–328. Reprinted with permission.

velopment of the fistula or proximal vein thrombosis not related to the laser welding process. Histology of the fistulae (see Fig. 24) at time of revision demonstrated good healing, similar to that observed in long-term canine models.

A second clinical series is underway using combined argon laser fusion and absorbable sutures. White's group has also begun a clinical study of laser fusions of the distal anastomosis of femoral-popliteal bypasses.

Primary welding has shown a modest advantage. Operative time is somewhat reduced. The effect of intimal hyperplasia and subsequent stenosis is unclear. Aneurysm rate is increased. Strength is borderline since multiple stay sutures are required. This was especially true for larger diameter, higher pressure applications such as distal arterial bypass.

Sealing of prosthetic vascular grafts to native vessels has been attempted. This has not been possible with native tissue welding, but some success has been produced with laser soldering. This is particularly useful for reducing leakage from anastomoses and from the pores of the graft material itself (Fig. 26). In one study [93], mean blood loss was reduced from 55.7 g to 9.4 g and operative time to achieve hemostasis was reduced by 10–15 minutes, compared with thrombin-soaked Gelfoam® in canine femoral artery polytetrafluoroethylene (PTFE) bypass grafts. Oz et al. [94] also demonstrated reduced blood loss in human PTFE arteriovenous fistulae sealed with solder compared with thrombin soaked Gelfoam®.

Blood loss can produce hematoma, which can promote thrombosis, or infection and dehiscence. Excessive blood loss may also require transfusion.

Vascular anastomosis is the most arduous test of laser welding's capabilities. A vascular repair is put under tremendous dynamic stress starting immediately after surgery. With each cycle of the heart, pressure varies substantially, stretching the repair ~100 times a minute. For this, reason, laser welding for vascular anastomosis may be one of the *least* favorable early applications. If strength can be greatly improved to eliminate the need for stay sutures, there may be enough advantage to make laser welding the predominate technique for smaller vascular anastomosis. This would include distal arterial bypass in the lower extremity, arteriovenous fistula creation, coronary artery bypass grafting, and microvascular (replantation and free flap) surgery. Large vessel anastomosis is reasonably easy and reliable with suture techniques leaving less need for improvements. As discussed above, LaPlace's law predicts that the wall stress on these larger anastomoses is very much greater. The moderate strength of laser welds makes this technique less suitable for these vessels.

As opposed to primary anastomosis, sealing applications to reduce blood loss offer tremendous potential for use in vascular surgery. They can reduce operative time at a competitive cost to other hemostatic techniques. This could be useful in lower extremity arterial bypass, to seal prosthetic femoral or aortic grafts, and to seal leakage from needle holes and grafts of patches (especially prosthetic) placed during carotid endarterectomy.

Laser welds are more compliant and hence mechanically more compatible with the rest of the arterial wall than are sutured repairs (Fig. 27) [95,96]. Being more compliant, laser welds may reduce the incidence or rate of progression of myointimal hyperplasia, atherosclerosis, turbulence, and thrombotic events, but this is a theoretical conclusion and has not been experimentally or clinically verified.

Thoracic Surgery

Air leaks after lung biopsy or wedge resection can be sealed with laser energy [97] or laser solder. Bronchial stump leaks can be sealed in a similar fashion [98]. Although fibrin glue has been used, strength with laser soldering is superior. There has also been a report of sealing patches of PTFE to bronchial fistulae to seal them temporarily and promote healing [99].

The potential exists to produce hemostasis after median sternotomy without creating necrosis of the bone. Low power, dye-enhanced laser techniques would appear to be particularly appropriate for this application.

Dermatology

Skin closure could be improved in several ways by laser welding. Advantages include improved cosmesis without the need to return for suture removal. Faster healing and immediate watertightness would also result. This approach has been tested in experimental models with CO_2, argon, 1.06 μm and 1.3 μm Nd:YAG [100]. In general, better cosmetic results are obtained with all of these lasers compared to epidermal sutures. Initially the concentration of collagen was lower in the laser wounds compared to sutures, but by week 2, collagen concentrations were similar in both sutured and laser-welded groups.

Indocyanine green dye-enhanced alexandrite laser skin closure was reported by Anderson's group at the Wellman Laboratory [101]. The near infrared alexandrite laser was chosen since it provides an adequate depth of penetration into guinea pig dermis. The indocyanine green dye was found to bind to the outer 25 μm of the dermis. This work indicated that there was an optimum range of laser irradiances at which strong welds were produced with thermal damage confined to the immediate weld site (i.e., the region where the indocyanine green dye was bound).

Experimentally, dye-enhanced solder has been shown to improve the results both in terms of strength and tissue injury without producing

tattooing from the dye. Wider et al. [81] evaluated two dye-enhanced fibrinogen solder models (argon laser-fluorescein isothiocyanate and 808 nm diode laser-indocyanine green). By 15 days, both argon and diode laser solder systems showed superior collagen production compared to sutured controls.

The significance of collagen content is unclear. The amount of collagen does not correlate directly with wound strength. The organization and cross-linking of collagen fibers is responsible for the strength of the wound. For clinical application, skin closure presents a heterogenous set of challenges. Dermis thickness varies from 0.1 mm in the eyelid to >3 mm in the back. The amount of underlying vasculature is also quite variable, which has an impact on the ability of the skin to handle the thermal load of the welding process. In facial areas little tension is placed on the closure during animation, but high tension is produced over the extensor surface of joints such as the knee and elbow. In addition, there is significant variation in levels of skin pigmentation due to diverse factors such as race, location on the body, geographical location of the patient, and even seasonal variation.

A clinical trial is underway of the ProClosure® system for closure of breast biopsy incisions.

A superior cosmetic result is claimed as the principle advantage to laser skin closure. The principal disadvantage (besides strength) is increased time to completion of the closure compared with suturing, since in most situations sutures can be placed quickly with an acceptable cosmetic result. In addition, metal skin staples can even further reduce the time required for mechanical skin closure. However, for some very fine closures such as the eyelid, time may actually be somewhat reduced by use of laser techniques.

The principle risk of laser closure is dehiscence since the tensile strength is less than that of a suture closure. This risk has not been significant, although the rate is higher than suture closure. Both experimentally and in early clinical results, if precise coaptation is obtained, a fine line scar can be produced that is comparable or superior to sutured repairs (Fig. 28). However, if edges are not carefully coapted, a wider scar results. Whether the rate of abnormal scar production such as hypertrophic and keloid scarring will be increased or decreased compared to suture closure is unknown.

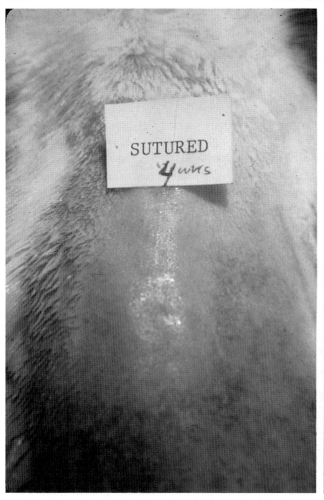 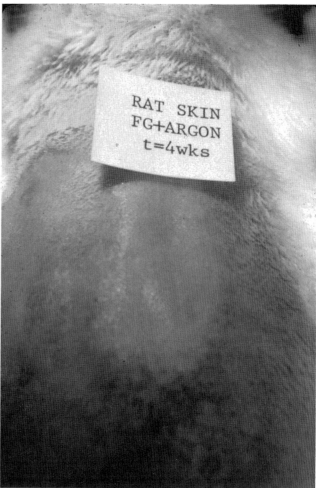

Fig. 28. Gross examination of (**a**) suture and (**b**) argon ion laser closures at 4 weeks. Note the typical cross hatched markings in the suture specimen. The argon scar is finer. From Wider TM, Libutti SK, Greenwald DP, Oz MC, Yager JS, Treat MR, Hugo NE. Skin closure with dye-enhanced laser welding and fibrinogen. Plast Reconstr Surg 1991; 88(6): 1018–1025. Reprinted with permission.

At least experimentally, the rate of healing of laser closed skin incisions is faster than that of sutured controls. It is also possible, experimentally, to incorporate exogenous growth factors into laser solder to enhance the rate and quality of skin wound healing.

Laparoscopic and Endoscopic Surgery

Endoscopic suturing is time-consuming and difficult. For example, although it is possible with current techniques to explore the common bile duct via a choledochotomy as would be done in open surgery, the technical demands of endoscopic repair of the common bile duct cannot be overstated [102]. Despite modest advances in the instrumentation and technique of laparoscopic suturing, there is general agreement over the need for technically easier methods of tissue closure.

In using laparoscopic instruments, the "fulcrum effect" is caused by the fact that the instruments must pivot about the point where they cross the abdominal wall. As the instrument is moved in or out of the abdominal cavity, the position of that fulcrum point changes relative to the shaft of the instrument. The amount of motion obtained at the tip of the instrument relative to a given displacement of the handle depends on the location of the fulcrum point along the length of the shaft of the instrument. This effect produces difficulties in suturing efficiently or in applying staples. The lack of depth perception also significantly impairs such contact techniques as suturing.

Stapling devices can be laparoscopically delivered; limitations exist on the ability to miniaturize these devices. Laser welding is a noncontact technique that can be readily performed endoscopically. Laser fibers or cannulae to apply solder are easy to deliver via even very narrow ports (Fig. 29) [103]. The principal challenge to endoscopic welding is tissue coaptation. This can be produced by traction with forceps for most applications or placement of stay sutures or tacking staples to produce approximate positioning of the structures to be welded.

Mesh repair of hernias and fascial defects could use laser welding or soldering to seal the mesh into place since fibrosis during healing provides the ultimate fixation for mesh and not the sutures. Although laser welding strength is low compared with sutures, the large cross-sectional area of the contact provides a high overall weld strength, particularly to shear forces. This could also greatly speed fixation of mesh during laparoscopic herniorrhaphy and avoid the problem of nerve entrapment by staples.

The potential of welding to solve the tissue joining problems currently faced in endoscopic surgery offers the exciting prospect of greatly expanding the number and type of procedures that can be performed through minimal access.

General (Nonendoscopic) Surgery

The principle applications in general surgery are for the watertight closure of low-tension structures like bile ducts. Unlike blood, bile has no intrinsic mechanism for clotting and sealing a leak. Also, leakage of bile can be clinically detrimental, producing infectable bile collections ("biloma") or even generalized peritonitis. These real clinical concerns often result in the use of T-tube drainage of a sutured bile duct closure and/or the use of drains placed in the vicinity of the duct. Using laser techniques, bile ducts can be sealed to achieve time zero leakage pressures, which greatly exceed those even in a completely obstructed bile duct. This would eliminate the need for T-tube or other forms of peritoneal drainage. Experimentally, it was found that canine choledochotomies could be laser soldered with an immediate leakage pressures of 264 mm Hg, which is well above maximum obstructed bile duct pressure (~40 mm Hg) (see Fig. 30) [85].

Many other gastrointestinal structures treated by the general surgeon are also subject to a real risk of leakage. Several experimental studies have demonstrated the feasibility of gastrointestinal laser welding. Representative examples of such studies using a variety of lasers are discussed below.

Mercer et al. [104] showed that in a rabbit small intestine model, the initial bursting (leakage) strength of the noncontact lasered 0.5 cm linear enterotomies was roughly comparable to that of the sutured repairs. These workers noted a tendency for the higher energies to yield (initially) stronger repairs. The highest laser energy tested produced bursting pressures equal to that of the sutured controls, but there was a significant amount of charring and desiccation of tissue adjacent to the repair. Long-term healing results were satisfactory, with ultimate bursting pressures similar to that of sutured control and with no evidence of stricture at the lasered site. The results obtained in this study at the midrange of the energy levels were similar to results obtained earlier in a CO_2 laser-rabbit intestine model by Sauer [105].

In a rat model, Dempsey et al. [106] used a CO_2 laser to weld 1.5 cm linear gastrotomies. Compared to the sutured controls, the lasered repairs were somewhat weaker on postoperative day 1 but contained more hydroxyproline. By day 11, both groups had achieved the bursting pressures of unwounded stomach.

Vlasak et al. [107], in a rabbit intestinal model, closed 1 cm longitudinal enterotomies with CO_2 and argon lasers. The immediate bursting pressure of both laser-welded groups was not statistically significantly different from that of sutured controls. However, there was a trend toward weaker closures in the laser-welded groups.

In all of the above examples of *linear enterotomies* closure, the pressures obtained by the laser-welded closures were significantly higher than pressures normally encountered in the gastrointestinal tract. The first report of a sutureless laser-welded, end-to-end anastomosis was by Sauer in 1989 [108]. In this experiment, a biocompatable intraluminal stent was employed in an ileal rabbit model in conjunction with a Nd:YAG laser.

Laser-Assisted Tissue Sealing

Complete reliance of laser techniques for closure of intestinal and other anastomoses is meeting with slow acceptance due to justifiable concerns about the high morbidity or even mortality of laser closure failure. Regulatory barriers also

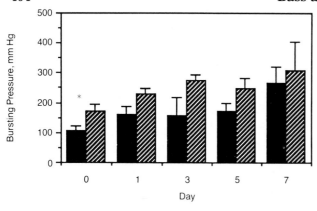

Fig. 31. Appendiceal bursting pressures from time 0–7 days following the creation of an anastomosis. The sutured (black bars) and laser-welded (hatched bars) groups; bursting pressures are significantly different immediately after creation (asterisk; $P < 0.05$). From Moazami N, Oz MC, Bass LS, Treat MR. Reinforcement of colonic anastomoses with a laser and dye-enhanced fibrinogen. Arch Surgery 1990; 125:1452–1454. Reprinted with permission.

have been a significant obstacle. An alternative and probably more acceptable initial approach is laser-activated tissue sealing, or *reinforcement* of sutured or stapled repairs with laser solder, providing the strength and security of sutures and the watertightness of solder. This "belt and suspenders" approach presents low or no additional risk and adds little to overall operative time. Using a low-powered, solid-state diode laser system, the cost of this laser reinforcement is likely to be low. It can be convincingly argued that the economic benefits of preventing even an occasional leak far outweigh the cost of routine laser reinforcement. In this scenario, laser-activated tissue sealing could be used in *high-risk anastomoses,* or emergency cases where the known dehiscence rate is significant.

Experimental work in the area of reinforcing or sealing gastrointestinal anastomoses was done by the Columbia group [109,110]. Their technique used an 810 nm diode laser and indocyanine green dye-enhanced fibrinogen to reinforce colonic anastomoses in a rabbit model. In this study, there was a statistically significant increase in bursting (leakage) pressures at time 0 in the lasered anastomoses compared to sutured controls (Fig. 31). This difference was reduced at further follow-up times. The laser-solder reinforcement technique may be of value in reducing the incidence of early postoperative leaks and associated clinical complications. A similar result was obtained in a canine tracheal esophageal anastomo-

sis model using an indocyanine green/albumin/hyaluronate solder in conjunction with the 810 nm diode laser. Both studies noted minimal foreign body reaction to the solder, which was eventually resorbed completely.

Some clinical examples of this include esophageal anastomoses, colorectal repairs below the peritoneal reflection, pancreaticojejunostomy, tracheobronchial anastomoses, and major urinary tract closures. The clinical validity of this approach is suggested by the early results obtained at Columbia with solder reinforcement of high risk, leaky anastomoses in humans [111]. In a series of 12 solder reinforced pancreaticojejunostomies, no clinical leaks occurred [112].

Gynecology

Fallopian tube repairs are possible using laser welding, but experimental results, at least with the CO_2 laser, have been mixed. A less than satisfactory outcome in terms of rate of pregnancy was reported by Fayez [113] in a rabbit model using a CO_2 laser. Other earlier reports confirmed the lack of success with the CO_2 laser in the rabbit model [114,115]. Choe et al. [116] reported a decrease in peritubular and generalized adhesions when the CO_2 laser was used to incise rabbit uterine horns for suture repair, compared to scalpel or electrocautery incision. However, they were unable to weld with the CO_2 laser in this study. Yet, Shapiro et al. [117] reported that, in a rat model, the CO_2 laser-welded tubal reanastomoses were superior to sutured controls in terms of the amount of inflammatory response.

The difficulties even in heating with the CO_2 laser, as discussed above, may well explain the cause of the failures with fallopian tubes/uterine horns, which are even thicker walled than microvessels. The use of a low-powered diode laser in conjunction with dye-enhanced protein solder has not yet been explored for tubal reanastomosis. Other technical refinements, such as careful parameter control with more favorable wavelengths, absorbable stents, and specialized coaptation devices, may also make tubal welding or soldering feasible. The situation with tubal reanastomosis, the use of dye-enhanced solder, and other technical adjuncts may result in tubal anastomoses that are superior to those obtained with conventional suture techniques.

For open tubal surgery, these advantages could result in higher fertility rates. Laparoscopic tubal procedures have been extremely tedious and time-consuming. Laser welding could allow expeditious laparoscopic reanastomosis of fallopian tubes.

Neurosurgery

Extensive studies evaluating laser welding of peripheral nerves have been performed. These have used most laser wavelengths (CO_2, argon, Nd:YAG, diode). These studies have demonstrated nerve regeneration with results in some respects superior to suture repair. For example, Fischer et al. [118] compared CO_2 laser rat sciatic nerve anastomosis to 10-0 nylon epineural sutured repairs. Although 87% of the lasered repairs remained intact at 60 days postoperatively compared to 100% of the sutured repairs, 85% of the lasered repairs had action potentials detectable across the anastomosis compared to 78% of the sutured group. In addition, morphological studies revealed that the sutured group exhibited a greater degree of disorientation of the regenerating fibers as well as perianastomotic narrowing from scarring. In a follow-up study [119], this group observed that the density of myelinated nerve fibers in segments distal to the laser-anastomosed regions was slightly higher than in the sutured group. Based on this observation, they suggested that the regenerating capacity in the laser-treated nerves would be slightly enhanced compared to the sutured nerves.

In general, the various experimental studies show that laser repair is as functionally effective as standard microsurgical suture technique even in animal models that are a more rigorous test of nerve healing such as a primate model [120]. Also, there appears to be a technical advantage to the lasered repairs in terms of speed and ease of construction of the anastomosis [121]. However, the dehiscence rate is substantially higher, ranging from 12 to as high as 60% in various studies [122]. The work of Maragh et al. [123] suggests that the dehiscence problem stems from lower initial (time 0) tensile strength of the laser repairs and may not be an issue by the end of the first postoperative week. Kim et al. [124] were able to reduce the dehiscence rate of CO_2 lasered repairs of rat sciatic nerve to zero by using the periepineural sheath as a structural adjunct while maintaining electrophysiologic and morphometric values comparable to those of sutured repairs.

Bass et al. [125] have investigated the use of lasered dye-enhanced solder for rat sciatic nerve repair. In this study the dehiscence rate was reduced to zero and nerve conduction values and axon counts were no different than in sutured repairs. Morphologic analysis did reveal a greater proportion of large diameter myelinated axons in the laser-soldered group. Menovsky et al. [126] recently reported on the use of a lasered dried-albumin solder, which substantially enhanced the strength of nerve repairs. These results were in contrast to the 80% dehiscence rate observed in nonlasered fibrin glue repairs [127].

The principle barriers to success in nerve repair are malalignment and scar formation that blocks regenerating axons. Both of these effects reduce the ability of regenerating nerve fibers to successfully find the appropriate locale on the other side of the nerve gap. Sutures produce torsion and distortion of tissue when tightened, shifting the nerve ends from proper alignment. The tissue trauma of needle passage and the foreign body response of the suture material itself all act to increase scar formation. Sutureless laser nerve repairs are associated with an apparent decrease in nerve escape and entrapment of axons [128] and promises to circumvent these difficulties.

Laser soldering has reduced the high dehiscence rate that has been a troublesome point with nonreinforced laser nerve repairs. Laser solder repair would be particularly applicable in situations where access is limited such as where nerves exit bony canals. Examples of this include avulsed stumps of the brachial plexus and division of the facial nerve where it exits the stylomastoid foramen. Further, it could allow endoscopic nerve repair and nerve grafting in the forearm and during skull base surgery.

Dura is repaired or replaced in neurosurgery. A watertight seal is desirable to prevent leakage of cerebrospinal fluid. A spinal drain or shunt is often placed to reduce CSF pressure preventing leakage. Laser welding or soldering could reduce time for repair compared with suturing and prevent leakage. It would also allow sealing of leakage in hard to reach places. Heiferman et al. [129] showed experimentally that a milliwatt CO_2 laser could be used to obtain a watertight dural closure, although the tensile strength of these repairs was low. It can be anticipated that solder closure of dura might overcome limitations in terms of tensile strength.

Ophthalmology

Conventional cataract incision closure using sutures may be subject to postoperative astigmatic refractive errors, even in the hands of a skilled operator. Sutureless closure would over-

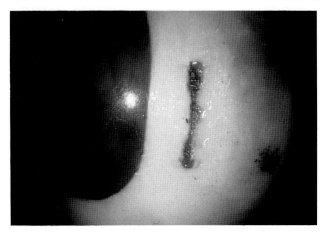

Fig. 32. Porcine eye after laser solder incision closure. Solder produces a strong, watertight bond with no shrinkage or distortion of the surface. The technique is rapid and less skill intensive than suture closure and tunneling incision techniques. Courtesy of A.M. Eaton, M.D.

come this problem. A thrombin-activated fibrin glue preparation Tisseel™ (Immuno, Vienna, Austria) has been used to close scleral tunnel incisions [130], but this pooled, human serum blood product is not available in the United States. Moreover, the strength of fibrin glue is somewhat limited. Native tissue welding can produce unwanted tissue shrinkage adjacent to the closure and can also lead to astigmatic refractive errors. Laser solder closure of incisions in sclera and cornea has been studied by Eaton et al. [131] at Columbia using mixtures of albumin/hyaluronate and albumin/hyaluronate/chondroitin sulfate. In this study, the thixotropic (low viscosity at high shear rates and high viscosity at low shear rates) handling characteristic of these solders were of value. At the high shear rates encountered in delivery of the glue via a syringe and small gauge needle, the glues flow easily and are easily directed into the scleral incision. After being deposited in the tissues, the shear forces drop to near zero and the viscosity increases correspondingly, preventing the spread of glue to unwanted areas such as the cornea or the anterior chamber (Fig. 32). Bonding of synthetic collagen epikeratoplasty lenticles to the cornea surface may also be possible with laser welding [132].

Oral Surgery

Gingiva often needs to be repaired or repositioned during procedures in the oral cavity. This material is quite friable, allowing sutures to tear out. Laser welding would allow bonding of gingiva without the point forces of sutures.

Oral mucosa is noted for rapid healing. This is sometimes facilitated in gaping lacerations by placement of several sutures to loosely approximate tissue. This could be replaced by laser welding. Because closure of oral incisions is often needed to protect exposed bone, bone grafts or prosthetic implants, a watertight closure technique would be greatly preferable to prevent exposure to saliva and reduce risk of infection.

The ability to laser bond mineral matrix to bone or tooth exists. The clinical applicability of these techniques is questionable as fusion of these materials takes place at unphysiologic temperatures (e.g., several hundred degrees). This would produce unacceptable cell death. The loose adhesions created at temperatures currently used in laser welding would provide grossly inadequate strength for the stresses found in these applications.

Orthopedics

Welding of bone is being investigated, but there are several problems associated with this application. The temperatures at which mineral matrix materials fuse are totally unphysiologic. Acceptable bone healing will not take place if the periosteum and viable bone cells are killed during welding. An innovative approach has been attempted that mimics soft tissue welding [133]. Bone ends were acid-treated prior to laser exposure to remove calcium mineral matrix from a thin layer of the joint surface. The demineralized bone ends were then approximated in compression, and welding was done with either a Nd:YAG laser or an indocyanine green dye-albumin solder in conjunction with an 810 nm diode laser. The tensile strengths of the resulting bonds in both groups were well below what would be required clinically, given the tremendous forces to which bones are subject in vivo, even in the immobilized patient. Nonetheless, the technique described is quite interesting and may point the way for further refinement of the process.

Another potential use of laser welding in orthopedics is repair of tendons. The time zero tensile strength obtained by laser welding of rat tail tendon using indocyanine-enhanced protein solder with a diode laser is in the range of 160 g/cm^2. Time zero strength in the range of 4,000 g/cm^2 has been obtained by heating bovine tendon in a water bath under compression [38]. Tendon is almost exclusively (>90%) type I collagen. Structures that contain other compounds in the extracellular matrix such as blood vessels can achieve higher weld strengths, up to 7,400 g/cm^2 in holmium: YAG welding of rabbit aorta [63]. Because of the significant stress to which tendons are subjected immediately after repair even in the immobilized patient, there appears to be only limited potential for application of existing welding techniques.

Meniscus tears could also be repaired. Existing repairs are less successful in the avascular portion of the meniscus, and partial meniscectomy is needed, which leads to subsequent degenerative effects in the joint. Preliminary experiments with fibrinogen solder repairs show low initial strength, which would be unacceptable unless protracted immobilization was used. The solder did, however, provide a biologic scaffold that is compatible with reparative cell migration and proliferation, resulting in cartilage formation with the biomechanical properties of native meniscus rather than the fibrocartilage that is produced after conventional repair [134]. The use of synthetic biopolymers seeded with chondrocytes and bonded to the native cartilage by laser may be another way of promoting regeneration of normal cartilage [60].

Otolaryngology

Possible applications of laser welding or soldering include the fixation of flaps to vocal cords or other mucosal flaps. In addition, the microvascular and nerve techniques discussed elsewhere would be applicable.

Pediatric Surgery

Pediatric surgery presents several problems such as structures that are small compared with adults. Precise tissue handling and minimal tissue injury are essential to a good outcome. A unique problem in pediatric surgery is that the repaired structures need to grow, which often limits the performance of sutured repairs. In a miniswine femoral artery end-to-end anastomosis study, Frazier et al. [17] compared the outcome of conventional interrupted sutured vascular anastomoses with CO$_2$ lasered anastomoses. Miniswine were selected because of their rapid growth and vascular properties, which are similar to those of humans. In the 13 weeks over which these miniswine were followed, the animals had increased their body weight by 350% and their normal (unoperated) arteries grew 80%. Many of the sutured anastomoses were nonpatent or strictured at the end of the study period, whereas the

lasered anastomoses were all patent and had grown an amount similar to the unoperated arteries. These workers attributed the superiority of the lasered results to a relative lack of foreign body response and fibrotic reaction.

Plastic Surgery

Plastic surgeons handle many body tissues with the requirement of rapid healing with minimal scarring. Often these tissues are partially devitalized, and it is critical to keep the surgical tissue injury to an absolute minimum. Plastic surgical techniques are of interest to all surgeons, since these technically refined and sophisticated approaches often have application in many other specialties.

Cosmetic Surgery

Cosmetic closure of skin incisions is obviously of great concern. The uses of a laser skin welding system to obtain improved cosmesis is discussed under Dermatology.

Microvascular Anastomosis

Microvascular anastomosis is used for replantation and free tissue transfer and has far-ranging applications in many other specialties. Conventional microsurgical suture techniques are certainly reliable and of time-tested value. However, as noted above, there are certain drawbacks to sutures that laser anastomotic techniques may be able to address.

Laser microvascular anastomosis offers moderately reduced operative time [14,17,135–137], reduced skill requirements, faster healing [84], ability to grow [17], and possibly reduced intimal hyperplasia [18]. These advantages must be contrasted with the cost of laser purchase, maintenance and training, the need for as many as three or four sutures (a conventional suture anastomosis has 9 or 10), and increased aneurysm rate [14,15,84,135–137]. This technique has been feasible in experimental animals using many lasers (see Table 3) [14–17,49,84,135–141].

Laser microvascular anastomosis may be done by a variety of related techniques that are designed to produce accurate coaptation of the vessel edges involved in the weld. A simple arteriotomy may be repaired by using two forceps or two stay sutures at the ends of the arteriotomy. Traction on the forceps or sutures will bring the vessel edges into apposition for laser exposure. An end-to-end laser microvascular anastomosis relies on a stay suture triangulation technique similar

TABLE 3. Selected Microvascular Anastomosis Studies

Author	#	Pow den	Time	Patency	F/U	Aneurysms	Stay sutures	Burst press	Notes
Arteries		W/cm 2	min	%	Week s	%		mm Hg	
CO_2			L/S	L/S		L/S		L/S	
Serure 14	32	396	5/15	100/100	9	6/0	3	—	
Frazier 17	9	?	20/30*	100/40	13	0/0	3	—	miniswine suture grew 15%, laser 81%
Quigley 138	32	396	—	—	3	—	3	606/691 ns	
Neblett 135	212	453	16/27*	95/96	3	7/13	3	—	
Quigley 15	125	396	—	—	12	30/0	3	—	
Vale 84	43	318	—	93/98	26	29/8	3	>300/>300	laser-variable coaptation
Fried 139	23	318	—	78/84	6	0/0	3	—	
McCarthy 136	24	75	5–10 min diff	100/100	52	22/4*	4	—	rabbit
Flemming 137	160	?849	11/12	90/97*	12	38/14*	3	—	
Ruiz-Razura 16	42	80 mw ? spot	—	100/100	5	2/0	3	500/620	
Argon Kreuger 49	9	750 mw ? spot	—	67/—	6	75	0	—	blood bonding
Diode Lewis 140	24	955	—	100/100	12	—	3	—	contact weld
Reali 141	29	30 mw	—	100/100	12	0/0	2	—	
Veins Fried 139	21	283	—	86/81	6		4	—	
Flemming 137	105	?679	12/16	83/98*	12		3	—	
Kreuger 139	8	750 mw	—	75/—	6		0	—	blood bonding
Lewis 140	24	955	—	100/100	12	0	4	—	contact weld

to that used in conventional repairs. The stay sutures are placed on traction bringing the vessel edges into apposition. Two to four stay sutures have been used. Instead of stay sutures, intraluminal stents may be used to obtain proper coaptation. Dissolvable stents have the advantage of not requiring a counterincision for withdrawal once the anastomosis is completed [71,72]. Dissolvable stents capable of withstanding increased temperatures during welding have been used experimentally [73]. Specially designed mechanical coaptation devices may also be employed to approximate and hold the vessel edges in optimum position. An advantage of mechanical coaptation devices is that they can be designed to hold the tissues together with a predefined amount of force. As discussed above, optimum weld strength does depend on the force used to appose the tissues during the welding process.

Once vessel edge coaptation has been achieved, laser light is then applied using a hand-held laser fiber or micromanipulator mounted on the operating microscope. Shrinkage, whitening, or desiccation of the edges is used as the visual endpoint for welding (Fig. 33). Laser light is usually applied in one area at a time until the changes are observed. As discussed above, there is much work currently being done on thermal and optical feedback methods to automate the welding process and eliminate the imprecision of relying on a visual endpoint.

Soldering techniques rely on the laser energy to produce activation or fixation of the solder to the vessel edges and also to the adventitial surface of the vessel adjacent to the actual anastomosis. In this way, a sleeve type of joint is formed by the solder, which is mechanically much stronger than a simple edge to edge joint (see Figs. 3d, 10). One of the earliest reports of a solder technique used blood that was laser coagulated to form an adherent sleeve around the end-to-end anastomosis [49,13]. More recently, protein-based solders have been used [52]. Mean immediate bursting pressures of 515 mm Hg have been obtained in sutureless rat carotid end-to-end anastomoses (142), which is in the range of values found in suture repairs [16,138]. In addition to being mechanically stronger, laser soldering techniques may be more technically forgiving than nonsolder techniques since the solder may be able to bridge small gaps in coaptation that would otherwise produce a lead-point for separation of the weld and may reduce or eliminate the need for stay sutures. Solder also may be beneficial in that it can protect the underlying vessel wall from the damaging thermal affects seen with nonsolder techniques [142]. Thermal damage to the internal elastic lamella may be responsible for the rela-

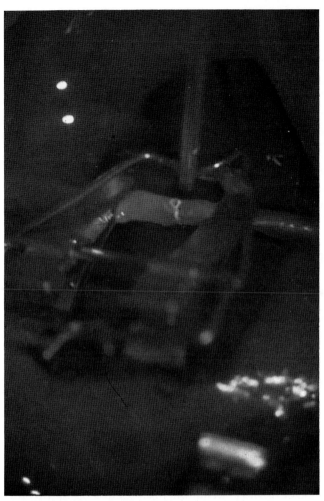

Fig. 33. After vessel edges are coapted using an approximator clamp and intraluminal stent, solder is sealed across the cut edges using laser light.

tively high occurrence of aneurysms in previous reports.

The earliest clinical report of laser microvascular anastomosis was by Jain in a remarkable pioneering work [13]. He performed an extraintracranial arterial bypass on five patients with occlusive cerebrovascular disease. Jain constructed an end-to-side anastomosis of a branch of the superficial temporal artery to a cortical branch of the middle cerebral artery, using a Nd: YAG laser operating at 18 watts with 0.1 second single applications. The lensed laser handpiece, mounted on a micromanipulator, provided a spot size of 0.3 mm. Using the micromanipulator, the handpiece was advanced from one spot application to the next. The site of the anastomosis was covered with a thin layer of blood, which was also exposed to the laser. Jain [13] reported that all of

these patients had uneventful postoperative courses with angiographic evidence at 6–9 months of patent, nonaneurysmal anastomoses. The time for these anastomoses was <5 minutes compared to ~15 minutes for the suture technique.

In 1992, Kiyoshige et al. [143] reported on the use of CO_2 laser-stay suture technique to perform 16 microvascular anastomoses in six patients. Their clinical cases included posttraumatic revascularization/reimplantation involving digital arteries and veins. Based on preclinical animal studies, the group noted that the laser repairs were characterized by greater speed and ease, equivalent patency rate, and less tissue inflammatory response compared to sutured anastomoses. There was no significant difference in the immediate or follow-up *bursting* pressures of the lasered versus the sutured vessels. This group stressed the importance of creating a tension-free condition for the repair, since they did observe that the lasered anastomoses were significantly weaker with regard to *tensile* strength than the sutured controls.

Compared to medium-size vessels such as major peripheral arteries, great reduction in wall stress due to the small diameter of microvessels is favorable to tissue welding or soldering techniques. With the right adjunctive support in terms of dissolvable intravascular stents, mechanical coaptation devices, and optimized tissue solders, laser anastomotic techniques will likely replace sutures for microvascular anastomosis.

Peripheral nerve repair and nerve grafting with laser welding is another microsurgical application that is a potential clinical application. This subject is discussed in detail under Neurosurgery.

The success of grafts and flaps relies on good adherence to the underlying wound bed. Laser welding can provide several advantages in these applications. Most of these are significantly enhanced by use of solder. Hemostasis of the wound can be assured during the welding or soldering process. Rather than fixation of skin, skin/muscle, and muscle flaps and skin grafts in place at the borders, the entire surface area is fixed in place. The improved contact that results between the graft and the irregular topography of the wound surface speeds healing, reduces seroma, hematoma, and therefore infection. This could readily function as a replacement for fibrin glue for these applications.

Bone and cartilage grafts can be fixated using welding instead of sutures or wires. This reduces the foreign material in the wound and potentially improves flap fixation. As discussed earlier in the Orthopedic section, laser-welded cartilage may be able to act as a biological scaffold for the regeneration of normal cartilage.

Trauma and Combat Care

Trauma care is predicated on early delivery of therapeutic services, which means that treatment is generally delivered in the field by medical personnel with less than average experience. Early hemostasis and closure or sealing of wounds can improve outcome. Blood and fluid loss can be reduced and bacterial exposure limited by early closure. Because of the reduced skill requirements and the potential for an almost automatic process with controlled laser parameters, field sealing of open wounds and combat treatment of more complex injuries may be possible with prefabricated laser units configured specifically for these applications. There may be application for a type of laser-activated biological dressing incorporating not only a protein solder but also other factors designed to improve healing.

Urology

Urology has many specialized needs that can be served by laser welding. Most urinary tract closures must be watertight to prevent leakage of urine and resulting infection or fistula formation. Stenosis may result from the inflammation caused by subclinical leakage through the suture line and the foreign body reaction of the sutures themselves. Suture closures have a certain inherent leakage rate that can be minimized only by meticulous technique. Unlike blood, urine has no intrinsic clotting mechanism to seal up small leaks in the suture line. Consequently, suture technique in the urinary tract tends to be relatively technically demanding and time-consuming. The suture material itself can act as a nidus for stone formation. Tissue-welding techniques can overcome these obstacles and potentially expand the number of procedures that can be performed endoscopically or laparoscopically.

Laser welding or soldering can be applied to closure of ureter, ureteroneocystostomy, urethra, and bladder (see Fig. 34). This has been investigated using several wavelengths and techniques [144–147]. Leakage rates can be reduced and leakage pressures increased using laser solders. This was first demonstrated by Poppas et al. [50] using egg white albumin. In this work, a CO_2 la-

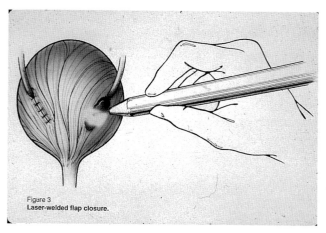

Figure 3
Laser-welded flap closure.

Fig. 34. Ureteroneocystostomy can be performed using laser solder after the placement of two stay sutures. Watertightness is improved and operating time is reduced. Endoscopic soldering is possible. From Kirsch AJ, Dean GE, Oz MC, Libutti SK, Treat MR, Nowygrod R, Hensle TW. Preliminary results of laser tissue welding in extravesical reimplantation of the ureters. J Urol 1994; 151:514–517. Reprinted with permission.

ser was used to repair a partial transection of the rat urethra. The combined use of the egg albumin solder with the CO_2 laser resulted in an overall success rate of 90%, compared to ~50–58% for the sutured controls and the nonsoldered CO_2 group. There were no urinary fistulas noted in the soldered group, although fistulas did occur in both the sutured and nonsoldered groups. These results are quite interesting, particularly in light of the 10–30% occurrence of urethrocutaneous fistula in patients undergoing urethral repair. In principle, fistulas could be sealed using laser welding. There have been no publications to our knowledge documenting this in humans or experimental animals, but it is a theoretically useful application. These studies have been extended by Kirsch et al. [148] using a diode laser and the solder of Bass et al. [57] and by Poppas using a diode laser and albumin with ICG [149].

The laser welding application most thoroughly tested in humans is vasovasostomy. There is an extensive experimental literature in the use of various lasers [150–152] in animal models, with generally good results. The CO_2, Nd:YAG, and more recently the 810 nm diode lasers have found proponents.

A number of small clinical series have recently appeared. Gilbert and Beckert [153] in Germany described their results with four patients who underwent Nd:YAG vasovasostomy over a 6-0 proline suture stent. Technically, the procedures were successful and compared very favorably to suture repair in terms of time for the repair. Their clinical results in terms of sperm counts were mixed, with two of the patients having normal counts. The largest series so far reported is by Shanberg et al. [154], who used the CO_2 laser in 50 patients demonstrating comparable fertility compared with suture repairs. Operative time was approximately halved with the laser technique. Further reports using solder techniques are expected. Very recently, Kirsch et al. at Columbia University have employed the indocyanine green-albumin-hyaluronate solder to perform urethroplasty in five patients as well as pyeloplasty with good initial results [155].

Veterinary

Laser welding may be useful for applications that have a high leakage rate. Intestinal closure in horses is prone to a much higher leakage rate than in comparable human repairs. Although this has not been experimentally demonstrated, the value of such techniques must be considered.

Summary

Laser welding provides tremendous promise for improved tissue joining in all surgical fields. It will not replace sutures in all applications, but it will solve many existing problems with tissue repair, including greater ease and speed, improved watertightness, and reduced tissue injury and inflammatory response. The potential to convert many current open procedures to the endoscopic approach is extremely exciting. Refinements in the welding technique that will greatly improve reliability are on the verge of entering clinical testing. Over the next few years, laser welding will likely become the preferred technique for an increasing number of applications. Laser welding, in combination with other surgical technology advances, will provide the precise control over tissue effects that we believe will be the hallmark of surgery in the twenty-first century.

REFERENCES

1. Seki S. Techniques for better suturing. Br J Surg 1988; 75(12):1181–1184.
2. Templeton JL, McKelvey STD: Low colorectal anastomoses: An experimental assessment of two sutured and two stapled techniques. Dis Colon Rectum 1985; 28(1):38–41.
3. Houston KA, Rotstein OD. Fibrin sealant in high-risk colonic anastomoses. Arch Surg 1988; 123:230–234.
4. Rapaport SI, Zivelin A, Minow RA, Hunter CS, Donnelly K. Clinical significance of antibodies to bovine and human thrombin and factor V after surgical use of bovine thrombin. Am J Clin Path 1992; 97:84–91.
5. Toriumi DM, Raslan WF, Friedman M, Tardy ME. Histotoxicity of cyanoacrylate tissue adhesives: A comparison study. Arch Otololaryngol Head Neck Surg 1990; 116:546–550.
6. Thompson DF, Letassy NA, Thompson GD. Fibrin glue: A review of its preparation, eficacy and adverse effects as a topical hemostat. Drug Intelligence and Clinical Pharmacy 1988; 22:946–951.
7. Hardy TG Jr., Pace WG, Maney JW, Katz AR, Kaganov AL. A biofragmentable ring for sutureless bowel anastomosis. Dis Colon Rectum 1985; 28(7):484–490.
8. Lanzetta M, Owen ER. Long-term results of 1-mm arterial anastomosis using the 3M Precise Microvascular Anastomotic System. Microsurgery 1992; 13:313–320.
9. Bass LS, Popp HW, Oz MC, Treat MR. Anastomosis of biliary tissue with high-frequency electrical diathermy. Surg Endosc 1990; 4:94–96.
10. Sigel B, Acevedo FJ. Vein anastomosis by electrocoaptive union. Surg Forum 1962; 13:291.
11. Jain KK, Gorisch W. Repair of small blood vessels with the Neodymium-YAG laser: A preliminary report. Surgery 1979; 85:684–688.
12. Strully KJ, Yahr WZ. The effect of laser on blood vessel wall: a method of non-occlusive vascular anastomosis. In: Donaghy RMP, Yasargil MG, eds. "Micro-Vascular Surgery." Stuttgart: Thieme, 1967, pp. 135–138.
13. Jain KK. Sutureless extra-intracranial anastomosis by laser. Lancet 1984; 8406:816–817.
14. Serure A, Withers EH, Thomsen S, Morris J. Comparison of carbon dioxide laser-assisted microvascular anastomosis and conventional microvascular sutured anastomosis. Surg Forum 1983; 34:634–636.
15. Quigley MR, Bailes JE, Kwaan HC, Cerullo LJ, Brown JT. Aneurysm formation after low power carbon dioxide laser-assisted vascular anastomosis. Neurosurgery 1986; 18:292–299.
16. Ruiz-Razura Amado, Lan Ma, Hita CE, Khan Z, Hwang NHC, Cohen BE. Bursting strength in CO_2 laser-assisted microvascular anastomoses. J Reconstr Microsurg 1988; 4(4):291–296.
17. Frazier OH, Painvin A, Morris JR, T Sharon, Neblett CR. Laser-assisted microvascular anastomoses: angiographic and anatomopathologic studies on growing microvascular anastomoses: Preliminary report. Surgery 1985; 97(3):585–589.
18. Quigley MR, Bailes JE, Kwaan HC, Cerullo LJ, Block S. Comparison of myointimal hyperplasia in laser-assisted and suture anastomosed arteries. J Vasc Surg 1986; 4:217–219.
19. Bayly JG, Kartha VB, Stevens WH. The absorption spectra of liquid phase H2O, HDP and D2O from 0.7 μm to 10 μm. Infrared Phys 1963; 3:211–223.
20. Curcio JA, Petty CC. The near infrared absorption spectrum of liquid water. J Opt Soc Am 1951; 41(5):302–315.
21. Pribil S, Powers SK. Carotid artery end-to-end anastomosis in the rat using the argon laser. J Neurosurg 1985; 63:771–775.
22. Godlewski S, Rouy S, Dauzat M. Ultrastructural study of arterial wall repair after argon laser micro-anastomosis. Lasers Surg Med 1987; 7:258–262.

23. Ulrich F, Durselen R, Schober R. Long-term investigations of laser-assisted microvascular anastomoses with the 1.318-μm Nd:YAG laser. Lasers Surg Med 1988; 8:104–107.

24. Niijima KH, Yonekawa Y, Handa H, Taki W. Nonsuture microvascular anastomosis using an Nd-YAG laser and a water-soluble polyvinyl alcohol splint. J Neurosurg 1987; 67:579–583.

25. Esterowitz L, Hoffman CA, Tran DC, Levin K, Storm M, Bonner RF, Smith P, Leon M. Angioplasty with a laser and fiberoptics at 2.94 μm. Proc SPIE 1986; 605:32–36.

26. White RA, Kopchok G, Donayre C, White G, Lyons R, Fujitani R, Klein ST, Uitto J. Argon laser-welded arteriovenous anastomoses. J Vasc Surg 1987; 6:447–53.

27. Cespanyi E, White RA, Lyons R, Kopchok G, Abergel RP, Dwyer RM, Klein ST. Preliminary report: A new technique of enterotomy closure using Nd:YAG laser welding compared to suture repair. J Surg Res 1987; 42(2):147–152.

28. White RA, White GH, Fujitani RM, Vlassak JW, Donayre CE, Kopchok GE, Peng SK. Initial human evaluation of argon laser-assisted vascular anastomoses. J Vasc Surg 1989; 9(4):542–547.

29. White RA, Kopchok GE. Laser vascular fusion: development, current status and future perspectives. J Clin Laser Med Surg 1990; 8:47–54.

30. Caro CG, Pedley TJ, Schroter RC, Seed WA. "The Mechanics of the Circulation." Oxford: Oxford University Press, 1978, p 207.

31. Dew DK: Review and status report on laser tissue fusion. Lasers in Medicine Proc SPIE 1986; 712.

32. Bass LS, Treat MR, Dzakonski C. Sutureless microvascular anastomosis using the THC:YAG laser: A preliminary report. Microsurgery 1989; 10:189–193.

33. Kung RTV, Stewart RB, Zelt DT, L'Italien GJ, LaMuraglia GM. Absorption characteristics at 1.9 micron: Effect on vascular welding. Lasers Surg Med 1993; 13:12–17.

34. Schober R, Ulrich T, Sander, H Durselen, Hessel S. Laser induced alteration of collagen substructure allows microsurgical tissue welding. Science 1986; 232:1421–1422.

35. White RA, Kopchok GE, Donayre CE, Peng Shi-Kaung, Fujitani RM, White GH, Uitto Jouni. Mechanism of tissue fusion in argon laser-welded vein-artery anastomoses. Lasers Surg Med 1988; 8:83–89.

36. Kopchock GE, White RA, White GH, Fujitani R, Vlasak J, Dykhovsky L, Grundfest WS. CO_2 and argon laser vascular welding: acute histologic and thermodynamic comparison. Lasers Surg Med 1988; 8:584–588.

37. Lemole GM, Anderson RR, DeCoste S. Preliminary evaluation of collagen as a component in the thermally-induced "weld": Proc SPIE 1991; 1422:116–122.

38. Solhpour S, Weldon E, Foster TE, Anderson RR. Mechanism of thermal tissue "welding" (Part I). (Abstract) Lasers Surg Med Supplement 1994; 6:56.

39. Anderson RR, Lemole GM Jr., Kaplan R, Solhpour S, Michaud N, Flotte T. Molecular mechanisms of thermal tissue welding (Part 2). (Abstract) Lasers Surg Med Supplement 1994; 6:56.

40. Murray LW, Su L, Kopchok GE, White RA. Crosslinking of extracellular matrix proteins: A preliminary report on a possible mechanism of argon laser welding. Lasers Surg Med 1989; 9:490–496.

41. Helmsworth TF, Wright CB, Scheffter SM, Schlem DJ, Keller SJ. Molecular surgery of the basement membrane by the argon laser: Lasers Surg Med 1990; 10:576–583.

42. Bass LS, Moazami N, Pocsidio J, Oz MC, LoGerfo P, Treat MR. Changes in type I following laser welding. Lasers Surg Med 1992; 12:500–505.

43. Deckelbaum LI, Isner JM, Donaldson RF, Laliberte SM, Clarke RH, Salem DN. Use of pulsed energy delivery to minimize tissue injury resulting from CO_2 laser irradiation of cardiovascular tissues. J Am Coll Cardiol 1986; 7(4):898–900.

44. Carslaw HS, Jaeger JC. "Conduction of Heat in Solids." Oxford: Oxford University Press, 1959, p 259.

45. Walsh JT Jr., Flotte TJ, Anderson RR, Deutsch TF. Pulsed CO_2 laser tissue ablation: effect of tissue type and pulse duration on thermal damage. Lasers Surg Med 1988; 8:108–118.

46. Anderson RR, Parrish JA. Selective photothermolysis: precise microsurgery by selective absorption of pulsed radiation. Science 1983; 220:524–527.

47. Welch AJ. The thermal response of laser irradiated tissue. IEEE J Quant Elect 1984; QE-20(12):1471–1480.

48. Visuri SR, Cummings JP, Walsh JT Jr. Dynamics of the absorption coefficient of water using 2.1 micron laser radiation. (Abstract) Lasers Surg Med Supplement 1993; 5:3.

49. Krueger RR, Almquist EE. Argon laser coagulation of blood for the anastomosis of small vessel. Lasers Surg Med 1985; 5:55–60.

50. Poppas DP, Schlossberg SM, Richmond IL, Gilbert DA, Devine CJ. Laser welding in urethral surgery: Improved results with a protein solder. J Urology 1988; 139:415–417.

51. Wang S, Grubbs PE, Basu S, Robertazzi RR, Thomsen S, Rose DM, Jacobowitz IJ, Cunningham JN, Jr. Effect of blood bonding on bursting strength of laser-assisted microvascular anastomoses. Microsurgery 1988; 9:10–13.

52. Grubbs PE, Wang S, Corrado M, Basu S, Rose DM, Cunningham JN, Jr. Enhancement of CO_2 laser microvascular anastomoses by fibrin glue. J Surg Res 1988; 45:112–119.

53. Cikrit DF, Dalsing MC, Weinstein Ts, Palmer K, Lalka SG, Unthank JL. CO_2-welded venous anastomosis: enhancement of weld strength with heterologous fibrin glue. Lasers Surg Med 1990; 10(6):584–590.

54. Oz MC, Bass LS, Chuck RS, Johnson JP, Parangi S, Nowygrod R, Treat MR. Urokinase modulation of weld strength in laser vascular anastomosis. Laser Surg Med 1990; 10:393–395.

55. Oz MC, Chuck RS, Johnson JP, Parangi S, Bass LS, Nowygrod R, Treat MR. Indocyanine green dye enhanced vascular welding with the near infrared diode laser. Vasc Surg 1990; 24(8):564–570.

56. Oz MC, Johnson JP, Parangi S, Chuck RS, Marboe CC, Bass LS, Nowygrod R, Treat MR. Tissue soldering using indocyanine green dye enhanced fibrinogen with the near infrared diode laser. J Vasc Surg 1990; 11(5):718–25.

57. Bass LS, Libutti SK, Eaton AM. New solders for laser welding and sealing. (Abstract) Lasers Surg Med Supplement 1993; 5:63.

58. Bass LS, Libutti SK, Kayton ML, Nowygrod R, Treat MR. Soldering is a superior alternative to fibrin sealant.

In: Current Trends In Surgical Tissue Adhesives, Technomic Publishing Co., Inc., Lancaster, PA, in press.

59. Himel HN. In: Symposium on Surgical Tissue Adhesives, Atlanta, Oct 1993.

60. Vacanti CA, Langer R, Schloo, Vacanti JP. Synthetic polymers seeded with chondrocytes provide a template for new cartilage formation. Plastic Reconstr Surg 1991; 88(5):753–759.

61. Soltz BA, Watters RD, Tihanyi PL, Hill DS. High power laser diodes and applications. Proc SPIE 1988; 1878: 203–209.

62. Dew DK, Hsu TM, Hsu LS, Halpern SJ, Michaels CE. Laser-assisted skin closure at 1.32 microns: the use of a software driven medical laser system. Proc SPIE 1991; 1422:111–115.

63. Bass LS, Moazami N, Libutti SK, Treat M, Romney CA, Dailey BD, Thomsen S. Laser vascular welding: biomechanical properties and temperature/time profiles. (Abstract) Lasers Surg Med Supplement 1993; 5:62.

64. Badeau AF, Lee CE, Morris JR, Thompson S, Malk EG, Welch AJ. Temperature response during microvascular anastomosis using milliwatt CO_2 laser. Lasers Surg Med 1986; 6:179.

65. Torres JH, Springer TA, Welch AJ, Pearce JA. Limitations of a thermal camera in measuring surface temperature of laser irradiated tissues. Lasers Surg Med 1990; 10:510–523.

66. Shenfeld O, Eyal B, Goldwasser B, Katzir A. Temperature monitoring and control of CO_2 laser tissue welding in the urinary tract using a silver halide fiber optic radiometer. Proc SPIE 1993; 1876:203–209.

67. Stewart RB, LaMuraglia GM, Kung RTV. Controlled heating of vascular tissue with a 1.9 micron laser. (Abstract) Lasers Surg Med Supplement 1994; 6:55.

68. Thomsen SL, Cheong W, Pearce JA. Changes in collagen birefringence: a quantitative histologic marker of thermal damage in skin. Proc SPIE 1991; 1422:34–42.

69. Pearce JA, Thomsen SL, Vijverberg H, McMurray TJ. Kinetics for birefringence changes in thermally coagulated rat skin collagen. Proc SPIE 1993; 1876:180–186.

70. Vijverberg H, Huang R, Jacques S, Schwartz J, Thomsen S. Optical property changes in thermally coagulated rat skin. (Abstract) Lasers Surg Med Supplement 1993; 5:63.

71. Kamiji T, Maeda M, Matsumoto K, Nishioka K. Microvascular anastomosis using polyethylene glycol 4000 and fibrin glue. Br J Surg 1989; 42:54–58.

72. Cong Z, Nongxuan T, Changfu Z, Yuanwei X, Tongde W. Experimental study on microvascular anastomosis using a dissolvable stent support in the lumen. Microsurgery 1991; 12:67–71.

73. Moskovitz MJ, Bass LS, Siebert JW. A new stent for laser microanastomosis. Proc SPIE 1994; 2128:489–494.

74. Sauer JS, McGuire KP, Hinshaw JR. Exoscope update: Automated laser welding of circumferential tissue anastomoses. Proc SPIE 1989; 1066:53–57.

75. Judy MM, Matthews JL, Boriack RL, Burlacu A, Lewis DE, Utecht RE. Heat-free photochemical tissue welding with 1,8-naphthalimide dyes using visible (420 nm) light. Proc SPIE 1993; 1876:175–179.

76. Judy MM, Fuh L, Matthews JL, Lewis DE, Utecht R. Gel electrophoretic studies of photochemical cross-linking of Type I collagen with brominated 1,8-napthalimide dyes and visible light. Proc SPIE 1994; 2128:506–509.

77. Thomsen S. Pathological analysis of photothermal and photomechanical effects of laser-tissue interactions. Photochem Photobiol 1991; 53:825–835.

78. Castro DI, Abergel RP, Johnston KJ, Adomian GE, Dwyer RM, Uitto J, Lesavoy MA. Wound healing: Biological effects of Nd: YAG laser on collagen metabolism in pig skin in comparison to thermal burn. Ann Plast Surg 1983; 11:131–140.

79. Moreno RA, Hebda PA, Zitelli JA, Abell E. Epidermal cell outgrowth from CO_2 laser- and scalpel- cut explants: Implications for wound healing. J Dermatol Surg Oncol 1984; 10:863–868.

80. Green HA, Burd E, Nishioka NS, Bruggemann, Compton CC. Middermal wound healing. Arch Dermatol 1992; 128:639–645.

81. Wider TM, Libutti SK, Greenwald DP, Oz MC, Yager JS, Treat MR, Hugo NE. Skin closure with dye-enhanced laser welding and fibrinogen. Plast Reconstr Surg 1991; 88(6):1018–1025.

82. Abergel RP, Meeker CA, Dwyer RM, Lesavoy MA, Uitto J. Nonthermal effect of Nd: YAG laser on biological functions of human skin fibroblasts in culture. Lasers Surg Med 1984; 3:279–286.

83. White RA, Abergel RP, Lyons R, Klein SR, Kopchok G, Dwyer RM, Uitto J. Biological effects of laser welding on vascular healing. Lasers Surg Med 1986; 6:137–141.

84. Vale BH, Frenkel A, Trenka-Benthin S, Matlaga BF. Microsurgical anastomosis of rat carotid arteries with the CO_2 laser. Plast Reconstr Surg 1986; 77(5):759–766.

85. Bass LS, Libutti SK, Oz MC, Rosen J, Williams MR, Nowygrod R, Treat MR. Canine choledochotomy closure with diode laser-activated fibrinogen solder. Surgery 1994; 115(3):398–401.

86. Ashworth EM, Dalsing MC, Olson JF, Hoagland WP, Baughman S, Glover JL. Large-artery welding with a milliwatt carbon dioxide laser. Arch Surg 1987; 122: 673–677.

87. White RA, Kopchok G, Donayre DC, Lyons R, White G, Klein SR, Pizzuro D, Abergel RP, Dwyer RM, Uitto J. Large vessel sealing with the argon laser. Lasers Surg Med 1987; 7:229–235.

88. Oz MC, Libutti SK, Ashton RC, Lontz JF, Lemole GM, Nowygrod R. Comparison of laser-assisted fibrinogen-bonded and sutured canine arteriovenous anastomoses. Surgery 1992; 112(1):76–83.

89. Weng G, Williamson WA, Aretz HT, Pankratov MM, Shapshay SM. Diode laser activation of indocyanine green dye-enhanced albumin for in vitro internal mammary artery anastomosis. (Abstract) Lasers Surg Med Supplement 1994; 6:57.

90. Okada M, Shimizu K, Ikuta H, Horii H, Nakamura K. An alternative method of vascular anastomosis by laser: Experimental and clinical study. Lasers Surg Med 1987; 7(3):240–248.

91. Okada M, Ikuta H, Shimizu K, Horii H, Tsuji Y, Yoshida M Nakamura K. Experimental and clinical studies on the laser application in the cardiovascular surgery: Analysis of clinical experience of 112 patients. Nippon Geka Gakkai Zasshi 1989; 90(9):1589–1593. (in Japanese)

92. Oz MC, Bass LS, Williams MR, Libutti SK, Benvenisty AI, Hardy M, Treat MR, Nowygrod R. Clinical experi-

ence with laser enhanced tissue soldering of vascular anastomoses. (Abstract) Laser Surg Med Supp 1991; 3:74.

93. Auteri JS, Libutti SK, Oz MC, Bass LS, Treat MR. Reduced blood loss in canine PTFE-femoral anastomoses using a dye enhanced laser activated protein solder. (Abstract) *Symposium on Surgical Tissue Adhesives.* Atlanta, Oct 1993.

94. Oz MC, Bass LS, Williams MR, Benvenisty A, Hardy M, Treat MR, Nowygrod R. Initial clinical experience with laser assisted solder bonding of human vascular tissue. Proc SPIE 1991; 1422:147–151.

95. Ashton RC, Oz MC, Lontz JF, Matsumae M, Taylor R, Lemole GM Jr., Shapira N, Lemole GM. Laser-assisted fibrinogen bonding of vascular tissue. J Surg Res 1991; 51:324–328.

96. Dalsing MC, Packer CS, Kueppers P, Griffith SL, Davis TE. Laser and suture anastomosis:passive compliance and active force production. Lasers Surg Med 1992; 12(2):190–198.

97. Lo Cicero J 3rd, Frederiksen JW, Hartz RS, Kaufman MW, Michaelis LL. Experimental air leaks in lung sealed by low-energy carbon dioxide laser irradiation. Chest 1985; 87(6):820–822.

98. Oz MC, Williams MR, Moscarelli R, Kaynar M, Fras CI, Libutti SK, Smith H, Setton AJ, Treat MR, Nowygrod R. Laser-assisted solder closure of bronchial stumps. Proc SPIE 1992; 1643:191–194.

99. Arai T, Tanaka S, Kikuchi M. Investigation of possible mechanism of laser welding between artificial film and bronchial tissue. Proc SPIE 1994; 2128:510–516.

100. Abergel RP, Lyons R, Dwyer R, White RA, Uitto J. Use of lasers for closure of cutaneous wounds: Experience with Nd:YAG, argon and CO_2 lasers. J Dermatol Surg Oncol 1986; 12(11):1181–1185.

101. De Coste SD, Farinelli W, Flotte T, Anderson RR. Dye-enhanced laser welding for skin closure. Lasers Surg Med 1992; 12(1):25–32.

102. Swanstrom LL. Common bile duct exploration. In: Hunter JF, Sackier JM, eds. "Minimally Invasive Surgery." New York: McGraw-Hill, 1993, pp 231–244.

103. Bass LS, OZ MC, Auteri JS, Williams MR, Rosen J, Libutti SK, Eaton AM, Lontz J, Nowygrod R, Treat MD. Laparoscopic application of laser-activated tissue glues. Proc SPIE 1991; 1421:164–168.

104. Mercer CD, Minich P, Pauli B. Sutureless bowel anastomosis using Nd:YAG laser. Lasers Surg Med 1987; 7(6):503–506.

105. Sauer JS, Rogers DW, Hinshaw JR. Bursting pressures of CO_2 laser welded rabbit ileum. (Abstract) Lasers Surg Med 1985; 5:149.

106. Dempsey DT, Showers D, Valente P, Sterling R, White JV. Tissue fusion of the rat stomach with the CO_2 laser. Surgical Forum 1987; 38:118–120.

107. Vlasak JW, Kopchok GE, White RA. Closure of rabbit ileum enterotomies with the argon and CO_2 lasers: Bursting pressures and histology. Lasers Surg Med 1988; 8:527–532.

108. Sauer JS, Hinshaw JR, McGuire KP. The first sutureless, laser-welded, end-to-end bowel anastomosis. Lasers Surg Med 1989; 9:70–73.

109. Moazami N, Oz MC, Bass LS, Treat MR. Reinforcement of colonic anastomoses with a laser and dye-enhanced fibrinogen. Arch Surgery 1990; 125:1452–1454.

110. Auteri JS, Oz MC, Sanchez JA, Bass LS, Jeevanandam V, Williams M, Smith CR, Treat MR. Preliminary results of laser assisted sealing of hand sewn canine esophageal anastomoses. Proc SPIE 1991; 1421:182–184.

111. Libutti SK, Bessler M, Chabot J, Bass LS, Oz MC, Auteri JS, Kirsch AJ, Nowygrod R, Treat MD. Reinforcement of high risk anastomoses using laser activated protein solders: A clinical study. Proc SPIE 1993; 1876: 164–167.

112. Libutti SK, Chabot J. Early results with reinforcement of pancreaticojejunostomies using dye-enhanced laser activated solder, (pers. comm.), 1994.

113. Fayez JA, Jobson VW, Lentz SS, Payne DG, Westra DF, Martin DK. Tubal microsurgery with the carbon dioxide laser. Am J Obstet Gynecol 1982; 146(4):371–373.

114. Baggish MS, Chong AP. Carbon dioxide laser microsurgery of the uterine tube. Obstet Gynecol 1981; 58:111–116.

115. Klink F, Grosspietzsch R, Klitizing L, et al. Animal in vivo studies and in vivo experiments on human tubes for end to end anastomotic operation by CO_2 laser technique. Fertil Steril 1978; 30:100–102.

116. Choe JK, Dawood MY, Bardawil WA, Andrews AH. Clinical and histologic evaluation of laser reanastomosis of the uterine tube. Fertil Steril 1984; 41(5):754–760.

117. Shapiro AG, Carter M, Ahmed A, Sielszak MW. Conventional reanastomosis versus laser welding of rat uterine horns. J Obstet Gynecol 1987; 156:1006–1009.

118. Fischer DW, Beggs JL, Kenshalo DL, Shetter AG. Comparative study of microepineural anastomoses with the use of CO_2 laser and suture techniques in rat sciatic nerve: Part 1: Surgical technique, nerve action potentials, and morphological studies. Neurosurgery 1985; 17:300–308.

119. Beggs JL, Fischer DW, Shetter AG. Comparative study of rat sciatic nerve microepineural anastomoses made with carbon dioxide laser and suture techniques: Part 2: A morphometric analysis of myelinated nerve fibers. Neurosurgery 1986; 18:266–269.

120. Bailes JE, Cozzens JW, Hudson AR, Kline DG, Ciric I, Gianaris P, Bernstein LP, Hunter D. Laser-assisted nerve repair in primates. J Neurosurg 1989; 71:266–272.

121. Huang TC, Blanks RHI, Berns MW, Crumley RL. Laser vs. suture nerve anastomosis. Otolaryngol Head Neck Surg 1992; 107:14–20.

122. Korff M, Bent SW, Havig MT, Schwaber MK, Ossoff RH, Zeaalear DL. An investigation of the potential for laser welding. Otolaryngol Head Neck Surg 1992; 106:345–350.

123. Maragh H, Hawn RS, Gould JD, Terziz JK. Is laser nerve repair comparable to microsuture coaptation? J Reconstr Microsurg 1988; 4(3):189–195.

124. Kim DH, Kline DG. Peri-epineural tissue to supplement laser welding of nerve. Neurosurgery 1990; 26:211–216.

125. Bass LS, Moazami N, Avellino A, Trosaborg W, Treat MR. Feasibility studies for laser solder neurorrhaphy. Proc SPIE 1994; 2128:472–475.

126. Menovsky T, Beek JF, van Gemert MJC. CO_2 laser nerve welding: Optimal laser parameters and the use of solders in vitro. Microsurgery 1994; 15:44–51.

127. Cruz NI, Debs N, Fiol RE. Evaluation of fibrin glue in

rat sciatic nerve repairs. Plast Reconstr Surg 1986; 78: 369–373.

128. Eppley BL, Kalenderian E, Winkelmann T, Delfino JJ. Facial nerve graft repair: Suture versus laser-assisted anastomosis. J Oral Maxillofac Surg 1989; 18(1):50–54.

129. Heiferman KS, Quigley MR, Cerullo LJ et al. Dural welding with CO_2 laser. (Abstract) Lasers Surg Med 1986; 6:207.

130. Henrick A, Gaster RN, Silverstone PJ. Organic tissue glue in the closure of cataract incisions. J Cat Ref Surg 1987; 13:551–553.

131. Eaton AM, Bass LS, Libutti SK, Schubert HD, Treat M. Sutureless cataract incision closure using laser activated tissue glues. Proc SPIE 1991; 1423:52–57.

132. Gailitis RP, Thompson KP, Ren QS, Morris J, Waring GO 3rd. Laser welding of synthetic epikeratoplasty lenticules to the cornea. Refract Corneal Surg 1990; 6(6): 430–436.

133. Mourant JR, Anderson GD, Biglio IJ, Johnson TM. Laser welding of bone: Successful in vitro experiments. Proc SPIE 1994; 2128:484–488.

134. Forman SK, Oz MC, Lontz J, Treat M, Kiernan H. Laser assisted fibrin clot bonding of human meniscus. (Abstract) Lasers Surg Med Supplement 1991; 3:51.

135. Neblett CR, Morris JR, Thomsen S. Laser-assisted microsurgical anastomosis. Neurosurgery 1986; 19:914–934.

136. McCarthy WJ, LoCicero J, Hartz RS, Yao JST. Patency of laser-assisted anastomoses in small vessels: One-year follow-up. Surgery 1987; 102(2):319–325.

137. Flemming AFS, Colles MJ, Guillianotti R, Brough MD, Bown SG. Laser assisted microvascular anastomosis of arteries and veins: Laser tissue welding. Br J Plastic Surg 1988; 41:378–388.

138. Quigley MR, Bailes JE, Kwaan HC, Cerullo LJ, Brown JT, Fitzsimmons J. Comparison of bursting strength between suture- and laser-anastomosed vessels. Microsurgery 1985; 6:229–232.

139. Fried MP. Microvascular anastomoses. Arch Otolaryngol Head Neck Surg 1987; 113:968–973.

140. Lewis JW, Uribe A. Contact diode laser microvascular anastomosis. Laryngoscope 1993; 103:850–853.

141. Reali UM, Gelli R, Giannotti V, Gori F, Pratesi R, Pini R. Experimental diode laser-assisted microvascular anastomosis. J Reconstr Microsurg 1993; 9:203–218.

142. Bass LS, Oz MC, Libutti SK, Treat MR. Alternative wavelengths for sutureless laser microvascular anasto-

mosis: A preliminary study on acute samples. J Clin Laser Med Surg 1992; 10(3):207–210.

143. Kiyoshige Y, Tsuchida H, Hamasaki M, Takayanagi M, Watanabe Y. CO_2 laser-assisted microvascular anastomosis: Biomechanical studies and clinical applications. J Reconstr Microsurg 1991; 7(3):225–230.

144. Burger RA, Gerharz CD, Bunn H, Engelmann UH, Hohenfellner R. Laser assisted urethral closure in the rat: Comparison of CO_2 and neodymium-YAG laser techniques. J Urol 1990; 144:1000–1003.

145. Mininberg DT, Sosa RE, Neidt G, Poe C, Somers WJ. Laser welding of pedicled flap skin tubes. J Urol 1990; 142:623–625.

146. Merguerian PA, Seremetis G, Becher MW. Hypospadias repair using laser welding of ventral skin flap in rabbits: Comparison with sutured repair. J Urol 1992; 148: 667–670.

147. Merguerian PA, Rabinowitz R. Dismembered nonstented ureteroureterostomy using the carbon dioxide laser in the rabbit: Comparison with suture anastomosis. J Urol 1986; 136:229–231.

148. Kirsch AJ, Dean GE, Oz MC, Libutti SK, Treat MR, Nowygrod R, Hensle TW. Preliminary results of laser tissue welding in extravesical reimplantation of the ureters. J Urol 1994; 151:514–517.

149. Poppas DP, Rooke CT, Schlossberg SM. Optimal parameters for CO_2 laser reconstruction of urethral tissue using a protein solder. J Urol 1992; 148:220–224.

150. Lynne CM, Carter M, Morris J, Dew D, Thomsen S, Thomsen C. Laser-assisted vas anastomosis: A preliminary report. Lasers Surg Med 1983; 3:261–263.

151. Lowe BA, Poage MD. Vasovasostomy in the murine vas deferens: Comparison of the Nd:YAG laser at 1.06 microns and 1.318 microns to the CO_2 laser. Lasers Surg Med 1988; 8:377–380.

152. Alefelder J, Philipp J, Engelmann UH Senge T. Stented laser-welded vasovasostomy in the rat: Comparison of Nd:YAG and CO_2 lasers. J Reconstr Microsurg 1991; 7:317–320.

153. Gilbert PTO, Beckert R. Laser-assisted vasovasostomy. Lasers Surg Med 1989; 9:42–44.

154. Shanberg A, Tansey L, Baghdassarian R, Sawyer D, Lynn C. Laser-assisted vasectomy reversal: Experience with 32 patients. J Urol 1990; 143:528–530.

155. Kirsch AJ, Miller MI, Chang DT, Olsson CA, Hensle TW, Connor JP. Laser tissue soldering in urinary tract reconstruction. First Human Experience. J Urol, in press.

Chapter 13

Lasers in Urology

Krishna M. Bhatta, MD

Redington Fairview General Hospital, Skowhegan, Maine

INTRODUCTION

In 1968, Mulvany [1] described the use of the ruby laser in attempting to fragment urinary calculi. In 1973, attempts were made to use the carbon dioxide laser as an adjunct to partial nephrectomy [2]. The endoscopic applications of first argon and later Nd:YAG (neodimium:yttrium aluminum garnet) lasers were reported by Staehler and associates in 1973 [3]. Applications of lasers in urology have since expanded to include laser lithotripsy, laser treatment of benign prostatic hypertrophy (BPH), photodynamic therapy, and laser destruction of bladder tumors. Urological applications of laser welding and various diagnostic capabilities using autofluorescence techniques are under investigation. Laser applications for superficial lesions have also been described. During the first decade (1984–1994) in which lasers have been available for clinical use in urology, this technology has achieved an im-portant place in our urologic surgical armamentorium.

Two features relating to laser applications in urology are of note. First, because of recent improvements in endourology, nephroscopy, laparoscopy, pelviscopy, perinephroscopy, and retroperitoneopscopy, almost all the urologic organs are visually accessible. Thus all these areas become accessible via fiberoptic laser delivery. Second, water (fluid medium) is a common medium where laser tissue or laser stone interaction takes place. Water is an essential element for laser lithotripsy and for hemostatic laser cutting and coagulating procedures. Moreover, laser applications have led to improvements in instrumentation for endourology, e.g., miniscopes, and developments of competing technology, e.g., electromechanical impactor [4] and pulseguard [5].

This article reviews current laser applications in urology. Possible future uses of lasers in urology are also discussed.

TABLE 1. Description of Different Types of Laser

Laser (type)	Wavelength (nm)	Delivery	c.w./Pulsed	Max power (watts)
Solid-state lasers				
Nd:YAG	1,064	SiO_2	c.w.	100
			pulsed	10 (average)
				10^5–10^8 (peak)
Ho:YAG	2,060	SiO_2(low OH)	pulsed	20–50 (average)
				10^4 (peak)
Er:YAG	2,900	ZrF4	pulsed	1–10 (average)
				10^5 (peak)
Ruby	694.3	articulated-arm & SIo_2	pulsed	10^6 (peak) (10^9Q-Switch)
Titanium sapphire	660–1,160	SiO_2	c.w.	3 (average)
			pulsed	10^5 (peak)
Gas lasers				
CO_2	10.6 μm	Halide fiber	c.w.	100
		Hollow waveguide	ultra pulse	10^3–10^6
Ar-ion	351	SiO_2	c.w.	2
	488–514.5	SiO_2	c.w.	20
Dye lasers				
Dye	400–1,000	SiO_2	c.w.	20
			pulsed	10^7
	350–1,000		pulsed	10^3–10^8
Diode lasers				
Semiconductor	800–1,100	SiO_2	c.w.	1–100
			pulsed	

LASER TISSUE INTERACTION IN PRESENCE OF WATER

Photothermal effects are a product of laser light absorption by a certain tissue. As the laser energy is increased, removal of tissue occurs, and the point at which this starts can be termed "ablation threshold." This property is used clinically for making laser incisions or evaporating lesions. A laser power that is suitable for cutting is not that suitable for hemostasis. A lower power is generally better, which is why typically a defocused beam is used for coagulation by backing the laser fiber away from the tissue, thereby reducing the power density.

Presence of water shifts the ablation threshold to a higher laser energy. Thus a higher laser wattage is required to achieve an efficient ablation of the same tissue under water than in air. Water serves to (1) cool the surface of the tissue thereby preventing surface ablation of the tissue, (2) allow light to penetrate deeper and permit light absorption at subsurface level, making possible a larger coagulation area, and (3) cool the laser fiber, thus allowing a larger wattage to be delivered without damage to the quartz fiber. A detailed study in ablation threshold in air and water has not been reported, but from clinical and experimental re-

sults, the author and coworkers have observed that 20 watts of Nd:YAG laser power can be transmitted via a 600-μm laser fiber and be used for contact or noncontact cutting in air. The hemostasis is not complete and a defocused mode is used for coagulation. In presence of water, 60 watts of laser is used for coagulation of prostatic tissue. Only minimal evaporation occurs at this power level. A higher wattage of 80–100 watts has been used by some urologists primarily to evaporate prostate tissue. They have reported that bleeding is noticeable at 100 watts of power [6].

Effect of surface irrigation on thermal response of tissue during laser irradiation has been reported recently by Anvari et al. [7]. They primarily studied the influence of temperature and flow rate of irrigation fluid on resulting temperature distribution and coagulation depths. Nd:YAG laser was used on bovine muscle tissue. Higher temperature and deeper coagulation depths were achieved as the temperature of the irrigation fluid was increased. Cold irrigation showed prevention or delay in tissue carbonization. Beyond a critical irradiance and exposure time, use of cold irrigation did not prevent tissue charring. Flow rate changes did not affect temperature distribution and coagulation depths.

They concluded that the dominating mechanism of heat transfer during laminar irrigation is thermal diffusion [7].

TYPES OF LASERS

Table 1 lists common medical lasers that are presently or potentially available for urological application. The four basic lasers used for cutting, coagulating, and evaporating purposes in urological surgery are carbon dioxide, neodymium-yttrium aluminum garnet (Nd:YAG), Nd:YAG passed through a potassium-titenyl-phosphate (KTP) crystal, and holmium:YAG laser. The lasers used for lithotripsy are the pulsed dye, alexandrite, and Ho:YAG.

The tissue interactions produced by each laser depend on laser wavelength, output power, and whether the laser is pulsed or continuous (cw). For example, the CO_2 and Ho:YAG laser output in the far infrared is absorbed by water, whereas the visible light emitted by the KTP or argon lasers will transmit directly through water and is absorbed by hemoglobin. The near-infrared Nd:YAG laser is absorbed poorly by water, tissue proteins, and blood. Therefore, this laser produces highly tissue-penetrating radiation. In summary, the tissue reaction to the laser depends not only upon the power density of the laser and the duration of exposure but also on the water content and color of the tissue.

CO_2 Laser

The CO_2 laser, which has an invisible infrared wavelength of 10.6 μm, is usually coupled to a visible helium-neon beam for guidance and can ablate tissue or make precise incisions by vaporizing high water density tissues. Although the depth of CO_2 laser absorption is <0.1 mm, heat conduction to adjacent tissue occurs and thermal coagulation necrosis of ~0.5 mm is typical. The CO_2 beam is directed through an articulating arm by a series of mirrors and is then focused on the tissue to be vaporized. Waveguides recently have been introduced to deliver the CO_2 beam through the laparoscope, which alleviates focusing difficulties and allows the surgeon rapidly to defocus the beam for improved hemostasis [8]. Some disadvantages of the CO_2 laser include production of plume with vaporization, which may contain viral particles [9] and may cause a potential health hazard [10], poor coagulative properties for vessels of 1.0 mm, and the development of oxidized char tissue, which may impede vaporization of underlying tissues.

Argon Laser

The argon laser produces wavelengths in the blue-green portion of the spectrum, which are absorbed by pigmented molecules such as hemoglobin. Because the argon laser will pass through clear peritoneal tissues, it becomes an excellent tool to vaporize pigmented endometriotic lesions. Although the argon laser output can be transmitted through a flexible quartz fiber, an aiming beam is often necessary for accurate direction. Advantages include the versatility allowed by transmission through a flexible fiber, paucity of plume with vaporization, and excellent coagulative capabilities. Disadvantages are that the argon laser requires a water hookup for cooling and tinted filters to protect the eyes of those in the operating room.

Neodymium:Yttrium Aluminum Garnet (Nd:YAG) Laser

The Nd:YAG is a solid-state laser that utilizes a crystal seeded with neodymium ions to furnish the active medium. The beam, which is in the near-infrared portion of the light spectrum and requires a helium aiming beam for direction, also can be guided through fluid and is absorbed by soft tissues to a depth of 3–5 mm. It has good hemostatic capabilities, although perhaps not as effective as the argon laser. The use of the sapphire tip, introduced by Daikuzono and Joffe [11], not only limits the laser backscatter but enhances the laser's cutting properties through a touch technique. However, caution should be used when using the sapphire tip because of its extremely high temperatures. A potential disadvantage of the Nd:YAG laser is its relatively high degree of penetration depth (up to 5 mm).

Potassium-Titanyl Phosphate (KTP) Crystal Laser

The KTP crystal laser is generated by passing a rapidly pulsed Nd:YAG beam through a crystal, which doubles the frequency and halves the wavelength to 532 nm. This beam, like the Nd:YAG and the argon lasers, can be passed through the laparoscope and hysteroscope. Unlike the Nd:YAG, however, the KTP laser has a bright green, clearly visible beam. This beam has coagulative properties similar or identical to the argon laser, but compared with Nd:YAG laser, there is a shallow depth of penetration (0.3–1 mm).

Semiconductor Lasers

Semiconductor lasers are smaller, potentially cheaper, and much more efficient than traditional lasers. Diode lasers have the potential to provide a "second revolution" of laser medical uses. Fibers easily transmit diode laser radiation, which can be pulsed or continuous. There is some possibility to tune (change the wavelength) by adding aluminum or indium.

Low power diode lasers have been used for dye-enhanced tissue welding using indocyanine green dye [12]. Diode lasers have had limited clinical applications in urology until recently when a 25 watt diode laser operating at 805 nm (Diomed, Cambridge, UK) was introduced. Because of the low power limit of 25 watts, this laser was practical only for contact evaporation of prostate tissue and that also has been slow [13].

Diode lasers can be better understood by comparison to a light emitting diode. A current is passed via an appropriate semiconductor and spontaneous light is emitted, which is called LED (light emitting diode). A laser light is produced by using the same principles but adding reflecting mirrors to form a resonator where a stimulated light can reflect back and forth, allowing only a certain wavelength to be emitted. The wavelength is determined by the active compound used. The 805 nm wavelength is obtained by using AlGaAs, whereas 1,000 nm is obtained by using InGaAs as the active compound.

A new 50 watt 1000 nm Diode laser, Photofome (Cynosure Inc., Bedford, MA), has recently been introduced. A spectroscopic analysis was performed with photofome and compared to the standard 1,064 nm Nd:YAG wavelength on a piece of chicken breast and bovine liver tissue [14]. The ratio of absorption coefficient at 1,000 nm and 1,064 was found to be 1.05. This means that the absorption by the two tissues described were fractionally higher for the diode laser than the Nd:YAG. Laser tissue interaction were also examined by using beef liver, beef kidney, chicken breast, and calf bladder. These were similar to that of Nd:YAG effects.

Dye Lasers

The active medium is an organic liquid dye, which has to be optically excited by another light source (e.g., another laser or flash lamp). Liquid dyes are brightly colored and have complex sets of electronic and vibrational energy levels, and the wavelength emitted depends on the type of dye used. Their main advantage is that their emission covers a whole range of wavelengths in the visible part of the spectrum, between 0.4 and 0.7 μm, and they can be tuned, i.e., the emission wavelength can be changed. Pulsed dye lasers are currently used for laser lithotripsy of urinary calculi in urology, for vascular lesion treatment in dermatology, and potentially for the ablation of arterial thrombus in cardiology. They can also operate in the continuous mode.

The dye in these lasers must be changed at regular intervals, and the use of dyes typically makes these lasers difficult and expensive to maintain when compared to solid-state lasers.

Ruby Laser

Synthetic ruby was the first material to be used for a laser. It was made by doping aluminum oxide with 0.01–0.5% chromium. Normally, ruby rods are 3–25 mm in diameter, and up to ~20 cm long. The laser produces red pulses at 694.3 nm wavelength. Because its laser properties degrade rapidly with increasing temperature, it must be operated at low repetition rates (typically no more than a few pulses per second) to prevent heat buildup. This limits its use to pulsed operations at low repetition rates. It can be "Q-switched" to produce short pulses (a few billionths of a second), packing energies of a few joules. Ruby lasers are less efficient than lasers commonly used today, and this inefficiency therefore limits current use. However, Q-switched ruby lasers have recently been authorized for removal of tattoos and pigmented lesions from skin with little or no scarring. Nearly ideal selective absorption by melanin at 694 nm allows highly selective treatment for pigmented skin lesions.

Titanium-Sapphire Laser

A potentially valuable new system with no present medical applications, the titanium-doped sapphire laser has two major advantages: wide tunability and good material characteristics. It produces light at wavelengths ranging from a visible red wavelength of 660 nm to the near-infrared wavelength of 1,160 nm. In addition, it can operate in pulses or continuous mode waves.

Erbium Yttrium Aluminum Garnet (Er:YAG) Laser

Erbium, a rare earth element, can be used to create laser light at a wavelength of 2.94 μm, which is the strongest peak of the absorption curve of water. This limits its depth of penetration to 1 μm, and therefore thermal damage is minimal. This in turn limits its coagulative property. This laser normally operates in the pulsed mode with pulses of ~200 ms. Er:YAG laser radiation is usually transmitted using reflecting mirrors, but it can be transmitted using reflecting mirrors, but it can be transmitted via low-OH silica fibers. In a study examining Er:YAG laser cutting effect upon rabbit ovaries, explosive effects, bleeding, and poor coagulation were observed [15]. Er:YAG lasers may be developed in ophthalmology for corneal surgery, due to its minimal thermal damage property. Unlike most other lasers, Er:YAG can clearly cut bone. Although it produces minimal thermal damage, it is not a good general cutting tool due to its poor coagulative properties. It therefore has not generally been proposed for urologic applications.

Holmium Yttrium Aluminum Garnet (Ho:YAG) Laser

Holmium is a rare-earth element, which when doped in YAG can emit laser radiation at a wavelength of $2.1 \mu m$ with normal pulse duration of 250 ms. The absorption depth in water is ~400 m, and therefore thermal tissue damage is moderate with good hemostasis when used in a pulsed mode at low pulse repetition rates. The laser can be transmitted through low OH (low water content) silica fibers. Recently, this laser has obtained approval from the Food and Drug Administration for use in laparoscopic cholecystectomy.

Alexandrite Laser

The alexandrite is a vibronic solid-state laser with a composition of chromium-doped $BeA_{1}2O_{4}$ (mineral known as alexandrite). Its wavelength ranges from 380 nm to 830 nm, with the strongest laser emission between 700–830 nm. This provides the possibility of a tuning range. It can operate both in continuous and pulsed modes, and the average power can reach up to 100 watts. The laser light is absorbed well by melanin and has been used for laser lithotripsy, removal of tattoos, and for dye-enhanced welding of skin, using indocyanine green, which has a similar wavelength in comparison to the alexandrite laser. Recently this laser has been used for laser lithotripsy procedures. When a 250 ns-pulse duration was used, the laser fiber was found to fragment easily and was a limiting factor in its clinical use. A 1 ms pulse duration has been found to be much better for the laser fiber and for stone fragmentation as well. However, pale stones are difficult to fragment with this laser [16].

LASER LITHOTRIPSY

As already noted, laser energy was first used to fragment stones by Mulvaney in 1968 [1]. Using a ruby laser, he was able to ablate the calculi, but this method generated excessive heat and hence was not suitable for clinical use. However, his work resulted in specific contributions: the first was the observation that surrounding the calculus with fluid, confining the laser energy, improved laser induced fragmentation, and the second was that the level of laser light energy absorption of the stone was determined by the color of the stone and the selective absorption by the stone of the laser light wavelength. Further investigations were carried out by Anderholm [17]. He addressed the issue of how to create a shock wave strong enough to break the stone without tissue-damaging heat production. He demonstrated that by confining the laser-induced plasma between a transparent solid and the target, the stress wave could be increased significantly. Anderholm was able to create 34 kilobar of pressure by this technique. By comparison, the pressure at the secondary focus of ESWL is ~1 kilobar. In 1974, Yang [18] further refined Anderholm's technique and described a simple method for generating 1–20 kilobar pressure using a 20 ns pulsed Q-switched ruby laser.

In 1983, Watson [19] investigated the Q-switched Nd:YAG laser, and although the Nd:YAG laser at 1,064 nm wavelength and an energy of 1 joule per 15 ns pulse duration could fragment calculi, this could not be passed down a quartz fiber without causing disintegration and destruction of the fiber. Since Watson's initial experiments, Thomas et al. [20], using an improved laser focusing technique, has successfully used the ns pulsed Nd:YAG laser to clinically fragment urinary calculi. The Nd:YAG laser is used at a 10 ns pulse duration, and since it produces a very high power density that destroys smaller fibers, a large diameter (600 μm) quartz fiber is required to transmit the laser light. The optomechanical coupler investigated was a metal bar; the Nd:YAG laser was directed at a .5 mm bar; the metal on the bar vaporized, creating a plasma and subsequent shock wave. Thus fragmentation of calculi by the 1,064 nm Nd:YAG no longer depended on the absorption of laser light by the stone as the shock wave was being formed before, not at, the stone. The diameter of the optomechanical coupler device is 5.7F, and it needs to be placed visually and be in direct contact with the stone. However, the disadvantage of this device is that it requires a large working channel in the uretero-scope similar to that of an ultrasonic probe. As a result of these drawbacks, this clever innovation has been abandoned by its proponents in favor of the pulsed dye laser, which, because of direct absorption by the stone, has more effective fragmentation and may be used through miniaturized instruments.

In 1985, Watson [21] carried out laboratory investigations with pulsed dye lasers in the Wellman Laboratories of Photomedicine at the Massachusetts General Hospital. The advantages of using pulsed dye lasers is that they can be tuned to produce a specific wavelength for varying pulse duration. The wavelength 504 nm, obtained by using coumarin green dye, was found to be selectively absorbed by calculi and hemoglobin. For effective stone fragmentation, the optimum pulse duration was found to be 1 ms, the fiber diameter 200 μm, and the pulse energy 60 mJ. The laser is operated at 5–10 pulses per second (5–10 Hz.). The laser is kept in the operating room, requires a cold water inflow for cooling, and 220 volt current. The laser delivery fiber is sterilized by soaking in gluteraldehyde and is coiled in a sterile basin.

Mechanism of Action

Photoacoustic process. Rapid heating, thermal expansion and/or steam formation leads to rapid expansion and a high pressure acoustic effect. This may be associated with a laser-induced plasma, a gaseous collection of charged particles (ions and gases) (like an electric spark), and occurs in response to short pulse lasers. This process, along with photothermal phenomena, may be involved in tissue damage from the Ho:YAG laser. Tissue damage occurs as a result of shock waves or cavities of steam generated by laser absorption. This is also the mechanism behind laser lithotripsy, in which the shock waves fragment the calculi.

The discharge of laser energy on the stone produces a focus of microscopic heating and results in thermal expansion. Further heating causes vaporization of material. Rapid heating and vaporization lead to ionization of stone material and a plasma formation that is seen as a bright flash of white light distinct from the green laser light. Water is essential for confining the plasma and enhances fragmentation rates by ~10 times [22]. A cavitation bubble is created (Fig. 1a–d) and this first expands and then collapses. Shock waves are registered with both expansion and collapse of the bubble and contribute to fragmentation of the stone.

Stone Fragility

Studies with ESWL have shown that stone fragility [23] depends on stone composition, and that this distinction should be considered when managing patients with ureteral or renal stones. Predominantly calcium oxalate dihydrate (COD), struvite/apatite, and uric acid stones are relatively fragile and can be fragmented easily with either ESWL or laser. Predominantly calcium oxalate monohydrate (COM) and brushite are less fragile and harder to fragment with both ESWL and laser energy. Cystine calculi do not absorb 504 nm laser light, do not produce a plasma resultant shock wave, and hence are not fragmented with the pulsed dye laser.

Safety Considerations

It should be understood that the safety of pulsed dye laser (504 nm) is not primarily due to its wavelength, which is readily absorbed by the hemoglobin and in a continuous wave mode will cut and coagulate tissue similar to a frequency doubled KTP:YAG laser, which operates at 532 nm wavelength. The safety has to do with the pulse duration, which at 1 μs is minimal for a small amount of hemoglobin present in the tissue to absorb the small amount of total light. In presence of blood, however, this can be significant and can cause damage to the ureteral wall [24]. Safety is also related to the fact that laser is placed directly in contact with the stone away from the ureter under direct visualization. Alexandrite laser is absorbed much less by the pigment hemoglobin and is therefore safer for the tissue compared to the 504 nm laser, which is found to be useful for darker calcium oxalate stones but has difficulty fragmenting a pale struvite-apatite stone [16].

The Ho:YAG laser is a laser that is primarily used for cutting and coagulating purposes but is also able to fragment urinary calculi. Since it is used in direct contact with the stone away from the ureter, it has been reported to be safe for laser lithotripsy. The problem with Ho:YAG laser is that it drills holes in the stones rather than actually fragments them [25, 26]. Stones can be fragmented by making several drill holes or by making a drill hole and then placing an EHL probe to explode the stone into smaller pieces, especially in less fragile stones (John Denstedt, pers. comm.).

As described earlier, the pulsed dye laser (504 nm) operated at 1 μs is not absorbed by the normal ureter and hence does not cause significant direct injury. Injury due to heating is unlikely. Approximately 500 pulses (50 mJ at 10Hz.) are the average required to fragment a ureteral stone. Even if all of this energy is converted to heat, it will raise 1 ml of water by only 6.25°C. This heat can be removed effectively by an irrigation rate of only 4 mls/minute and still limit the temperature rise to <2°C. Therefore, it is apparent that the pulsed laser does not create enough heat to cause thermal injury. Initial studies showed that tissue injury was minimal and was confined to microscopic patches of inflammation and purpura limited to the lamina propria of a pig ureter [21]. Studies from Lubeck [20] have demonstrated that the laser discharge (50 mJ/pulse), in direct contact with the ureter, caused craterlike damage of the urothelium and minor hemorrhage to a depth of only 20–40 μm. Blood seemed to enhance this process probably due to enhanced laser light absorption by hemoglobin. Perforation of the ureteral wall may occur because the fiber is sharp and may be pushed through the wall. However, no adverse reports have occurred from fiber perforation.

A yellow filter is used over the eyepiece of the ureteroscope to absorb the 504 nm light. Yellow goggles may be used but are more cumbersome. When operating from the video system, watching the television screen, no protective glass is necessary. The principles of laser safety dictate that others in the operating room wear protective eye goggles and the patient's eyes also be protected during use of laser discharge.

Clinical Results

The pulsed laser (504 nm wavelength) using 1 μs pulses at 60 mJ pulse energy (high peak power) has been used clinically successfully to fragment urinary calculi [27–30]. The laser energy is transmitted through a 200–320-μm quartz fiber [29]. The success rate of laser lithotripsy alone was 77% and 84%, respectively [30]. When the laser was used in conjunction with other endourologic techniques and ESWL, 98–99% of the ureteral calculi were successfully treated without surgery. No major complications relating to laser lithotripsy have been observed. Further developments allowing application of laser energy for stone fragmentation using optical feedback signals [31] or by effectively enclosing the quartz fiber in a spring metal cap [32] have been performed in an attempt to perform blind laser lithotripsy. Although these studies were able to detect presence of stone from ureter wall

and blood clots, the technique was not successful clinically in blind lithotripsy.

Initially, the instrument used for ureteroscopic laser lithotripsy was a 9.5F rigid ureteroscope with a 5F channel. A 7.2F semirigid ureteroscope (Candela Corp., Wayland, MA) was reported [33] to be used as the instrument of first choice for laser lithotripsy in the distal ureter in males and in the entire ureter in females. This semirigid instrument was developed specifically for use with laser lithotripsy; it has two 2.1F working channels, one for the 200-μm core diameter quartz fiber and the other for irrigation. This instrument allows ~2″ of flexure without causing half-moon loss of the visual field (seen when a conventional ureteroscope is bent). It has flexible optical fibers in a metal sheath. It is 7.2F at its tip and gradually enlarges to 11F at the base of the shaft. Several miniscopes have since been developed. The fact that the instrument has flexibility and is semirigid does encourage overenthusiastic handling of the instrument. When trying to negotiate the pelvic curve of the ureter in males, it may be easily damaged. However, the advantage of the 7.2F semirigid ureteroscope is that one rarely needs to dilate the ureter to advance this instrument. Thus ureteroscopy is minimally traumatic. Flexible, steerable ureteroscopes of 8.5–10.8F are used in the upper ureter, in tortuous ureters, and for the occasional use of the laser in antegrade ureteroscopy for the selected patient who requires intrarenal laser lithotripsy. The working channel of the flexible ureteroscopes will easily accommodate the 250-μm silica-coated quartz fiber and leave considerable room for irrigation.

The results of 227 (155 males and 72 females) consecutive cases of ureteral laser lithotripsy performed at the Massachusetts General Hospital have been reported [30, 34]. Five were patients with steinstrasse who were treated successfully by laser disimpaction of the lead fragments and treatment completed using an ultrasonic probe. Of the 222 ureteral calculi treated by the pulsed dye laser, 141 (63.5%) were totally fragmented by the laser alone to spontaneously passable fragments; 30 (13.5%) were partially fragmented and basket extracted; 29 (13%) had intentional disimpaction by laser; and in four (2%) others, the impacted stone inadvertently migrated during ureteroscopy, and all these patients had ESWL; 18 (8%) of 222 had failed laser fragmentation and required other treatment.

Ureteroscopic lasertripsy of 120 cases with a success rate of 84% using laser alone has been

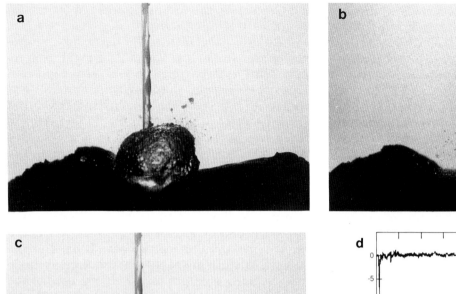

Fig. 1. Cavitation bubble after a pulsed dye laser (1 μs-pulse duration, 504 nm wavelength) discharge via a 320 micoron quartz fiber. **a:** After 450 μs. **b:** After 600 μs. **c:** After 800 μs of a laser discharge on a stone. Note the expansion and collapse of the bubble. **d:** Two shock waves measured via a hy- drophone after laser discharge on a stone, the first associated with initial expansion of the cavitation bubble, and the second with collapse of the cavitation bubble. Note the shock wave from collapse is greater than at the beginning.

reported by Copcoat et al. [35]. A further 14% were treated with ESWL following laser and only 2% required open ureterolithotomy. Blind laser- tripsy was attempted in 13 cases. The authors de- pended on the characteristic acoustic response of fragmentation to determine when they were on the stone. They passed the laser fiber in a ureteral catheter without a ureteroscope. They found it safe, but not efficient, and were successful in only 23% of cases. They concluded that the acoustic feedback is not a reliable indicator of laser dis- charge on stones and do not recommend blind la- ser lithotripsy using this method.

Dickson et al. [16] in 1993 reported clinical results of using an alexandrite laser for litho- tripsy in nine patients. The laser energy was transmitted via a 300-μm quartz fiber, and the laser was operated at 10 Hz and a power of 90 mJ. Complete fragmentation was noted in 89% of the cases and no complications were found.

Conclusions

Laser lithotripsy is safe and effective in frag- menting urinary calculi. The prices of the lasers used are prohibitive for smaller hospitals, al- though recent trends of lower prices are encour- aging. A mobile laser lithotripsy unit is available for renting in some areas. Some urologists believe that laser lithotripsy is not necessarily better than improved EHL devices and does not provide any advantages for ureteral stone management to justify the higher cost [36].

LASER APPLICATIONS FOR BENIGN PROSTATIC HYPERTROPHY

Benign prostatic hyperplasia (BPH) is one of the most common conditions in men and can lead to acute or chronic retention, which inevitably re- quires surgical intervention. The gold standard in surgical treatment for over the last 50 years has been the transurethral resection of prostate (TURP) using an electrocautery loop. This was popularized by Nesbit et al. [37] following the introduction of hot wire and a 30° telescope in 1943. TURP is not without morbidity. An 18% immediate postoperative morbidity and a 0.2% perioperative mortality rate have been reported by an AUA co-operative study [38]. Retrograde ejaculation is likely to develop in the majority of cases and ~20% of patients have persistent urinary symptoms [37, 38]. Moreover, individuals who are presently willing to accept the risks inherent with a TURP might initially opt for an alternative, albeit less effective, therapy, if available.

Laser prostatectomy with Nd:YAG laser using side firing lasers have been reported to be as effective as TURP for symptomatic BPH patients with fewer risks and reduced cost. Although these are not long-term results, the significant reduction in morbidity and a shorter learning curve associated with this procedure have attracted urologists to start doing this procedure for their patients. Blood loss and fluid absorption are negligible, and this dramatically minimizes acute patient morbidity typically associated with a standard TURP. The procedure can be performed under local anesthesia, on a patient taking coumadin, and can be performed in supine position if required [39].

Treatment options intended to replace TURP must ultimately be compared to TURP in properly designed clinical trials so that relative safety, efficacy, and cost can be acertained.

Development of Laser Prostatectomy

Several investigators have performed animal studies using Nd:YAG laser since 1986. Roth and Aretz [40] in 1991 reported the use of an ultrasound guided Nd:YAG laser system to ablate the canine prostate. They were encouraged by the degree of tissue ablation and suggested the possible role of this approach in human prostate ablation. Also in 1991, Johnson et al. [41] performed initial canine feasibility studies in the United States with the Urolase right-angle laser delivery fibers. They could create large prostatectomy defects with four quadrant irradiation of canine prostate using 60 watts of Nd:YAG laser power for 60 seconds each. Kandel et al. [42] have reported that a large prostatectomy defect could be created in canine prostate using 70–100 watts of Nd:YAG laser energy, where evaporation predominates and coagulation is sufficient.

Costello et al. [43, 44], in Australia, performed the first laser prostatectomy in a human

patient. In 1992, they reported their initial clinical experience in 17 patients treated with 60 watts of power. No adverse effects were reported in any of these studies. They showed significant improvements in symptom scores and a lesser extent of improvement in flow rates.

Lasers

Nd:YAG (1064 nm) laser, because of its deep optical penetration in tissue, has been the laser of choice for contact or free beam application in BPH treatments. A high power (40 watts), frequency-doubled YAG (KTP = 532 nm) laser has been used to supplement Nd:YAG laser application used mainly for surface ablation of the prostatic tissue. Because of its limited tissue penetration, the laser can be safely used in areas where a deep penetration would be undesirable. A 25 watt diode laser (Diomed, Cambridge, UK) has been used for contact evaporation of prostatic tissue, especially in smaller glands. The author and co-workers have used a 50-watt diode laser called Phototome (Cynosure, Bedford, MA) operating at 1,000 nm wavelength for contact and noncontact applications for BPH patients. Three clinical cases were performed using the Phototome diode laser. Two patients had retention of urine and one had bladder neck stenosis (BNS). A 1 mm quartz fiber was used to incise the BNS using watts of laser power (Fig. 2). A ball tip contact prostatectomy was performed for one retention (Fig. 3) and a side firing laser was used for the other retention patient, followed by a limited TURP. All three were discharged home the day after surgery and were catheter-free after 2 days except for the last patient, in whom the catheter was removed after 5 days. Apart from being small, compact, portable, and less noisy, the no warm-up time was a great advantage of the diode laser when compared to Nd:YAG laser. Results are early and the numbers are fairly small. More clinical results will need to be analyzed before this can be compared to Nd:YAG laser or to a TURP result.

Johnson et al. [45] reported results of transurethral incision of prostate using holmium:YAG laser in canine prostate and concluded that this laser warranted further evaluation for applications in prostate tissue.

Laser Tissue Interaction

Presence of a water medium is the key to achieving coagulation necrosis when the prostate is irradiated with high wattage of Nd:YAG laser energy. Water allows the high wattage to be tolerated by the laser probe, cools the surface of the prostate tissue, and shifts the ablation threshold to a higher wattage. The laser light penetrates deeper without causing surface ablation and thereby causes deeper coagulation. This is much like boiling a potato as compared with putting it directly on a flame.

The author believes that apart from the sloughing related defect, there is a consistency change in BPH tissue after the laserthermia procedure. In addition there is a possibility of alpha adrenergic receptor damage and damage to smooth muscles contributing to the pliability of the prostate. All these combined factors may lead to a decrease in the outflow resistance.

Laser energy can be delivered to the prostate by a free beam or with the use of contact tips. Free-beam lasers can be delivered via a conventional quartz fiber or with a side firing probe where the light traveling via a quartz fiber is reflected by a mirror to fire from the side of the probe. Although several investigators now recommend multiple firings of 15–60 watts for 60–180 s [41, 42, 46–48], the optimal setting for a human prostate has not been scientifically validated. It is inherently a difficult task since not only does the human prostate differ from that of a dog prostate, but there are differences among human prostates. A BPH prostate of one patient may have predominantly glandular tissue, which may melt away at 60 watts of Nd:YAG laser, whereas that of another patient may be mostly fibrotic tissue and the optical and thermal properties may be entirely different.

A significant difference between the VLAP procedure and conventional TURP procedure is the lack of acute tissue removal. This in turn causes lack of immediacy of effect after the VLAP procedures. There is some surface evaporation of tissue by the Nd:YAG laser, but key to the success of this procedure is believed to be deeper tissue ablation by means of coagulative necrosis, followed by much slower sloughing of the affected tissue. Kabalin et al. [47] have noted that significant improvement after laser procedure did not occur for up to 2–3 months, similar to the author's observation in the retention patients [39]. However, cystoscopies done up to 6 months later have revealed presence of residual albeit nonobstructive BPH tissue.

Specific Laser Procedures for BPH

Currently there are several lasers and laser delivery systems being evaluated for prostate sur-

gery. These include the TULIP procedure (transurethral laser-induced prostatectomy), various side firing free-beam fibers, and contact tips. The latter two systems have also been applicable to general urologic procedures.

Transurethral Ultrasound-Guided, Laser-Induced Prostatectomy

The transurethral ultrasound-guided, laser-induced prostatectomy (TULIP) procedure is performed by a novel delivery device where the laser probe is placed in the prostatic urethra using a real-time 7.5HZ ultrasound transducer to visualize the prostate. The probe tip consists of the ultrasound transducer, a right-angle microprisma, and a pressure balloon. The inflated balloon serves to secure the position of the probe and provides a constant laser tissue distance as well as a medium for transmission of the ultrasound waves. The balloon material is transparent to Nd:YAG light. The laser is activated under continuous real-time ultrasound imaging and slowly pulled along the prostatic urethra at various positions, thereby inducing prostatic damage. The proposed advantage of ultrasound imaging is the accurate application of laser energy to where the adenoma is largest [40].

McCullough [49] has recently reported the TULIP national human co-operative study results. The interim analysis included 63 patients followed for 6 months. The peak urinary flow rate improved 78% (baseline 6.7 ml/s; 6 months follow-up 11.9 ml/s) and the mean total symptom score improved 68% (baseline 18.8; 6 months follow-up 6.1). The estimated blood loss was only 17 ml. No incontinence or impotence was reported. The incidence of retrograde ejaculation, stricture, and bladder neck contracture was <1%; 21% of patients developed urinary tract infection (UTI); six underwent TURP, four of which were performed early in the study and may have been related to learning the technique. Although the results are encouraging, this technology has not become popular probably because of the additional cost of the ultrasound and the balloon in conjunction with an expensive laser.

Side-Firing, Free-Beam Lasers

Laser ablation of prostate, commonly known as VLAP (visual laser ablation of prostate), has been more commonly performed. There are increasing numbers of fibers available that deflect the laser beam at various angles. Although most have not been well studied, reported results have

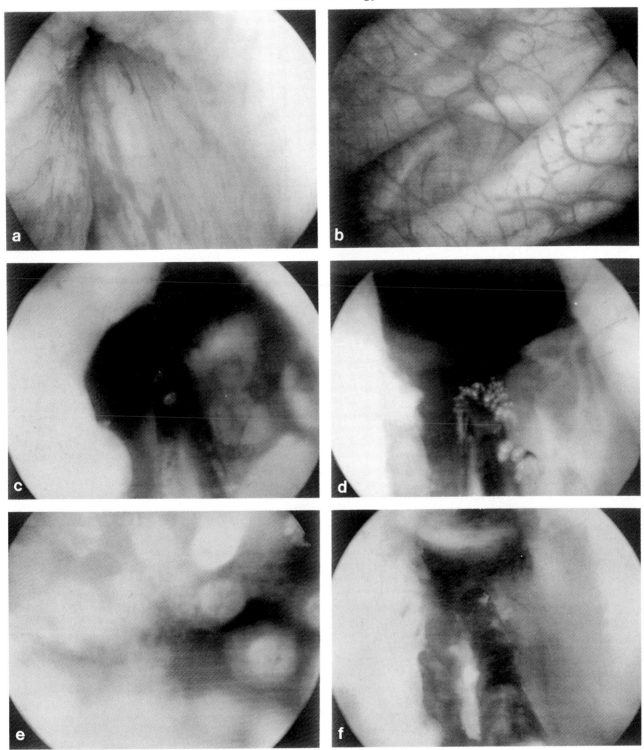

Fig. 2. Sequence of events during a typical laser ablation procedure for BPH with an ADD (Laserscope) using 60 watts of Nd:YAG lasing for 60 seconds in four quadrants. **a** shows the prostate gland; **b** shows trabeculations and pseudodiverticula of the bladder; **c** shows ADD with a helium neon beam ready to ablate that side; the other side has been ablated; **d** shows microbubbles on the probe tip during laser ablation; **e** shows blurring of view that is not uncommon; **f** shows a nearly burnt out probe. Good flow of irrigation in our experience was crucial for preventing the probe burn and for good visualization. See insert for color representation.

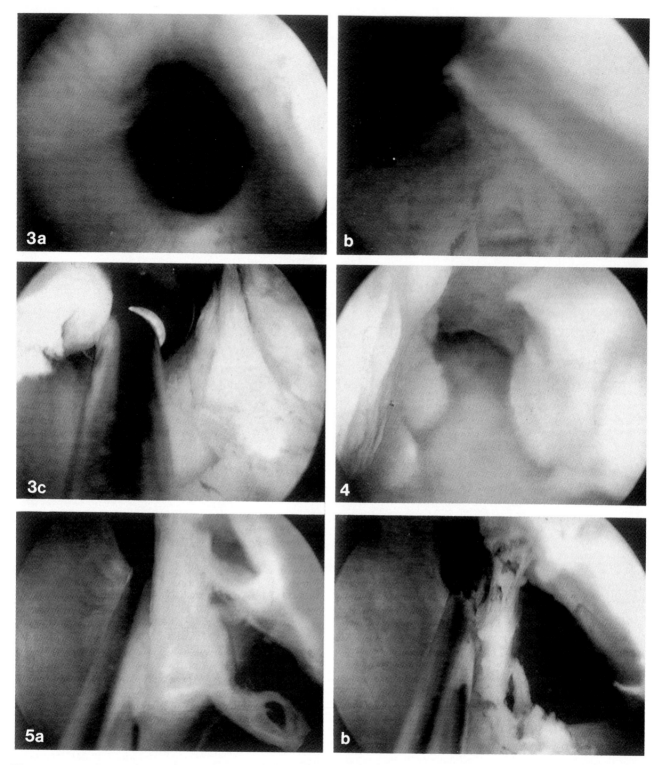

Fig. 3. **a:** An endoscopic view of a bladder neck stenosis following a TURP procedure in the past. **b:** 1 mm laser fiber delivering 30 watts of 1000 mm wavelength Phototome diode laser (Cynosure Inc.) power for incising a bladder neck stenosis. **c:** 3.5 mm Ball tip laser delivery fiber for contact prostatectomy using 30 watts of diode laser power in this case. See insert for color representation.

Fig. 4. Typical prostatic cavity 6 months after initial VLAP procedure. There is necrotic tissue seen attached to both sides of the prostatic fossa. Histologic examination confirmed it to be necrotic tissue. The bladder neck in this case appears to be

remarkably intact. The patient had concomitant papillary transitional cell carcinoma of bladder which allowed us to monitor his prostatic fossa at the time of his check cystoscopies. See insert for color representation.

Fig. 5. **a:** Interprostatic bridge following a previous TURP several years earlier causing irritative symptoms to the patient. **b:** The bridge was dealt with by contact laser cutting with the ADD fiber (Laserscope) with full irrigation and then resection of the remaining tissue with electrocautery loop. Note the presence of a passage above and below the bridge. See insert for color representation.

not shown much difference in the outcome of the procedure. A helium-neon aiming beam is used to direct the location of the beam. The delivery probes can be passed through a 21F cystoscope, although the author prefers to use a continuous flow resectoscope or, if available, a continuous flow cystoscope. A cystoscope is available (ACMI, MA) with an additional flange to keep the probe from touching the prostate tissue on the contralateral side of the laser procedure site. The author and co-workers did not find it to offer much advantage compared to a regular cystoscope. During laser application, the probe is held in one position in the prostatic urethra to maximize the ablation and coagulation effect. The fiber is positioned under direct vision preferably on a television screen, and the procedure is performed using 40–60 watts of power from a Nd:YAG laser; 60 watts for 60 s in one place are used. Other protocols suggested and used are 45 watts for 90 s [47]. A regimen of 15 watts for 3 min is also being proposed [46]. The laser application is repeated at various positions in the prostatic urethra. Exact techniques vary according to the urologists using it. Generally, it has been learned that human prostatic tissue behaves differently from canine prostatic tissue and that the defects found in canine prostate with laser coagulation have not been reproduced in human prostates.

Costello et al. [44] have reported their initial experience using lateral firing Nd:YAG laser to treat 17 patients with BPH. Mean symptom scores (Madsen-Iverson) improved from 15 to 4 at 6 weeks. The mean flow rates improved from 5 ml/s to 9 ml/s at 6 weeks. In two patients the procedure failed and required further intervention.

A multicenter prospective, randomized study comparing TURP vs. VLAP sponsored by C.R. Bard has been completed. The subjects—123 men >50 years of age—were candidates for TURP due to bladder outlet obstruction secondary to BPH. They were enrolled at five participating centers, and laser prostatectomy was performed using a 40-watt power setting. Laser energy was applied for 60 seconds to each lateral lobe at the 3 and 9 o'clock positions and 30 seconds to the 6 and 12 o'clock positions. If the prostatic urethra was >3.5 cm, two series of four quadrant circumferential laser burns were performed. The outcome parameters included changes in AUA symptom scores, peak urinary flow rates, and postvoid residuals. Although details of the results are not available at present, they are reported to be encouraging with a follow-up process of 1 year.

TABLE 2. VLAP Vs. TURP

	Kabalin N = 25	Dixon and Lepor N = 46
Qmax		
TURP		
Baseline	9.0	8.8
6 months	22.9	15.4
% change	154	75
VLAP		
Baseline	8.5	9.2
6 months	20.5	14.3
% change	141	58
AUA score		
TURP		
Baseline	18.8	20.5
6 months	5.7	7.3
% change	−70	−64
VLAP		
Baseline	20.9	17.9
6 months	4.1	11.9
% change	−78	−34

Kabalin [47] randomized 25 patients in this multicenter study and published a subset analysis of his 6-month follow-up data. The mean operative time for VLAP vs. TURP was 24 and 58 minutes, respectively. The outcome assessment for TURP and VLAP are presented in Table 2. The differences between the changes in symptom scores and peak urinary flow rates were not clinically or statistically significant. A total of 15% of the patients failed the initial VLAP procedure, and these treatment failures were censored from the outcome assessment. One patient undergoing TURP required a blood transfusion and another developed hyponatremia and mild confusion. In summary, the 6-month interim analysis reported by Kabalin suggests that both VLAP and TURP are safe and effective treatments for BPH.

Dixon et al. [50] have reported their interim results, and the 6-month outcome measures are summarized in Table 3. The level of improvement in the symptom scores was greater for the TURP group compared to the VLAP group. The difference was not statistically significant. The percentage of subjects exhibiting marked symptom improvement in the TURP and VLAP groups were 77% vs. 38%, respectively. The discrepancy between the Kabalin and Dixon/Lepor interim subset analyses could be due to single vs. double-blind study design, or the differences in surgical technique. The authors agree, however, that the safety profile of the VLAP procedure appeared to be superior to that of TURP. They feel that safety

TABLE 3. Laser Delivery Systems

Vendor	Fiber	Cost	Angle	Directing mechanism
C.R.Bard	Urolase	$850	90°	Gold reflecting dish
Cytocare	Prolase II	$700	90	Quartz refraction
Laserscope	ADD	$550	90	Quartz prism
Lasersonics ACMI	Ultraline	$595	80	Reflecting prism
Myriadlase	side-fire	$650	105	Gold mirror
SLT (contact)	MTRL	$225	—	Synthetic sapphire

favors VLAP procedure, whereas effectiveness favors TURP.

Bhatta [39] has reported results of VLAP in 21 consecutive patients with retention of urine. Twelve of these had spinal anesthesia, eight had local anesthesia, and one had general anesthesia. Seventeen had acute retention; 13 from BPH, one due to carcinoma of prostate, and three due to bladder neck stenosis (BNS). Four had chronic retention; three due to BPH and one due to BNS. A Nd:YAG/KTP laser was used and the laser light was delivered via angle delivery device (ADD). All 13 patients in acute retention due to BPH became catheter-free after a mean catheter time of 8 days (range 1–22 days); the three patients with acute retention due to BNS were catheter-free the next day after the laser incision of the BNS and the patient with acute retention from carcinoma of prostate required a TURP after 45 days of initial laser irradiation. Of the four patients with chronic retention, three with BPH required a TURP procedure after waiting over a month. The patient with chronic retention with BNS was catheter-free after 7 days of his laser procedure. It was concluded that visual laser ablation of prostate works well for patients with acute retention of urine and especially so when the cause of the retention is BNS, and in high risk patients, e.g., in patients with advanced COPD where the procedure can be performed under local anesthesia. Results on chronic retention of urine have not been good in the author's experience.

Contact Laser Ablation of the Prostate

Contact tips have been used to vaporize prostatic tissue under direct visualization using a standard cystoscope. These tips are placed in contact with the tissue to vaporize the prostatic tissue, thereby opening up the obstructing tissue immediately. This is usually a slower process compared to VLAP and therefore suitable for smaller prostates generally under 35–40 grams. The newer tips are larger so that tissue could be removed faster. The other advantage with contact

tip forward prostatectomy is that a lower wattage of laser can be used. A 25-watt diode laser has been used and Watson et al. [13] have reported encouraging results in smaller prostates. The author and co-workers have used this technique using a 50-watt diode laser (Phototome, Cynosure, Bedford, MA) operating at 30 watts with good results in a limited number of patients [14]. Daughtry and Rodan [51] have reported their experience in 25 patients using an SLT contact laser system with 3mm and 6 mm contact tips. Fifteen of the 25 patients were reported to have achieved good clinical outcome. None of the patients developed treatment related morbidity.

Other Techniques

Sacknoff [52] has popularized a combination of VLAP and a limited TURP techniques. He presented his results in 40 patients and concluded that the results as assessed on AUA symptom score, flow rates, sexual function, and return to normal activity, were similar to that of reported TURP results. He believes that a turpette or a limited TURP of the coagulated tissue facilitates earlier relief of the irritative and obstructive symptoms of the patients, which is typically associated with a VLAP procedure. However, in his report, 15% of the patients required a second procedure because of either obstruction or bleeding.

To achieve the same goal of immediacy of effects, Childs [48] used high power Nd:YAG laser of 80–95 watts primarily to vaporize the obstructing prostate tissue. He reported results in 50 patients where the AUA symptom scores improved from 19 to 7 and peak flow rates improved from 7.6 to 19.2 at 6-month intervals. Complications included dysuria syndrome, bladder neck contracture (2 patients), impotence (2 patients), and retrograde ejaculation.

Interstitial laser coagulation, or laser-induced thermal therapy by specially constructed laser fibers, either transurethrally under direct endoscopic vision or percutaneously through the perineum under ultrasound guidance, is a new and evolving procedure for the treatment of BPH [53–56]. Muschter et al. [53] reported first clinical results in 15 cases in 1993 and noted excellent clinical results. They used a percutaneous approach for lateral lobes and transurethral apraoch for median lobes. The prostate was irradiated with Nd:YAG laser for 10 minutes at 5 watts power output per application. They reported significant reduction in subjective symptom scores, a reduction of residual urine volume from a mean of 206 ml to 38 ml, and an improvement of peak urinary flow rate from a mean of 6.6 ml to 15.2 ml/s. No severe side effects were reported. Orovan and Whelan [54] have reported similar results in 16 patients using 7 watts of Nd:YAG laser irradiation for 10 minutes per treatment delivered by transurethral approach. They feel that interstitial laser therapy for BPH has the advantage of preseving the urothelium and is not associated with sloughing of prostate tissue after the procedure.

The lack of acute tissue removal remains to be addressed before a no bleeding, no catheter, no fluid absorption procedure can be performed. Contact laser surgery and high wattage use of Nd:YAG laser are steps in that direction. The author and co-workers are attempting to achieve a bloodless prostatic chip by combining laser and electrocautery in one device [57]. This is still experimental but appears promising in animal studies.

Futures of Lasers in BPH

As is obvious from the literature, there is no one agreed upon approach for using lasers in BPH patients. It is also clear that there are definite interest and potential advantages in using laser for this condition. It is probable that a single technique may not be suitable for every BPH patient, or put differently, every technique described above may have a place in certain types of prostate disease and individual patients. It is possible that contact laser surgery or high power laser evaporation may be suitable for patients with BPH under 35–40 grams weight, multiple quadrant VLAP for larger prostates, and a turpette for patients with significant median lobe enlargement. Several questions remain to be answered, but laser has found a place in the management of BPH. Whether or not it will replace TURP is not clear. A bloodless chip may be the future.

Lasers in Bladder Carcinoma

Johnson, in 1994, used Holmium:YAG laser in the treatment of 52 recurrent superficial bladder tumors [58]. At follow-up cystoscopy 3 months after initial laser treatment, four patients (27%) were free of tumor, eight patients (52%) had out of field recurrence, and three patients (20%) had infield recurrence. They concluded that laser treatment of bladder tumors has the advantage of not requiring anesthesia or an indwelling catheter. Other lasers used for recurrent superficial bladder carcinoma are Nd:YAG, argon, and KTP [59]. Although Hofstetter [60] had suggested that there was a decrease in the number of expected recurrences, this has not been found by other investigators. Beisland and Seland [61] reported no significant differences in tumor recurrences following conventional transurethral resection and laser photoirradiation. Laser treatment of invasive bladder cancer has frequently been reserved for elderly patients or in those with poor overall health, making results difficult to evaluate [62]. Application of photodynamic therapy has been extensively studied. In the bladder, HPD is retained preferentially by the malignant cells but is also retained by dysplastic and inflammatory cells. Several light delivery systems have been developed. PDT remains an investigational procedure with limited clinical data available. Prout and co-workers [63] in 1987 reported the results of 19 patients treated with PDT for superficial bladder cancer (Ta to T1). Complete tumor ablation was observed in nine patients (47%), whereas nine had partial response. However, its role is limited by competing and less invasive modes of therapies. PDT remains a potentially exciting treatment of bladder neoplasm. Photosensitizers tagged on monoclonal antibodies that can be targeted to malignant cells only is an attractive field of research in this field [64].

Condylomata Acuminata

Human paillomavirus (HPV) is the most common sexually transmitted viral disease [65]. Both the overt, grossly visible and the covert, clinically invisible (subclinical aceto-white) condylomata are well-known mucocutaneous manifestations of genital HPV infection. The association of certain HPV viruses with carcinoma of the cervix and perhaps carcinoma of the penis has increased the significance of this lesion.

Excellent results have been obtained with CO_2, KTP-532, and ND:YAG laser treatment of grossly identifiable condyloma acuminatum [66]. Gross recurrences are relatively unusual. Cosmetic and therapeutic results are often superior to alternative treatments. Fifteen to 20 watts of laser power output is generally used when a Nd:YAG laser is employed, whereas 5–10 watts are used with a KTP 532 laser. Muschter and Dann, in 1990, treated 161 patients with urogenital warts using a Nd:YAG laser [67]. With a mean follow-up of 16 months, 80% of treated patients were free of recurrence. Carpinello et al. [68] earlier reported results in 127 men with biopsy-proven, subclinical HPV infection and treated with CO_2 laser. A 6% recurrence rate was reported with a mean follow-up of 4 months. Thus with microscopic subclinical lesions, the recurrence rate is high even after adequate destruction of detected lesions.

Carcinoma of the Penis

The incidence of squamous cell carcinoma (SCCA) of the penis is 1 per 100,000 and poses a 50% higher risk for nonwhite men than for white men [69]. Lasers have been found to provide effective local control for selected penile cancers. Patients chosen for primary laser therapy should have only superficially invasive tumors. Cosmetic and therapeutic results are usually excellent. Malloy et al. [70] reported 16 patients with carcinoma of the penis treated with Nd:YAG laser. Five had Tis, nine had T1, and two had T2 carcinoma. All five patients with Tis were free of tumor. Of the nine with T1 disease, six were free of tumor. The two men with T2 tumor had reduction in the tumor mass but were not cured. Malek et al. [71] reported their experience in 34 white men with obvious or suspected penile lesions. They feel that laser therapy has evolved into an attractive penis sparing treatment for patients with low stage squamous cell carcinoma (SCCA) of the penis [72]. However, a review of the recent literature indicates no significant difference in the rate of local recurrence after conservative surgical procedures versus laser treatment, unless laser energy is applied not only to the visible lesion but also to the entire biopsy-proven, HPV-related, aceto-white field of change associated with the lesion. Smith and Dixon [66] feel that Nd:YAG laser is preferable in tumor ablation procedures. Bandiermonte and associates [73] have reported a series of 15 patients treated with CO_2 laser for glans lesions. Cosmetic and functional results were excellent.

Urethral Condyloma Acuminatum

Urethral condyloma acuminatum frequently occurs at the meatus and fossa navicularis. Lesions at the meatus are amenable to treatment with CO_2, Nd:YAG, argon, and KTP-532 lasers. CO_2 laser energy cannot be delivered via a fiber and hence is not suitable for more proximal lesions. Krogh et al. [74] have reported results in 74 men with condyloma of the urethral meatus with a follow-up of 18 months. Of these 78% had no recurrence. The recurrence rate was higher if the patient had co-existing lesions on the external skin. Six cases of meatal stenosis and one case of urethral stricture were observed more than 3 months after treatment.

Urethral Strictures

Lasers have been used in the treatment of benign strictures of the urethra. Because of delivery problems, the greatest experience is available with Nd:YAG laser. Initially, the reported technique involved cicumferential treatment of the stricture. A total of 24 patients were treated by this method and reported by Smith and Dixon in 1984 [75]. Although good early results were achieved without complications, recurrence was observed in 13 patients after 6 months. It was concluded that this technique offered no advantage over internal urethrotomy. Several series of laser urethromies have been reported using the Nd:YAG or KTP-532 laser. Undoubtedly, urethromy is feasible with a laser. However, reported results are difficult to interpret and have not been uniformly favorable.

Bladder Hemangioma

Hemangioma is a rare benign tumor of the bladder. A transurethral resection of the tumor is inadvisable because of the possibility of excessive bleeding. Laser offers an excellent means of treatment in such cases. In 1990, Smith reported results in 13 patients with hemangioma of the bladder treated with Nd:YAG laser for recurrent bleeding [76]. A power output of 20–35 watts was used. No complications were noted. The results were excellent.

Interstitial Cystitis

Lasers have been reported to be effective in the treatment of interstitial cystitis (IC). The mechanism for this remains uncertain. This may be related to ablation of sensitive nerve endings in the bladder wall around the inflammatory lesions of IC. Bowel perforations have been reported in a disproportionate number of patients, and this may be related to the proximity of the bowel to the dome of the bladder where most of the IC occurs in women. Shanberg and Malloy [77] reported their experience in 39 patients (33 females) with IC treated with Nd:YAG laser. A total of 19 patients had Hunner's ulcer and 17 of these had rapid relief of pain with a demonstrable increase in functional bladder capacity. Recurrent symptoms were noted in 12 of 17 patients between 6–8 months posttreatment.

Carcinoma of the Ureter and Renal Pelvis

Endoscopic access to the ureter or renal pelvis can be achieved with either the ureteroscope or the percutaneous aproach to the kidney. A transitional cell carcinoma (TCC) of the ureter or the renal pelvis is amenable to treatment with Nd:YAG or KTP laser energy. This may be especially true for patients with solitary kidneys. Favorable results have been reported for lesions of intramural ureter from several centers. Experience is limited in mid and upper ureteral lesions. Hoffstetter [78] reported good results in 14 patients with mid ureter tumors. No ureteral perforations or strictures were noted. Smith [79] used a ND:YAG laser to treat a renal pelvis tumor with a percutaneous access. Five of eight patients were free of recurrence at the follow-up.

The overall indications of laser treatment of the ureter are limited, and appropriate patient and treatment selection are necessary.

Carcinoma of Prostate

Currently, research efforts are being devoted to the destruction of prostatic carcinoma by three laser techniques [80]: 1) endoscopic laser applications (ELC), 2) interstitial laser coagulations (ILC), and 3) photodynamic therapy. Lasers have been used in conjunction with an extended TURP since the early 1980s [81, 82]. Clinical and ultrasonic assessment and staging is followed by an extended TURP. The purpose of this is to debulk the prostate gland under ultrasound control, aiming to remove all adenoma and to leave a residual rim of prostate tissue approximately 6 mm of less in depth. The results of this technique have been reported in 22 patients with a follow-up for a mean of 53 months. Eighteen of the 22 had no clinical evidence of disease on repeated biopsy and ultrasonic examination. The authors felt that, although this method is interstitial laser coagulation [83], it may be used in animal model and may have a role in carcinoma of the prostate in the future.

Other Laser Applications

Lasers have been used to weld tissue and clinical vasovasostomy procedures have been performed using various lasers [84]. Lasers have also been used for vaporizing Peyronie's disease [85], treating lichen sclerosus et atrophicus [86], and performing partial nephrectomy procedures [87], with mixed results.

Conclusions

In 10 years, the use of lasers in urology has become well established. Laser lithotripsy is safe and effective, particularly for lower ureteral stones. Laser applications in prostate have resulted in a bloodless procedure with its obvious advantages. Studies are underway to achieve a no bleeding, no anesthesia, no catheter prostatectomy procedure. Laser applications for superficial skin lesions are also well established. Photodynamic therapy and laser welding, although experimental at present, show promise for the future. Autofluoresence may have diagnostic applications in urological malignancies. Diode lasers in the 50-watt output range already are available and both solid-state and diode combination lasers are being developed (e.g., Nd:YAG and Ho:YAG combinations). Lasers have already made a significant contribution to the practice of urology. Their probable greater future role is just beginning to be investigated.

ACKNOWLEDGMENTS

The author thanks Norman S. Nishioka, M.D., for his valuable contribution, including the high-speed photographs of laser stone interaction taken in the Wellman Laboratories of Photomedicine, Massachusetts General Hospital, Boston. The author also thanks Lekha Bhatta, M.D., for her help in manuscript preparation, Alan Ball for coordination in editing the final aspects of the manuscript, and Wendy J. Parlin for secretarial assistance.

REFERENCES

1. Mulvany WP, Beck CR. The laser beam in urology. J Urol 1968; 99:112.
2. Breitweiser PH, Hebrich HD, Noske HD, et al. CO_2 laser alsoperation instrument in der experimentellen. Urologic Biomed Technik 1973; 18:6.
3. Staehler G, Hofstetter A, Gorisch W, et al. Endoscopy in experimental urology using an argon laser beam. Endoscopy 1976; 8:1.
4. Dretler SP, Bhatta KM, Rosen DI. Conversion of the electrohydraulic electrode to an electromechanical impactor: Basic studies and a case report. J Urol 146:746–50.
5. Bhatta KM, Mantel R. A new irrigating electrode for

safer electrohydraulic lithotripsy: In-vitro studies. J Urol 1993; 149:750A.

6. Childs SJ. Extended transurethral resection and Nd: YAG laser ablation of the prostate (TURLAP) for carconoma: A pilot study. International Society for Optical Engineering (SPIE): Proceedings of Lasers in Urology, Gynecology, and General Surgery, 1993; 1879:94–102.

7. Anvari B, Motamedi M, Torres J, Rastegar S, Orihuela E, et al. Effects of surface irrigation on the thermal response of tissue during laser irradiation. Lasers Surg Med 1994; 14:386–95.

8. Baggish MS, Sze E, Badawy S, Choe J. Carbon dioxide laser laparoscopy by means of a 3.0 mm diameter rigid wave guide. Fertil Steril 1988; 50:419–24.

9. Ferenczy A, Bergeron C, Richart RM. Human papillomavirus DNA in CO2 laser-generated plume of smoke and its consequences to the surgeon. Obstet Gynecol 1990; 75:114–118.

10. Baggish MS, Elbakry M. The effects of laser smoke on the lungs of rats. Am J Obstet Gynecol 1987; 156:1260.

11. Daikuzono N, Joffe SN. Artificial sapphire probe for contact photocoagulation and tissue vaporization with the Nd:YAG laser. Med Instrum 1985; 19:173–178.

12. Oz MC, Bass LS, Chuck RS, Johnson JP, Parangi S, Nowygrod R, Treat M. Strength of Laser Vascular Fusion: Preliminary observation on the role of thrombus. Lasers Surg Med 1990; 10:393–395.

13. Watson G. Use of semi-conductor diode laser in urology. SPIE Proc 1994; 2129:121–128.

14. Cho G, Bhatta K, Boll J, et al. A new high power (50 watts) diode laser with wavelength of 1 micron: Introvitro and initial clinical results. New England Section American Urological Association, 63rd Annual Meeting, Southampton, Bermuda.

15. Bhatta N, Isaacson K, Flotte T, Schiff I, Anderson R, et al. Injury and adhesion formation following ovarian wedge resection with different thermal surgical modalities. Lasers Surg Med 1993; 13:344–52.

16. Dickson CT, Clark PJ, Preminger GM. Alexandrite laser lithotripsy: Basic and clinical studies. J Urol 1993; 149:748A.

17. Anderholm NC. Laser generated stress waves. Applied Physics Letter 1970; 16:113–115.

18. Yang LC. Stress waves generated in thin metallic fibers by a Q-switched ruby laser. J Appl Physics 1974; 45:2601–2605.

19. Watson GM, Wickham GEA, Mills TN, Bown SG, Swain P, Salmon PR. Laser fragmentation of renal calculi. Br J Urol 1983; 55:613–616.

20. Thomas S, Pensel J, Engelhardt R, Meyer W, Hofstetter AG. The pulsed dye laser versus the Q-Switched Nd:YAG laser-induced shock wave lithotripsy. Lasers Surg Med 1988; 8:363–370.

21. Watson GM, Murray S, Dretler SP, Parish JA. The pulsed dye laser for fragmenting urinary calculi. J Urol 1987; 138:195–198.

22. Nishioka NS, Teng P, Deutsch TF, Anderson RR. Mechanism of laser-induced fragmentation of urinary and biliary calculi. Lasers Life Sci 1987; 1:231–245.

23. Dretler SP. Stone fragility: A new therapeutic distinction. J Urol 1988; 139:1124–1127.

24. Bhatta KM, Rosen DI, Flotte T, Nishioka NS. Effects of shielded and unshielded laser and electrohydraulic lithotripsy on rabbit bladder. J Urol 1990; 143:857–60.

25. Olchewski R, Hartung S, Haupt G, Englemann U. A new holmium:YAG laser for lithotripsy: In vitro stone disintegration and tissue effects. J Urol 1993; 149:744cA.

26. Hastie K, Hamdy F, Davis M, Stamp J. Initial assessment of the holmium:YAG laser in the treatment of ureteric calculi. J Urol 1993; 149:737a.

27. Dretler SP, Watson G, Parrish JA, Murray S. Pulsed dye laser fragmentation of ureteral calculi: Initial clinical experience. J Urol 1987; 137:386–389.

28. Dretler SP. Laser lithotripsy: A review of 20 years of research and clinical applications. Lasers Surg Med 1988; 8:341–356.

29. Dretler SP, Bhatta KM. Clinical experience with high power (140 mj, larger fiber (320 micron) pulsed dye laser lithotripsy. J Urol 1991; 146:1228–1231.

30. Bhatta KM, Dretler SP. Laser lithotripsy. Problems In Urology 1989; 3:435–448.

31. Bhatta KM, Rosen DI, Watson GM, Dretler SP. Acoustic and plasma guided lasertripsy (APGL) of urinary calculi. J Urol 1989; 142:433–437.

32. Bhatta KM, Rosen DI, Dretler SP. Plasma shield lasertripsy: In-vitro studies. J Urol 1989; 142:1110–1112.

33. Dretler SP, Cho G. Semi-rigid ureteroscopy: A new genre. J Urol 1989; 141:1314.

34. Dretler SP. An evaluation of ureteral laser lithotripsy: 225 consecutive patients. J Urol 1990; 143:267–272.

35. Copcoat MJ, Ison KT, Watson G, Wickham JEA. Lasertripsy for ureteric stones in 120 cases: lessons learned. Br J Urol 1988; 61:487–489.

36. Fuchs JF. Editorial: Interventional urinary stone management. J Urol 1994; 151:668–669.

37. Nesbit RM. "Transurethral Prostatectomy." Springfield, IL: Charles C. Thomas, 1943.

38. Mebust WK, Hotgrewe HL, Cockett ATK, Peters PC and Writing Committee. Transurethral prostatectomy: Immediate and postoperative complications. A cooperative study of 13 participating institutions evaluating 3,885 patients. J Urol 1989; 141:243.

39. Bhatta KM. Visual laser ablation of prostate (VLAP) for patients with retention of urine: Personal experience. SPIE Proc 1994; 2129:42–48.

40. Roth RA, Aretz HT. Transurethral ultrasound-guided laser-induced prostatectomy (TULIP procedure): a canine prostate feasibility study. J Urol 1991; 146:1128.

41. Johnson DE, Levinson AK, Greskovich FJ, Cromeens DM, Ro JY, Costello AJ, Wishnow JI. Transurethral laser prostatectomy using a right-angle delivery system. SPIE Proc 1991; 1421:36.

42. Kandel LB, Harrison LH, McCullough DL, Woodruff RD, Dyer RB. Transurethral laser prostatectomy in the canine model. Lasers Surg Med 1992; 12:33.

43. Costello AJ, Johnson DE, Bolton DM. Nd:YAG laser ablation of the prostate as a treatment for benign prostatic hypertrophy. Lasers Surg Med 1992; 12:121.

44. Costello AJ, Bowsher WG, Bolton DM, Braslis KG, Burt J. Laser ablation of the prostate in patients with benign prostatic hypertrophy. Brit J Urol 1992; 69:603.

45. Johnson DE, Cromeens DM, Price RE. Transurethral incision of prostate using the holmium:YAG Laser. Lasers Surg Med 1992; 12:354–369.

46. Orihuela E, Motamedi M, Pow-Sang M, Cammack TJ, Warren MM. Nd:YAG thermal effect in the prostate: application to laser treatment of benign prostatic hyperplasia. SPIE Proc 1994; 2129:19–24.

47. Kabalin JN. Laser Prostatectomy performed with a right angle firing neodymium:YAG laser fiber at 40 watts power setting. J Urol 1993; 150:95–99.

48. Childs SJ. High power density prostate cavitation. Lasers Surg Med 1994; Supplement 6 313A.

49. McCullough DL, Roth RA, et al. Transurethral ultrasound-guided laser induced prostatectomy. J Endocrinol Urol 1992; 5:145–149.

50. Dixon C, Machi C, Lepor H. A prospective double-blind randomized study comparing laser ablation of the prostate and transurethral prostatectomy for the treatment of BPH. J Urol 1993; 149:215A.

51. Daughtry JD, Rodan BA. Transurethral laser resection of the prostate. J Clin Laser Med Surg 1992; 10:269.

52. Sacknoff EJ. Laser prostatectomy with a turpette: Evolution of a new technique. Lasers Surg Med 1994; Supplement 6:312A.

53. Muschter R, Hofstetter A, Hessel S, Keiditsch E, Schneede P. Interstitual laser prostatectomy: Experimental and first clinic results (abstract). J Urol 1993; 149: 346.

54. Orovan WL, Whelan JP. Nd:YAG Laser treatment of BPH using interstitial thermotherapy: A transurethral approach. J Urol 1994; 150:230A.

55. Muschter R, Hofstetter A, Hessel S, Keiditsch E, Rothenberger K, Schneede P, Frank F. Hi-tech of the prostate: Interstitial laser coagulation of benign prostatic hyperplasia. SPIE 1643. Laser Surgery: Advanced Characterization. Therapeutic and Systems, 1992; III: 25–34.

56. Muschter R, Hoftstetter A, Hessel S, Keiditsch E, Rothenberger K, Schneede P. Interstitial laser coagulation of the prostate. Lasers Surg Med 1992; Suppl 4:25.

57. Bhatta KM, Perlmutter A. Laser assisted TURP: Animal experiments. J Endourology 1993; 7(suppl 1):IV-14.

58. Johnson JE. Use of holmium:YAG (Ho:YAG) laser for treatment of superficial bladder carcinoma. Lasers Surg Med 1994; 14:213–218.

59. von Eschenbach AC. Superficial bladder carcinoma. In: Smith JA, Stein BS, Bensen RC, eds. "Lasers in Urologic Surgery." Chicago: Year Book Medical, 1983, pp 57–66.

60. Hoffstetter AF. Laser use in Urology. In: Dixon, JA ed. "Surgical Applications of Laser." Chicago: Year Book Medical, 1983, pp 146–162.

61. Beisland HO, Seland PA. A prospective randomized study on neodymium:YAG laser irradiation versus TUR in the treatment of urinary bladder cancer. Scand J Urol Nephrol 1986; 20:29–212.

62. Smith JA Jr. Laser treatment of invasive bladder cancer. J Urol 1986; 135:55–57.

63. Prout GR, Lin C, Bensen RC, et al. Photodynamic therapy with hematoporphyrin derivative in the management of superficial papillary transitional cell carcinoma of the bladder. N Eng J Med 1987; 317:1251–1255.

64. Bachor R, Hautmann R, Hasan T. Comparison of two routes of photosensitizer administration for photodynamic therapy of bladder cancer. Urol Res 1994; 22:21–23.

65. Reid R, Campion MJ. The biology and significance of human papillomavirus infection in the genital tract. Yale J Biol Med 1988; 61:307–325.

66. Smith JA. Urologic laser surgery. In: Walsh CP, Retik AB, Stamey TA, Darracott Vaughn E Jr, eds: "Campbells Urology." Philadelphia: W.B. Saunders, 1992.

67. Muschter R, Dann TF. Laser coagulation of urogenital condylomata acuminata. J Endourol 1990; 4:549.

68. Carpiniello VL, Zderie SA, Malloy TR, Sedelacek TV. Carbon dioxide laser therapy of subclinical condyloma found by magnified penile surface scanning. Urology 1987; 24:608–610.

69. Thompson IM, Fraley WR. Penile carcinoma. AUA update series 1990; 9(1):1–7.

70. Malloy TR, Wein AJ, Carpiniello VL. Carcinoma of the penis treated with a Nd:YAG laser. Urology 1988; 31:26–29.

71. Malek RS, Goelner JR, Smith TF, Espy MJ, Cupp MR. Human papillomavirus infection and intraepithelial, in situ, and invasive carcinoma of penis. Urology 1993; 42: 159–170.

72. Malek RS. Laser treatment of premalignant and malignant squamous cell lesions of the penis. Lasers Surg Med 1992; 12:246–253.

73. Bandiearamonte A, Monte G, Lepera P, Marchesini R, et al. Laser microsurgery for superficial lesion of the penis. J Urol 1987; 138:315–319.

74. Krogh J, Beauke HP, Miskowiak J, et al. Long term results of carbon dioxide laser treatment of meatal condylomata acuminata. Br J Urol 1990; 65:621–623.

75. Smith JA Jr, Dixon JA. Neodymium:YAG laser treatment of benign urethral strictures. J Urol 1984; 131:655.

76. Smith JA Jr. Laser treatment of bladder hemangioma. J Urol 1990; 143:282–284.

77. Shanberg AM, Malloy TR. Treatment of interstitial cystitis with a Nd:YAG laser. Urology 1987; 24:31–33.

78. Hoffstetter A. Laser application for destroying ureteral tumors. Lasers Surg Med 1984; 3:152.

79. Smith AD. Percutaneous laser use in the upper tract. In Smith JA Jr, ed. "Lasers in Urologic Surgery." Chicago: Year Book Medical, 1989.

80. Smith JA, ed. "Lasers in Urologic Surgery," Ed 3. St. Louis: Mosby, 1989.

81. Sander S, Beisland HO. Laser in the treatment of localized prostate cancer. J Urol 1984; 132:280–281.

82. Samdal F, Brevik B. Laser combined with TURP in the treatment of localized prostatic cancer. Scand J Urol Nephrol 1990; 24:175–177.

83. McNicholas TA, Stegar AC, Charing C, et al. Interstitial laser coagulation of the prostate: An experimental study. Br J Urol 1993; 71:439–444.

84. Gilbert P, Beckert R. Laser-assisted vasovasostomy. Lasers Surg Med 1989; 9:42–44.

85. Costello RT. Laser vaporization of Peyronie's plaques. Lasers Surg Med 1993; 13:246–247.

86. Windahl T, Hellston S. Carbon dioxide laser treatment of lichen sclerosus et atrophicus. J Urol 1993; 150:868–870.

87. Johnson D, Wishnow K, von Eschenbach A, Grignon D, Ayala A. Partial nephrectomy using the Nd:YAG laser: A comparison of the 1.06μ and 1.32μ lasers employing different delivery systems. Lasers Surg Med 1988; 8:241–247.

Index

possible patch TO WILEY